Neuronal Mechanisms of Memory Formation

Concepts of Long-Term Potentiation and Beyond

Long-term potentiation (LTP) is by far the most dominant model for neuronal changes that might encode memory. LTP is an elegant concept that meets many criteria set up by theoreticians long before the model's discovery, and it also fits anatomical data of learning-dependent synapse changes. Since the discovery of LTP, the question has remained about how closely LTP produced *in vitro* by artificial stimulation of neurons actually models putative learning-induced synaptic changes.

A number of recent investigations have tried to correlate synaptic changes observed after learning with changes produced by artificial stimulation of neurons. These studies have failed to find a correlation between the two forms of synaptic plasticity.

In this book, an international group of neurobiologists and psychologists discuss their latest ideas and data. The results of experiments using electrophysiological techniques *in vitro* are discussed and compared with the results of *in vivo* experiments. Learning experiments are also discussed. Theoretical models, such as the Hebb theory of synaptic changes during learning, are compared to different models that do not predict upregulation of synaptic transmission. A wide approach is taken, and research and models in different brain areas such as the neocortex and the basal brain are discussed.

Christian Hölscher is a research fellow in the Department of Experimental Psychology at the University of Oxford.

NEURONAL MECHANISMS OF MEMORY FORMATION

Concepts of Long-Term Potentiation and Beyond

Edited by

CHRISTIAN HÖLSCHER
University of Oxford

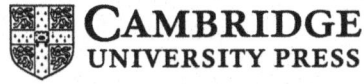

CAMBRIDGE
UNIVERSITY PRESS

CAMBRIDGE UNIVERSITY PRESS
Cambridge, New York, Melbourne, Madrid, Cape Town, Singapore, São Paulo

Cambridge University Press
The Edinburgh Building, Cambridge CB2 2RU, UK

Published in the United States of America by Cambridge University Press, New York

www.cambridge.org
Information on this title: www.cambridge.org/9780521770675

First published 2001
This digitally printed first paperback version 2005

A catalogue record for this publication is available from the British Library

Library of Congress Cataloguing in Publication data

Neuronal mechanisms of memory formation: concepts of long-term potentiation
and beyond / edited by Christian Hölscher.
    p. cm.
  ISBN 0 521 77067 X (hardback)
    1. Memory. 2. Neural transmission—Regulation. I. Hölscher, Christian.

  QP406.N486 2000
  612.8′2—dc21   00-036768

ISBN-13 978-0-521-77067-5 hardback
ISBN-10 0-521-77067-X hardback

ISBN-13 978-0-521-01803-6 paperback
ISBN-10 0-521-01803-X paperback

Contents

Contributors

Wickliffe C. Abraham
Department of Psychology and Neuroscience Research Centre
University of Otago
Dunedin, New Zealand

Donald P. Cain
Department of Psychology and Graduate
Program in Neuroscience
University of Western Ontario
London, Ontario, Canada

Paul F. Chapman
University of Wales
Cardiff, United Kingdom

Yoon H. Cho
CNRS UMR 5907
University of Bordeaux I
Talence Cedex, France

Sabrina Davis
Neurobiol De L'Apprentissage et de la Memoire URA-1491
CNRS-Universite Paris-SUD
Orsay, France

David M. Diamond
Departments of Psychology and Pharmacology
University of South Florida
Tampa, FL

Howard B. Eichenbaum
Department of Psychology
Boston University
Boston, MA

Christian Hölscher
University of Oxford
Department of Experimental Psychology
Oxford, United Kingdom

Yan-You Huang
Center for Neurobiology and Behavior
College of Physicians and Surgeons of Columbia University
New York, NY

Kathryn J. Jeffery
Department of Anatatomy and Developmental Biology
University College London
London, United Kingdom

Ole Jensen
Helsinki University of Technology
Low Temperature Laboratory
Helsinki, Finland

Michael Kahana
Department of Biology and Volen Center for Complex System
Brandeis University
Waltham, MA

Eric R. Kandel
Center for Neurobiology and Behavior
College of Physicians and Surgeons of Columbia University
New York, NY

Serge Laroche
Lab. de Neurobiologie de l'Apprentissage, de la Mémoire et de la Communication
Universite Paris Sud
Orsay, France

Joseph E. LeDoux
Center for Neural Science
New York University
New York, NY

John E. Lisman
Department of Biology and Volen Center for Complex Systems
Brandeis University
Waltham, MA

Stephen A. Maren
Department of Psychology and Neuroscience Program
University of Michigan
Ann Arbor, MI

Mouna Maroun
Laboratory for behavioral Neuroscience
Department of Psychology
University of Haifa
Haifa, Israel

Louis D. Matzel
Department of Psychology and Center for Neuroscience
Rutgers University
Piscataway, NJ

Jill C. McEachern
Department of Physiology
University of British Columbia
Vancouver, Canada

Neil McNaughton
Department of Psychology
University of Otago
Dunedin, New Zealand

Sturla Molden
Department of Psychology
Norwegian University of Science and Technology
Trondheim, Norway

Edvard I. Moser
Department of Psychology
Norwegian University of Science and Technology
Trondheim, Norway

Matthias H.J. Munk
Department of Neurophysiology
Max Planck Institute for Brain Research
Frankfurt, Germany

Collin R. Park
Department of Psychology and Neuroscience Program
University of South Florida
Tampa, FL

Ole Paulsen
MRC Anatomical Neuropharmacology Unit
University Department of Pharmacology
Oxford, United Kingdom

Fanella Pike
MRC Anatomical Neuropharmacology Unit
University Department of Pharmacology
Oxford, United Kingdom

Michael J. Puls
Department of Psychology and Neuroscience Program
University of South Florida
Tampa, FL

Gal Richter-Levin
Laboratory for Behavioral Neuroscience
Department of Psychology
University of Haifa
Haifa, Israel

Michael T. Rogan
Center for Neurobiology and Behavior
College of Physicians and Surgeons of Columbia University
New York, NY

Edmund T. Rolls
Department of Experimental Psychology
University of Oxford
Oxford, United Kingdom

Gregory M. Rose
Memory Pharmaceuticals Corporation
New York, NY

Christopher A. Shaw
Department of Physiology, Ophthalmology and Neuroscience
University of British Columbia
Vancouver, Canada

Tracey Shors
Department of Psychology and Center for Neuroscience
Rutgers University
Piscataway, NJ

Marc G. Weisskopf
Center for Neural Science
New York University
New York, NY

Dan Yaniv
Laboratory for Behavioral Neuroscience
Department of Psychology
University of Haifa
Haifa, Israel

Long-Term Potentiation as a Model for Memory Mechanisms

The Story So Far

Christian Hölscher

What Is LTP?

At present, long-term potentiation (LTP) of synaptic transmission is the most widely studied model for neuronal change that occurs during learning and that stores information in the brain. When Bliss and Lømo discovered the phenomenon of LTP 30 years ago, it must have been a very exciting moment (see Bliss and Lømo, 1996, for a detailed account). The finding was an important step in the long ongoing search for the neuronal basis of memory formation in the nervous system. Even though anatomists such as Exner showed changes in neuronal connections that were induced by exposure to rich environments as early as 1884 (Exner, 1884), it was by no means clear how exactly neurons change in order to store information. Exner and others (Hebb, 1949; Hinton, 1992; Jodar and Kaneto, 1995) proposed activity-dependent, selective plastic changes in the connections between neurons that could "freeze" the pattern of activity of the neurons and therefore preserve information. The theoretical basis for LTP existed for a long time, and when LTP was described by Bliss and Lømo in a full paper (Bliss and Lømo, 1973), researchers in the field were more than ready for the actual empirical evidence that neuronal network processes might be used in the brain.

The basic principle of every neuronal net is that connections between neurons can change in a defined, use-dependent way thereby storing information. Such a system has certain attributes such as pattern completion, parallel processing, and self-instructing learning properties, all of which are characteristics of activity in working brains (Hinton, 1992; Jodar and Kaneto, 1995).

At present, the concept that LTP is the basis for memory formation is the main theory in the field. Additionally, the lack of a rival theory that is backed by a similar amount of supporting empirical evidence makes it compelling to many people. However, the final proof for this theory remains to be found. Although there is evidence in support of the theory (Rogan et al., 1997; Wilson and Tonegawa, 1997; Moser et al., 1998) there is also equally strong evidence to the contrary (Moser, 1995; Saucier and Cain, 1995; Nosten-Bertrand et al., 1996; Hölscher et al., 1997b; Meiri et al., 1998). In reaction to this situation, a number of researchers that work in the area of LTP and memory formation have come together to present their ideas and to discuss mechanisms of memory formation.

The aim of this book is to discuss in detail what conclusions we can draw from the published results, what alterations or additions we might have to make to the theory of LTP, and what alternative concepts are feasible and are worth investigating.

In this introductory section, the developments in the research of LTP and memory formation are briefly presented to set the stage for the individual chapters in which the different authors present their work, their ideas, and concepts for the present and the future.

Properties of LTP

LTP is a selective, use-dependent increase or facilitation of synaptic transmission in neuronal circuits. The postulated requirements for LTP in order for it to act successfully in memory storage include the following:

> Use-dependency; synapses that are active and are part of information processing should change, and they should only change if they had been successful in driving the postsynaptic neuron (Hebb, 1949); and
>
> Selectivity of change, which requires that changes are limited to active synapses and do not affect inactive synapses in the vicinity

These properties are crucial for a system to store information. Only if selective changes occur in a use-dependent way would a neuronal net be able to store memory.

Both properties are found in empirical studies of LTP. However, some discussion has arisen as to what degree LTP is restricted to active synapses only and does not spread to nearby synapses. Some studies have shown that there can be a spread to neighboring synapses (Bonhoeffer et al., 1989; Hartell, 1996). Such a local spread of synaptic change might make the network more reliable, since synapses show a certain amount of failure (Malenka and Nicoll, 1997).

Furthermore, LTP also shows the important property of associativity. When stimulating neurons via two independent pathways, LTP can be induced in a low-frequency stimulation (LFS) in one pathway if the stimulation is paired synchronously with high-frequency stimulation (HFS) in the second pathway. LFS alone would not induce LTP, and asynchronous pairing of stimulation of more than 100 ms via the two pathways does not either (Gustafsson et al, 1987; Stanton, 1996). This demonstrates that this is not a simple additive effect but a true "computation" of inputs, similar to an "and" gate in electronic engineering. A change will only occur if the neuron receives the correct simultaneous inputs. Synchronicity appears to be an important aspect, as it can be assumed that synchronous activity might be related and be part of the same information processing, while asynchronous activity might not be.

These properties have made LTP a very attractive memory model for scientists. However, there needs to be proof and not just a good model. As we will see, there are a number of caveats that need to be kept in mind when interpreting LTP research results.

Techniques for Measuring LTP

■ **LTP *In Vivo*.** LTP was first discovered in the hippocampus (Lømo, 1966; Bliss and Lømo, 1973), a structure known to be involved in learning processes (Zola-Morgan et al., 1986). It was made in an *in vivo* preparation by lowering electrodes into the perforant path and the dentate (Figure 1) of a rabbit. Recording can be done on anesthetized (Bliss and Lømo, 1973; Doyle et al., 1996) or freely moving animals (Moser et al., 1993). There are advantages to this technique. The brain is kept intact as much as possible and only local damage to tissue by the electrodes has to be taken into account. However, more detailed studies such as intracellular recordings or even patch clamp recordings of neurons are virtually impossible under these conditions, and field recordings have to be done "blind," without the benefit of knowledge of the precise anatomic location of the electrodes during the experiment. Consequently, a different technique that allows the direct and controlled access to selective neurons was developed for the investigation of cellular mechanisms of synaptic plasticity, such as LTP.

■ **LTP *In Vitro*.** One reason for the success of LTP research is that it is possible to slice the hippocampus without cutting the main connections between the dentate and the cornu ammonis (CA) areas, and to keep the slice alive for many hours in artificial cerebrospinal solution. The efferent and afferent connections as well as intrinsic connections of the hippocampus are arranged in layers in a topologic order from dorsal to ventral (Blackstad, 1956). Cutting along the layers produces slices in which the connections via the entorhinal cortex to the dentate gyrus, to the area CA3, and further to the area CA1 remain intact. All three synaptic connections are capable of LTP and this trisynaptic pathway is considered to be the main information processing pathway of the hippocampus. However, many more connections exist that are usually cut during the preparation (Braitenberg and Schütz, 1983) and these might be of major importance for hippocampal functions and information processing.

LTP, Long-Term Depression, and Depotentiation of Responses

Electrical stimulation of a neuron produces a response in the neuron to which it projects. This response can be measured in the form of an excitatory postsynaptic response (EPSP) of either whole populations of neurons (field EPSPs) or a single

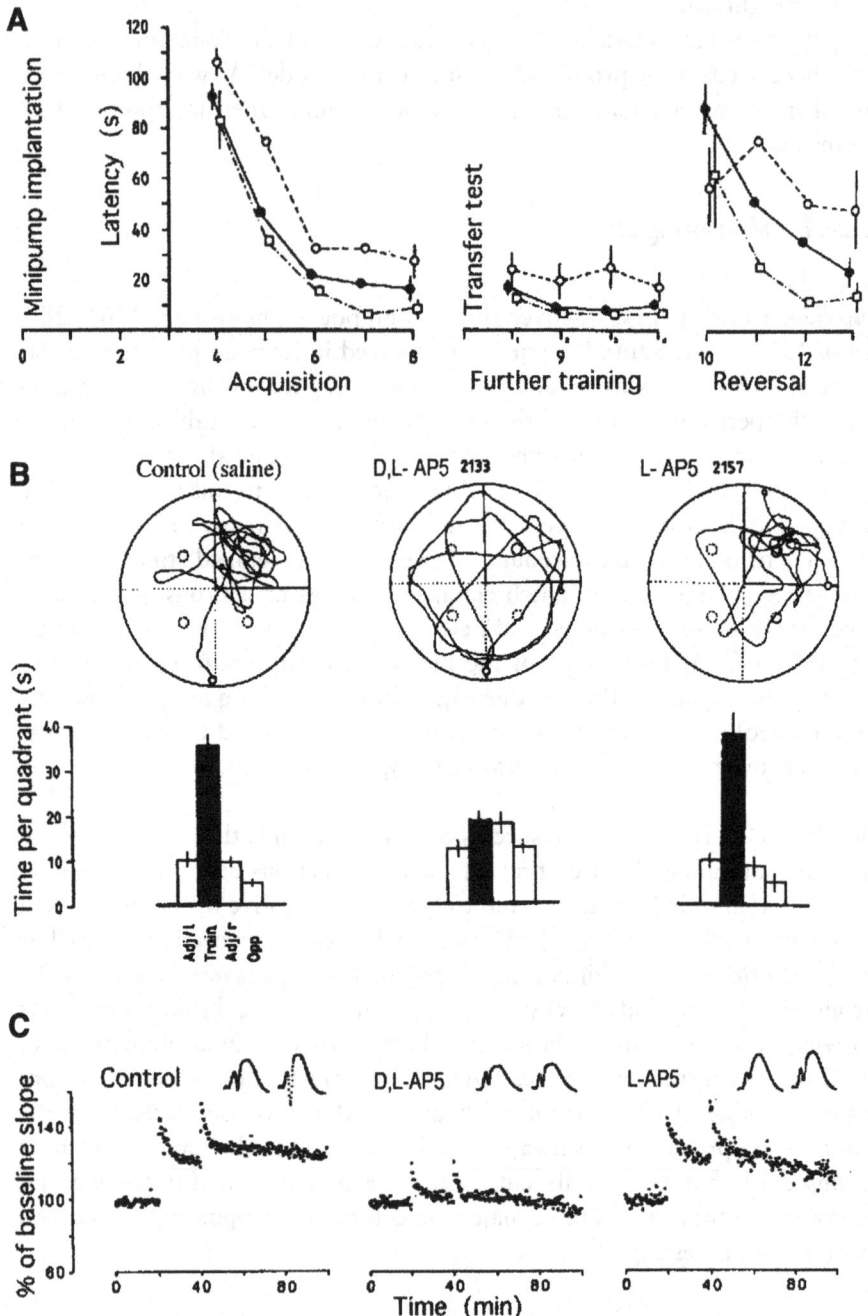

neuron. It is also possible to record population spikes, which measure summed action potentials of neurons rather than membrane potentials. A widely used technique for inducing LTP is by HFS, usually around several hundred pulses at 100 to 400 Hz. Such trains of pulses are a quick and reliable protocol to elicit LTP *in vitro* or *in vivo*.

A different type of synaptic plasticity is depotentiation (DP). In DP, field EPSPs that have been potentiated previously can be depotentiated back to baseline values by applying long trains of LFS (around 1 to 10 Hz). DP can be obtained *in vitro* (Selig et al., 1995; Huerta and Lisman, 1996) as well as *in vivo* (Stäubli and Lynch, 1990; Doyle et al., 1996) by applying LFS for 1 second. Again, the drawback of such a protocol is that no such prolonged and uniform firing patterns have been observed in the working hippocampus. DP is the reduction of previously potentiated EPSPs and should not be confused with long-term depression (LTD), which is a reduction of baseline EPSPs. DP and LTD appear to be different processes, as some researchers can induce DP readily but not LTD (Stäubli and Lynch, 1990; Doyle et al., 1996; Hölscher et al., 1997a).

LTD of the EPSP has also been described in the hippocampal slice by many groups (Stanton and Sejnowski, 1989; Christofi et al., 1993; Cummings et al., 1994; Selig et al., 1995). While LTD appears to be observed relatively easily in the hippocampal slice, it is more difficult to induce *in vivo*. One study found LTD *in vivo* only in extremely young animals with immature hippocampi (Errington et al., 1995). This suggests that LTD might be a developmental mechanism that is not involved in learning in mature brain areas. A study that did show LTD induction *in vivo* used sodium pentobarbital, an anesthetizing agent that is known to alter GABA inhibition (Thiels et al., 1995), which could explain the observed result (Heynen et al., 1996). Other studies using the same stimulation protocol, but employed urethane to anesthetize the rats, did not find any LTD (Stäubli and

---

Figure 1. The first study to show a correlation between LTP inducibility and learning abilities in animals showed that blocking LTP in the dentate gyrus using a blocker of NMDA receptors also impaired learning of a spatial water maze task. This study greatly supported and promoted the theory of LTP as a model for learning mechanisms and was extensively cited in following LTP studies. (A) Shown are the mean values of the time needed by rats to find a submerged platform in a water maze pool. The NMDA receptor antagonist D,L-AP5 was delivered by implanting osmotic pumps 4 days before start of the training The mean latencies of animals and the standard error of means are shown. A control group was infused with saline. As a second control, the inactive isomer L-AP5 was infused in a third group. The D,L-AP5 group was slower in learning the task. •, control; □, L-AP5; ○, D,L-AP5. (B) In a test of memory retrieval (transfer test), animals were left to explore the pool for 60 seconds with no platform present. The swim paths were analyzed and compared. Both control groups spent a lot more time in the quadrant that previously contained the platform compared with the other quadrants. Typical swim paths are shown. The D,L-AP5 group did not prefer the target quadrant over the other quadrants. (C) Block of LTP by D,L-AP5 on HFS in the dentate gyrus. Shown are the group mean normalized slope values of field EPSPs. HFS induced LTP in the saline control and also in the L-AP5 control group. No LTP was induced in the group that received D-AP5 infusions. For details see Morris et al. (1986). © Nature, reprinted with permission.

Lynch, 1990; Errington et al., 1995). Another study was able to induce LTD in area CA1 using a customized stimulation protocol (200 pairs of pulses at 0.5 Hz with an interpulse interval of 25 ms) and found LTD in area CA1 of the anesthetized rat (Thiels et al., 1995). These results were confirmed in a study with freely moving rats, using the same stimulation protocol. Here, LTD was found in area CA1, but not in the dentate (Doyère et al., 1996). A reliable method to induce LTD *in vivo* is to work with stressed animals. When stressed, the neuronal network appears to switch from an LTP-favoring system to a LTD favoring one. Numerous studies have shown that LTP is reduced in stressed rats, and some studies report the inducibility of LTD (Shors et al., 1989, 1990; Diamond et al., 1994a, 1994b, 1996; Pavlides et al., 1995; Xu et al., 1998). One of the factors governing this switch is the level of adrenal steroids present. Activation of mineralocorticoid type I receptors facilitates LTP, and when glucocorticoid type II receptors are activated, LTP is suppressed and LTD induction is facilitated (Bennett et al., 1991; Diamond et al., 1992; Pavlides et al., 1996; see also Section Four in this book). This mechanism of synaptic plasticity control suggests a physiologic role for enhancement or suppression of synaptic activity. However, if LTD is only inducible in stressed animals it is questionable that it plays a direct role in memory formation processes.

Advantages and Disadvantages of the Hippocampal Slice Preparation

One of the reasons for the great success of the LTP theory is the development of the hippocampal slice technique. Every year large numbers of articles are being published using this technique. Clearly, the slice preparations offer possibilities not found in *in vivo* preparations. It is possible to record from defined neurons, to fill neurons with tracers or enzyme inhibitors, to directly measure intracellular calcium changes with image analysis techniques, or even to record from isolated receptors or ion channels by means of patch-clamp recording. The important discoveries of the roles of receptors or enzymes in synaptic transmission are legion, for example, the role of the NMDA receptor (Cotman and Iversen, 1987) and the role of protein kinase C (Fagnou and Tuchek, 1995) to name just two. Furthermore, it is possible to identify the effect of novel drugs on isolated receptors or ion channels and investigate their precise mode of action, and the exact concentration of the drugs present in the slice buffer is known. Manipulations such as complete inhibition of GABAergic neurons are possible, which would not be feasible *in vivo*.

A price has to be paid for accessing these new areas of investigation. When cutting a slice one cuts off basal brain projections such as the cholinergic innervation by the nucleus basalis (involved in the development of theta rhythm), the noradrenergic projection from the locus coeruleus, the serotonergic afferences from the raphe nuclei, or modulation by neurotrophic agents, steroids, neuropeptides, hormones, and so forth. Disconnecting neurons from these modulating factors greatly alters the response characteristics of neurons in the slice, such as the probability to fire action potentials or to change in their synaptic responses. Furthermore, when cutting slices, cells get damaged and release very high concentrations of glutamate, a neurotoxic transmitter. Also, a slice is kept in a bath at temperatures usually much lower than 37°C, and when working in the dentate high doses of GABA antagonists are often added to facilitate LTP induction.

Another problem is that after HFS different components of the EPSP can be measured to determine whether LTP has occurred, and there is no general agreement between researchers about which variable is preferable. This problem has been addressed by others (Bliss and Lynch, 1988; Barnes, 1995) but with little success so far. For instance, the mechanisms that underlie changes of the population spike amplitude are quite distinct from the ones that regulate changes in the slope or amplitude of the EPSP (Bliss and Lynch, 1988).

It is therefore not surprising that the results obtained with slice preparations differ extremely between laboratories. For example, the metabotropic glutamate receptor (mGluR) group I and II agonist 1S,3R-ACPD evoked depression of the EPSP in the slice in one study (O'Mara et al., 1995), produced slow-onset potentiation of the EPSP without depression in another laboratory (Bortolotto and Collingridge, 1992), and yet produced potentiation with initial depression of the EPSP in a third study (Chinestra et al., 1994). Since the drug has agonistic effects on presynaptic receptors that cause depression of the baseline, and on postsynaptic receptors that can cause potentiation (Glaum et al., 1992), it is possible that the contradictory results are the product of slight differences between the different experimental setups, some of which might favor the depressing or the exciting property of the drug.

There has been similar confusion among reports of the effects of inhibitors of nitric oxide synthase (NOS) on LTP induction in the slice. In some studies, LTP induction in the CA1 field of rat hippocampal slices was prevented by NOS inhibitors (Böhme et al., 1991; O'Dell et al., 1991; Schuman and Madison, 1991; Bon et al., 1992). In contrast, other groups were able to inhibit LTP formation with NOS inhibitors only under particular conditions. Williams et al. (1993) were able to prevent LTP induction in the hippocampal slice with NOS inhibitors only under low temperatures (24°C) and not under more physiologic temperatures (30°C). It is important to note that the block under 24°C was highly specific and fully reversible with the NOS substrate L-arginine, showing that the effect is not a side effect of the inhibitor acting elsewhere. Why this selective effect suddenly disappeared at higher temperatures remains to be investigated. To make things even more complicated, HFS in the hippocampal slice showed LTP formation that could not be blocked by NOS blockers in a low stimulation protocol, but was blockable in a strong stimulation protocol (Gribkoff and Lum-Ragan, 1992; Lum-Ragan and Gribkoff, 1993). The opposite result was observed in other studies: Weak expression of LTP was blocked, but the drug did not impair stronger LTP induced by prolonged HFS (Chetkovich et al., 1993; Haley et al., 1993; Musleh et al., 1993). This shows that results obtained in the slice preparation should be taken cautiously, and ideally one would aim to confirm the results in *in vivo* studies.

Correlating LTP With Learning: Sometimes You See It, Sometimes You Don't

The studies of LTP induced in the hippocampal slice or *in vivo* in the hippocampus produced a large number of impressive and exciting findings. However, it is clearly of importance to investigate whether LTP-like processes are involved in learning and memory and therefore if LTP induced artificially could be considered as a model for learning mechanisms. Studies that correlate such synaptic changes with synaptic responses in learning animals are of great interest. There are several strategies how one could go about this task.

Recording of EPSPs in the Hippocampus During Learning

One strategy to investigate if LTP is involved in learning is to record EPSPs from learning animals and to see whether the response changes after the learning experience. This approach is the most straightforward but has turned out to be fraught with pitfalls. Initial reports that there is an increase of the EPSP in the dentate gyrus of the rat after exploring a novel environment (Green and Greenough, 1986) were later shown to be an artifact produced by temporary temperature increases in the brain following locomotion (Moser et al., 1993). More recent data suggest that after subtracting the effects of temperature, motor activity, handling, and so forth, an upregulation of the field EPSP in the dentate still remains for about 15 minutes after exposure of the rats to a novel environment (Moser, 1996). Yet 15 minutes is not a long time and cannot account for long-term memory formation. Also, as the author stated, field EPSP recording is not the ideal way to analyze possible changes in synaptic efficacy. If the changes are small or only few synapses change after learning, they might be obscured by the large group of synapses that were recorded from but did not potentiate. In fact, some neuronal network models do predict a distributed change of only a few synapses in the network to increase storage capacity (sparse synapse weight changes) (Marr and Vaina, 1982; Simmen et al., 1996; see also Section Three in this book). Furthermore, if some synapses are downregulated while others are upregulated, the overall sum of changes could be zero. Finally, the dentate might not be the ideal location to record long-term changes related to memory formation. It has been suggested by several authors that the dentate is only a gate for information filtering and passing on to area CA3 and CA1 for further processing. Measuring neuronal activity in the dentate showed that this activity is fairly nonspecific and more generally related to novelty of stimuli (Vinogradova, 1975; Deadwyler et al., 1981). Complex spike activity in area CA1, however, is related to specific stimuli and seems to encode defined information rather than to detect just novelty (Heit et al., 1988; Mizumori et al., 1989). The area CA1 may therefore be a more suitable location to look for learning-specific changes in the EPSP.

Behavioral Pharmacologic Studies

Another approach is to try to correlate the effect of drugs that inhibit LTP formation with the effect of these drugs on learning. Correlations are always indirect proof and cannot be seen as hard evidence for LTP-like effects during learning, since disturbing LTP and blocking learning with the same drug does not necessarily mean that both effects are based on the same mechanism. On the other hand, if it can be shown that animals learn while LTP induction in the hippocampus is blocked by a drug it would suggest that mechanisms that underlie LTP are not required for learning.

One of the first groups of researchers to follow this approach were Morris and colleagues, who conducted exhaustive studies on the effects of AP5, a drug that blocks the NMDA glutamate receptor. A famous and often cited study that seemed to support the assumption that LTP in the hippocampal slice is a good model for synaptic plastic changes during learning investigated the effect of AP5 on LTP and learning abilities. Doses of AP5 that blocked LTP induction *in vitro* and *in vivo* also impaired learning of a spatial water maze task (Morris et al., 1986; Morris, 1989; see also Figure 1). Recent studies, however, have shown that if the rats are pretrained in a spatial task in the water maze without drug application and then trained in a spatial task in another room, AP5 did not block learning even though it blocked induction of LTP (Bannerman et al., 1995; see Figure 2). A different study found that nonspatial pretraining in the water maze is sufficient to prevent the amnestic effect of NMDA antagonists in a subsequent spatial water maze task (Saucier and Cain, 1995; see also Chapter 13). The authors interpret the effect such that the animals first have to learn how to cope with drug-induced motor impairments and then are able to learn the task.

Studies with other drugs that act on mGluRs such as L-AP4 seem to show a correlation between LTP inducibility and learning. The same dose of L-AP4 reduced LTP formation *in vivo* (Manahan-Vaughan and Reymann, 1995) and impaired spatial learning (Hölscher et al., 1996).

Different studies that were testing the effects of mGluR drugs, however, did not show such a correlation. Injecting the mGluR agonist 1S,3S-ACPD did not impair learning of spatial or nonspatial tasks in the water maze or the radial arm maze. LTP in area CA1 measured *in vivo*, however, was obliterated completely (Hölscher et al., 1997b). Furthermore, using the mGluR agonist tADA that acts on different receptor subtypes than 1S,3S-ACPD, it was shown that LTP in the dentate gyrus measured *in vivo* was increased, while spatial learning abilities of rats were impaired (Riedel et al., 1995a, 1995b).

Such a lack of correlation between learning abilities of rats and the ability to block LTP *in vitro* or *in vivo* indicates that the concept of HFS-induced LTP being a good model for cellular processes that underlie learning processes is too simplistic.

Synapse Saturation Experiments

A different approach to study whether LTP is essential for learning is to try to saturate all synapses in the hippocampus by electrical stimulation, assuming that the upregulation of all synapses should make learning impossible. The first studies reported that after saturation of synapses, animals were not able to learn a spatial task normally, while learning in animals in which LTP was induced but allowed to decay was not impaired (Castro et al., 1989). This result was seen as evidence in

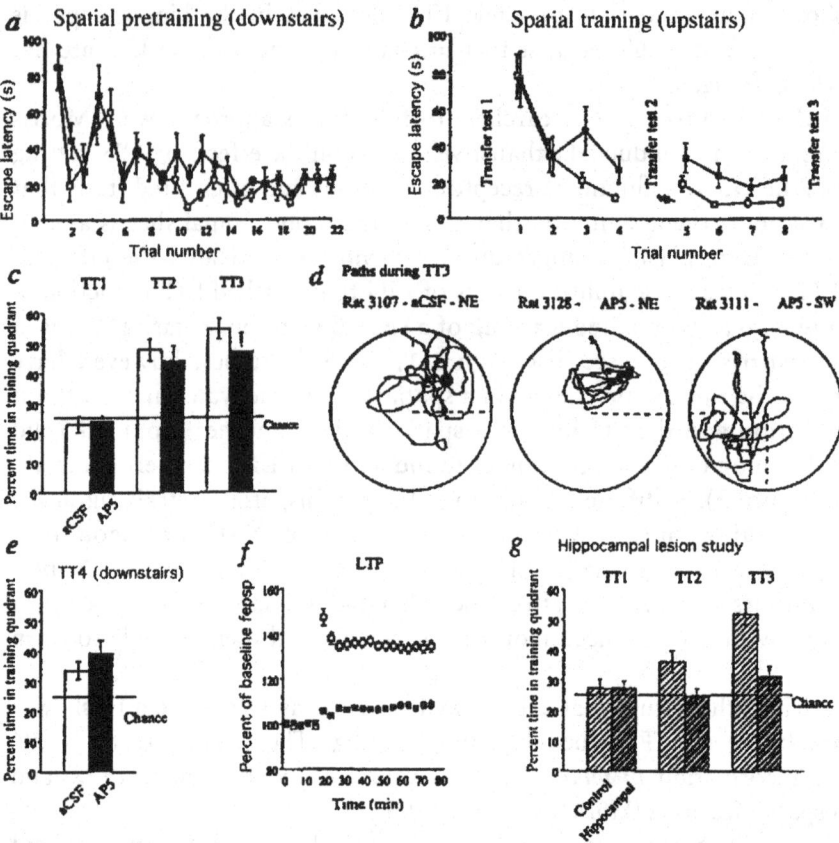

Figure 2. A follow-up study in the same laboratory showed that blocking HFS-induced LTP in the dentate gyrus does not necessarily impair learning of a spatial water maze task. (a) Shown are the mean times needed by animals in two groups to find a submerged platform. No drug was given in this spatial pretraining. The reduction of acquisition times after 22 trials was not different in both groups. (b) After having implanted osmotic pumps that delivered D-AP5 (■) or artificial cerebrospinal fluid (□). In a spatial training task in a different pool located in a different room, a difference between groups was recorded. (c) In the 60-second transfer task without a platform, both groups had no preference for the target quadrant before acquisition of the task (first pair of bars), but both groups had a clear preference for the target quadrant after acquisition of the task after trial 4 (second pair of bars) and 8 (last two bars). (d) Typical swim paths of rats in the third transfer task. (e) A fourth transfer task was conducted in the first room in which the pretraining took place. No difference in quadrant preference was seen. (f) Mean percentage slope potentiation of dentate field EPSPs showed near complete blockade of LTP in the AP5-treated group. (g) For comparison, the experiment was repeated with animals with hippocampal lesions or sham operations. The lesioned animals did not spend more time in the target quadrant before and after acquisition trials. Sham operated animals developed a preference for the target quadrant after the training protocol. For details see Bannerman et al. (1995). © Nature, reprinted with permission.

favor of the LTP theory. However, further investigations by other groups (Robinson, 1992; Jeffery and Morris, 1993; Sutherland et al., 1993) could not replicate these findings, and successive work by Barnes et al. (1994) showed that the initial studies were flawed and saturation of all synapses was probably never achieved.

In a different correlation study in which LTP was induced prior to learning a water maze, the surprising result was that animals that showed more LTP after HFS treatment learned the task better. This is the opposite of what one would expect from the saturation hypothesis, although it is not known how long saturation was maintained in the hippocampus (Jeffery and Morris, 1993). Further studies showed a more complex relationship between LTP inducibility and learning abilities. When inducing LTP in good learners, the input-output curve showed a small increase in EPSPs when stimulating weakly but large LTP when stimulating strongly. In poor learners this correlation was reversed, and LTP of EPSPs was large after HFS when giving a weak test stimulus but small when giving a strong test stimulus (Jeffery, 1995).

In a later study, a different technique was used to ensure saturation of synapses in the dorsal hippocampus. Using a multielectrode array, LTP had been induced by HFS, and using different electrodes, it was determined whether LTP was inducible in a different part of the dorsal hippocampus. The authors found that when synapses were saturated by this criterion, animals were impaired in learning a spatial water maze task. However, other animals that still displayed a small amount of LTP (more than 10 percent) at the site of the "naive" electrodes did learn the task (Moser et al., 1998). This result was later drawn into question. In experiments in which the animals were pretrained in one water maze, stimulated, and then trained in a different water maze, synapse saturation did not impair their spatial learning abilities (Otnaes et al., 1999).

It is interesting to note that in the initial Moser et al. (1998) study, the inducibility of only 10 percent LTP appeared to be sufficient to preserve the learning abilities of the animals, the same value found in a mouse strain that does not express the glycoprotein Thy-1 (Errington et al., 1997). If a 10 percent change in EPSPs of synapses is sufficient to encode stable memory, LTP studies that do not show a reduction of LTP below the 10 percent level would not be considered to be of any relevance for memory formation. However, it is not clear whether the 10 percent increase in field EPSPs was due to a large increase in few synapses or a small increase in all synapses.

Experiments With Gene Deletion (Knock-Out) or Transgenic Mice Strains

Mutant mice strains that do not express a defined gene for a protein that has been shown to be crucial for LTP induction have been used to compare their ability to learn spatial or nonspatial tasks, and to analyze whether LTP can be elicited in the hippocampus. Again, a correlation between learning impairments and reduced or blocked LTP formation does not directly prove that the same mechanisms are involved. Knocking out a gene that is essential for neuronal activity might well impair LTP and learning without being directly involved in both. More serious problems arise from the fact that the animals have to develop and mature until their learning abilities can be tested. Obviously, if the deleted gene is essential for normal development the organism cannot mature normally and might show impaired learning abilities or LTP inducibility. On the other hand, redundant mechanisms might compensate for the lack of a gene and no changes in adult animals would be seen when compared with wild-type animals. Other problems arise from the techniques that are involved in creating gene deletion of transgenic animals. For example, null mutant mice of gene targeting studies are often hybrids of two mouse strains, and such hybrids are genetically different from their control litter mates, not only at the locus of the targeted gene but also at other loci (Gerlai, 1996).

In an experiment that employed a strain of mutant mice that does not express the α-isoform of CaMkinase II, an enzyme that was found to be of importance in LTP formation (Malenka et al., 1989), the ability to develop LTP in slices taken from this strain was impaired. The changes in response after stimulation were located mostly presynaptically, while the properties of NMDA receptors appeared to be unchanged (Silva et al., 1992b). The same strain was tested in water maze tasks. The mutant mice took longer to learn a nonspatial cue task with a visible platform than control mice, indicating that the animals were impaired in a more general way. The mutants did not learn spatial orientation tasks with a submerged platform or learned only after several days of training, while the control animals memorized the location of the platform after a few trials (Silva et al., 1992a). This is an encouraging result for the LTP theory.

In a similar study that involved a specific tyrosine kinase found on the *fyn* gene, LTP was deficient in area CA1 and learning difficulties in a hidden platform water maze task were apparent. However, the anatomy of the hippocampus showed abnormalities that might be due to developmental deficits and could well explain the impairment of LTP and learning (Grant et al., 1992). More detailed analysis of the learning abilities of the animals, however, showed that they are able to learn spatial tasks if the right conditions are chosen, and that the inability to learn a water maze task is more associated with increased fear responses of the animals (Miyakawa et al., 1996). Furthermore, the animals displayed altered swimming behavior that interfered with the learning of a water maze task (Huerta et al., 1996).

To the great surprise of many scientists working in the field of LTP, a study of gene deletion mice strains that do not express the glycoprotein Thy-1 showed that these mice did not express LTP in the dentate *in vivo* in the anesthetized preparation (while LTP in CA1 was unaffected) yet the animals were able to learn a spatial task in the water maze (Nosten-Bertrand et al., 1996). In the same study it was found that LTP in the dentate was not blocked in hippocampal slice preparation. Further investigations showed that the reason for inhibition of LTP formation is a much greater inhibition of the dentate *in vivo* by GABAergic interneurons. Since it is necessary in slice studies of LTP in the dentate to block GABAergic inhibition to facilitate expression of LTP, it was not surprising that the slice studies showed "normal" LTP. This result shows two important things: that slice studies of the dentate are conducted under extremely unrealistic conditions, which makes any result of such studies rather questionable, and that LTP in the dentate, as elicited by standard stimulation protocols, is a poor model for learning mechanisms.

In further studies in freely moving mice, LTP was inducible to about 110 percent of baseline value, small LTP compared with 160 percent in control mice (Errington et al., 1997). This result shows that results obtained in anesthetized animals are not always identical with results from awake animal studies. It is not known whether the 10 percent increase is due to a 10 percent LTP in all synapses involved or to much higher LTP in a small subpopulation of synapses. If the latter is the case, one might assume that it is sufficient for memory formation to occur if only a small percentage of neurons can be upregulated, as predicted in sparse encoding neuronal network theories. If that is the case, the previously reported results of the blocking of LTP by selective drugs have to be reevaluated. If the study still shows a greater than 10 percent LTP after application of the drug, one cannot assume that the block would impair memory formation *in vivo*.

Another study revealed that "knock out" mice strains that do not express either a regulator or a catalytic subunit of neuronal protein kinase A (PKA) show no LTP selectively in the dentate mossy fiber terminals in area CA3 but do learn spatial and nonspatial tasks (Huang et al., 1995; see Figure 3). The associational-commissural pathways were unaffected by the gene deletion. The stimulation protocols used to elicit LTP were standard protocols (100 Hz for 1 s at 10-s intervals) used in many slice studies. It might be possible that LTP could have been induced in these mice using a very different protocol. However, since most researchers use such a protocol of trains of 100 to 400 Hz stimulation, and this protocol failed to elicit LTP while learning remained unimpaired, it questions the validity of results of dentate LTP studies *in vivo* or *in vitro*. Interestingly, a study of a mice strain with a gene deletion of the *Steel* factor showed normal LTP at the mossy fiber pathway in CA3 but impaired performance in a spatial water maze task (Motro et al., 1996). This suggests that LTP in the mossy fiber pathway is not needed for normal performance in the water maze task.

Apart from creating knock-out mice strains that do not express a specific protein, or transgenic mice that express a protein that has been inserted into the genome, a different technique is in use by researchers to test the roles of specific genes in LTP and learning. In a study using such an approach, oligonucleotides that bind to known gene sequences (antisense oligonucleotides) are injected into an animal, and the expression of the protein encoded by that gene is inhibited by binding to the target gene and preventing the transcription process. The advantage of this technique is that neuronal activity is not impaired or altered during development by a lack of or addition of proteins in the system, which could lead to secondary deficits that show up in tests after maturation. In one study, the role of the presynaptic A-type voltage-dependent K+ channel mKv1.4 in both learning and LTP in CA1 was investigated. Antisense oligodeoxyribonucleotides to the mKv1.4 gene were injected intraventricularly into rat brains. This antisense "knockdown" had no effect on spatial learning, but eliminated both early- and late- phase LTP in

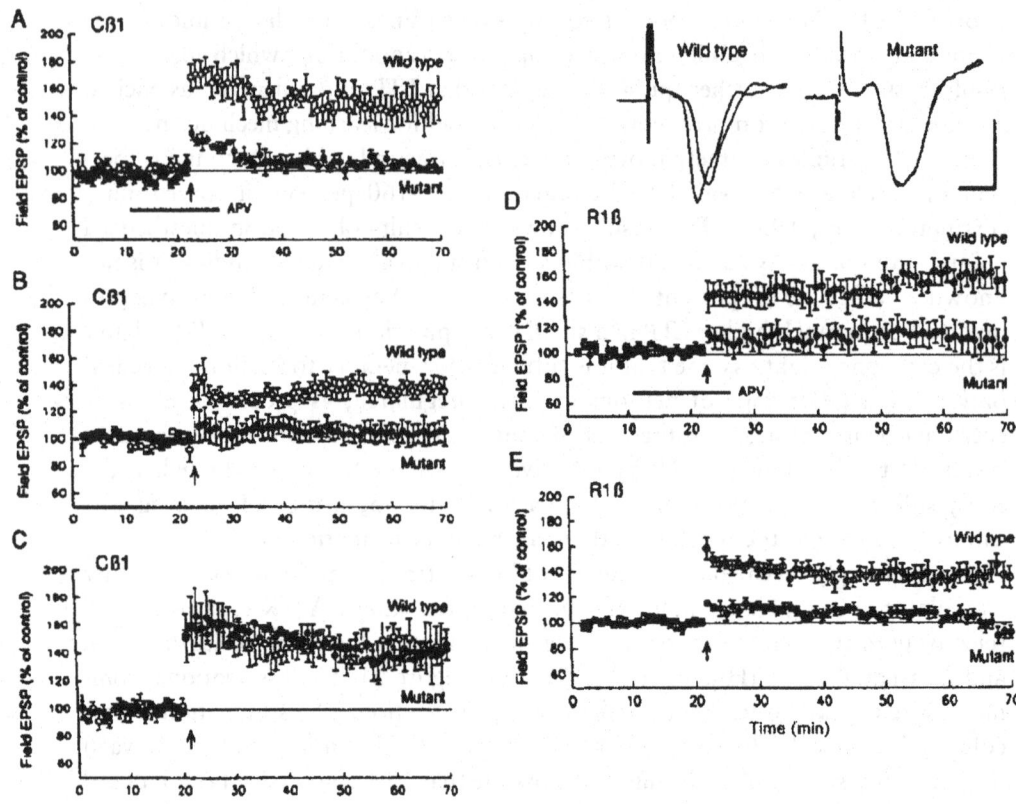

Figure 3. Correlating spatial learning abilities of genetically altered mice with LTP inducibility in area CA3 and CA1. Two strains were tested, one that has a deletion of the Cβ$_1$ catalytic subunit of protein kinase A (PKA) and a second with the deletion of the regulatory RIβ isoform of PKA. (a) Effect of HFS on mossy fiber Section (A) shows lack of mossy fiber LTP after HFS in area CA3 in Cβ$_1$ mutants. Two trains of HFS induced robust LTP in the presence of AP5 in wild-type controls. B: The same experiment in the absence of AP5 did no induce LTP in mutant mice either. C: LTP is intact in Cβ$_1$ mutants in the associational-commissural pathway. D: In mice with RIβ gene deletion, HFS did not induce LTP of the mossy-fiber pathway in the presence of AP5. Inset traces show EPSP 10 minutes before and 45 minutes after HFS in controls (**left**) and mutant mice (**right**). E: No LTP was observed in the absence of AP5 in the same pathway. In contrast, wild-type control animals developed robust LTP. (b) Performance of mice in the Morris water maze task and in fear conditioning tasks. A: Time required by animals to reach the hidden platform in a spatial water maze task by RIβ mutants and wild-type control. No difference in acquisition was observed. B: No difference was seen in time spent in the pool quadrants during the transfer task. TQ, target quadrant. C: Number of times RIβ mutants and control mice crossed the location where the platform was in the target quadrant or the equivalent location in the other quadrant during the acquisition trials. No difference between groups was seen. D–I: Contextual and cued fear conditioning tasks. D: Freezing responses following an unconditioned stimulus (US) were not different between Cβ$_1$ and control groups. E: Freezing responses 24 hours after training were not different between groups. F: Cued fear conditioning tasks did not reveal a difference between groups. G–I show results of the same experiments as D–F, testing fear conditioning responses of RIβ mutant mice. No significant difference to responses of wild-type mice were observed. For details see Huang et al. (1995). © Cell Press Ltd, reprinted with permission. (*Figure continues.*)

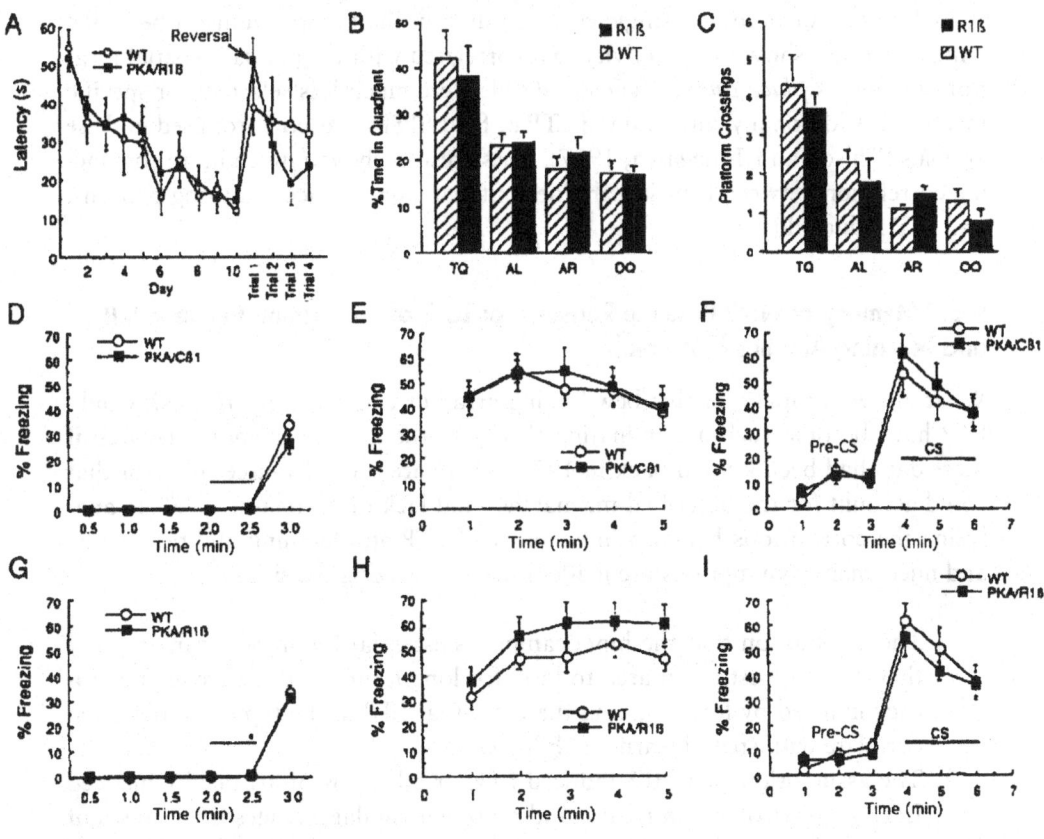

Figure 3 *Continued*

CA1 pyramidal neurons without affecting dentate gyrus LTP. The authors concluded that this Kv1.1 knockdown experiment demonstrates that LTP in CA1 is neither necessary nor sufficient for rat spatial memory (Meiri et al., 1998). In a different experiment, antisense reduction or elimination of mKv1.1 K$^+$ channels showed the opposite result. Now, learning of a spatial water maze was impaired, but LTP in area CA1 was unimpaired. Again, the authors concluded that LTP in CA1 is neither necessary nor sufficient for rat spatial memory (Meiri et al., 1997; see Alkon, 1999, for details).

Selective NMDA Receptor Knock-Out in Area CA1 of Transgenic Mice

The techniques of deleting defined genes in mice strains have been refined. In one study the area of altered gene expression was confined to a limited brain area only. The expression of NMDA receptors was selectively repressed in area CA1 of the hippocampus. Clearly, any unwanted indirect effects caused by lack of NMDA receptors in other parts of the brain, or any developmental impairments in the brain that could result in compromised learning abilities of animals, are avoided in such a surgical knock-out technique. These mice were impaired in learning spatial tasks. Furthermore, single cell recording in the hippocampus in behaving animals did not show firing activity that correlated with the animal's spatial location (known as *place cells*). Their place cells were much less selective for specific locations. Additionally, induction of LTP of field EPSPs was compromised in these animals (Wilson and Tonegawa, 1997). These results show a much more convincing correlation between learning abilities of the animals, space cell firing patterns, and LTP inducibility.

Is LTP Memory or Not? Possible Reasons for Lack of Correlation Between LTP and Learning Abilities in Animals

What are we to make of this bewildering array of contradictory results? Would LTP have become such a dominating theory in the area of memory research if these data had been known back in 1973? There are several sources of error that could account for the described mismatches and lack of correlations. When analyzing the correlations between inducibility of LTP and learning abilities of rats and mice, many assumptions are made prior to analyzing the situation:

1. The assumption that the hippocampus is essential for spatial learning, and that it is the best brain area to look for long-term changes in synaptic efficacy induced by learning, and therefore that LTP in the hippocampus must correlate with spatial learning abilities.
2. The assumption that HFS-induced LTP, or all forms of artificially induced LTP, are physiologic in nature and represent similar changes in synapses of neurons that process and encode information.
3. Most studies use the water maze as a learning task and assume that learning a spatial water maze task tests predominantly (if not exclusively) spatial learning skills.

Is the Hippocampus the Correct Area?

All of these assumptions have to be fulfilled if the previously reported correlations between learning abilities in animals and inducibility of LTP can be seen as supporting evidence for the theory that LTP is a model for memory formation. Point No. 1 has been shown to be incorrect by several experimental results that show that animals with lesions in the hippocampus are still able to learn the water maze task (Jarrard et al., 1984; Whishaw and Jarrard, 1996). There may be impairments, but by no means is the ability of learning such a task completely blocked. Jarrard concludes that a pronounced block of spatial learning capacity of rats can only be observed if the entire hippocampus together with an associated structure such as the fimbria fornix or the subiculum are lesioned. On a similar note, Schenk et al. (1995) found that hippocampal lesions render rats far from incapable of learning spatial tasks if the correct conditions are chosen. Perhaps the block of LTP in the hippocampus is by no means sufficient to prevent spatial learning in rats and mice, because LTP occurs in other areas.

As indicated previously, an important assumption that many researchers make is that the study of one subsection of the hippocampus (e.g., the dentate gyrus) is sufficient to analyze memory processes, and that the block of LTP in that section will prevent memory formation. This concept of a strictly linear information flow through the hippocampus involves only three synapses: input from the entorhinal cortex to the dentate, connecting then to area CA3 and then to CA1. According to this concept interruption of the "data flow" anywhere in the chain should disrupt memory formation altogether.

However, since there are many additional pathways in the hippocampus, this might not be a realistic concept. There are, for example, direct connections between the entorhinal cortex and area CA1. In this way, information could "circumvent" the dentate gyrus and the system could still function properly and process and memorize information. The concept of parallel connections or decentralized distribution of information processing and memory storage in the brain is far from new. Anatomic evidence for parallel connections of the entorhinal cortex with the dentate, with the areas CA3 and CA1 directly, or with the subiculum was described some time ago and could explain the recent findings in studies of gene deletion mice strains (Blackstad, 1956; Steward, 1976; Schwerdtfeger, 1984). Evidence that these multiple connections play a functional role in information processing and memory formation has been given in a large number of reports on the effect of localized lesions or pharmaceutical inhibitions within the hippocampus or the associated structures. Lesioning the entorhinal cortex, the major cortical afference to the hippocampus, only produced mild impairments of spatial learning abilities in rats (Schenk and Morris, 1985; Hölscher and Schmidt, 1994). Lesions of the fimbria-fornix pathway did impair the animals to some extent yet they were able to learn a spatial task (Whishaw et al., 1995). Lesioning defined areas within the hippocampus with neurotoxic agents that spare axons running through the lesioned areas showed that lesioning, for example, the dentate or area CA3 showed only mild impairments in spatial tasks in a radial arm maze (Jarrard, 1983; Jarrard et al., 1984). Axon-sparing lesions of the hippocampus caused rats to make more errors when learning spatial tasks but again they were far from being totally incapable of learning spatial tasks (Jarrard, 1986, 1995; Kesslak, 1986).

Hence, a block of LTP in a single brain area with a selective drug cannot be seen as a decisive result that proves the involvement of the receptor or enzyme in question in memory formation. The anatomic connections would make it possible that only small synaptic changes take place in many areas that are functionally connected. The sum of all minor changes would then encode memory. Measuring naturally evolving LTP *in vivo* could therefore be an even more difficult project than expected.

Additionally, it is unlikely that memory is processed or stored only in the hippocampus. The reason why the hippocampus has been chosen as a potential seat of memory is historically founded. Lesioning of the hippocampus along with other temporal lobe brain areas in the textbook case H.M., a patient who had been treated for severe epilepsy by bilateral temporal surgery (Scoville and Milner, 1957), or the case of R.B., who suffered hypoxia-induced loss of pyramidal neurons selectively in area CA1 (Zola-Morgan et al., 1986) or other similar cases (Rempel-Clower et al., 1996) showed that the hippocampal formation is of great importance in human memory formation and in the consolidation of long-term memory. However, previously established long-term memory was not strongly impaired in these people (Warrington, 1996). Animals with hippocampal lesions showed similar symptoms. Memory that had been formed before the lesion is still available to the animals in postsurgical tests (Jarrard, 1983; Barnes, 1988; Whishaw and Jarrard, 1996). Instead, short-term or working memory (Olton et al., 1979; Rawlins, 1985; Butelman, 1990), and the consolidation of long-term memory appear to be affected (Jarrard, 1995; Eichenbaum, 1996; Vnek and Rothblat, 1996).

The question is if the hippocampus is the ideal brain area to study when analyzing long-term memory formation. It is possible that the hippocampus is of importance in enabling consolidation of long-term memory. If this was the case, searching for long-term changes in the hippocampus (e.g., naturally occurring LTP after learning) might be futile. Other brain areas that are involved in long-term memory storage could be better areas to investigate.

LTP in Brain Areas Other Than the Hippocampus

■ **LTP in the Thalamus-Amygdala Pathway *In Vitro* and *In Vivo*.** The amygdala plays a major role in the development of emotional memory formation. Animals with lesions in the amygdala will not learn fear conditioning tasks that contain an element of punishment (e.g., bright light, electric shock, water) very well. Therefore, the role of the amygdala in these tasks has been under considerable investigation. In two studies it was shown that the projection from the thalamus to the lateral amygdala shows synaptic plasticity after learning a fear conditioning task. When measuring field potentials in the lateral nucleus of the amygdala that were evoked by auditory stimuli in freely moving animals it was found that after a fear conditioning training protocol, field potentials were increased (Rogan et al., 1997). Investigating this type of LTP further using *in vitro* slice techniques, it was found that the projection of the medial geniculate nucleus to the lateral amygdala nucleus showed a presynaptic facilitation of AMPA receptor mediated transmission in evoked EPSCs in whole cell recording (McKernen and Shinnick-Gallagher, 1997; see also Chapter 2). This novel observation of naturally occurring increases of EPSPs is very encouraging and supports the suggestion that the hippocampus might not be the ideal brain area in which to study long-term memory formation, since naturally occurring upregulation of field EPSPs after learning has not been found there (yet).

■ **LTP in the Cortex.** LTP has been described in the neocortex. Since long-term memory is encoded in different neocortical areas, perhaps investigating the role of LTP in the cortex is a more promising approach. A disadvantage is the fact that fiber connections are more diffuse and of relatively short length and not as neatly organized in defined pathways as in the hippocampus. This makes it technically challenging to record from neurons in the cortex. LTP has been studied in some defined areas, for example, the somatosensory cortex. Synaptic plasticity and developmental processes in the somatosensory areas that process whisker sensory input in rodents (the "barrel cortex") have been under considerable investigation. During development the fiber connections in the barrel cortex are remodeled in a highly flexible fashion depending on the sensory input from the whiskers. The removal of one whisker will lead to a dramatic remodeling of the topographic fiber projections within the cortical area that previously processed sensory input from that whisker. Furthermore, deprivation of sensory input through whisker activation plastically alters the neuronal response properties of cortical neurons in the barrel cortex (Glazewski et al., 1998a,b).

To investigate if LTP-like changes occur in the neocortex after learning a spatial water maze task, posterior parietal cortex field EPSPs were evoked through transcallosal stimulation. After intensive training the animals learned the task, but transcallosal evoked field potentials were not changed. Administering HFS induced LTP of field potentials, showing that the fiber connections were capable of developing LTP (Beiko and Cain, 1998). Again, the possibility remains that very few synaptic connections actually develop LTP during learning that cannot be picked up in field recordings, or no LTP develops at all in the neocortex during learning. LTP appears to be more difficult to induce in the cortex compared to the hippocampal formation. In a chronic recording study, LTP in callosal-neocortical field EPSPs was only inducible after potent stimulation that extended over days. The induction of LTP occurred after 5 days of administrating thirty HFS trains per day. Once induced, however, the observed LTP lasted for 4 weeks (Racine et al., 1995). It is questionable that this stimulation can be called physiologic, but the persistence of the LTP induced at least harbors the promise that LTP-like processes can be used as a basis for long-term memory in the cortex.

How Many Types of LTP Are There?

Assumption number 2 is that all types of LTP are equal and all are modeling synaptic changes that occur during learning. We already know that there are a number of different types of LTP. LTP at mossy fiber synapses in area CA3 is quite different from LTP in area CA1 or in the dentate gyrus. LTP in CA3 appears to be NMDA receptor independent and preferentially induced at the presynaptic site (Johnston et al., 1992; Langdon et al., 1995), while in area CA1 there are changes at the postsynaptic site and possible presynaptic site (Kullmann et al., 1996). The distribution of mGluRs and NMDA glutamate receptors is different in area CA1 and CA3. In CA1, NMDA receptors are high in density, whereas mGluRs are relatively low (Cotman and Iversen, 1987; Ohishi et al., 1995). In CA3, this relation is reversed (Ohishi et al., 1995; Blümcke et al., 1996). Furthermore, there are chemically induced forms of LTP, such as slow-onset potentiation (Chinestra et al., 1994). Are all of these types of LTP identical? Once LTP has been induced, are there differences between LTP induced by HFS or by chemical agents?

Additionally, there are differences in stimulation protocols used by researchers. Usually, a protocol is used that has been empirically shown to produce stable LTP. While the standard protocol consists of trains of HFS (trains of ca. 100 to 400 Hz), more sophisticated protocols are sometimes in use that have been shown to induce LTP easier and in a more reliable way. For example, a theta-patterned type of stimulation protocol has been developed. In this type of protocol, a train of HFS is interrupted by an intertrain interval of around 50 to 200 ms (Rose and Dunwiddie, 1986; Stäubli and Lynch, 1987). This protocol mimics theta frequency activity that is observed in electroencephalographic (EEG) measurements and represents membrane depolarization in the 5 to 10 Hz area. If different protocols have different effects on field EPSPs, does this mean that the resulting LTP is different, or is it simply the same LTP induced differently?

In conclusion, a lack of correlation between LTP inducibility and learning abilities in animals could therefore be due to the fact that the wrong stimulation protocol has been applied. HFS might not induce LTP, but rather a different stimulation protocol that nobody has thought of yet. In addition, the type of LTP induced by HFS might be genuinely different from LTP induced by learning processes or theta-patterned stimulation. Such an LTP might be induced differently (e.g., activation of different voltage-gated calcium channel subtypes) and is consolidated by different second messenger systems and upregulation of different receptor subtypes.

Hence, even if it was proven that one form of LTP is underlying memory formation, it would not prove that all forms are. Conversely, if one can prove that a particular type of LTP does not correlate with memory formation, it does not rule out the possibility that other forms of LTP might be related to learning processes.

What Kind of Memory Does LTP Encode?

A simple but important question that needs to be addressed is what type of memory could be encoded by LTP-like processes. Although LTP can last for months (Bliss and Lynch, 1988; Stäubli and Lynch, 1990) it is often measured only for 30 minutes to 1 hour, which makes it questionable whether a true LTP had been induced in the experiment. More to the point, a long-term, stable memory trace after a single event is not what is observed in everyday life. Clearly, learning and memory formation is a dynamic process that involves processing, deleting, fading (forgetting), and so forth. Psychologists differentiate between long-term, short-term, and working memory, which can be of varying length governed entirely by the length of the tasks that require working memory (Baddeley and Hitch, 1974; Olton, 1977). If LTP lasts forever, how is forgetting achieved? Could the mechanisms for forgetting be depotentiation of LTP, a form of active erasing of memory as discussed by Wilshaw and Dayan (Willshaw and Dayan, 1990)? There is no reason why memory must be an upregulation of EPSPs. Downregulations alone as seen in the cerebellum (Aiba et al., 1994) could account for memory storage.

Therefore, an upregulation of the amplitude of the EPSP that lasts forever might not be a good model for memory formation. Upregulations of EPSPs that decay over time have much more potential to explain observed dynamics in memory formation in humans and animals. It has been suggested that different forms of EPSP potentiation might exist that last only a defined period of time (McNaughton, 1983) and that these periods underlie defined biochemical processes that modulate LTP consolidation (Nguyen et al., 1994; Hölscher, 1995). Such mechanisms could account for memory that lasts different periods of time (see also Chapter 1 on this issue). However, most researchers studying the mechanisms of LTP induction and consolidation do not seem to be interested in decaying or short-lasting upregulations of the EPSP, or in differences in the amplitude or slope of LTP, and instead focus mainly on long-lasting changes. Hence, one could imagine that "natural" LTP induced in synapses during learning is not permanent and might only be a fraction of the magnitude of LTP induced by HFS.

Beyond LTP: The Influence of Naturally Occurring Facilitating Mechanisms in the Working Brain – Theta and Gamma Rhythms

■ **Theta Rhythm in the Hippocampus.** HFS protocols induce LTP in a robust and reliable way, a reason that explains their popularity. However, such stimulation patterns are quite different from naturally occurring firing patterns of neurons. Endogenous neuronal firing patterns such as complex spike activity are observed in CA1 as high-frequency bursts of about two to seven spikes (Buzsáki, 1986; Muller and Kubie, 1989; Otto et al., 1991). Furthermore, HFS stimulates large populations of neurons simultaneously and nonselectively, while neuronal activation in the living brain is limited to groups of neurons that are involved in processing a task (Burgess et al., 1996; Moser, 1996).

In addition, when cutting a hippocampal slice, numerous projections from the basal brain are severed. The serotonergic projection from the raphe nuclei, noradrenergic projections from the locus coeruleus, acetylcholinergic projections from the septal nuclei, and dopaminergic projections from the substantia nigra modulate neuronal activity in the working brain. The importance of such modulators is shown in vivid detail in Parkinson's disease. The dopaminergic projection from the substantia nigra to the basal ganglia activates neuronal networks and enables the processing of input. In the absence of dopamine the neuronal networks are inhibited and motor activity ceases in these patients.

The importance of serotonin and noradrenaline in modulation of neuronal activity has been investigated in detail (Richter-Levin et al., 1991; Everitt and Robbins, 1997; Izquierdo and Medina, 1997; Myslivecek, 1997). The acetylcholinergic projection from the septal nuclei to the hippocampal formation appears to play a special role.

EEG recordings of the brain show oscillations that reflect rhythmic membrane depolarizations. Theta rhythm is a slow wave oscillation that occurs in the EEG of moving animals or in animals that are sensory stimulated, and correlates with alertness or arousal of the brain (Winson, 1972; Fox et al., 1983; Vanderwolf and Leung, 1983; Buzsáki, 1986). Theta in the awake rat occurs around 7 Hz whereas in the anesthetized rat it is found at around 4 Hz after sensory stimulation (Vanderwolf and Leung, 1983; Buzsáki, 1986; Green and Greenough, 1986). Theta oscillations represent to a large extent modulation of inhibition by interneurons. Since a large percentage of septal and entorhinal projections terminate at interneurons, local inhibition in the hippocampus is greatest at the peak of theta activity. After the peak of theta activity inhibition of excitatory neurons is very much reduced (Buzsáki, 1997; Lisman, 1997; Kamondi et al., 1998). Furthermore, neuronal loops in corticothalamic networks are implicated in inducing coherent oscillations in the theta range. In such loops, cortical neurons are excited by thalamic afferences and project back to the stimulating neurons in specific thalamic nuclei (Steriade, 1999).

One strategy to induce LTP in a perhaps more physiologic way and to take advantage of this intrinsic facilitatory network property is to give short bursts of stimuli with an interburst interval of around 200 ms, the previously mentioned theta-patterned stimulation protocol. Such high-frequency bursts of around five pulses resemble complex spike activity that occurs predominantly on the positive or negative phase of theta rhythm (Buzsáki, 1986; Otto et al., 1991; Stewart et al., 1992; Jeffery et al., 1996). The interburst interval of around 200 ms during theta-patterned stimulation is supposed to mimic theta-type activity. A 200-ms interburst interval therefore mimics theta-type activity, and interneuron inhibition is greatly altered at that time, facilitating the induction of LTP (Larson et al., 1986; Stäubli and Lynch, 1987; Diamond et al., 1988). However, such patterned stimulation only imitates theta rhythm on the input axons and does not make use of naturally occurring theta activity that can affect the target cells. A more physiologic protocol would be stimulating neurons during theta rhythm that has been reported to facilitate the induction of LTP both *in vitro* and *in vivo*. LTP can be obtained by a single burst of four pulses at 100 Hz if given on the positive phase of theta rhythm in the hippocampal slice. The same burst on the negative phase induces depotentiation of previously potentiated EPSPs (Huerta and Lisman, 1995). Studies in anesthetized rats showed a similar result: Stimulation with bursts of five pulses on the positive phase of theta rhythm induced LTP in the dentate gyrus (Pavlides et al., 1988) or CA1 (Hölscher et al., 1997a) while stimulation on the negative phase of theta with ten bursts reversed this LTP. Similar results were obtained in freely moving rats. Here, five trains of four pulses at 100 Hz, separated by 200 ms, produced reliable LTP that lasted at least 16 days (Stäubli and Lynch, 1987).

Using such a novel stimulation protocol, which is not only within the physiologic range of natural neuronal activity but also takes advantage of the reduction of inhibition by intrinsic modulatory oscillations, could be used as a potentially more realistic model of putative synaptic changes during learning. How realistic this model is remains to be investigated (see also Section Two in this book).

■ **Gamma Rhythm in the Neocortex.** In the cortex, similar EEG oscillations can be recorded as in the hippocampus. In detailed investigations of this activity, the gamma frequency range of around 40 Hz has been found to be of particular interest. In one single cell recording study in the visual cortex, neuronal firing of several recorded neurons was synchronized in the 40-Hz range. This phase-locked neuronal synchronization only occurred when the neurons involved processed the same visual stimulus and neurons that processed different stimuli were not phase-locked in their activity at any frequency. In field recordings of different cortical areas in the cat, it was found that in an appetitive conditioning task, synchronization occurred between areas of the visual and parietal cortex, and between areas of the parietal and motor cortex. When the animals responded to a sudden change in a visual pattern, neuronal activity in cortical areas exhibited synchrony without time lags between areas that processed related functions. Without the correct visual stimulation synchrony disappeared, and no synchronization was seen between areas that were not functionally related (Roelfsema et al., 1997). Single cell recording in the retina showed that neurons fired phase-locked with high-frequency oscillation from 60 to 120 Hz. This phase-locked firing pattern was also found in the lateral geniculatum to which retina neurons project, and further on in the visual cortex. In the cortex, secondary oscillations in the 30 to 60 Hz range were also observed. Again, phase-locked neuronal firing was only observed when neurons in the retina processed the same visual stimulus. If independent stimuli were processed, no phase locking of neuronal activity was observed (Neuenschwander and Singer, 1996).

Gamma-activity can be observed in the working brain. In one study, 40-Hz EEG activity was observed in other cortical regions known to be involved in visual processing when the subjects were shown pictures in which patterns can be recognized, such as a face. Only when the subjects recognized the face were 40-Hz oscillations seen in the visual processing areas (Rodriguez et al., 1999). In another study, subjects learned an associative task between a visual and tactile stimulus. EEG recording showed a marked increase of gamma activity after the visual stimulus was presented. There was also a selective increase of gamma synchronization between the visual cortex and the sensor-cortical areas that represent the hand that received the tactile stimulus. When a visual stimulus was shown that the subject had not been conditioned to, no gamma frequency activity was observed (Miltner et al., 1999). Interestingly, reticular stimulation enhanced the occurrence of gamma frequency phase-locked neuronal activity in the visual cortex after visual stimulation. Importantly, this 40-Hz phase locking of neuronal activity with gamma oscillation is not induced in a static fashion but is plastic and adaptable and is perhaps achieved by modulation of the synaptic transmission of selective connections (Munk et al., 1996; see also Section Two in this book).

Oscillating membrane depolarizations appear to play several roles: modulating local inhibition that focuses neuronal firing on discrete time windows of low inhibition and thereby increases the signal-to-noise ratio, and perhaps facilitation of synaptic plasticity; and synchronization of neuronal activity of neurons that are involved in processing the same information, thereby solving the "binding problem" of how information processed by individual neurons that analyze the same object is combined to perception of a complete image (Singer, 1994).

EEG oscillations change the system properties significantly. In the context of correlation between LTP inducibility and learning ability in animals, it is conceivable that in learning animals, LTP-like processes can develop in the presence of theta or gamma oscillation, while HFS is not capable of inducing LTP in transgenic or drug-infused animals.

Conditions of Learning: How Do Animals Learn?

Correlations between the inducibility of LTP with the ability of animals to learn spatial tasks are based on the assumption that the tasks are suitable to test predominantly spatial learning ability (assumption number 3). The water maze task has been developed as a convenient and reliable task for assessing spatial learning in animals (Morris et al., 1982; Morris, 1984). The ability to remember orientation in space and the position of a submerged platform in a pool clearly is a spatial task. However, recent analysis of the factors that determine learning of spatial water maze tasks show that a number of additional factors play crucial roles in the acquisition of this task.

It has been shown that stress impairs learning abilities in animals. Since the water maze is a stressful task (as are all other tasks to some degree), one has to be aware of this confounding variable. As mentioned earlier, in some transgenic mice strains the altered response to stressful situations led to impairments in learning a spatial water task and showed a correlation between the inducibility of LTP and learning abilities (Miyakawa et al., 1996). Furthermore, stress impaired performance in spatial water maze tasks or other tasks (Diamond et al., 1994a, 1996; Miyakawa et al., 1996; Hölscher, 1999), and steroids released in stress responses greatly affected synaptic plasticity (Diamond et al., 1992; Pavlides et al., 1996; Xu et al., 1997; see the chapters in Section Four on the influence of stress and arousal on learning). As described above, in a detailed study of *fyn*-deficient mice strains that previously had been reported to show reduced LTP in area CA1 and impaired spatial learning in the water maze task (Grant et al., 1992), it was shown that these mice were greatly altered in their fear conditioning behavior. The knock-out mutants showed increased anxiety in an elevated maze task. In a spatial radial arm maze task, a task that is considerably less stressful than a water maze task, the knock-out mutants scored equally well compared with non–knock-out littermates (Miyakawa et al., 1996). In other words, exposing animals to a stressful situation can alter their learning ability, and any experimental procedure such as drug application, lesion, or transgenic modification could influence the stress response of animals. If this is the case, performance in the water maze will be greatly altered in the test group compared with the control group, even though spatial learning might not be changed in any way.

Therefore, correlating performance in spatial tasks with the inducibility of LTP in hippocampal areas might produce false positives. One should keep in mind that the hippocampus is part of the limbic system and plays important roles in habituation to stress and control of anxiety (Gray, 1982). Our knowledge of how animals actually learn tasks is not sufficient to allocate a brain area to the learning of a particular task. More research in the area of animal behavior and spatial learning is of vital importance if we want to correlate any neuronal activities or mechanisms of synaptic plasticity to learning processes.

Conditions of Learning: What Do Animals Have to Learn?

The water maze task has been developed as a spatial task, and the ability to remember the position of a submerged platform in a pool clearly is a spatial task. However, additional factors have to be learned by animals in order to be able to perform such a task. Laboratory rats usually grow up in relatively small cages and have never experienced swimming before. Therefore, the animals have to learn to coordinate their motor activity during swimming, depending on the extent of pre-training in the water maze. Also, the fine-tuning of the coordination between sensory input (seeing the external cues in the room) and the orientation of the swimming movements and motor coordination will have to be learned. Finally, the rats will have to learn to mount the platform and stay on it until taken out of the pool, a task not easily achieved by all rats. This poses the question as to what percentage improved performance in the water maze is dependent on spatial learning ability.

In several experiments it has been shown that spatial or even nonspatial pre-training in a water maze influenced the animals' ability to learn a spatial water maze task. Infusing an NMDA antagonist at concentrations that block LTP in the dentate gyrus did not impair learning of a spatial task as previously shown (Bannerman et al., 1995; Saucier and Cain, 1995; see also Figures 1 and 2). Further analysis by Cain et al. showed that learning of a spatial water maze task involves learning and improvement of specific motor tasks and of sensory-motor coordination, and other aspects that are not part of the spatial learning segment of the task (Cain and Saucier, 1996; Cain et al., 1996; Saucier et al., 1996; Cain, 1997; see also the Chapter 13).

Hence, performance in a spatial water maze task might not correctly reflect the animals' ability to learn spatial tasks. Perhaps the intact ability to perform in a water maze task in transgenic mice or in animals that have been treated with drugs could be due to intact nonspatial learning abilities to perform well in a water maze task even though their spatial learning is compromised. Impairments in learning a spatial water maze task do not necessarily have to be due to an impairment in spatial learning abilities.

Conclusions

There are a number of confounding variables one has to be aware of when comparing the inducibility of LTP using standard HFS protocols with spatial learning abilities in water maze tasks, which can produce false negatives:

1. There are several types of LTP, depending on brain area, type of induction (chemical vs. electrical), type of stimulation protocol, and so forth, and

research so far has shown that these types of LTP are different and do not equally correlate with learning abilities of animals or constitute models of learning processes equally well.

2. Most research of LTP has been conducted in the hippocampus, which might not be the area that encodes all forms of long-term memory. Results of LTP studies of the thalamus-amygdala pathway are more encouraging and might lead to a better understanding of neuronal processes that underlie memory formation.

3. Experiments conducted in slice preparations are subject to a large number of variables that influence the results to a great extent, and might not represent physiologic conditions.

4. Learning experiments are also subject to numerous confounding variables. Spatial learning tasks involve a number of nonspatial components (motor control or stress factors) that are not hippocampal-dependent and can influence the results. A correlation between the inducibility of LTP and memory formation can be biased this way.

5. Some stimulation protocols are more physiologic than others, and the use of intrinsic facilitating mechanisms such as theta or gamma rhythm could be put to use to develop more realistic models of memory formation.

6. The technique of recording neuronal activity in behaving animals has several advantages, and observation of plastic changes of firing activities in learning animals could teach us more about neuronal network activity in the brain.

REFERENCES

Aiba, A., Kano, M., Chen, C., Stanton, M.E. et al. (1994). Deficient cerebellar long-term depression and impaired motor learning in mGluR1 mutant mice. *Cell* 79: 377–388.

Alkon, D.L. (1999). Ionic conductance determinants of synaptic memory nets and their implications for Alzheimer's disease. *J. Neurosci. Res.* 58: 24–32.

Baddeley, A.D., and Hitch, G.J. (1974). *Working Memory.* New York: Oxford University Press.

Bannerman, D.M., Good, M.A., Butcher, S.P., Ramsay, M. et al. (1995). Distinct components of spatial learning revealed by prior training and NMDA receptor blockade. *Nature* 378: 182–186.

Barnes, C.A. (1988). Spatial learning and memory processes: The search for their neurobiological mechanisms in the rat. *Trends Neurosci.* 11: 163–169.

Barnes, C.A. (1995). Involvement of LTP in memory: Are we "searching under the street light"? *Neuron* 15: 751–754.

Barnes, C.A., Jung, M.W., McNaughton, B.L. et al. (1994). LTP saturation and spatial-learning disruption—effects of task variables and saturation levels. *J. Neurosci.* 14: 5793–5806.

Beiko, J., and Cain, D. (1998). The effect of water maze spatial training on posterior parietal cortex transcallosal evoked field potentials in the rat. *Cereb. Cortex* 8: 407–414.

Bennett, M., Diamond, D., Fleshner, M., and Rose G. (1991). Serum corticosterone level predicts the magnitude of hippocampal primed burst potentiation and depression in urethane-anesthetized rats. *Psychobiology* 19: 301–307.

Blackstad, T.W. (1956). Commissural connections of the hippocampal region in the rat with special reference to their mode of termination. *J. Comp. Neurol.* 105: 417–537.

Bliss, T., and Lømo, T. (1973). Long-lasting potentiation of synaptic transmission in the dentate area of the anaesthesised rabbit following stimulation of the perforant path. *J. Physiol. London* 232: 331–356.

Bliss, T., and Lømo, T. (1996) Discovering LTP. In M. Bear, B. Connors, and M. Paradiso (Eds.), *Neuroscience—exploring the brain* (pp. 563–564). Baltimore: Williams & Wilkins.

Bliss, T.V.P., and Lynch, M.A. (1988). Long-term potentiation of synaptic transmission in the hippocampus: Properties and mechanisms. In *Long-term potentiation: From biophysics to behavior* (pp. 3–72). New York: Alan R. Liss.

Blümcke, I., Behle, K., Malitschek, B., Kuhn, R. et al. (1996). Immunohistochemical distribution of metabotropic glutamate receptor subtypes mGluR1b, mGluR2/3, mGluR4a and mGluR5 in human hippocampus. *Brain Res.* 736: 217–226.

Böhme, G.A., Bon, C., Stutzmann, J.-M., Doble, A. et al. (1991). Possible involvement of nitric oxide in long-term potentiation. *Eur. J. Pharmacol.* 199: 379–381.

Bon, C., Böhme, G.A., Doble, A., Stutzmann, J.-M. et al. (1992). A role for nitric oxide in long-term potentiation. *Eur. J. Neurosci.* 4: 420–424.

Bonhoeffer, T., Staiger, V., and Aertsen A. (1989). Synaptic plasticity in rat hippocampal slice cultures: Local "Hebbian" conjunction of pre- and postsynaptic stimulation leads to distributed synaptic enhancement. *Proc. Natl. Acad. Sci. USA* 86: 8113–8117.

Bortolotto, Z.A., and Collingridge, G.L. (1992). Activation of glutamate metabotropic receptors induces long-term potentiation. *Eur. J. Pharmacol.* 214: 297–298.

Braitenberg, V., and Schütz A. (1983). Some anatomical comments on the hippocampus. In W Seifert (Ed.), *Neurobiology of the hippocampus* (Chapter 2). London: Academic Press.

Burgess, N., Recce, M., and O'Keefe, J. (1996). A model of hippocampal function. *Neuronal Networks.* 7: 1065–1081.

Butelman, E.R. (1990). The effect of NMDA antagonists in the radial arm maze task with an interposed delay. *Pharmacol. Biochem. Behav.* 35: 533–536.

Buzsáki, G. (1986). Generation of hippocampal EEG patterns. In R. Isaacson and K. Pribram (Eds.), *The hippocampus.* (pp. 137–167). New York: Plenum Press.

Buzsáki, G. (1997). Functions for interneuronal nets in the hippocampus. *Can. J. Physiol. Pharmacol.* 75: 508–515.

Cain, D.P. (1997). Prior non-spatial pretraining eliminates sensorimotor disturbances and impairments in water maze learning caused by diazepam. *Psychopharmacology (Berl.)* 130: 313–319.

Cain, D.P., and Saucier, D. (1996). The neuroscience of spatial navigation: Focus on behavior yields advances. *Rev. Neurosci.* 7: 215–231.

Cain, D.P., Saucier, D., Hall, J., Hargreaves, E.L. et al. (1996). Detailed behavioral analysis of water maze acquisition under APV or CNQX: Contribution of sensorimotor disturbances to drug-induced acquisition deficits. *Behav. Neurosci.* 110: 86–102.

Castro, C.A., Silbert, L.H., McNaughton, B.L., and Barnes C.A. (1989). Recovery of spatial-learning deficits after decay of electrically induced synaptic enhancement in the hippocampus. *Nature* 342: 545–548.

Chetkovich, D.M., Klann, E., and Sweatt, J.D. (1993). Nitric oxide synthase independent long-term potentiation in area CA1 of hippocampus. *NeuroReport* 4: 919–922.

Chinestra, P., Diabira, D., Urban, N.N., Barionuevo, G. et al. (1994) Major differences between long-term potentiation and ACPD-induced slow onset potentiation in hippocampus. *Neurosci. Lett.* 182: 177–180.

Christofi, G., Nowicky, A.V., Bolsover, S.R., and Bindman, L.J. (1993). The postsynaptic induction of nonassociative long-term depression of excitatory synaptic transmission in rat hippocampal slices. *J. Neurophys.* 69: 219–227.

Cotman, C.W., and Iversen, L.L. (1987). Excitatory amino acids in the brain—focus on NMDA receptors. *Trends Neurosci.* 10: 263–265.

Cummings, J.A., Nicola, S.M., and Malenka, R.C. (1994). Induction in the rat hippocampus of long-term potentiation (LTP) and long-term depression (LTD) in the presence of a nitric oxide synthase inhibitor. *Neurosci. Lett.* 176: 110–114.

Deadwyler, S.A., West, N.O., and Robinson, J.H. (1981). Entorhinal and septal inputs differentially control sensory-evoked responses in the rat dentate gyrus. *Science* 211: 1181–1183.

Diamond, D., Bennett, M., Fleshner, M., and Rose, G. (1994a). Stress impairs LTP and hippocampal-dependent memory. In *Brain corticosteroid receptors,* Vol. 746, *Ann. NY Acad. Sci.*

Diamond, D., Fleshner, M., and Rose, G. (1994b). Psychological stress repeatedly blocks hippocampal primed burst potentiation in behaving rats. *Behav. Brain Res.* 62: 1–9.

Diamond, D.M., Bennett, M.C., Fleshner, M., and Rose, G.M. (1992). Inverted U-relationship between the level of peripheral corticosterone and the magnitude of hippocampal primed burst potentiation. *Hippocampus* 2: 421–430.

Diamond, D.M., Dunwiddie, T.V., and Rose, G.M. (1988). Characteristics of hippocampal primed burst potentiation *in vitro* and in the awake rat. *J. Neurosci.* 8: 4079–4088.

Diamond, D.M., Fleshner, M., Ingersoll, N., and Rose, R.M. (1996). Psychological stress impairs spatial working memory: Relevance to electrophysiological studies of hippocampal function. *Behav. Neurosci.* 110: 661–672.

Doyère, V., Errington, M.L., Laroche, S., and Bliss, T.V.P. (1996). Low-frequency trains of paired stimuli induce long-term depression in CA1 but not in dentate gyrus of the intact rat. *Hippocampus* 6: 52–57.

Doyle, C., Hölscher, C., Rowan, M.J., and Anwyl, R. (1996). The selective neuronal NO synthase inhibitor 7-nitro-indazole blocks both long-term potentiation and depotentiation of field EPSPs in rat hippocampal CA1 *in vivo*. *J. Neurosci.* 16: 418–426.

Eichenbaum, H. (1996). Memory: Old questions, new perspectives. *Curr. Biol.* 7: R53–R55.

Errington, M.L., Bliss, T.V.P., Richter-Levin, G., Yenk, K. et al. (1995). Stimulation at 1–5 Hz does not produce long-term depression or depotentiation in the hippocampus of the adult rat *in vivo*. *J. Neurophysiol.* 74: 1793–1799.

Errington, M.L., Bliss, T.V.P., Morris, R.J., Laroche, S. et al. (1997). Long-term potentiation in awake mutant mice. *Nature* 387: 666–667.

Everitt, B., and Robbins, T. (1997). Central cholinergic systems and cognition. *Annu. Rev. Psychol.* 48: 649–684.

Exner, S. (1884). *Entwurf zu einer physiologischen Erklärung der psychischen Erscheinungen*. Leipzig u. Wien: Franz Deutike Verlag.

Fagnou, D.D., and Tuchek, J.M. (1995). The biochemistry of learning and memory. *Mol. Cell. Biochem.* 149–150: 279–286.

Fox, S.E., Wolfson, S., and Ranck, J.B. (1983). Investigating the mechanisms of hippocampal theta rhythms: Approaches and progress. In: W. Seifert (Ed.), *Neurobiology of the hippocampus* (pp. 303–319). London: Academic Press.

Gerlai, R. (1996). Gene-targeting studies of mammalian behavior: Is it the mutation or the background genotype? *Trends Neurosci.* 19: 177–180.

Glaum, S.R., Slater, N.T., Rossi, D.J., and Miller, R.J. (1992). Role of metabotropic glutamate (ACDP) receptors at the parallel fiber-Purkinje cell synapse. *J. Neurophysiol.* 68: 1453–1462.

Glazewski, S., Herman, C., McKenna, M., Chapman, P.F. et al. (1998a). Long-term potentiation in vivo in layers II/III of rat barrel cortex. *Neuropharmacology* 37: 581–592.

Glazewski, S., McKenna, M., Jacquin, M., and Fox K. (1998b). Experience-dependent depression of vibrissae responses in adolescent rat barrel cortex. *Eur. J. Neurosci.* 10: 2107–2116.

Grant, S.G.N., O'Dell, T.J., Karl, K.A., Stein, P.A. et al. (1992). Impaired long-term potentiation, spatial learning, and hippocampal development in *fyn* mutant mice. Science 258: 1903–1910.

Gray, J.A. (1982). *The Neuropsychology of Anxiety*. New York: Clarendon Press.

Green, E.J., and Greenough, W.T. (1986). Altered synaptic transmission in dentate gyrus of rats reared in complex environments: Evidence from hippocampal slices maintained *in vitro*. *J. Neurophysiol.* 55: 739–750.

Gribkoff, V.K., and Lum-Ragan, J.T. (1992). Evidence for nitric oxide synthase inhibitor sensitive and insensitive hippocampal synaptic potentiation. *J. Neurophysiol.* 68: 639–642.

Gustafsson, B., Wigstrom, H., Abraham, WC, and Huang, Y.Y. (1987). Long-term potentiation in the hippocampus using depolarizing current pulses as the conditioning stimulus to single volley synaptic potentials. *J. Neurosci.* 7: 774–780.

Haley, J.E., Malen, P.L., and Chapman P.F. (1993). Nitric oxide synthase inhibitors block long-term potentiation induced by weak but not strong tetanic stimulation at physiological brain temperatures in rat hippocampal slices. *Neurosci. Lett.* 160: 85–88.

Hartell, N.A. (1996). Strong activation of parallel fibers produces localized calcium transients and a form of LTP that spreads to distant synapses. *Neuron* 16: 601–610.

Hebb, D.O. (1949). *The Organization of Behavior.* New York: John Wiley & Sons.

Heit, G., Smith, M.E., and Halgren, E. (1988). Neural encoding of individual words and faces by the human hippocampus and the amygdala. *Nature* 333: 773.

Heynen, A.J., Abraham, W.C., and Bear, M.F. (1996). Bidirectional modification of CA1 synapses in the adult hippocampus *in vivo. Nature* 381: 163–166.

Hinton, G.E. (1992). How neuronal networks learn from experience. *Sci. Am.* 251: 105–127.

Hölscher, C. (1995). Inhibitors of cyclooxygenases but not lipoxygenases have amnestic effects in the chick. *Eur. J. Neurosci.* 7: 1360–1365.

Hölscher, C. (1999). Stress impairs performance in spatial water maze tasks. *Behav. Brain Res.* 100: 225–235.

Hölscher, C., and Schmidt, W.J. (1994). Quinolinic acid lesion of the rat entorhinal cortex pars medialis produces selective amnesia in allocentric working memory (WM), but not in egocentric WM. *Behav. Brain Res.* 63: 187–194.

Hölscher, C., Anwyl, R., and Rowan, M. (1997a). Stimulation on the positive phase of hippocampal theta rhythm induces long-term potentiation which can be depotentiated by stimulation on the negative phase in area CA1 *in vivo. J. Neurosci.* 17: 6470–6477.

Hölscher, C., McGlinchey, L., Anwyl, R., and Rowan, M.J. (1997b). HFS-induced long-term potentiation and depotentiation in area CA1 of the hippocampus are not good models for learning. *Psychopharmacology* 130: 174–182.

Hölscher, C., McGlinchey, L., and Rowan, M.J. (1996). L-AP4 (L-(+)-2-amino-4-phosphonobutyric acid) induced impairment of spatial learning in the rat is antagonized by MAP4 ((S)-2-amino-2-methy 1-4-phosphonobutanoic acid). *Behav. Brain Res.* 81: 69–79.

Huang, Y.Y., Kandel, E.R., Varshavsky, L., Brandon, E.P. et al. (1995). A genetic test of the effects of mutations in PKA on mossy fiber LTP and its relation to spatial and contextual learning. *Cell* 83: 1211–1222.

Huerta, P.T., and Lisman, J.E. (1995). Bidirectional synaptic plasticity induced by a single burst during cholinergic theta oscillation in CA1 in vitro. *Neuron* 15: 1053–1063.

Huerta, P.T., and Lisman, J.E. (1996). Synaptic plasticity during the cholinergic theta-frequency oscillation in vitro. *Hippocampus* 6: 58–61.

Huerta, P.T., Scearce, K.A., Farris, S.M., Empson, R.M. et al. (1996). Preservation of spatial learning in fyn tyrosine kinase knockout mice. *NeuroReport* 7: 1685–1689.

Izquierdo, I., and Medina, J.H. (1997). The biochemistry of memory formation and its regulation by hormones and neuromodulators. *Psychobiology* 25: 1–9.

Jarrard, L.E. (1983). Selective hippocampal lesion and behavior. Effects of kainic acid lesions on performance of place and cue tasks. *Behav. Neurosci.* 97: 873–889.

Jarrard, L.E. (1986). Selective hippocampal lesions and behavior. Implications for current research and theorizing. In R. Isaacson and K. Pribram (Eds.), *The hippocampus* (pp. 93–126). New York: Plenum Press.

Jarrard, L.E. (1995). What does the hippocampus really do? *Behav. Brain Res.* 71: 1–10.

Jarrard, L.E., Steward, O., Ozwald, F.T., Okaichi, H. et al. (1984). On the role of hippocampal connections in the performance of place and cue tasks: Comparisons with damage to hippocampus. *Behav. Neurosci.* 98: 946–954.

Jeffery, K. (1995). Paradoxical enhancement of long-term potentiation in poor learning rats at low test-stimulus intensities. *Exp. Brain Res.* 104: 55–69.

Jeffery, K.J., and Morris, R.G.M. (1993). Cumulative long-term potentiation in the rat dentate gyrus correlates with, but does not modify, performance in the water maze. *Hippocampus* 3: 133–140.

Jeffery, K.J., Donnett, J.G., and O'Keefe, J. (1996). Medial septal control of theta-correlated unit firing in the entorhinal cortex of awake rats. *NeuroReport* 6: 2166–2170.

Jodar, L., and Kaneto, H. (1995). Synaptic plasticity: Stairway to memory. *Jpn. J. Pharmacol.* 68: 359–387.

Johnston, D., Williams, S., Jaffe, D., and Gray, R. (1992). NMDA-independent long-term potentiation. *Annu. Rev. Physiol.* 54: 489–505.

Kamondi, A., Acsady, L., Wang, X.J., and Buzsaki, G. (1998). Theta oscillations in somata and dendrites of hippocampal pyramidal cells in vivo: Activity-dependent phase-precession of action potentials. *Hippocampus* 8: 244–261.

Kesslak, J.P. (1986). Recovery of spatial alternation deficits following selective hippocampus destruction with kainic acid. *Behav. Neurosci.* 100: 280–283.

Kullmann, D.M., Erdemli, G., and Asztely, F. (1996). LTP of AMPA and NMDA receptor-mediated signals: Evidence for presynaptic expression and extrasynaptic glutamate spillover. *Neuron* 17: 461–474.

Langdon, R.B., Johnson, J.W., and Barrionuevo, G. (1995). Posttetanic potentiation and presynaptically induced long-term potentiation at the mossy fiber synapse in rat hippocampus. *J. Neurobiol.* 26: 370–385.

Larson, J., Wong, D., and Lynch, G. (1986). Patterned stimulation at the theta frequency is optimal for the induction of hippocampal long-term potentiation. *Brain Res.* 368: 347–350.

Lisman, J.E. (1997). Bursts as a unit of neural information: Making unreliable synapses reliable. *Trends Neurosci.* 20: 38–43.

Lømo, T. (1966). Frequency potentiation of excitatory synaptic activity in the dentate area of the hippocampal formation. *Acta Physiol. Scand.* 68(Suppl. 277): 128.

Lum-Ragan, J.T., and Gribkoff, V.K. (1993). The sensitivity of hippocampal long-term potentiation to nitric oxide synthase is dependent upon the pattern of conditioning stimulation. *Neuroscience* 57: 973–983.

Malenka, R.C., and Nicoll, R.A. (1997). Silent synapses speak up. *Neuron* 19: 473–476.

Malenka, R.C., Kauer, J.A., Perkel, D.J., and Nicoll, R.A. (1989). The impact of postsynaptic Ca^{2+} on synaptic transmission—its role in LTP. *Trends Neurosci.* 12: 444–450.

Manahan-Vaughan, D., and Reymann, K.G. (1995). Regional and developmental profile of modulation of hippocampal synaptic transmission and LTP by AP4-sensitive mGluRs *in vivo*. *Neuropharmacology* 34: 995–1005.

Marr, D., and Vaina, L. (1982). Representation and recognition of the movements of shapes. *Proc. R. Soc. Lond. (B)* 214: 501–524.

McKernen, M., and Shinnick-Gallagher, P. (1997). Fear conditioning induces a lasting potentiation of synaptic currents in vitro. *Nature* 390: 607–611.

McNaughton, B.L. (1983). Activity dependent modulation of hippocampal synaptic efficacy: Some implications for memory processes. In: W. Seifert (Ed.), *Neurobiology of the hippocampus* (Chap. 13). London: Academic Press.

Meiri, N., Ghelardini, C., Tesco, G., Galeotti, N. et al. (1997). Reversible antisense inhibition of Shaker-like Kv 1.1 potassium channel expression impairs associative memory in mouse and rat. *Proc. Natl. Acad. Sci. US* 94: 4430–4434.

Meiri, N., Sun, M.K., Segal, Z., and Alkon, D.L. (1998). Memory and long-term potentiation (LTP) dissociated: Normal spatial memory despite CA1 LTP elimination with Kv1.4 antisense. *Proc. Natl. Acad. Sci. USA* 95: 15037–15042.

Miltner, W., Braun, C., Arnold, M., Witte, H., and Taub, E. (1999). Coherence of gamma-band EEG activity as a basis for associative learning. *Nature* 397: 434–436.

Miyakawa, T., Yagi, T., Kagiyama, A., and Niki, H. (1996). Radial maze performance, open field and elevated plus-maze behaviors in Fyn-kinase deficient mice: Further evidence for increased fearfulness. *Mol. Brain Res.* 37: 145–150.

Mizumori, S.J.Y., McNaughton, B.L., Barnes, C.A., and Fox, K.B. (1989). Preserved spatial coding in hippocampal CA1 pyramidal cells during reversible suppression of CA3c output—evidence for pattern completion in hippocampus. *J. Neurosci.* 9: 3915–3928.

Morris, R. (1984). Developments of a water-maze procedure for studying spatial learning in the rat. *J. Neurosci. Meth.* 11: 47–60.

Morris, R.G.M. (1989). Synaptic plasticity and learning: Selective impairment of learning in rats and blockade of long-term potentiation *in vivo* by the N-methyl-D-aspartate receptor antagonist AP5. *J. Neurosci.* 9: 3040–3057.

Morris, R.G.M., Garrud, P., Rawlins, J.N.P., and O'Keefe, J. (1982). Place navigation impaired in rats with hippocampal lesions. *Nature* 297: 681–683.

Morris, R.G.M., Anderson, E., Lynch, G.S., and Baudry, M. (1986). Selective impairment of learning and blockade of LTP by a NMDA receptor antagonist, AP5. *Nature* 319: 774–776.

Moser, E.I. (1995). Learning-related changes in hippocampal field potentials. *Behav. Brain Res.* 71: 11–18.

Moser, E.I. (1996). Altered inhibition of dentate granule cells during spatial learning in an exploration task. *J. Neurosci.* 16: 1247–1259.

Moser, E., Mathiesen, I., and Andersen, P. (1993). Association between brain temperature and dentate field potentials in exploring and swimming rats. *Science* 259: 1324–1326.

Moser, E., Krobert, K., Moser, M.-B., and Morris, R. (1998). Impaired spatial learning after saturation of long-term potentiation. *Science* 281: 2038–2042.

Motro, B., Wojtowicz, J.M., Bernstein, A., and Van der Kooy, D. (1996). Steel mutant mice are deficient in hippocampal learning but not long-term potentiation. *Proc. Natl. Acad. Sci. USA* 93: 1808–1813.

Muller, R.U., and Kubie, J.L. (1989). The firing of hippocampal place cells predicts the future position of freely moving rats. *J. Neurosci.* 9: 4101–4110.

Munk, M., Roelfsema, P., König, P., Engel, A. et al. (1996). Role of reticular activation in the modulation of intracortical synchronization. *Science* 272: 271–274.

Musleh, W.Y., Shahi, K., and Baudry, M. (1993). Further studies concerning the role of nitric oxide in LTP induction and maintenance. *Synapse* 13: 370–375.

Myslivecek, J. (1997). Inhibitory learning and memory in newborn rats. *Prog. Neurobiol.* 53: 399–430.

Neuenschwander, S., and Singer, W. (1996). Long-range synchronization of oscillatory light reponses in the cat retina and lateral geniculate nucleus. *Nature* 379: 728–733.

Nguyen, P.V., Abel, T., and Kandel, E.R. (1994). Requirement of a critical period of transcription for induction of a late phase of LTP. *Science* 265: 1104–1107.

Nosten-Bertrand, M., Errington, M.L., Murphy, K.P.S.J., Tokugawa, Y. et al. (1996). Normal spatial learning despite regional inhibition of LTP in mice lacking Thy-1. *Nature* 379: 826–829.

O'Dell, T.J., Hawkins, R.D., Kandel, E.R., and Arancio, O. (1991). Tests of the roles of two diffusible substances in long-term potentiation: Evidence for nitric oxide as a possible early retrograde messenger. *Proc. Natl. Acad. Sci. USA* 88: 11285–11289.

O'Mara, S., Rowan, M.J., and Anwyl, R. (1995). Metabotropic glutamate receptor-induced homosynaptic long-term depression and depotentiation in the dentate gyrus of the rat hippocampus *in vitro*. *Neuropharmacology* 34: 983–989.

Ohishi, H., Akazawa, C., Shigemoto, R., Nakanishi, S. et al. (1995). Distributions of the mRNAs for L-2-amino-4-phosphonobutyrate-sensitive metabotropic glutamate receptors, mGluR4 and mGluR7, in the rat brain. *J. Comp. Neurol.* 360: 555–570.

Olton, D.S. (1977). Spatial Memory. *Sci. Am.* 236: 82–93.

Olton, D.S., Becker, J.T., and Handelmann, G.E. (1979). Hippocampus, space and memory. *Behav. Brain Sci.* 2: 313–365.

Otnaes, M.K., Brun, V.H., Moser, M.-B., and Moser, E.I. (1999). Pretraining prevents spatial learning impairment following saturation of hippocampal long-term potentiation. *J Neurosci.* 19: RC49.

Otto, T., Eichenbaum, H., Wiener, S., and Wible, C. (1991). Learning-related patterns of CA1 spike trains parallel stimulation parameters optimal for inducing hippocampal long-term potentiation. *Hippocampus* 1: 181–192.

Pavlides, C., Greenstein, Y.J., Grudman, M., and Winson, J. (1988). Long-term potentiation in the dentate gyrus is induced preferentially on the positive phase of θ-rhythm. *Brain Res.* 439: 383–387.

Pavlides, C., Watanabe, Y., Magarifios, A.M., and McEwen, B.S. (1995). Opposing roles of type I and type II adrenal steroid receptors in hippocampal long-term potentiation. *Neuroscience* 68: 387–394.

Pavlides, C., Ogawa, S., Kimura, A., and McEwen, B.S. (1996). Role of adrenal steroid mineralocorticoid and glucocorticoid receptors in long-term potentiation in the CA1 field of hippocampal slices. *Brain Res.* 738: 229–235.

Racine, R.J., Chapman, C.A., Trepel, C., Teskey, G.C. et al. (1995). Post-activation potentiation in the neocortex. IV. Multiple sessions required for induction of long-term potentiation in the chronic preparation. *Brain Res.* 702: 87–93.

Rawlins, J.N.P. (1985). Association across time: The hippocampus as a temporary memory store. *Behav. Brain Sci.* 8: 479–496.

Rempel-Clower, N.L., Zola, S.M., Squire, L.R., and Amaral, D.G. (1996). Three cases of enduring memory impairment after bilateral damage limited to the hippocampal formation. *J. Neurosci.* 16: 5233–5255.

Richter-Levin, G., Segal, M., and Sara, S. (1991). An alpha 2 antagonist, idazoxan, enhances EPSP-spike coupling in the rat dentate gyrus. *Brain Res.* 540: 291–294.

Riedel, G., Manahan-Vaughan, D., Kozikowski, A., and Reymann, K. (1995a). Metabotropic glutamate receptor agonist trans-azetidine-2,4-dicarboxylic acid facilitates maintenance of LTP in the dentate gyrus in vivo. *Neuropharmacology* 34: 1107–1109.

Riedel, G., Wetzel, W., Kozikowski, A.P., and Reymann, K.G. (1995b). Block of spatial learning by mGluR agonist tADA in rats. *Neuropharmacology* 34: 559–561.

Robinson, G.B. (1992). Maintained saturation of hippocampal long-term potentiation does not disrupt acquisition of the eight-arm radial maze. *Hippocampus* 2: 389–395.

Rodriguez, E., George, N., Lachaux, J.-P., Martinerie, J. et al. (1999). Perception's shadow: Long-distance synchronization of human brain activity. *Nature* 397: 430–433.

Roelfsema, P., Engel, A., König, P., and Singer W. (1997). Visuomotor integration is associated with zero time-lag synchronization among cortical areas. *Nature* 385: 157–161.

Rogan, M., Stäubli, U., and LeDoux, J. (1997). Fear conditioning induces associative long-term potentiation in the amygdala. *Nature* 390: 604–607.

Rose, G.M., and Dunwiddie, T.V. (1986). Induction of hippocampal long-term potentiation using physiologically patterned stimulation. *Neurosci. Lett.* 69: 244–248.

Saucier, D., and Cain, D.P. (1995). Spatial learning without NMDA receptor-dependent long-term potentiation. *Nature* 378: 186–189.

Saucier, D., Hargreaves, E.L., Boon, F., Vanderwolf, C.H. et al. (1996). Detailed behavioral analysis of water maze acquisition under systemic NMDA or muscarinic antagonism: Nonspatial pretraining eliminates spatial learning deficits. *Behav. Neurosci.* 110: 103–116.

Schenk, F., and Morris R.G.M. (1985). Dissociation between components of spatial memory in rats after recovery from the effects of retrohippocampal lesions. *Exp. Brain Res.* 58: 11–28.

Schenk, F., Grobéty, M.C., Lavenex, P., and Lipp, H.-P. (1995). Dissociation between basic components of spatial memory in rats. In E. Alkva et al. (Eds.), *Behavioural brain research in naturalistic and semi-naturalistic settings* (pp. 277–300). New York: Kluwer Academic Publishers.

Schuman, E.M., and Madison D.V. (1991). A requirement for the intercellular messenger nitric oxide in long-term potentiation. *Science* 254: 1503–1506.

Schwerdtfeger, W.K. (1984). *Structure and Fiber Connections of the Hippocampus. A Comparative Study.* Heidelberg: Springer Verlag.

Scoville, W.B., and Milner, B. (1957). Loss of recent memory after bilateral hippocampal lesion. *J. Neurol. Psychiatry* 20: 11–21.

Selig, D.K., Lee, H.K., Bear, M.F., and Malenka, R.C. (1995). Re-examination of the effects of MCPG on hippocampal LTP, LTD, and depotentiation. *J. Neurophysiol.* 74: 1075–1082.

Shors, T., Seib, T., Levine, S., and Thompson, R. (1989). Inescapable versus escapable shock modulates long-term potentiation in the rat hippocampus. *Science* 244: 224–226.

Shors, T., Levine, S., and Thompson, R. (1990). Opioid antagonist eliminates the stress-induced impairment of long-term potentiation. *Brain Res.* 506: 316–318.

Silva, A.J., Paylor, R., Wehner, J.M., and Tonegawa, S. (1992a). Impaired spatial learning in α-calcium-calmodulin kinase II mutant mice. *Science* 257: 206–211.

Silva, A.J., Stevens, C.F., Tonegawa, S., and Wang, Y. (1992b). Deficient hippocampal long-term potentiation in α-calcium-calmodulin kinase II mutant mice. *Science* 257: 201–206.

Simmen, M.W., Treves, A., and Rolls, E.T. (1996). Pattern retrieval in threshold linear associative nets. Network-computation in neural systems. *Network Comp. Neur. Sys.* 7: 109–122.

Singer, W. (1994). Time as coding space in neocortical processing: A hypothesis. In Buzsáki, G. (Ed.), *Temporal Coding in the Brain* (pp. 51–79). Berlin: Springer Verlag.

Stanton, P.K. (1996). LTD, LTP, and the sliding threshold for long-term synaptic plasticity. *Hippocampus* 6: 35–42.

Stanton, P.K., and Sejnowski, T.J. (1989). Associative long-term depression in the hippocampus induced by Hebbian covariance. *Nature* 339: 215–218.

Stäubli, U., and Lynch, G. (1987). Stable hippocampal long-term potentiation elicited by 'theta' pattern stimulation. *Brain Res.* 435: 227–234.

Stäubli, U., and Lynch, G. (1990). Stable depression of potentiated synaptic responses in the hippocampus with 1–5 Hz stimulation. *Brain Res.* 513: 113–118.

Steriade, M. (1999). Coherent oscillations and short-term plasticity in corticothalamic networks. *Trends Neurosci.* 22: 337–345.

Steward, O. (1976). Topographic organization of the projections from the entorhinal area to the hippocampal formation of the rat. *J. Comp. Neurol.* 167: 285–314.

Stewart, M., Luo, Y., and Fox, S.E. (1992). Effects of atropine on hippocampal theta cells and complex-spike cells. *Brain Res.* 591: 122–128.

Sutherland, R.J., Dringenberg, H.C., and Hoesing, J.M. (1993). Induction of long-term potentiation at perforant path dentate synapses does not affect place learning or memory. *Hippocampus* 3: 141–147.

Thiels, E., Barrionuevo, G., and Berger, T. (1995). Excitatory stimulation during postsynaptic inhibition induces long-term depression in hippocampus *in vivo*. *J. Neurophysiol.* 72: 3009–3116.

Vanderwolf, C.H., and Leung L.-W.S. (1983). *Hippocampal Rhythmical Slow Activity: A Brief History and the Effects of Entorhinal Lesions and Phencyclidine.* London: Academic Press.

Vinogradova, O.S. (1975). Functional organization of the limbic system in the process of registration of information: Facts and hypotheses. In R.L. Isaacson and K.H. Pibram (Eds.), *The hippocampus: 2. Neurophysiology and behavior* (pp. 1–70). New York: Plenum Press.

Vnek, N., and Rothblat, L.A. (1996). The hippocampus and long-term object memory in the rat. *J. Neurosci.* 16: 2780–2787.

Warrington, E.K. (1996). Studies of retrograde memory: A long-term view. *Proc. Natl. Acad. Sci. USA* 93: 13523–13526.

Whishaw, I.Q., and Jarrard, L.E. (1996). Evidence for extrahippocampal involvement in place learning and hippocampal involvement in path integration. *Hippocampus* 6: 513–524.

Whishaw, I.Q., Cassel, J.C., and Jarrard, L.E. (1995). Rats with fimbria-fornix lesions display a place response in a swimming pool—a dissociation between getting there and knowing where. *J. Neurosci.* 15: 5779–5788.

Williams, J.H., Errington, M.L., Li, Y.-G., Nayak, A. et al. (1993). The supression of long-term potentiation in rat hippocampus by inhibitors of nitric oxide synthase is temperature and age dependent. *Neuron* 11: 877–884.

Willshaw, D., and Dayan, P. (1990). Optimal plasticity form matrix memories: What goes up must come down. *Neural Comput.* 2: 85–93.

Wilson, M.A., and Tonegawa, S. (1997). Synaptic plasticity, place cells and spatial memory: Study with second generation knockouts. *Trends Neurosci.* 20: 102–105.

Winson, J. (1972). Interspecies differences in the occurrence of theta. *Behav. Biol.* 7: 479–487.

Xu, L., Anwyl, R., and Rowan, M.J. (1997). Behavioural stress facilitates the induction of long-term depression in the hippocampus. *Nature* 387: 497–500.

Xu, L., Hölscher, C., Anwyl, R., and Rowan, M.J. (1998). Glucocorticoid receptor and protein/RNA synthesis-dependent mechanisms underlie the control of synaptic plasticity by stress. *Proc. Natl. Acad. Sci. USA* 95: 3204–3208.

Zola-Morgan, S., Squire, L.R., and Amaral, D.G. (1986). Human amnesia and the medial temporal region: Enduring memory impairment following a bilateral lesion limited to CA1. *J. Neurosci.* 6: 2950–2967.

Long-Term Potentiation *In Vitro* and *In Vivo*

How Can We Fine-Tune the Current Models for Memory Formation?

CHAPTER ONE

Persisting with Long-Term Potentiation as a Memory Mechanism

Clues from Variations in Long-Term Potentiation Maintenance

Wickliffe C. Abraham

SUMMARY

Studies of long-term potentiation (LTP) induction and persistence in awake animals have revealed intriguing regional differences. LTP and heterosynaptic LTD in the dentate gyrus both inevitably appear to be decremental in nature, with the time constant of decay related to the strength of the induction stimulus. On the other hand, nondecremental LTP can be induced in area CA1 with a very mild stimulus that, when given in the dentate gyrus, evokes little or no LTP at all. CA1 synapses can also exhibit decremental LTP. LTP in neocortex has so far been observed only after multiple, spaced tetanization episodes, but this LTP can then be quite long-lasting. These data indicate intriguing differences in the pattern of LTP persistence across brain regions that may reflect different contributions to the memory or information storage process in behaving animals.

The dentate gyrus and CA1 appear to differ in a number of ways at molecular, cellular, and network levels that could account for the apparent differences in LTP persistence. These include the ability to produce voltage-dependent calcium channel (VDCC)-dependent LTP, the contribution by catecholamines to the persistence of LTP, the pattern of constitutive gene expression, and the pattern of tetanic stimulation commonly used to study LTP in these two regions. Few of these features appear to strongly differentiate the two hippocampal regions, however, making it conceivable that the dentate gyrus has the inherent capacity for nondecremental LTP, if only the right induction conditions could be met. Indeed, apparently nondecremental LTP has been reported for perforant path synapses in studies that have employed electroconvulsive shocks. Whether more subtle synaptic activation, as would occur during learning, can effect such changes remains

The research and preparation of this manuscript were supported by the Health Research Council of New Zealand. I thank Assoc. Prof. N. McNaughton and Dr. D. Bilkey for helpful discussions and comments made on drafts of this manuscript.

to be seen. Given the data that are available, however, one can at least conclude that CA1 has a much lower threshold for nondecremental LTP than
the dentate gyrus, but the mechanisms underlying this difference remain to
be delineated.

What is the significance of differentially induced nondecremental LTP between
CA1 and the dentate gyrus? The absence of a consensus description of what these
structures are doing in a cognitive or behavioral sense makes it difficult to answer
this question. However, the commonly held perception of the hippocampus as a
temporary memory store appears to clash with the capacity of CA1 to show
apparently permanent LTP. It is proposed that models or theories of hippocampal
function that allow for the establishment and storage of relatively permanent representations, combined with a capacity for experience to flexibly modify these
representations, would appear to best suit the existing data on the persistence of
LTP in this key brain structure.

Introduction

For over 25 years, the intriguing characteristics of long-term potentiation (LTP)
have led many researchers toward the belief that it is a critical mechanism underlying learning and memory storage in the brain. Notable features of LTP include
rapid induction by brief periods of high-frequency afferent activity, persistence
over a period of time that is many orders of magnitude greater than the duration
of the induction stimulus, synapse specificity, cooperativity/associativity between
active inputs, and associativity between presynaptic activity and postsynaptic
depolarizations. The fact that these properties were important components (either
explicitly or implicitly) of the physiological learning rule hypothesized by Hebb
(1949) added gloss to the LTP effect. Later, the phenomenon was found widely
throughout the central nervous system, and appeared to correlate well with learning and memory in initial behavioral studies, suggesting that the vision held by the
pioneers, Bliss, Lømo, and Gardner-Medwin of LTP as a memory mechanism was
well justified.

In recent years, the refinement of physiological techniques and behavioral paradigms plus the development of new technologies such as transgenic animals has
led to a questioning of the fundamental beliefs about the role(s) played by LTP in
nervous system functioning (e.g., Shors and Matzel, 1997; other chapters in this
book). Much of this debate has arisen from studies examining the behavioral
effects of manipulating LTP, but alongside these efforts the fundamental properties of LTP have also come under renewed scrutiny. In some instances, the outcome of this reevaluation has been enhanced support for LTP as a memory
mechanism, such as the findings that postsynaptic action potential firing may be
more vital to LTP induction than indicated by previous experiments (Linden,
1999). The need for conjunctive presynaptic activity and postsynaptic cell firing is
specifically required in Hebb's theory. On the other hand, the supposed strict

synapse specificity of LTP has been challenged in recent times (Engert and Bonhoeffer, 1997).

The purpose of this chapter is to reconsider the paramount feature of LTP if it is to serve as a long-term memory mechanism (i.e., its persistence). Data regarding the persistence of LTP will be reviewed, and the possibility that there are regional variations will be considered. Potential mechanisms underlying such regional differences in LTP persistence will then be discussed, along with their significance for behavioral studies and certain network models. The material presented in this chapter will focus on LTP in the hippocampus, but on occasion LTP in other brain areas such as neocortex will also be discussed, as will long-term depression (LTD).

How Persistent *Should* LTP Be?

A mechanism that lasts only minutes or hours, while clearly suitable for mediating memory storage over a limited period of time, nonetheless does not appear sufficient for underpinning long-term memory, the understanding of which has been a holy grail in this literature. It has generally been assumed that synaptic changes must persist over days, months, or even years to account for the persistence of long-term memories that can be observed behaviorally. It is reasonable, therefore, to inquire whether LTP can in fact last for such lengthy periods of time. Before doing so, however, two caveats to the basic presumption that it *ought* to be able to last so long will be presented.

First, memories may be held for differing periods of time in different brain regions. For example, the hippocampus and associated medial temporal lobe structures have long been considered to be intermediate memory stores rather than long-term stores, since remote memories of all kinds remain relatively intact following medial temporal lobe lesions (reviewed, for example, by Squire, 1986). Posterior cortical lesions, on the other hand, appear to be able to produce pronounced nontemporally graded retrograde amnesias, sometimes of a very specific nature. Accordingly, there have been various proposals that the hippocampus may serve as a rapid but temporary store that, through repeated reactivation and feedback, promotes longer term storage in the relevant cortical areas (Marr, 1971; Milner, 1989; McClelland et al., 1995; see below). It is reasonable to expect, therefore, that there may be regional variations in the requirements for information storage, medium term in the hippocampus and long-term or permanent in the neocortex. Thus, LTP persistence mechanisms may have evolved to suit the storage requirements for particular cell types in particular brain areas. Milner (1989), for example, distinguished between "soft" and "hard" synapses, proposing that the hippocampus contains soft synapses that change quickly and robustly but transiently, while in contrast, the neocortex contains hard synapses that change in small increments over repeated activation cycles, although these changes are very long-lasting if not permanent. Similar concepts can be found in other models (Marr, 1971; McClelland et al., 1995). Two potential variations on this theme, which will be discussed below, are (1) that the hard versus soft synapse distinction might even apply within the hippocampus, and (2) that a single synapse may be able to show both kinds of characteristics simultaneously.

The second caveat is that, in principle, it may not be the case that the extraordinary persistence of long-term memory has to be served by equally long-lasting synaptic changes following a single induction episode. For example, explicit or implicit rehearsal and reuse of information may restore a decaying synaptic trace (and the memory) back to the efficacy level attained during initial learning. Thus, a passively decaying synaptic memory could fulfill long-term memory persistence requirements if the memories were recalled periodically over time. Extending such reasoning further, it might be that full memory reactivation is not necessary for such synaptic retraining. If individual neurons and synapses contribute to multiple, related memories, then learning or retrieval of one memory could in principle update synaptic weights that participate in closely related memories (e.g., such as may occur during stimulus generalization). The extent to which this latter mechanism might come into play would depend on the sparseness of the coding pattern in the neuronal network involved.

How Long *Does* LTP Persist?

■ **LTP in the Dentate Gyrus.** The persistence of LTP over the time periods pertinent to long-term memory can only be studied in awake animals with chronically implanted electrodes. Such studies have been undertaken rarely, and mostly for perforant path–dentate gyrus synapses. The initial report by Bliss and Gardner-Medwin (1973) showed that LTP could last over days, and noted the important principle that LTP persistence was prolonged if multiple tetanization protocols were delivered. LTP persistence in this study was nearly always decremental, however, eventually decaying back to baseline within a few days, although in one animal the population spike was persistently enhanced for 16 weeks.

The extant data on the persistence of dentate gyrus LTP were summarized by Abraham and Otani in 1991, and the relatively few studies that have been published since then have not changed the essential conclusions. The decay of LTP in this brain region is clearly of a decremental nature, apparently no matter how many stimulus trains are delivered (Barnes and McNaughton, 1985; De Jonge and Racine, 1985; Abraham et al., 1993). This could be due to an insidious deterioration of the recording preparation that sometimes occurs in such studies, but exponentially decremental LTP was still observed even when stable recordings were maintained in a converging control pathway (Abraham et al., 1995). Interestingly, the decay rates of LTP across studies do not appear to be randomly distributed, but rather fall into three groups with average decay time constants of about 2 hours, 3.5 days, and 20 days (Figure 1.1). Using the terminology of Racine et al. (1983), the two shorter phases of LTP were termed LTP1 and LTP2, while the longer lasting phase of LTP, not observed by Racine et al., was termed LTP3 (Abraham and Otani, 1991; Abraham et al., 1993). Each of the LTP phases can be fit with a single negative exponential function. While LTP1 is additive with the

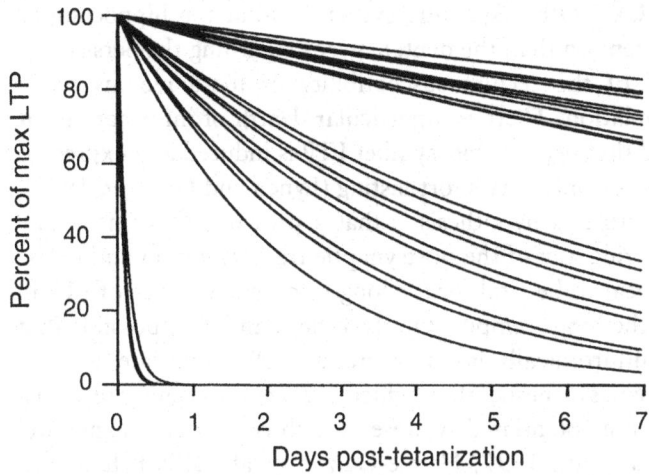

Figure 1.1. Families of dentate gyrus LTP decay curves obtained from a survey of the literature in 1991 by Abraham and Otani. The three families of curves have average decay time constants of 2.1 hours, 3.5 days, and 20.3 days, and were termed LTP1, LTP2, and LTP3, respectively. To date, nondecremental LTP has still not been reported to occur in the dentate gyrus following non–seizure-inducing stimulation. LTP1 is protein-synthesis independent, and corresponds to "early" LTP in a more commonly used terminology. The extent to which LTP2 and LTP3 require de novo transcription is not clear, but a variety of correlations between LTP3 and immediate early gene expression suggest that at least this latter phase does. (Data from Abraham and Otani, 1991, with permission.)

other two phases (Racine et al., 1983), LTP2 and LTP3 are not additive, and so may involve some common underlying mechanisms. These persistence characteristics are not confined to the dentate gyrus, since Racine et al. (1983) observed that pathways throughout the limbic forebrain exhibited decremental LTP in the forms of LTP1 and LTP2. [It should be noted that a terminology that is now more commonly used for LTP phases is early, intermediate, and late phase LTP (Matthies, 1989). LTP1 and early-LTP both refer to a protein-synthesis independent phase of LTP. LTP3 and late-LTP are both protein synthesis- and gene transcription-dependent, but there is still some question regarding the extent to which the later two phases in each terminology system are mechanistically related. The waters surrounding the intermediate phase(s) of LTP are rather murky.]

In a few experiments where electroconvulsive shocks (ECS) have been given to animals, a long-lasting increase in dentate evoked responses has been reported (Stewart and Reid, 1993; Stewart et al., 1994; Barnes et al., 1994). In some of these studies the response potentiation was observed to be nondecremental, and measured in one case to last up to 91 days post-ECS (Gombos et al., 1997). It is not clear, however, whether this seizure-induced potentiation reflects LTP induction, or activation of some other potentiation mechanism. If these response changes do represent LTP, then they suggest that synapses in the dentate gyrus may have the capacity to exhibit nondecremental LTP, even if special circumstances may be required for its induction and expression.

■ **LTP in Areas CA3 and CA1.** Other synaptic systems within the hippocampus have received much less attention than the dentate gyrus regarding the persistence of LTP, perhaps because of the seizure susceptibility of these regions when given high-frequency stimulation. There is a particular dearth of information for CA3. It has been proposed that because mossy fiber LTP is induced and expressed presynaptically, that it may be only very short-lasting (Lynch and Granger, 1992). An argument consistent with this hypothesis is that a presynaptic form of LTP might occur without triggering any of the postsynaptic transcriptional and translational responses that appear to be vital for the long-term maintenance of LTP in other synaptic systems in the hippocampus. On the other hand, it is possible that mossy fiber stimulation antidromically instructs granule cells to initiate de novo gene expression and protein synthesis, after which the new proteins are transported down the axons to the potentiated synapses and thus promote the maintenance of their LTP (Hicks et al., 1997; Helme-Guizon et al., 1998). It is also unfortunate that there is no information on the persistence of LTP at the recurrent excitatory synaptic connections between CA3 pyramidal cells, as these synapses are considered by many theorists to be a vital site of information storage in the hippocampus (see below).

Somewhat more effort has been expended on LTP at Schaffer collateral/commissural synapses in area CA1. Several studies have reported a decremental form of LTP here (Buzsáki, 1980; Leung et al., 1992; Leung and Shen, 1995), although in general, the LTP has only been followed for a few days, making it difficult in some cases to make a clear assessment. What has been remarkable, however, is the single report by Staubli and Lynch (1987) that LTP following theta-burst stimulation (TBS) of these synapses can be nondecremental; in 17 of 25 animals, TBS induced a stable, input-specific LTP. In most cases the recordings could not be maintained for more than 1 to 2 weeks, due to sudden response declines that probably reflected deteriorations in the preparation. Nonetheless, the authors noted that in three cases LTP was observed to remain stably potentiated for 3 to 5 weeks posttetanus. In four of the twenty-five animals, a decremental LTP was induced that lasted only a few days. It is vital that the finding of non-decremental LTP in CA1 be verified and extended to longer periods of time, as by the standards of some studies in the dentate gyrus that have followed LTP for months, 3 weeks of stable LTP is a relatively short time over which to assess whether LTP is non-decremental or not.

■ **LTP in the Neocortex.** Compared to the hippocampus, LTP in the neocortex has been difficult to obtain. While methods for generating its induction have improved dramatically over the years, the success has largely been in either slice preparations or anesthetized animals. Recently, however, Racine and colleagues have established extracellular stimulating and recording protocols that successfully produce LTP in awake animals (Racine et al., 1995). The key to success appears to be the use of multiple episodes of tetanization, spread across many days. Using such paradigms, LTP can be incrementally produced over the days of high-frequency stimulation, and it is then very long-lasting, having been measured up to 4 to 5 weeks after the last tetanization episode (Trepel and Racine, 1998). It is not entirely clear whether this LTP is decremental. The LTP values, when expressed as group averages over days, do appear to slowly decline, although exponential curve-fitting was not performed to quantitatively assess this. As shown by Staubli and Lynch (1987) and observed in our preliminary experiments in the hippocampus, however, one needs to assess the data for each animal individually to tell whether nondecremental LTP occurs in any given case. Given the shallow slope of the decay curves for some of Trepel and Racine's (1998) data, it does appear possible that LTP for at least some of the cortical recordings in nondecremental, or at least decaying to an asymptotic level well above the baseline value.

LTD in the Hippocampus

LTD may be another essential component in the learning process, either directly by contributing to the overall pattern of synaptic weight changes or by counteracting or reversing LTP that is residual from a prior learning episode. When LTP in CA1 is reversed by low-frequency stimulation, this effect appears to be permanent, that is, there is no recovery over 24 hours (Staubli and Lynch, 1990). However, there are no studies that systematically examine the persistence of homosynaptic LTD (i.e., depression expressed at activated synapses) when it is induced by low-frequency stimulation in naïve synapses. Such LTD can last for days (Doyére et al., 1996; Manahan-Vaughan and Braunewell, 1999), but beyond that there is no information. In the dentate gyrus, heterosynaptic LTD (i.e., depression expressed at inactive synapses when other synapses are activated) is robustly observed. When we measured the persistence of such depression, we found that like LTP, heterosynaptic LTD was exponentially decremental (Abraham et al., 1994; see also Krug et al., 1985). Furthermore, the LTD was as long-lasting on average as the simultaneous LTP in the tetanized synapses (measured over days and weeks).

Taken together, the above data are suggestive of substantial regional differences in the duration of LTP. However, a major caveat to this interpretation is that the synchronous stimulation used to elicit LTP in these studies may not activate the same mechanisms that are engaged by the actual patterns of activity occurring during learning. LTP, for example, can very easily be induced by a single tetanic episode in neocortical slices (Artola et al., 1990; Kirkwood and Bear, 1994). Thus neocortex clearly has the capacity for rapid LTP induction without the multiple episodes of stimulation given across days. Unfortunately, it is not yet known which tetanization paradigm most closely resembles learning-related patterns of activity in the cortex.

Possible Mechanisms for Regional Differences in LTP Persistence

Before considering in more detail the behavioral implications of regional differences in LTP persistence, some consideration will be given to possible mechanisms for the effect. Not only would regional differences in LTP mechanisms provide some backing to the general concept, but some of the mechanisms themselves may relate to behavior in interesting ways. Most of this section concentrates on differences in possible LTP-related mechanisms between CA1 and the dentate gyrus.

■ **Pattern of Stimulation.** It is possible that the regional difference in LTP persistence is merely an artifact of the stimulation protocol used. Nondecremental LTP was induced in CA1 using 40 pulses of TBS, while to achieve decremental LTP in the dentate gyrus, hundreds of pulses have often been delivered. In the latter experiments, different patterns and frequencies of high-frequency stimulation have been used, but like TBS, they typically have involved repeated, short bursts of pulses. Accordingly, we have begun to test identical protocols for both CA1 and the dentate gyrus (Hargreaves et al., 1998). Our data to date indicate that, in contrast to CA1, TBS is a remarkably unsuccessful paradigm for eliciting any LTP at all in the dentate gyrus of awake animals, much less nondecremental LTP.

■ **NMDA-Dependent Versus VDCC-Dependent LTP.** In CA1 slices, there is considerable evidence that two semi-independent forms of LTP can be elicited, one dependent on NMDA receptor activation and one dependent on activation of L-type VDCCs (Grover and Teyler, 1990). These two forms of LTP are optimally elicited by different frequencies of stimulation, but at a midrange frequency of 100 Hz, both forms of LTP can be simultaneously elicited, according to some reports (Grover and Teyler, 1995; but see Reymann et al., 1989). Recently, it has been reported that activation of L-type VDCCs, but not NMDA receptors, is required for the induction of the late phase of LTP (Impey et al., 1996). Consistent with this finding, the VDCC-dependent late phase of LTP, but not an NMDA-dependent decremental phase, was associated with an increase in gene expression driven by activation of the cAMP-dependent response element (CRE). In the case of TBS-induced LTP, however, NMDA receptor antagonists completely block its induction, both *in vitro* and *in vivo* (Larson and Lynch, 1988; Hargreaves et al., 1998). It is not known, however, what effects VDCC antagonists may have specifically on nondecremental LTP *in vivo*. Taken together, these data raise the possibility that nondecremental LTP in CA1 may be explained by its association with CRE-triggered gene expression. In contrast, while the slowly decrementing LTP3 in the dentate gyrus in vivo is associated with an increase in gene expression of various kinds, our preliminary findings to date show no effect of VDCC antagonists on either LTP induction or persistence (B. Logan and W.C. Abraham, unpublished observations) nor any association between LTP3 and CRE-binding protein (CREB) phosphorylation (Walton et al., 1999). It is interesting to note that contextual fear conditioning enhances CRE-mediated gene expression in CA1 but not the dentate gyrus, although the latter region can nonetheless exhibit the effect, as well as CREB phosphorylation, if animals are given passive avoidance training (Impey et al., 1998; Taubenfeld et al., 1999). Thus, it may be that a nondecremental LTP can be elicited in the dentate gyrus if the CRE mechanisms are properly brought into play.

Another pertinent regional difference within the hippocampus is that the constitutive expression of various genes varies quite widely across the subregions. For example, the protein levels of the inducible transcription factor zif/268 are relatively high in the basal state for CA1 but are virtually undetectable in the dentate gyrus immunohistochemically. On the other hand, the reverse situation is true for brain-derived neurotrophic factor (Tokuyama et al., 1998). It is possible, therefore, that area CA1 is primed for nondecremental LTP by virtue of its preexisting levels of crucial transcription factors or other gene products. It is interesting to note that some areas of cortex have a similar profile of constitutive gene expression to CA1 (e.g., Tokuyama et al., 1998).

■ **Catecholamines.** The catecholamines noradrenaline and dopamine widely innervate the hippocampus, and there is now considerable evidence that they play a vital role in the persistence of LTP. For example, D1/D5 receptor antagonists prevent the late phase of CA1 LTP both *in vitro* (Figure 1.2; Frey et al., 1990) and *in vivo* (Swanson-Park et al., 1999), even when the level of initial induction is not affected. It has been proposed that this is due to the coupling of such receptors to adenylyl cyclase and thus a cAMP-mediated cascade of gene expression and protein synthesis. The simplicity of this explanation, however, is challenged by the fact that antagonism of beta-adrenergic receptors, which also couple to adenylyl cyclase, does not affect the persistence of CA1 LTP. Furthermore, activation of beta-adrenergic receptors does not prolong LTP persistence, even though it can increase the level of LTP initially induced (Cohen et al., 1999). It remains to be seen whether nondecremental LTP requires D1/D5 receptor-mediated synaptic transmission.

Interestingly, the persistence of LTP in the dentate gyrus shows the converse dependence on catecholamines, that is, it is blocked by beta-adrenergic antagonists but not by D1/D5 antagonists (Figure 1.2; Swanson-Park et al., 1999). Furthermore, the persistence of LTP is enhanced in freely moving animals when they have access to a reinforcing stimulus near to the time of LTP induction, an effect that is blocked by a beta-adrenergic antagonist (Seidenbecher et al., 1997). There is no evidence, however, that such noradrenaline-enhanced LTP in the dentate gyrus can be nondecremental.

The reasons why noradrenaline and dopamine, the terminals and receptors for which are found throughout the hippocampus, play regionally specific roles in LTP persistence are not well understood. However, there may be behavioral significance to this dichotomy, since these catecholaminergic afferents are preferentially active during different behavioral situations. Neurons in the locus coeruleus, source of the noradrenergic innervation to the hippocampus, are phasically activated by both noxious and nonnoxious stimuli (Aston-Jones and Bloom, 1981b). They are also tonically inhibited during slow-wave sleep but show marked activation just prior to waking (Aston-Jones and Bloom, 1981a). For these and other reasons, the locus coeruleus has often been described as participating in behavioral arousal as well as orienting responses and attention (Amaral and Sinnamon, 1977; Aston-Jones and Bloom, 1981b) through its divergent modulation of multiple brain regions. Dopaminergic neurons in the

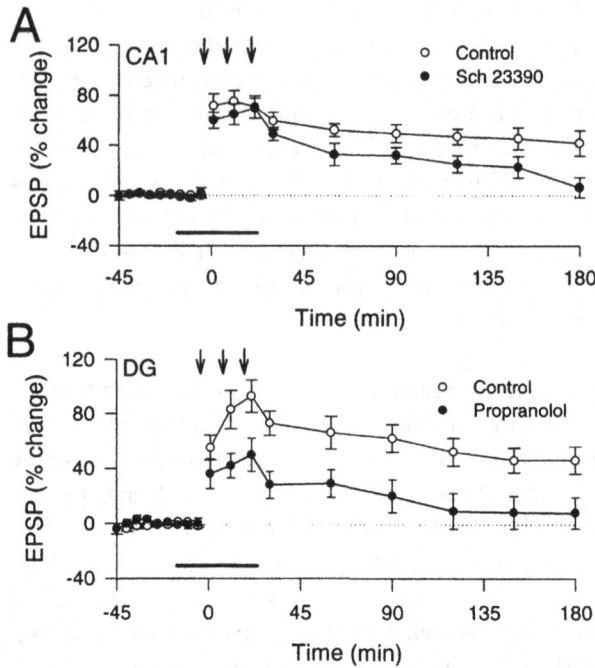

Figure 1.2. Double dissociation between areas CA1 and the dentate gyrus (DG) in the dependence of LTP persistence on catecholaminergic receptor activation. In CA1, LTP persistence is blocked by the dopamine D1/D5 receptor antagonist SCH-23390 (**A**), while dentate gyrus LTP persistence is blocked by the beta-adrenergic receptor antagonist propranolol (**B**). LTP in each area is not affected by the other antagonist (data not shown). The field potential data were taken from hippocampal slices, in which three bouts of 100-Hz tetanic stimulation were administered (**arrows**) to induce LTP. The period of drug administration is indicated by the thick line. The region-specific mechanisms responsible for this double dissociation of catecholaminergic contributions to LTP persistence remain to be established. (Data from Swanson-Park et al., 1999, with permission.)

ventral midbrain, on the other hand, are typically activated during the expectation or receipt of positive reward (Ljungberg et al., 1992; Schultz et al., 1992). These differences in neural responses to behavioral stimuli suggest that the consolidation of LTP will show regional variations in its dependence on the behavioral state of the animals. It still remains to be established, however, whether nondecremental LTP in CA1 is dependent on catecholamines and if so, which one(s).

■ **Depotentiation.** In principle, the persistence of LTP will be regulated by two general factors. First, the LTP may passively decay at some intrinsic rate as mediated, for example, by protein turnover, reversal of protein posttranslational modifications, or synaptic morphology changes until the original basal state is achieved. Alternatively, there may be active mechanisms for reversal of LTP through depotentiation or LTD processes. Nondecremental LTP in CA1 by definition does not appear to have a passive decay component, yet it can be actively depotentiated by homosynaptic low-frequency stimulation (LFS) if given within minutes of LTP induction (Staubli and Lynch, 1990). Other studies have also suggested that late-phase LTP in CA1 (whether decremental or nondecremental is not known) exhibits a period of consolidation for an hour or so posttetanus during which LFS-induced depotentiation is readily obtained, but that LFS applied after this time is much less effective (e.g., O'Dell and Kandel, 1994; but see Bashir and Collingridge, 1994). Furthermore, two recent studies have demonstrated that baseline rates of synaptic stimulation, if applied while an animal is exploring a novel environment or novel objects, will reverse LTP when given within an hour post-LTP induction, but are ineffective 24 hours later (Xu et al., 1998). Intriguingly, to date there is little evidence that LTP in CA1 can be significantly reversed by heterosynaptic stimulation (but see Muller et al., 1995), and none is available from *in vivo* studies.

Synapses in the dentate gyrus, in contrast, exhibit heterosynaptic LTD and depotentiation quite readily *in vivo*, while homosynaptic LTD or depotentiation has been particularly difficult to induce (Errington et al., 1995; Abraham et al., 1996). Early studies indicated that the crossed perforant path synapses can rapidly switch between LTP and depotentiation depending on whether activation of these synapses is paired (LTP) or not (depotentiation) with high-frequency stimulation of the ipsilateral perforant path (Levy and Steward, 1979). Ipsilateral medial and lateral perforant path synapses can also mutually depotentiate each other (Christie and Abraham, 1992; Doyére et al., 1997), and while there was an early indication that there may be a time dependence to the depotentiation (Abraham and Goddard, 1983), subsequent studies in both anesthetized and awake animals have shown that significant depotentiation can still be induced up to at least 24 hours post-LTP induction (Steward et al., 1988; Doyére et al., 1997).

The reasons underlying the regional differences in the ease of obtaining homosynaptic and heterosynaptic LTD or depotentiation are, once again, not clear. However, while these apparent differential properties may be simply artifacts of the experimental preparations used (Abraham, 1996), nonetheless they show an interesting relation to the regional variations in the persistence of LTP. Nondecremental LTP, such as seen in CA1, must not only be unaffected by intrinsic decay but it must also be immune from active depotentiation, at least after the initial period of consolidation. This accords well with the depotentiation properties described above for CA1. LTP in the dentate gyrus, being decremental, must suffer either passive decay or active depotentiation, or both. The apparent ease of heterosynaptic LTD and depotentiation in the dentate gyrus fits well at least with the latter possibility.

■ **Neurogenesis.** The dentate gyrus exhibits the unique property that new granule cells are born throughout life (Kaplan and Hinds, 1977). Moreover, the birth rate and survival rate both appear to be modifiable by experience, such as locomotor activity, learning hippocampal-dependent tasks, and exposure to enriched environments (van Praag et al., 1999; Gould et al., 1999), as well as by stress hormones and NMDA receptor-mediated mechanisms (Cameron et al., 1995). Some

of these cells differentiate into granule cells, migrate into the cell layer, express calbindin, and make apparent mossy fiber synapses in CA3. It is important in the
context of this review to emphasize that no other hippocampal neurons, and very
few cortical neurons, are born in adulthood (Kaplan and Hinds, 1977). What is
not understood at this time is whether the new neurons replace existing ones,
which may undergo apoptosis, or whether there is an expanding number of granule cells during adulthood, prior to the eventual net cell loss observed in aged animals. The facts that stable field potential recordings can be maintained in a
control nontetanized pathway for several months (Abraham et al., 1995) and that
the dentate gyrus volume does not change following experience-induced increases
in survival of newborn neurons (Gould et al., 1999; van Praag et al., 1999) suggest that there is little net change in neuron numbers. In contrast, one study has
reported that granule cell numbers change quite dramatically (24 percent increase)
in response to an NMDA receptor antagonist (Cameron et al., 1995), but this
finding needs to be verified using more sophisticated stereologic techniques.

Ongoing neurogenesis and neurodegeneration in the dentate gyrus could have
important implications for the measured persistence of LTP. First, if preexisting
neurons are lost at about the same rate as new ones come in, then the population
measure of LTP will decrease, assuming that among the cells that are lost are ones
with potentiated synapses and assuming that the synapses on the new cells are in
a nonpotentiated state. Thus, LTP could appear to be decremental, even if there
was in fact nondecremental LTP at individual surviving synapses. (The reverse
argument holds in principle for LTD.) Secondly, if the number of granule cells
gradually increases with age, the population measure of LTP might appear to be
more slowly decrementing than is actually the case. Determining which of these
scenarios is the case should make more accurate any decision as to whether nondecremental LTP is differentially present in the dentate gyrus and CA1.

Although neurogenesis of granule cells may represent a major difference
between the dentate gyrus and other brain regions, the importance of this unique
characteristic for LTP remains speculative because there are critical gaps of knowledge regarding some important details. In particular, information is required
regarding the change or stability of total granule cell numbers, the survival rates of
neurons born at different times over the life span, and the relative efficacy of
synapses on newly differentiated neurons. Nonetheless, the lesson from the dentate gyrus so far is that it has a more variable citizenry of cells and thus synapses
than other brain regions, and thus it is not unreasonable to expect that the stability of plasticity in this brain region will have different characteristics to that found
elsewhere in the brain.

Implications of Regional Differences in the Persistence of LTP

■ **Network and Computational Models of Hippocampal Function.** As alluded to
above, the hippocampus and surrounding medial temporal lobe structures are
conceived by many theorists to form an intermediate memory store, since lesions

to these structures can result in a temporally graded retrograde amnesia lasting from days to years, depending on the task and species being studied, while remote memories are spared (see McClelland et al., 1995, for a review). It has been commonly proposed, therefore, that medial temporal lobe structures provide a means for rapid but temporary storage of newly learned information, for example, using Milner's (1989) "soft synapses," but that readout of this information during repeated rehearsal or during either quiet waking or slow-wave sleep episodes causes the neocortical representations to be updated or elaborated using "hard synapses" (Marr, 1971; Willshaw and Buckingham, 1990; McClelland et al., 1995). The advantages of slow, multitrial learning in the neocortex, particularly for integrating the new information into the memory structure without loss of prior information, have been discussed elsewhere (O'Keefe and Nadel, 1978; McClelland et al., 1995; Rolls, 1996), and indeed there is evidence that hippocampal place cells, recently active in an explored environment, replay that activity during later behavioral quiescence (Pavlides and Winson, 1989; Wilson and McNaughton, 1994).

Within a number of theories, it is hypothesized that information proceeds by a series of synaptic steps through the temporal lobe into the hippocampus, each step compressing the signals, removing redundancy, and establishing orthogonal and sparse memory traces (Eichenbaum et al., 1996; Hasselmo et al., 1996; Rolls, 1996). The critical end point for this processing is area CA3 which, due to its relatively small number of cells, must represent the most compressed storage system. CA3, by virtue of its extensive excitatory recurrent collateral connections, may also be able to "autoassociate" and thereby form (via LTP) memory structures capable of re-creating the whole signal from a partial reactivation stimulus (Marr, 1971; McNaughton and Morris, 1987). The synaptic connections from CA3 to CA1 and on posteriorly through retrohippocampal cortex and thence neocortex have been described as decoding steps necessary for mapping the stored but compressed information back onto the cortical representations. The following discussion will consider the possible roles played by differentially persistent LTP and LTD in the storage of information in the hippocampus, taking the above summary sketch as one broad view of hippocampal function. It is recognized, however, that differences in detail between individual theories may be of great importance in correctly understanding the contribution of synaptic plasticity to hippocampal function.

The synaptic connections between the entorhinal cortex and the dentate gyrus have been proposed to be a key step in removing information redundancy and establishing the sparse representations necessary for efficient storage. It is interesting to note that although LTP is the prototypical mechanism for establishing these modifications to the information, heterosynaptic LTD may play a key role in keeping memories separate, or else erasing old memories and thereby preventing storage overload in the limited capacity CA3 (McClelland and Goddard, 1996; Rolls, 1996). Thus, there may be a competition between the entorhinal inputs to the dentate gyrus, that is, LTP at some synapses counterbalanced by heterosynaptic LTD at others, such that the net synaptic weight for a given cell is relatively constant (Rolls, 1996). This proposal is in striking accord with the data cited above that indicate that heterosynaptic LTD is relatively easily induced at perforant path synapses. Furthermore, our comparisons between the medial and lateral path inputs indicate that, on average, the magnitude of LTP at one set of synapses is relatively well matched by heterosynaptic LTD at the other set (Abraham et al., 1994). Because the dentate gyrus has been presumed to be required only for storage, but not retrieval, of memory from CA3, synaptic plasticity in the dentate gyrus is expected to be decremental over time, an idea consistent with the data reviewed above. (Retrieval from the autoassociative memory network in area CA3 may be triggered by the direct perforant path projection from the entorhinal cortex, thus bypassing the dentate gyrus.) Although a specific prediction has not been made in any model, to our knowledge, about the relative persistence of LTP and LTD, it appears to be sensible for the two to have equivalent time constants of decay, as has been shown (Abraham et al., 1994). This is particularly true if LTD is a part of the storage process, and not just a means of erasing old memories.

The Schaffer collateral afferents from CA3 to CA1 have been characterized as the first stage of decoding of the memory stored in CA3. Alternatively, CA1 neurons may serve to compare a memory (attractor state) from CA3 with the existing situation, as informed by the direct perforant path input to CA1 (Hasslemo et al., 1996). Either way, CA1 can then feed the relevant information back to cortex. It has been suggested that much information would be lost if the Schaffer collateral synapses were nonmodifiable (Rolls, 1996), and it is clear that these synapses can indeed be rapidly modified, particularly by LTP. The degree of LTP persistence for any collateral synapses, whether terminating in CA3 or CA1, should parallel the persistence of memory in the hippocampal formation, as detected by the retrograde amnesia gradient in behavioral studies employing hippocampal lesions. In fact, it has been noted that retrograde amnesia gradients in rats match closely with the LTP3 time constant (McClelland et al., 1995), and that the persistence of memory and LTP both decline with age (reviewed by Treves et al., 1996). What is curious about these correlations is that the LTP persistence values have been taken from studies in the dentate gyrus, a region that may not be involved in memory retrieval. It is important, therefore, to compare the duration of hippocampal memories with the duration of LTP in CA3 and CA1.

It is by no means clear how nondecremental LTP fits into the schema of the hippocampus as a temporary storage device. However, some theorists have suggested that the more stable the environment, the more stable the corresponding representations in the hippocampus (Rolls, 1996), particularly postdevelopment (McClelland and Goddard, 1996). Since animals used for LTP decay studies are typically exposed to extremely stable environments and have very few opportunities for new learning, synaptic weights might be expected in these animals to change little over time. Another possibility is that CA1 may be more neocortical-like than archicortical in its connections and properties of plasticity. Accordingly, a nondecremental LTP would not be out of place in CA1 (Granger et al., 1996), although it remains to be definitively shown that nondecremental LTP does indeed occur in the neocortex.

■ **Insights From Hippocampal Place Fields.** Recordings of the place field properties of hippocampal neurons have provided some interesting insights into the storage and persistence of spatial representations in the hippocampus. This is so even though place fields may reflect only a specialized subset of the information processing undertaken by the hippocampus. Pertinent to the present discussion, it is notable that the place field firing of CA1 pyramidal cells is extremely persistent over time for a given environment (Thompson and Best, 1990), and it is unaffected by exposure of the animal to other, new environments, even when those same cells are found to have place fields in the new environments. Place fields do not appear to be simply driven by the particular array of extrinsic stimuli, since removal or repositioning of one or more stimuli does not affect the field, up to some limit (reviewed by Muller, 1996). Furthermore, CA1 and CA3 place fields do not appear to be a simple copy of representations elsewhere in the brain since (1) the fields endure when the dentate gyrus is inactivated (McNaughton et al., 1989), (2) the fields are more spatially refined than the fields of afferent entorhinal cortical cells, which appear to be more closely aligned with the sensory features of the environment (Quirk et al., 1992), and (3) transgenic mice with a knock-down of the R1 subunit of the NMDA receptor confined specifically to the CA1 region show place cell firing that is less spatially selective, and less well correlated with other cells in this region, relative to wild-type controls (McHugh et al., 1996). Because the transgenic mice also show an impairment of LTP induction selective to CA1, these findings suggest that the place fields form, or are refined by, an LTP-like process. This is consistent with the finding that place fields develop over the first few minutes of exposure to a novel environment (Wilson and McNaughton, 1993). However, a more recent study has indicated that only the persistence, and not the initial establishment, of a new place field is modified by an NMDA receptor antagonist (acting globally in the brain) (Kentros et al., 1998). Thus, if LTP is indeed involved in the establishment of place fields, it appears to be through an NMDA-independent process.

A somewhat different model has been put forward to account for the various place field data (McNaughton et al., 1996). In this "path integration" model, the hippocampus is conceived to have a "set of quasi-independent spatial reference frame representations that are preconfigured within the synaptic matrix of the hippocampus and related structures, and which permit position and direction to be updated solely on the basis of idiothetic information" (p. 174). Navigation within a new environment involves acquiring various landmark information, and binding it to the location representations within the relevant reference frame through associative synaptic plasticity mechanisms. An intriguing aspect of this model is that one might infer from it that "hard" and "soft" synapses coexist in the same brain region (e.g., CA1 or CA3). Thus, reference frames could be hardwired, presumably during the course of development, through long-lasting (permanent) changes at hard synapses. The model has not specified, however, when the preconfiguration takes place, and it is reasonable to suggest that new reference frames may continue to be constructed into adulthood. Updating the reference frame with current landmark information would appear to involve more rapid and robust plasticity, but perhaps in a less permanent way given that key stimuli and landmarks may change; accordingly, this process may employ soft synapses. A logical extension of these considerations is that the same synapses in these hippocampal (or other) areas should be able to undergo both kinds of synaptic changes, in other words, nondecremental (hard) LTP as well as decremental (soft) LTP. Certainly the evidence is there that Schaffer collateral synapses can do both, but a specific test that synapses can superimpose the two has yet to be made.

It would appear to make sense for synapses in at least some regions of the hippocampus to exhibit both nondecremental and decremental LTP. If so, the hippocampus may not serve as a *tabula rasa,* simply taking in and storing information without reference to prior experience, as one might infer from some models. Although it has been shown that the hippocampus could in principle store many independent memories using sparse and orthogonal storage mechanisms (e.g., McNaughton and Morris, 1987), there appears to be merit in the concept that there is linkage of new information (required for working memory perhaps) to preexisting reference frames. The concept of reference frames appears to bear some similarity to the concept of reference memory, since both seem to refer to a relational map of permanent or slowly varying environmental stimuli (and perhaps reinforcement contingencies). Thus, it is perhaps not surprising that hippocampal damage can impair performance on spatial reference memory tasks (e.g., Morris et al., 1982).

Conclusion

The existing data indicate that while CA1 and the dentate gyrus have very similar induction mechanisms for LTP, CA1 has a much lower threshold for its LTP to be maintained nondecrementally than the dentate gyrus, if the latter region has the capacity for it at all. Since it is commonly believed that very long-lasting or even life-long memories are stored in neocortex, it is presumed that nondecremental synaptic plasticity must occur there as well. Firm evidence for this is still lacking, but at least the issue can be rigorously tested now that successful paradigms for the induction of neocortical LTP *in vivo* have been established. Neocortex aside, it is beginning to be possible to go beyond the general phenomenological research on the persistence of LTP, which has largely characterized the experimental efforts so far, to compare the regional variations in this property of LTP with those predicted by theories of the roles that different parts of the hippocampus and related structures play during learning and memory. If it can be established that the properties of LTP are tailored to the information storage requirements of particular brain regions, this could considerably strengthen the case that LTP is more than an epiphenomenon, and may instead be a vital mechanism for the normal function of these areas. It is recognized that these data remain very correlational in nature, but they would represent an important move away from simply noting the interesting fact that LTP can last over days or beyond. In the longer term, it will be interesting to learn if there are special mechanisms associated with nondecremental LTP, and what the behavioral consequences would be of selectively manipulating this form of plasticity.

In the more immediate future, some previously employed lines of research may be usefully retraced. One in particular that we are beginning to undertake is a reanalysis of the "prior learning" approach to the correlation of LTP and behavior (Morris and Baker, 1984). Exposure of animals to a novel enriched environment has been shown in studies over a decade old to cause an increase in evoked field potentials in the dentate gyrus (Green and Greenough, 1986; Sharp et al., 1987). Interestingly, these changes declined over time and were no longer apparent after several weeks, reminiscent of the slow but inevitable decay of tetanically evoked LTP in the dentate gyrus. Such changes are blocked by NMDA receptor antagonists (Croll et al., 1992), but whether they represent LTP has not been tested by, for example, saturation and occlusion experiments. Equally interesting, however, would be tests for response changes in CA1. Would any potentiation of the evoked responses be transient, or nondecremental, in nature? Importantly, would any evoked response changes correlate with altered performance on learning and memory tasks? Although still not definitive, any parallels or interactions between experience-dependent potentiation and tetanically evoked LTP that covaried on a regional basis would lend considerable support to the hypothesis that LTP is a mechanism for information storage in the brain. There appears to be a need, therefore, to further refine our understanding of the basic properties of LTP, such as its persistence, and to investigate how well they map onto the properties of memory itself, keeping in mind that these properties may vary across different brain regions.

REFERENCES

Abraham, W.C. (1996). Induction of heterosynaptic and homosynaptic LTD in hippocampal subregions in vivo. *J. Physiol. Paris* 90: 305–306.

Abraham, W.C., Christie, B.R., Logan, B., Lawlor, P. et al. (1994). Immediate early gene expression associated with the persistence of heterosynaptic long-term depression in the hippocampus. *Proc. Natl. Acad. Sci. USA* 91: 10049–10053.

Abraham, W.C., Demmer, J., Richardson, C., Williams, J. et al. (1993). Correlations between immediate early gene induction and the persistence of long-term potentiation. *Neuroscience* 56: 717–727.

Abraham, W.C., and Goddard, G.V. (1983). Asymmetric relations between homosynaptic long-term potentiation and heterosynaptic long-term depression. *Nature* 305: 717–719.

Abraham, W.C., Mason-Parker, S.E., and Logan, B. (1996). Low-frequency stimulation does not readily induce homosynaptic long-term depression or depotentiation in the dentate gyrus of awake rats. *Brain Res.* 722: 217–221.

Abraham, W.C., Mason-Parker, S.E., Williams, J., Dragunow, M. (1995). Analysis of the decremental nature of LTP in the dentate gyrus. *Mol. Brain Res.* 30: 367–372.

Abraham, W.C., and Otani, S. (1991). Macromolecules and the maintenance of long-term potentiation. In F. Morrell (Ed.), *Kindling and synaptic plasticity* (pp. 92–109). Boston: Birkhäuser.

Amaral, D.G., and Sinnamon, H.M. (1977). The locus coeruleus: Neurobiology of a central noradrenergic nucleus. *Prog. Neurobiol.* 9: 147–196.

Artola, A., Bröcher, S., and Singer, W. (1990). Different voltage-dependent thresholds for inducing long-term depression and long-term potentiation in slices of rat visual cortex. *Nature* 346: 69–72.

Aston-Jones, G., and Bloom, F.E. (1981a). Activity of norepinephrine-containing locus coeruleus neurons in behaving rats anticipates fluctuations in the sleep-waking cycle. *J. Neurosci.* 1: 876–886.

Aston-Jones, G., and Bloom, F.E. (1981b). Norepinephrine-containing locus coeruleus neurons in behaving rats exhibit pronounced responses to non-noxious environmental stimuli. *J. Neurosci.* 1: 887–900.

Barnes, C.A., Jung, M.W., McNaughton, B.L., and Korol, D.L. et al. LTP saturation and spatial learning disruption: Effects of task variables and saturation levels. *J. Neurosci.* 14: 5793–5806.

Barnes, C.A., and McNaughton, B.L. (1985). An age comparison of the rates of acquisition and forgetting of spatial information in relation to long-term enhancement of hippocampal synapses. *Behav. Neurosci.* 99: 1040–1048.

Bashir, Z.I., and Collingridge, G.L. (1994). An investigation of depotentiation of long-term potentiation in the CA1 region of the hippocampus. *Exp. Brain. Res.* 100: 437–443.

Bliss, T.V.P., and Gardner-Medwin, A.R. (1973). Long-lasting potentiation of synaptic transmission in the dentate area of the unanaesthetized rabbit following stimulation of the perforant path. *J. Physiol.* 232: 357–374.

Buzsáki, G. (1980). Long-term potentiation of the commissural-CA1 pyramidal cell response in the hippocampus of the freely moving rat. *Neurosci. Lett.* 19: 293–296.

Cameron, H.A., McEwen, B.S., and Gould, E. (1995). Regulation of adult neurogenesis by excitatory input and NMDA receptor activation in the dentate gyrus. *J. Neurosci.* 15: 4687–4692.

Christie, B.R., and Abraham, W.C. (1992). NMDA-dependent heterosynaptic long-term depression in the dentate gyrus of anaesthetized rats. *Synapse* 10: 1–6.

Cohen, A.S., Coussens, C.M., Raymond, C.R., and Abraham, W.C. (1999). Long-lasting increase in cellular excitability associated with the priming of LTP induction in rat hippocampus. *J. Neurophysiol.* 82: 3139–3148.

Croll, S.D., Sharp, P.E., and Bostock, E. (1992). Evidence for NMDA receptor involvement in environmentally induced dentate gyrus plasticity. *Hippocampus* 2: 23–28.

De Jonge, M., and Racine, R.J. (1985). The effects of repeated induction of long-term potentiation in the dentate gyrus. *Brain Res.* 328: 181–185.

Doyère, V., Errington, M.L., Laroche, S., Bliss, T.V.P. (1996). Low-frequency trains of paired stimuli induce long-term depression in area CA1 but not in dentate gyrus of the intact rat. *Hippocampus* 6: 52–57.

Doyère, V., Srebro, B., and Laroche, S. (1997). Heterosynaptic LTD and depotentiation in the medial perforant path of the dentate gyrus in the freely moving rat. *J. Neurophysiol.* 77: 571–578.

Eichenbaum, H., Schoenbaum, G., Young, B., Bunsey, M. (1996). Functional organization of the hippocampal memory system. *Proc. Natl. Acad. Sci. USA* 93: 13500–13507.

Engert, F., and Bonhoeffer, T. (1997). Synapse specificity of long-term potentiation breaks down at short distances. *Nature* 388: 279–284.

Errington, M.L., Bliss, T.V.P., Richter-Levin, G., Yenk, K. et al. (1995). Stimulation at 1-5 Hz does not produce long-term depression or depotentiation in the hippocampus of the adult rat in vivo. *J. Neurophysiol.* 74: 1793–1799.

Frey, U., Schroeder, H., and Matthies, H. (1990). Dopaminergic antagonists prevent long-term maintenance of posttetanic LTP in the CA1 region of rat hippocampal slices. *Brain Res.* 522: 69–75.

Gombos, Z., Mendonca, A., Racine, R.J., Cottrell, G.A. et al. (1997). Long-term enhancement of entorhinal-dentate evoked potentials following 'modified' ECS in the rat. *Brain Res.* 766: 168–172.

Gould, E., Beylin, A., Tanapat, P., Reeves, A. et al. (1999). Learning enhances adult neurogenesis in the hippocampal formation. *Nat. Neurosci.* 2: 260–265.

Granger, R., Wiebe, S.P., Taketani, M., Lynch, G. (1996). Distinct memory circuits composing the hippocampal region. *Hippocampus* 6: 567–578.

Green, E.J., and Greenough, W.T. (1986). Altered synaptic transmission in dentate gyrus of rats reared in complex environments: Evidence from hippocampal slices maintained in vitro. *J. Neurophysiol.* 55: 739–750.

Grover, L.M., and Teyler, T.J. (1995). Different mechanisms may be required for maintenance of NMDA receptor-dependent and independent forms of long-term potentiation. *Synapse* 19: 121–133.

Grover, L.M., and Teyler, T.J. (1990). Two components of long-term potentiation induced by different patterns of afferent activation. *Nature* 347: 477–479.

Hargreaves, E.L., Peters, M., Mason-Parker, S.E., and Abraham, W.C. (1998). Double dissociation of 400 Hz and theta-burst stimulation protocols on LTP persistence in the dentate gyrus & CA1 of the rat hippocampus. *Soc. Neurosci. Abstr.* 24: 1321.

Hasselmo, M.E., Wyble, B.P., and Wallenstein, G.V. (1996). Encoding and retrieval of episodic memories: Role of cholinergic and GABAergic modulation in the hippocampus. *Hippocampus* 6: 693–708.

Hebb, D.O. (1949). *The Organization of Behavior.* New York: John Wiley & Sons.

Helme-Guizon, A., Davis, S., Israel, M., and Lesbats, B. et al. (1998). Increase in syntaxin 1B and glutamate release in mossy fibre terminals following induction of LTP in the dentate gyrus: A candidate molecular mechanism underlying transsynaptic plasticity. *Eur. J. Neurosci.* 10: 2231–2237.

Hicks, A., Davis, S., Rodger, J., and Helme-Guizon, A. et al. (1997). Synapsin I and syntaxin 1B: Key elements in the control of neurotransmitter release are regulated by neuronal activation and long-term potentiation in vivo. *Neuroscience* 79: 329–340.

Impey, S., Mark, M., Villacres, E.C., and Poser, S. et al. (1996). Induction of CRE-mediated gene expression by stimuli that generate long-lasting LTP in area CA1 of the hippocampus. *Neuron* 16: 973–982.

Impey, S., Smith, D.M., Obrietan, K., and Donahue, R. et al. (1998). Stimulation of cAMP response element (CRE)-mediated transcription during contextual learning. *Nat. Neurosci.* 1: 595–601.

Kaplan, M.S., and Hinds, J.H. (1977). Neurogenesis in the adult rat: Electron microscopic analysis of light radioautographs. *Science* 197: 1092–1094.

Kentros, C., Hargreaves, E., Hawkins, R.D., and Kandel, E.R. et al. (1998). Abolition of long-term stability of new hippocampal place cell maps by NMDA receptor blockade. *Science* 280: 2121–2126.

Kirkwood, A., and Bear, M.F. (1994). Hebbian synapses in visual cortex. *J. Neurosci.* 14: 1634–1645.

Krug, M., Müller-Welde, P., Wagner, M., and Ott, T. et al. (1985). Functional plasticity in two afferent systems of the granule cells in the rat dentate area: Frequency-related changes, long-term potentiation and heterosynaptic depression. *Brain Res.* 360: 264–272.

Larson, J., and Lynch, G. (1988). Role of N-Methyl-D-aspartate receptors in the induction of synaptic potentiation by burst stimulation patterned after the hippocampal θ-rhythm. *Brain Res.* 441: 111–118.

Leung, S.L., and Shen, B. (1995). Long-term potentiation at the apical and basal dendritic synapses of CA1 after local stimulation in behaving rats. *J. Neurophysiol.* 73: 1938–1946.

Leung, S.L., Shen, B., and Kaibara, T. (1992). Long-term potentiation induced by patterned stimulation of the commissural pathway to hippocampal CA1 region in freely moving rats. *Neuroscience* 48: 63–74.

Levy, W.B., and Steward, O. (1979). Synapses as associative memory elements in the hippocampal formation. *Brain Res.* 175: 233–246.

Linden, D.J. (1999). The return of the spike: Postsynaptic action potentials and the induction of LTP and LTD. *Neuron* 22: 661–666.

Ljungberg, T., Apicella, P., and Schultz, W. (1992). Responses of monkey dopamine neurons during learning of behavioral reactions. *J. Neurophysiol.* 67: 145–163.

Lynch, G., and Granger, R. (1992). Variations in synaptic plasticity and types of memory in corticohippocampal networks. *J. Cog. Neurosci.* 4: 189–199.

56 Wickliffe C. Abraham

Marr, D. (1971). Simple memory: A theory for archicortex. *Phil. Trans. R. Soc. London B* 262: 23–81.

Matthies, H. (1989). In search of cellular mechanisms of memory. *Prog. Neurobiol.* 32: 277–349.

Manahan-Vaughan, D., and Braunewell, K.-H. (1999). Novelty acquisition is associated with induction of hippocampal long-term depression. *Proc. Natl. Acad. Sci. USA.* 20: 8739–8744.

McNaughton, B.L., and Morris, R.G.M. (1987). Hippocampal synaptic enhancement and information storage within a distributed memory system. *Trends Neurosci.* 10: 408–415.

Milner, P. (1989). A cell assembly theory of hippocampal amnesia. *Neuropsychologia* 27: 23–30.

McClelland, J.L., and Goddard, N.H. (1996). Considerations arising from a complementary learning systems perspective on hippocampus and neocortex. *Hippocampus* 6: 654–665.

McClelland, J.L., McNaughton, B.L., and O'Reilly, R.C. (1995). Why there are complementary learning systems in the hippocampus and neocortex: Insights from the successes and failures of connectionist models of learning and memory. *Psychol. Rev.* 102: 419–457.

McHugh, T.J., Blum, K.I., Tsien, J.Z., Tonegawa, S. et al. (1996). Impaired hippocampal representation of space in CA1-specific NMDAR1 knockout mice. *Cell* 87: 1339–1349.

McNaughton, B.L., Barnes, C.A., Gerrard, J.L., Gothard, K. et al. (1996). Deciphering the hippocampal polyglot: The hippocampus as a path integration system. *J. Exp. Biol.* 199: 173–185.

McNaughton, B.L., Barnes, C.A., Meltzer, J., and Sutherland, R.J. (1989). Hippocampal granule cells are necessary for normal spatial learning but not for spatially-selective pyramidal cell discharge. *Exp. Brain Res.* 76: 485–496.

Morris, R.G.M., and Baker, M. (1984). Does long-term potentiation/synaptic enhancement have anything to do with learning or memory? In L.R., Squire and N., Butters (Eds.), *Neuropsychology of memory* (pp. 521–535). New York: Guilford Press.

Morris, R.G.M., Garrud, P., Rawlins, J.N.P., and O'Keefe, J. (1982). Place navigation impaired in rats with hippocampal lesions. *Nature* 297: 681–683.

Muller, D., Hefft, S., and Figurov, A. (1995). Heterosynaptic interactions between LTP and LTD in CA1 hippocampal slices. *Neuron* 14: 599–605.

Muller, R.U. (1996). A quarter of a century of place cells. *Neuron.* 17: 813–822.

O'Dell, T.J., and Kandel, E.R. (1994). Low-frequency stimulation erases LTP through an NMDA receptor-mediated activation of protein phosphatases. *Learn. Mem.* 1: 129–139.

O'Keefe, J., and Nadel, L. (1978). *The Hippocampus as a Cognitive Map.* Oxford: Clarendon Press.

Pavlides, C., and Winson, J. (1989). Influences of hippocampal place cell firing in the awake state on the activity of these cells during subsequent sleep episodes. *J. Neurosci.* 9: 2907–2918.

Quirk, G.J., Muller, R.U., Kubie, J.L., and Ranck, G.B. (1992). The positional firing properties of medial entorhinal neurons: Description and comparison with hippocampal place cells. *J. Neurosci.* 12: 1945–1963.

Racine, R.J., Milgram, N.W., and Hafner, S. (1983). Long-term potentiation phenomena in the rat limbic forebrain. *Brain Res.* 260: 217–231.

Racine, R.J., Chapman, C.A., Trepel, C., Teskey, G.C. et al. (1995). Post-activation potentiation in the neocortex. IV. Multiple sessions required for induction of long-term potentiation in the chronic preparation. *Brain Res.* 702: 87–93.

Reymann, K.G., Matthies, H.K., Schulzeck, K., and Matthies, H.J. (1989). N-methyl-D-aspartate receptor activation is required for the induction of both early and late phases of long-term potentiation in rat hippocampal slices. *Neurosci. Lett.* 96: 96–101.

Rolls, E.T. (1996). A theory of hippocampal function in memory. *Hippocampus* 6: 601–620.

Schultz, W., Apicella, P., Scarnati, E., and Ljungberg, T. (1992). Neuronal activity in monkey ventral striatum related to the expectation of reward. *J. Neurosci.* 12: 4595–4610.

Seidenbecher, T., Reymann, K.G., and Balschun, D. (1997). A post-tetanic time window for the reinforcement of long-term potentiation by appetitive and aversive stimuli. *Proc. Natl. Acad. Sci. USA* 94: 1449–1499.

Sharp, P.E., Barnes, C.A., and McNaughton, B.L. (1987). Effects of aging on environmental modulation of hippocampal evoked responses. *Behav. Neurosci.* 101: 170–178.

Shors, T.J., and Matzel, L.D. (1997). Long-term potentiation: What's learning got to do with it? *Behav. Brain Sci.* 20: 597–655.

Squire, L.R. (1986). Mechanisms of memory. *Science* 232: 1612–1619.

Staubli, U., and Lynch, G. (1987). Stable hippocampal long-term potentiation elicited by 'theta' pattern stimulation. *Brain Res.* 435: 227–234.

Staubli, U., and Lynch, G. (1990). Stable depression of potentiated synaptic responses in the hippocampus with 1-5 Hz stimulation. *Brain Res.* 513: 113–118.

Steward, O., White, G., Korol, D., and Levy, W.B. (1988). Cellular events underlying long-term potentiation and depression in hippocampal pathways: Temporal and spatial constraints. In P.W. Landfield and S.A. Deadwyler (Eds.), *Long-term potentiation: From biophysics to behavior* (pp. 139–166). New York: Liss.

Stewart, C., and Reid, I. (1993). Electroconvulsive stimulation and synaptic plasticity in the rat. *Brain Res.* 620: 139–141.

Stewart, C., Jeffery, K., and Reid, I. (1994). LTP-like synaptic efficacy changes following electroconvulsive stimulation. *NeuroReport* 5: 1041–1044.

Swanson-Park, J.L., Coussens, C.M., Mason-Parker, S.E., and Raymond, C.R. et al. (1999). A double dissociation within the hippocampus of dopamine D1/D5 receptor and β-adrenergic receptor contributions to the persistence of long-term potentiation. *Neuroscience* 92: 485–497.

Taubenfeld, S.M., Wiig, K.A., Bear, M.F., and Alberini, C.M. (1999). A molecular correlate of memory and amnesia in the hippocampus. *Nat. Neurosci.* 2: 309–310.

Thompson, L.T., and Best, P.J. (1990). Long-term stability of the place-field activity of single units recorded from the dorsal hippocampus of freely behaving rats. *Brain Res.* 509: 299–308.

Tokuyama, W., Hashimoto, T., Li, Y.X., Okuno, H. et al. (1998). Highest trkB mRNA expression in the entorhinal cortex among hippocampal subregions in the adult rat: Contrasting pattern with BDNF mRNA expression. *Mol. Brain. Res.* 62: 206–215.

Trepel, C., and Racine, R.J. (1998). Long-term potentiation in the neocortex of the adult, freely moving rat. *Cereb. Cortex* 8: 719–729.

Treves, A., Skagges, W.E., and Barnes, C.A. (1996). How much of the hippocampus can be explained by functional constraints? *Hippocampus* 6: 666–674.

van Praag, H., Kempermann, G., and Gage, F.H. (1999). Running increases cell proliferation and neurogenesis in the adult mouse dentate gyrus. *Nat. Neurosci.* 2: 266–270.

Walton, M., Henderson, C., Mason-Parker, S., Lawlor, P. et al. (1999). Immediate early gene transcription and synaptic modulation. *J. Neurosc. Res.* 58: 96–106.

Willshaw, D.J., and Buckingham, J.T. (1990). An assessment of Marr's theory of the hippocampus as a temporary memory store. *Phil. Trans. R. Soc. London B* 329: 205–215.

Wilson, M.A., and McNaughton, B.L. (1993). Dynamics of the hippocampal ensemble code for space. *Science* 261: 1055–1058.

Wilson, M.A., and McNaughton, B.L. (1994). Reactivation of hippocampal ensemble memories during sleep. *Science* 265: 676–679.

Xu, L., Anwyl, R., and Rowan, M.J. (1998). Spatial exploration induces a persistent reversal of long-term potentiation in rat hippocampus. *Nature* 394: 891–894.

CHAPTER TWO

Long-Term Potentiation in the Amygdala

Implications for Memory

Michael T. Rogan, Marc G. Weisskopf, Yan-You Huang, Eric R. Kandel, and Joseph E. LeDoux

SUMMARY

Since the discovery that neurons connect to each other via synapses, it has been hypothesized that experience leads to modifications in these connections, and that memory is embodied in these changes. Application of the cellular-connection approach to the study of the plasticity of defense responses to sensory cues has proved to be a particularly fruitful means of studying the relation of learning to changes in synaptic transmission – first in *Aplysia*, and, more recently, in studies of classical fear conditioning in the rodent. The discovery of artificial means of inducing neural plasticity (long-term potentiation, LTP) has added an important tool for the examination of plasticity mechanisms in specific pathways identified through the successful application of the cellular-connection approach. The demonstration that sensory pathways to the amygdala critical for fear conditioning are susceptible to LTP induction has led to examination of the mechanisms underlying LTP in the amygdala, the ability of these mechanisms to modulate sensory transmission, and their relation to the learning-induced changes in sensory-evoked neural activity that accompany fear conditioning.

Introduction

Learning refers to the acquisition of new information about the world and memory to the storage of that information over time. In his Croonian lecture to the Royal Society in 1894, Ramon y Cajal suggested that learning involves alterations in the strength of connections between neurons, and that these alterations in synaptic strength might persist and underlie memory storage. Although subsequent demonstrations that certain synapses are capable of undergoing functional modification were not uncommon (e.g., Eccles, 1964), such changes were short lasting and not clearly related to the acquisition and storage of information.

In 1968, Kandel and Spencer proposed a strategy for determining the relation between synaptic changes and learning and memory. Their cellular-connection approach involved selection of a well-defined and easily measured behavioral response that changes with experience, identification of the circuits involved in the learning, analysis of the activity of neurons in that circuit during learning, and determination of the mechanisms that mediate the learning and storage (Kandel and Spencer, 1968). Following this strategy, Kandel and colleagues achieved the first success in relating learning and memory to changes in synaptic transmission in the early 1970s. They used the gill-withdrawal reflex in the *Aplysia,* an invertebrate with a simple nervous system in which neural activity in specific circuits could be related to stimulus-evoked modifications of the behavioral reflex. Initial studies showed that habituation of the gill-withdrawal reflex, a nonassociative form of learning, involved transient alterations in the strength of synapses that processed the eliciting stimulus (Castellucci et al., 1970; Kupfermann et al., 1970; Pinsker et al., 1970). Subsequently, they found that long-term memory for habituation involved persistent changes in synaptic transmission at that very synapse (Carew and Kandel, 1973) and a *loss* of synaptic connections (Bailey and Chen, 1983). Long-term sensitization of the reflex, another simple form of nonassociative learning, was then found to require an *increase* in the number of synaptic connections (Bailey and Chen, 1983). Classical conditioning of the reflex, an associative form of learning, turned out to involve synaptic changes similar to those occurring in sensitization (Walters et al., 1979; Carew et al., 1981). In subsequent studies, the molecular mechanisms of synaptic plasticity and their relation to learning and memory were characterized in detail in *Aplysia* and in *Drosophila.* Specifically, second messenger systems, gene induction, and protein synthesis were implicated in the formation and stabilization of associative and nonassociative forms of memory (Bailey et al., 1996; Martin et al., 1997).

Kandel and his colleagues had used a top-down approach: beginning with behavior, going on to a delineation of the neural circuitry, and finally an analysis of the neural activity while the behavior was being modified. In 1973, a new bottom-up approach to studies of synaptic plasticity in the mammalian brain emerged as a result of Bliss and Lomo's discovery that brief periods of electrical stimulation of input fibers could alter the efficiency of synaptic transmission (Bliss and Lomo, 1973). This was an attractive approach because it involved the hippocampus, a region of the brain known to be involved in memory. However, unlike the studies of *Aplysia* and other invertebrates, this approach bypassed questions of how plasticity relates to behavior. So-called long-term potentiation (LTP) became the paradigm of choice for studying synaptic plasticity in the mammalian brain, and numerous studies by many different investigators led to detailed understanding of the mechanisms involved in LTP induction and maintenance (e.g., Bortolotto et al., 1999; Klintsova and Greenough, 1999; Nicoll and Malenka, 1999). Interestingly, many of the same molecular mechanisms involved in plasticity in the *Aplysia* turned out to be involved in hippocampal LTP (Squire and Kandel, 1999).

Considerable effort has gone into attempts to relate hippocampal LTP to learning and memory (Eichenbaum, 1995; Morris and Frey, 1997; Silva et al., 1998). The hippocampus is known to be involved in a variety of learning tasks, especially spatial learning in rodents, and studies of genetically altered mice have established molecular links between LTP and spatial learning (Mayford et al., 1997; Silva et al., 1998). However, the interpretation of hippocampal-dependent learning and memory processes in terms of hippocampal synaptic physiology is limited by the poor understanding of the flow of sensory information in specific synaptic circuits within the hippocampus that might be involved in spatial learning and memory. As a result it has remained somewhat unclear how LTP at specific hippocampal synapses might explain learning or memory. Also, the induction procedures for LTP do not resemble in any obvious way the learning requirements in spatial tasks: LTP involves brief interactions between pre- and postsynaptic neurons, whereas spatial learning tasks typically require prolonged training over many trials, often over several days.

An alternative approach to relating synaptic mechanisms to memory in the mammalian brain involves the use of the cellular-connection approach outlined by Kandel and Spencer to identify circuits and neural changes involved in a specific learned behavioral task. One of the most successful applications of this approach in mammals has involved classical fear conditioning in rodents. In fear conditioning, an animal receives a neutral conditioned stimulus (CS) in conjunction with an aversive unconditioned stimulus (US). After a few pairings, as few as one under the right conditions, the CS acquires the capacity to elicit defensive behavioral responses and associated autonomic and endocrine changes. As will be detailed below, studies by several laboratories have led to a fairly detailed understanding of the neural circuits that mediate fear conditioning. Further, progress has been made in identifying loci within these circuits where cellular changes take place, and in elucidating some of the mechanisms involved. Another successful application of the cellular-connection approach to the study of the relation between synaptic plasticity and memory in the mammalian brain involving eyeblink conditioning will not be described here (for a review see Thompson et al., 1997).

Classical fear conditioning has much to offer as a behavioral approach to the general problem of how synaptic changes relate to learning and memory, as well as to the specific topic of how the synaptic alterations that constitute LTP relate to learning and memory. Convergence of CS and US inputs onto common postsynaptic neurons is believed to underlie classical conditioning. As a result, the weak CS, after association with the strong US, is able to activate postsynaptic cells on its own. Fear conditioning is therefore at least superficially similar to the associative form of LTP, in which the convergence of two afferents, one weak and one strong, onto postsynaptic neurons confers on the weak input the ability to activate the postsynaptic cells (see Barrionuevo and Brown, 1983). Given that a putative set of synapses required for the fear learning have been identified and that LTP occurs in these synapses (see Maren and Fanselow, 1996; Rogan and

LeDoux, 1996; Fanselow and LeDoux, 1999; LeDoux, 2000), fear conditioning would seem to offer a unique hope for relating synaptic changes to learning and memory in mammals.

It is particularly interesting that both the initial and the more recent application of the cellular-connection approach have involved studies of circuits through which defense responses come under the control of sensory stimuli through learning. Defense responses, whether in rats or snails, meet the criteria outlined by Kandel and Spencer for cellular analyses of learning. Defense responses can be modified by experience and can be evoked by a discrete and well-controlled stimulus with a sharp onset, and the neural processing of this stimulus can be tracked anatomically and physiologically from peripheral sensory transducers to behavioral effectors. Since learning about such a stimulus involves alterations in the neural activity evoked by that stimulus, identification of the processing pathways suggests candidate synapses at which learning-related plasticity may occur. The neurophysiologic analyses of learning then follow rather directly, with analysis of the time-locked neural activity and behavior evoked by the stimulus in the course of learning.

The key anatomic structure underlying fear (defense) conditioning in rodents is the amygdala, and the synapses that have been implicated in both fear conditioning and LTP are those made by pathways transmitting an acoustic CS from auditory processing areas in the thalamus and cortex to the lateral nucleus of the amygdala (LA) (Figure 2.1). The aim of this chapter is to review the evidence that LA and its sensory input synapses are involved in fear conditioning, and to show that physiologic changes similar to those occurring in LTP take place in the amygdala *in vivo* during fear conditioning. We then describe recent *in vitro* studies of amygdala slices that have begun to analyze the mechanisms of LTP in the two sensory input pathways to LA.

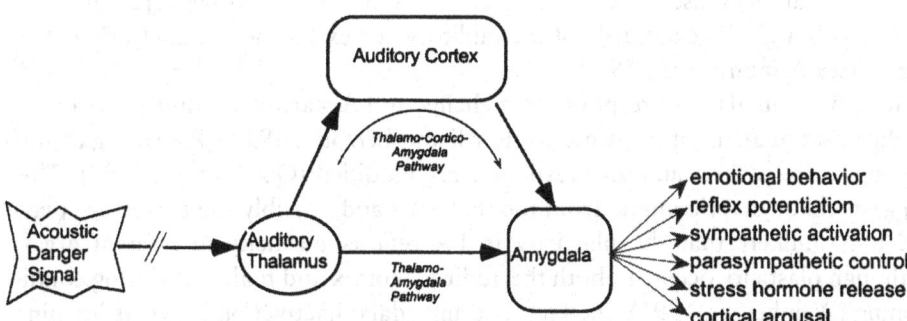

Figure 2.1. Schematic of a fear conditioning circuit. Auditory CS information is transmitted from the auditory thalamus to the lateral nucleus of the amygdala by way of two parallel pathways. The subcortical thalamo-amygdala pathway is monosynaptic, while the thalamo-cortico-amygdala pathway involves multiple synaptic connections. Through intraamygdala connections, the output of the lateral nucleus is transmitted to the central nucleus of the amygdala, which controls various effector systems involved in the expression of defense responses.

Contribution of the Lateral Amygdala to Fear Conditioning

Anatomic (LeDoux et al., 1990b; Turner and Herkenham, 1991; Amaral et al., 1992; Mascagni et al., 1993; Romanski and LeDoux, 1993; McDonald, 1998) and physiologic (Clugnet et al., 1990; Bordi and LeDoux, 1992, 1994a, 1994b; Bordi et al., 1993) studies have shown that LA is the major site within the amygdala of synaptic inputs from auditory processing areas in the thalamus and cortex. Accordingly, electrolytic and neurotoxic lesions of LA prevent the acquisition and expression of fear conditioning (LeDoux et al., 1990a; Campeau and Davis, 1995b). Further, temporary inactivation of the LA and adjacent amygdala regions during but not immediately after fear conditioning prevents learning from taking place (Willenski et al., 1998). Together, these findings suggest that processes occurring in LA or adjacent amygdala regions are sites of plasticity during fear conditioning.

Indeed, single unit recordings in freely behaving rats have shown that conditioning modifies the rate of firing of LA neurons during the CS (Quirk et al., 1995). Thus, the number of spikes elicited by the CS is greater after than before conditioning. Further, when the conditioned changes in unit activity in LA and fear behavior are evaluated on a trial by trial basis, the unit responses occur prior to or on the same trial as conditioned behavior (Repa et al., submitted). Synaptic changes involving LA neurons are therefore plausibly involved in the essential plasticity that underlies conditioned fear behavior. Recent fMRI studies in humans showing that functional activity increases in the amygdala during fear conditioning strongly suggest that the animal findings apply to the human brain (LaBar et al., 1998).

The two major sources of auditory synaptic input to LA are the auditory cortex and thalamus (e.g., Romanski and LeDoux, 1992). These two pathways are more or less interchangeable in their ability to mediate the acquisition of simple fear conditioning tasks involving a single tone that is paired with the US (Romanski and LeDoux, 1992). However, it appears that as the auditory processing demands of the task are increased, the auditory cortex comes to be involved (Jarrell et al., 1987), although the exact role of the auditory cortex has not been clearly determined (see Armony et al., 1994).

In naïve animals, unit responses are elicited in LA starting around 12 to 15 ms of the onset of an auditory stimulus (Bordi and LeDoux, 1992). Following conditioning, these earliest auditory responses are modified (Quirk et al., 1995). This suggests that synaptic inputs from the thalamus and possibly the cortex are plastic. It is unlikely that the plasticity in LA reflects plasticity in afferent areas. Although plasticity occurs in both the auditory cortex and thalamus during conditioning (Weinberger, 1995), the fact that amygdala inactivation prevents learning shows that these afferent structures alone are unable to mediate learning. Further, comparison of the latency of unit responses in auditory areas with LA is revealing. For example, while cells in the auditory cortex and LA both respond to a tone within 12 to 15 ms after onset, and conditioning modifies the earliest response in LA, the earliest response in auditory cortex is not modified (Quirk et al., 1997). Indeed, conditioned activity is not present in the auditory cortex spike train until around 30 to 40 ms after tone onset. Finally, some aspects of auditory cortex plasticity, especially late responses that anticipate the US, appear to depend on the amygdala (Armony et al., 1998).

Together, the various findings described suggest that LA is required for conditioning to take place and that physiologic changes occurring in LA contribute significantly to the acquisition of conditioned fear behavior. Further, the fact that the earliest auditory responses in LA are modified suggests that the input synapses are involved. Input synapses to LA would therefore seem to be excellent candidates for exploring the role of LTP in fear conditioning.

LTP in Sensory Pathways to the Amygdala *In Vivo:* The Relation to Fear Conditioning

In vivo studies of amygdala LTP began in 1990, with the demonstration that high-frequency electrical stimulation of the auditory thalamus led to LTP measured in the LA of the anesthetized rat (Clugnet and LeDoux, 1990). These studies, along with work done about the same time in the cortico-amygdala pathway in brain slices (Chapman et al., 1990, see below) added the amygdala to the still growing list of brain areas susceptible to LTP induction. However, the fact that auditory CS information is known to be transmitted over these pathways permitted a novel series of *in vivo* studies designed to bridge the gap between the artificial methods of LTP induction and learning-induced modification of sensory processing.

In an anesthetized rat preparation, high-frequency electrical stimulation of the thalamo-amygdala pathway led to LTP in LA, as assessed by electrical test stimulation, and a commensurate long-lasting potentiation of a field potential in LA elicited by a CS-like auditory stimulus delivered to the rat's ear (Rogan and LeDoux, 1995a). Physiologic and anatomic data indicated that these auditory evoked field potentials are generated in LA and reflect, in substantial part, the activation of thalamo-amygdala synapses. This demonstrated that natural information processing can make use of the physiologic mechanisms involved in LTP induction, and that such mechanisms are, at least, *available* for use by natural learning processes at critical synapses in LA.

The question remained – Are these mechanisms used during learning? To determine whether fear conditioning results in learning-related changes in CS processing similar to those caused by LTP induction in auditory CS pathways, Rogan et al. (1997b) used freely behaving rats to concurrently measure auditory CS-evoked field potentials and CS-evoked fear behavior for all presentations of the CS over several days: before, during, and after fear conditioning (Figure 2.2). Rats received either paired CS/US training, which leads to the acquisition of fear responses to the CS, or unpaired CS/US training, which does not result in fear of the CS. CS/US paired training led to an increase in the slope and amplitude of CS-evoked field potentials in LA, increases that are very similar to those that occur after artificial LTP induction in the CS pathway (Rogan et al., 1997b) (Figure 2.3). The changes parallel the acquisition of CS-elicited fear behavior, are enduring, and do not occur if the CS and US remain unpaired. Analyses of behavioral and electrophysiologic data discount the possible nonassociative effects of arousal or movement

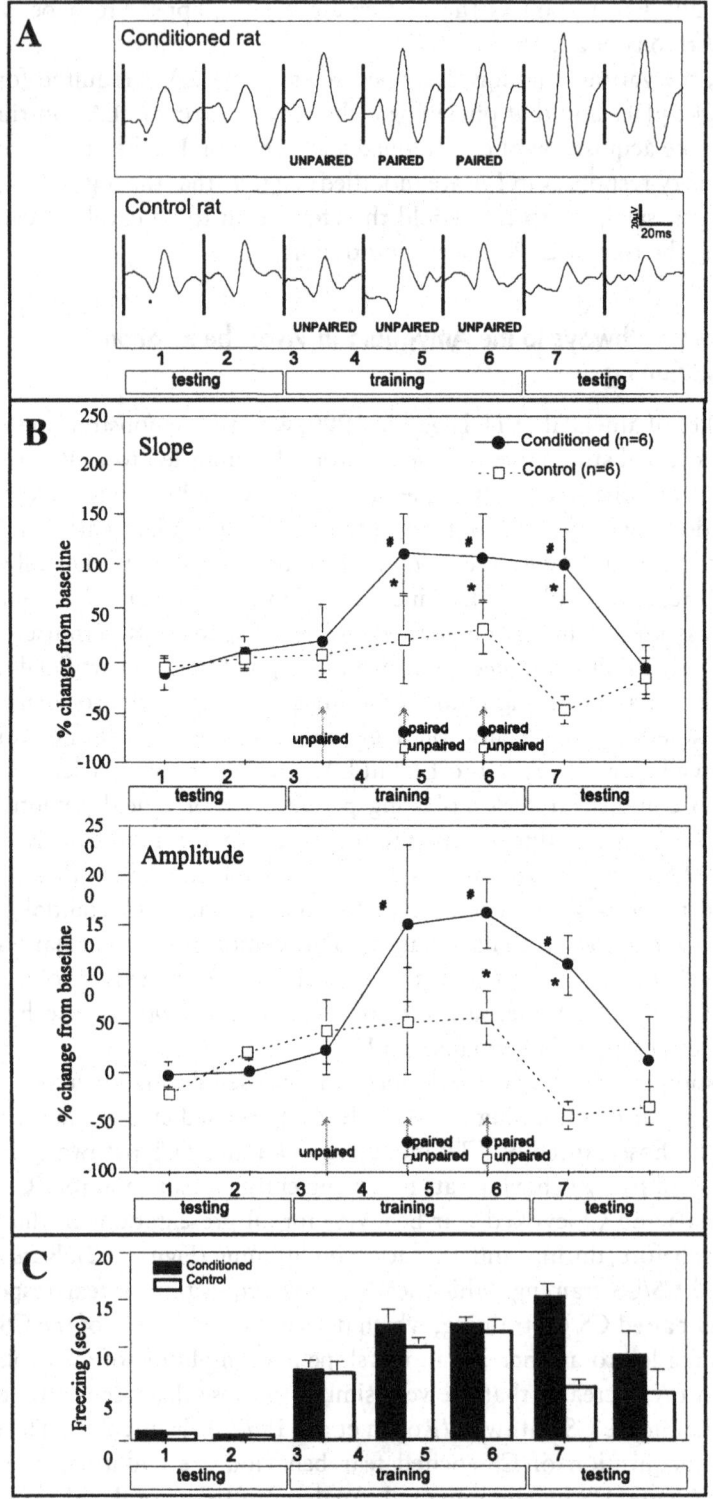

on field potential measures. These data suggest that fear conditioning results in an increase in efficacy of LA synapses involved in CS processing. It must be noted that fear conditioning is known to induce neural plasticity in the auditory cortex and auditory thalamus (Weinberger, 1995; Quirk et al., 1997); however, the latency of the plastic evoked responses measured in LA using field (Rogan and LeDoux, 1995a; Rogan et al., 1997b) and single unit responses (Quirk et al., 1995, 1997) specifically implicate thalamo-amygdala synapses in learning. This interpretation is supported by the finding that excitatory postsynaptic potentials evoked in LA by electrical stimulation of the thalamo-amygdala pathway in brain slices taken from fear-conditioned rats are enhanced compared to the same measures from rats who were not conditioned (McKernan and Shinnick-Gallagher, 1997).

Figure 2.2. The effect of paired and unpaired training on CS-evoked field potentials and on behavior. Sessions are numbered 1 to 7: One session occurred per day, except that sessions 3 and 4 occurred in one day. (**A**) CS-evoked field potentials from a Conditioned rat (**top**) and a Control (**bottom**) rat, covering the full time course of the experiment. Quantitative analysis was performed on the first negative (downward) going deflection (marked with "."). Our previous studies of these waveforms have concentrated on this feature, since it has the shortest latency, is reliably present, coincides with local evoked unit activity, shows experience-dependent plasticity, and reflects transmission from the auditory thalamus to the amygdala (Rogan and LeDoux, 1995a, 1995b). The other components of the waveform visible in these examples are not reliably present across trials and subjects, and little is known about their origin and mechanisms (Rogan and LeDoux, 1995a). (**B**) Fear conditioning increases the slope and amplitude of CS-EPs, while unpaired training does not. Slope and amplitude of the negative going potential are shown normalized as a percentage of the mean values before training (sessions 1 and 2). The normalized slope and amplitude of the evoked potentials were evaluated statistically with two-factor ANOVAs with group (Conditioned, Control) as the between-subjects factor and experimental session as within-subject factor. A significant group × session interaction was observed for both measures [slope: $F(6, 60) = 2.59, p < .05$; amplitude: $F(6, 60) = 2.70, p < .05$]. Significant differences of post hoc analyses are indicated (*Duncan, $p < .05$, between groups; # Duncan, $p < .05$, within group with respect to pretraining sessions 1 and 2). Error bars are in units of SEM. (**C**) Fear conditioning leads to associative conditioning of fear behavior. Freezing responses during the CS and pre-CS period were evaluated statistically with two-factor ANOVAs with group (Conditioned, Control) as the between-subjects factor and experimental session as within-subject factor. A significant group × session interaction was observed for CS freezing [$F(6, 60) = 5.23, p < .001$] but not for pre-CS freezing [$F(6, 60) = .42, p > .1$] (not shown). Significant difference of post hoc analysis is indicated (*Duncan, $p < .05$, between groups). Freezing in sessions in which US presentations occur (sessions 3–5) is not useful as a measure of fear conditioning, as behavior in these sessions is dominated by persistent responses to footshocks. Associative conditioning of freezing is best reflected in session 6, in which only the CS was presented. The reduction in freezing in session 7, relative to session 6, reflects extinction of the CS/US association. The small amount of freezing exhibited by the Control group after training (~5 seconds) reflects normal acquisition of freezing to the experimental context that extends into but that is not elicited by the CS (Phillips and LeDoux, 1992; Kim and Fanselow, 1992). Error bars are in units of SEM.

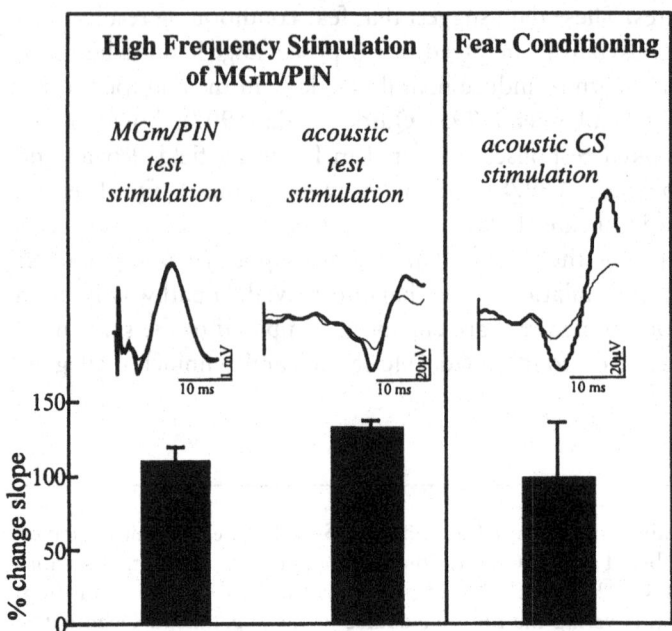

Figure 2.3. Comparison of the effect of LTP induction and fear conditioning on CS-evoked field potentials and transmission in CS pathways. **Left panel:** Two sets of data from the same animal before (thin line) and after (thick line) induction of LTP in the thalamo-amygdala CS pathway by high-frequency electrical stimulation of MGm/PIN (Rogan and LeDoux, 1995b). Both the field potentials evoked by electrical test stimulation of MGm/PI and field potentials evoked by CS-like acoustic stimuli are enhanced by this treatment. The bar graphs show the mean percentage change in slope derived from group data for each measurement (group data, $n = 7$; mean across 1 hour posttetanus period). **Right panel:** Example from an animal in the Conditioned group of a CS-evoked field potential (mean across 1 session) obtained during baseline measurement (thin line) superimposed on the potential from the same animal measured on the first test day after fear conditioning (thick line), showing a marked increase in slope and amplitude. Fear conditioning produced effects on CS-evoked activity in LA (group data, n = 6; mean percentage change in slope across first posttraining test session) similar to those produced by LTP induction in the thalamo-amygdala CS pathway by high-frequency electrical stimulation.

In Search of Mechanisms: *In Vitro* Studies of Amygdala LTP

The behavioral studies discussed above indicate that the lateral amygdala is required for fear conditioning to occur, and the single unit and field potential recordings show that some form of plasticity occurs in the lateral amygdala during fear conditioning. However, in order to achieve a more mechanistic account of the link between behavioral learning and physiologic plasticity, a detailed understanding of amygdala plasticity must be obtained. This has been pursued through *in vitro* studies of amygdala brain slices. Although various synapses have been studied *in vitro*, much of the research to date has focused on inputs to the basolateral complex of the amygdala, which includes the lateral nucleus (of interest as the recipient of sensory inputs to the amygdala and a presumed site of plasticity during fear conditioning) and the basal nucleus (of interest as the recipient of inputs from polymodal cortical areas, including the hippocampus) (e.g., Pitkanen et al., 1997).

■ **Cortico-Amygdala LTP.** Inputs from the cortex arrive in amygdala from the external capsule (EC). A number of studies have found that high-frequency stimulation of the EC leads to LTP in the basolateral complex (e.g. Chapman et al., 1990; Chapman and Bellavance, 1992; Gean et al., 1993; Huang and Kandel, 1998). A key issue in these studies has been whether LTP in this pathway depends on NMDA receptors. This is of critical interest because of the importance of NMDA receptors in the most extensively studied from of hippocampal LTP (Nicoll and Malenka, 1999) and because of the associated role of these receptors in hippocampal-dependent spatial learning (Morris and Frey, 1997; Steele and Morris, 1999). Further, the fact that behavioral studies have found that infusion of NMDA antagonists in the basolateral complex of the amygdala prevents fear conditioning from occurring (Miserendino et al., 1990; Kim et al., 1991; Gewirtz and Davis, 1997; Lee and Kim, 1998) makes analyses of the role of NMDA receptors in amygdala LTP particularly cogent.

Chapman and Bellevance found that LTP in the basolateral complex of the amygdala following EC stimulation occurred in the presence of NMDA antagonism. Although Gean found an NMDA-dependent from of LTP in the basolateral complex, these studies involved stimulation of the ventral endopyriform cortex and not the EC. Thus, this may be a distinct synapse from those in most other studies of cortico-amygdala inputs that stimulate the EC, and may not reflect the synapses that carry the most direct sensory information from cortex to amygdala.

The most thorough analysis of cortico-amygdala LTP to date was performed by Huang and Kandel (1998) (Figure 2.4). They found NMDA-dependent LTP in the lateral amygdala following stimulation of the EC. This LTP was dependent on postsynaptic calcium entry, as it could be prevented by chelating postsynaptic calcium. Moreover, they could also induce LTP by pairing lower frequency stimulation with a postsynaptic depolarizing current pulse. With this induction procedure, two forms of LTP were found, one that was NMDA-independent and the one that was NMDA-dependent. This suggests that different induction methods can lead to similar enhancements of synaptic transmission by way of NMDA receptor activation or some other means of calcium entry into the postsynaptic cell. However, although this LTP was initiated postsynaptically it was not completely expressed postsynaptically. A presynaptic contribution to LTP expression was suggested by the fact that protein kinase A (PKA) inhibitors blocked LTP, but only if applied in the bath and not in the postsynaptic cell. Consistent with the PKA activation requirement for LTP expression, Huang and Kandel also found that the adenylyl cyclase activator forskolin enhanced synaptic transmission and this occluded subsequent LTP induction by high-frequency stimulation. The necessity of both pre- and postsynaptic involvement in LTP expression indicates an aspect of associativity to this plasticity, which correlates with the associative nature of the behavioral learning. Presynaptic mechanisms also seem to be

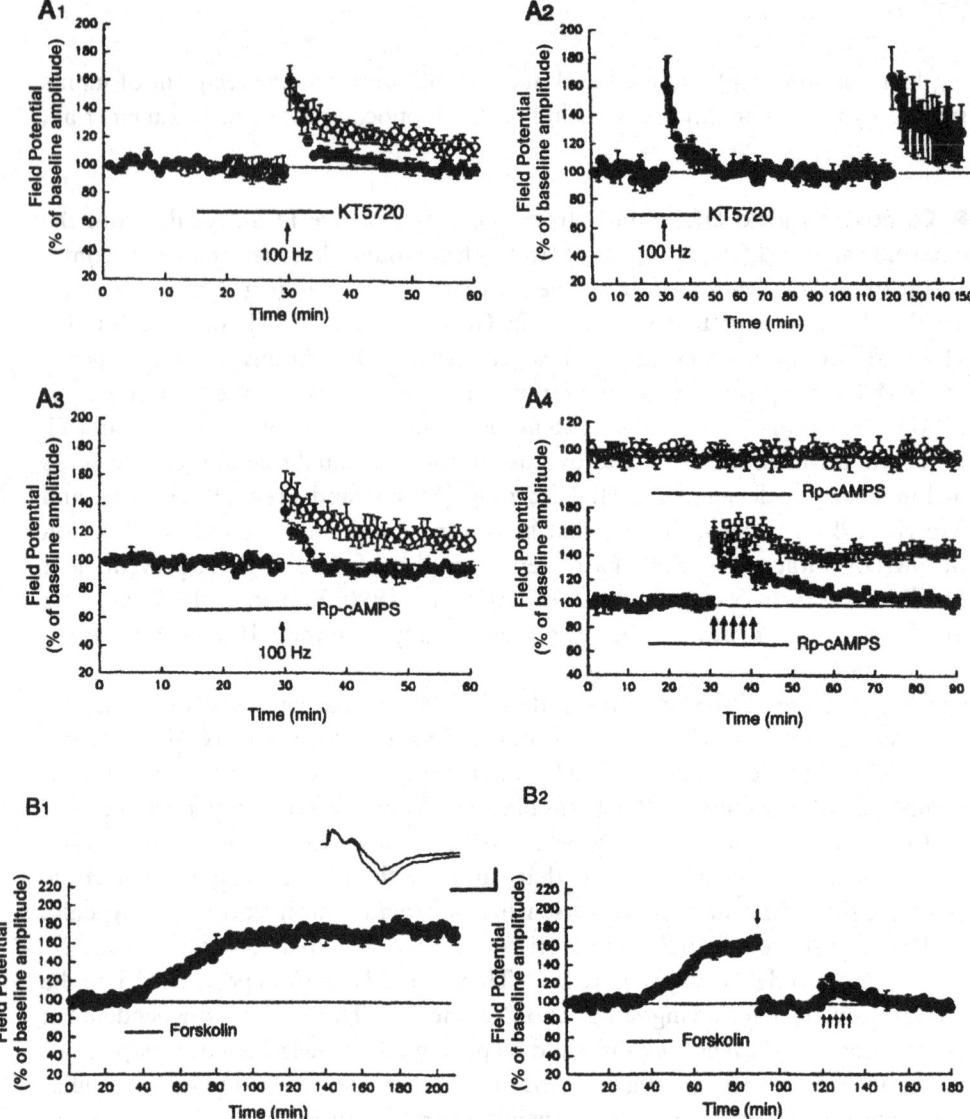

Figure 2.4. Cortico-amygdala LTP. **(A)** PKA inhibitors block LTP. **(A1)** Bath application of the PKA inhibitor KT5720 (1 μM) blocks LTP induced by a single train of tetanus (100 Hz, 1 second) (control, open circles; KT5720, $n = 7$, mean ± SEM, closed circles). **(A2)** The depression of LTP by KT5720 was reversible. LTP could be partially induced 90 minutes after washout of the drug (mean ± SEM, $n = 3$). **(A3)** Bath application of Rp-cAMPs (50 μM) blocks LTP induced by a single train of tetanus (control, $n = 9$, open circles; Rp-cAMPs, $n = 5$, mean ± SEM, closed circles). **(A4)** LTP induced by five trains of tetanus (100 Hz, 1 seconds 3 minute interval) was significantly depressed by bath application of Rp-cAMPs (50 μM) (control, $n = 5$, open squares; Rp-cAMPs, $n = 5$, mean ± SEM, closed squares). However, bath application of the PKA inhibitor Rp-cAMPs (50 μM) has no effect on the baseline field potentials (upper panel; $n = 5$). **(B)** Forskolin induces a long-lasting potentiation. **(B1)** Forskolin induces a long-lasting synaptic potentiation in lateral amygdala. Forskolin (50 μM) was perfused for 15 to 20 minutes, as indicated. Shortly after application of the drug, the field potential began to be enhanced, and this enhancement reached a stable level 60 to 90 minutes after drug application ($n = 6$, mean ± SEM). Data traces before and 90 minutes after forskolin are shown at the top of this figure. Calibration, 0.5 mV, 5 ms. **(B2)** Forskolin potentiation occludes tetanus-induced LTP. One hour after forskolin-induced potentiation, the stimulus intensity was reduced (down arrow) to match the baseline potential prior to forskolin. Five tetani (100 Hz, 1 second, 3 minute interval; up arrows) were then applied and failed to induce LTP ($n = 5$, mean ± SEM).

required for LTP expression since paired-pulse facilitation was reduced following LTP induction

■ **Thalamo-Amygdala LTP.** Fibers arriving in the lateral amygdala from the auditory thalamus enter medially from the ventral internal capsule (LeDoux et al., 1990b). Consistent with *in vivo* studies of thalamo-amygdala transmission (Li and LeDoux, 1995; Li et al., 1996) Weisskopf and LeDoux found that NMDA receptors contribute significantly to synaptic responses elicited in LA following stimulation of this medial (thalamic) pathway (Weisskopf and LeDoux, 1999) (Figure 2.5). In spite of the contribution of NMDA receptors to transmission, however, LTP could still be induced at this synapse in the presence of NMDA antagonism (Weisskopf et al., 1999). This was true regardless of whether the LTP was produced by pairing synap-

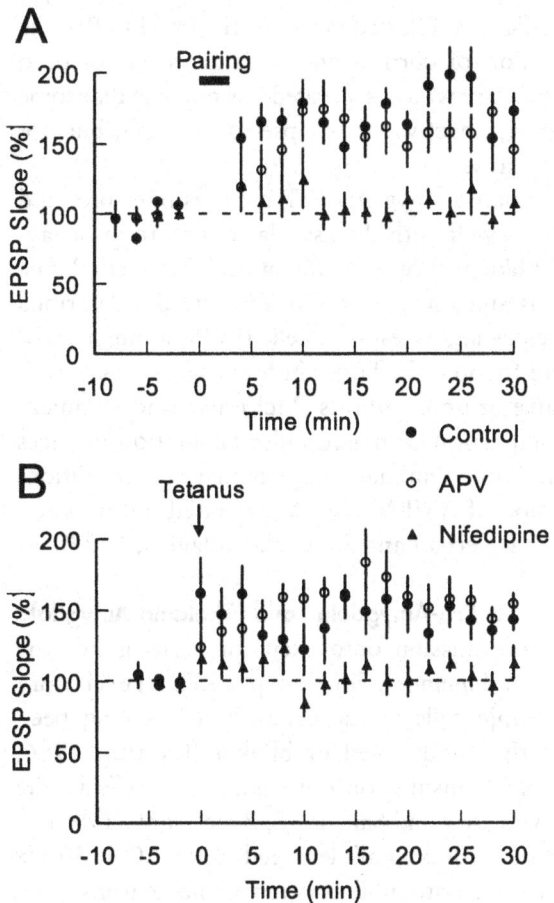

Figure 2.5. Thalamo-amygdala LTP. (A) Pairing a train of ten presynaptic stimuli delivered at 30 Hz with 1 nA, 5 ms depolarizations in the postsynaptic cell at the peak of each EPSP in the train induces LTP in control conditions (filled circles, $n = 7$), and in the presence of 50 μM D-APV (open circles, $n = 9$), but not in the presence of 30 μM nifedipine (triangles, $n = 8$). (B) Tetanization (100 Hz, 1 second, given four times at 20 second intervals), given while injecting DC current to depolarize the cell near to action potential discharge threshold (tetanus), induced LTP in control conditions (filled circles, $n = 6$), and in the presence of 50 μM D-APV (open circles, $n = 6$), but not in the presence of 30 μM nifedipine (triangles, $n = 7$).

tic input with postsynaptic action potentials or by combining high-frequency stimulation with constant postsynaptic current injection. Thalamo-amygdala LTP was dependent on postsynaptic calcium, as injection of a calcium chelator into the postsynaptic cell prevented LTP. Given that LTP could be induced in the presence of NMDA antagonists, calcium entry must have occurred through some other means, and indeed it was found that calcium entry occurred through L-type voltage gated calcium channels (VGCCs). L-type VGCCs are likely to be widely distributed over the dendritic arbors and are not dependent on synaptic activity for activation in the way NMDA receptors are, which raises questions about the synaptic specificity of such LTP. Nonetheless, when a cortical (EC stimulation) input was monitored simultaneously, LTP was found to be specific to the activated thalamic input. This suggests that some other synaptic factor may operate during induction to restrict this form of LTP to the activated synapses, perhaps a metabotropic glutamate receptor, which has been implicated in this role in some studies of LTP. However, it unclear what degree of synaptic specificity is reflected in the restriction of LTP to the stimulated pathway, as the distribution of cortical and thalamic synapses onto amygdala neurons is not known. If they are widely separated it is possible that some spread of potentiation to neighboring, unactivated synapses does occur, but not enough to be seen at a very distant synapse.

As with cortico-amygdala LTP, thalamo-amygdala LTP requires both pre- and postsynaptic activity, which correlates well with the associative nature of behavioral fear conditioning. That an LTP-like phenomenon might occur in the thalamic pathway during fear conditioning is suggested by the *in vivo* studies described above, as well as by a study in which synaptic responses elicited by stimulation of the medial (thalamic) pathway were found to be larger in brain slices taken from fear conditioned rats than from naïve or unpaired rats (McKernan and Shinnick-Gallagher, 1997). In this study, comparison of paired-pulse facilitation in slices taken from conditioned and unconditioned animals suggests that fear conditioning results in a presynaptic facilitation of AMPA receptor mediated transmission in the thalamo-amygdala pathway (McKernan and Shinnick-Gallagher, 1997).

■ **LTP at Inhibitory Synapses in Cortico-Amygdala and Thalamo-Amygdala Pathways.** Plasticity of excitatory transmission onto excitatory cells is not the only proposed substrate for learning and memory. For example, LTD of excitatory transmission onto (inhibitory) Purkinje cells in the cerebellum has long been known and proposed to underlie the conditioned eyeblink reflex (Ito, 1986; Thompson, 1988). LTP of excitatory transmission onto inhibitory cells in the amygdala also has been observed (Mahanty and Sah, 1998; Bauer et al., 1999).

Mahanty and Sah (1998) found that 100 stimuli delivered to the EC at 30 Hz led to calcium-dependent LTP at synapses onto inhibitory amygdala neurons, even though NMDA receptors were not present at these synapses. However, they showed that the AMPA receptors present at these synapses have a rectifying current-voltage relation and are inhibited by spermine, indicating that they are permeable to calcium. Therefore, this LTP is distinct from that discussed above not only in the type of synapse at which it occurs but also in terms of the induction mechanism, as neither cortical nor thalamic inputs onto excitatory amygdala neurons have calcium-permeable AMPA receptors (Mahanty and Sah, 1998; Weisskopf and LeDoux, 1999). Using the same procedures, Bauer et al. (1999) found evidence for an identical form of inhibitory LTP in the thalamo-amygdala pathway. Inhibitory LTP has also been found in *in vivo* studies. Li et al. (1998) recorded intracellularly from LA cells before and after tetanization of the auditory thalamus. The main change consistently observed was a facilitation of inhibitory postsynaptic potentials (IPSPs).

Although behavioral fear conditioning is believed to be mediated by increases in excitatory transmission, as discussed in the earlier sections, inhibitory LTP could play an important role in regulating the extent of excitatory LTP during conditioning. This could help tune the specificity of learning, and also might provide a means of eliminating plasticity at redundant or irrelevant synapses.

■ **Molecular Mechanisms of LTP in the Thalamo-Amygdala and Cortico-Amygdala Pathways.** One feature characteristic of conditioned fear is its persistence. Learning-induced changes in CS-evoked field potentials measured by Rogan and colleagues persisted over several days, returning to baseline levels with extinction training. Huang, Martin, and Kandel (submitted) have examined in brain slices the persistence of amygdala LTP and its dependence on gene expression and the synthesis of new protein. In both cortico-amygdala and thalamo-amygdala pathways they found that a single high-frequency train of stimuli induced a transient LTP (E-LTP), whereas five repeated high-frequency train stimuli induced a late phase of LTP (L-LTP), which is dependent on gene expression and on new protein synthesis. The late phase of LTP is mediated by PKA and mitagen-activated protein kinase (MAPK) in both pathways. The application of adenylyl cyclase activator forskolin induced an L-LTP in both pathways and this potentiation is blocked by inhibitors of protein synthesis and by inhibitors of MAPK. Immunocytochemistry studies show that both the repeated tetanization and the application of forskolin stimulate phosphorylation of cAMP-responsive element binding protein (CREB) in amygdala. The late phase of LTP is also importantly modulated by beta-adrenergic agonists and an application of a beta-adrenergic agonist induces L-LTP. Inhibitors of beta-adrenergic receptor blocked L-LTP. This agonist-induced L-LTP also is blocked both by inhibitors of PKA, MAPK, and mRNA synthesis. These results suggest that PKA and MAPK can modulate the expression of a persistent phase of LTP in the amygdala and that this late component requires the phosphorylation of CREB and the synthesis of new protein and mRNA. These findings from brain slices are completely consistent with the results of studies of fear conditioning in living animals. Thus, injection of inhibitors of MAPK, PKA, and of protein synthesis either in the lateral ventricles (Abel et al., 1997; Schafe et al., 1999) or directly into the amygdala (Nadel et al., 1999) blocks fear conditioning. Further, upregulation of CREB in the amygdala enhances fear conditioning (Josselyn et al., submitted). Behavioral and mechanistic studies are thus beginning to show remarkable convergence.

■ **LTP at Intrinsic Amygdala Synapses.** Pathways transmitting information between amygdala nuclei are likely to play an important role in the behavioral learning functions of the amygdala (see Pitkanen et al., 1997; LeDoux, 2000). Relatively little is known at present about the mechanisms of synaptic transmission or plasticity in these pathways. Studies by Pare and colleagues have found that communication between LA and the central nucleus mainly involves GABAergic inhibitory transmission (Smith and Pare, 1994). Studying LTP in the excitatory pathway from LA to the basal nucleus, Brambilla et al. (1997) found that high-frequency stimulation induced LTP in slices from control mice, but LTP did not occur in slices from mutant mice that lacked the neuronal specific guanine nucleotide exchange factor Ras-GRF. Thus, at this synapse, the G-protein signaling and the MAP kinase cascade were implicated in LTP (Brambilla et al., 1997). Obviously, much remains to be done in these and other intraamygdala pathways.

Conclusion

Research on the amygdala and its contribution to fear learning has paved the way for cellular and molecular analyses of the underlying synaptic mechanisms. In contrast to hippocampal LTP, which can be thought of as a well-characterized mechanism in search of a relation to behavior, studies of the amygdala have applied the techniques of LTP research to ask question about how synaptic plasticity is mediated in a behaviorally relevant set of circuits. Although much remains to be done before the circuits of fear conditioning are fully understood (see Cahill et al., 1999; Fanselow and LeDoux, 1999) and before synaptic plasticity in those circuits can explain the learning and memory functions that the circuits make possible, the rapid progress to date highlights the promise of this approach.

REFERENCES

Abel, T., Nguyen, P.V., Barad, M., Deuel, T.A. et al. (1997). Genetic demonstration of a role for PKA in the late phase of LTP and in hippocampus-based long-term memory. *Cell* 88: 615–626.

Amaral, D.G., Price, J.L., Pitkanen, A., and Carmichael, S.T. (1992). Anatomical organization of the primate amygdaloid complex. In J.P. Aggleton (Ed.), *The amygdala: Neurobiological aspects of emotion, memory, and mental dysfunction* (pp. 1–66). New York: Wiley-Liss.

Armony, J.L., Servan-Schreiber, D., and LeDoux, J.E. (1994). Effects of cortical lesions on generalization of learned fear responses. *Soc. Neurosci. Abstr.* 20, 1007.

Armony, J.L., Quirk, G.J., and LeDoux, J.E. (1998). Differential effects of amygdala lesions on early and late plastic components of auditory cortex spike trains during fear conditioning. *J. Neurosci.* 18: 2592–2601.

Bailey, C.H., and Chen, M. (1983). Morphological basis of long-term habituation and sensitization in Aplysia. *Science* 220: 91–93.

Bailey, C.H., Bartsch, D., and Kandel, E.R. (1996). Toward a molecular definition of long-term memory storage. *Proc. Natl. Acad. Sci. USA* 93: 13445–13452.

Barrionuevo, G., and Brown, T.H. (1983). Associative long-term potentiation in hippocampal slices. *Proc. Natl. Acad. Sci. USA* 80: 7347–7351.

Bauer, E.P., Weisskopf, M.G., and LeDoux, J.E. (1999). Excitatory and inhibitory LTP at thalamic input synapses to the lateral amygdala. *Soc. Neurosci. Abstr.* 25: 879.

Bliss, T.V.P., and Lømo, T. (1973). Long-lasting potentiation of synaptic transmission in the dentate area of the anaesthetized rabbit following stimulation of the perforant path. *J. Physiol.* 232: 331–356.

Bordi, F., and LeDoux, J. (1992). Sensory tuning beyond the sensory system: An initial analysis of auditory properties of neurons in the lateral amygdaloid nucleus and overlying areas of the striatum. *J. Neurosci.* 12: 2493–2503.

Bordi, F., and LeDoux, J.E. (1994a). Response properties of single units in areas of rat auditory thalamus that project to the amygdala. I. Acoustic discharge patterns and frequency receptive fields. *Exp. Brain Res.* 98: 261–274.

Bordi, F., and LeDoux, J.E. (1994b). Response properties of single units in areas of rat auditory thalamus that project to the amygdala. II. Cells receiving convergent auditory and somatosensory inputs and cells antidromically activated by amygdala stimulation. *Exp. Brain Res.* 98: 275–286.

Bordi, F., Clugnet, M.C., Pavlides, C., and LeDoux, J.E. (1993). Single unit activity in the lateral nucleus of the amygdala and overlying areas of the striatum in freely-behaving rats: Rates, discharge patterns, and responses to acoustic stimuli. *Behav. Neurosci.* 107: 757–769.

Bortolotto, Z.A., Fitzjohn, S.M., and Collingridge, G.L. (1999). Roles of metabotropic glutamate receptors in LTP and LTD in the hippocampus. *Curr. Opin. Neurobiol.* 9: 299–304.

Brambilla, R., Gnesutta, N., Minichiello, L., White, G. et al. (1997). A role for the Ras signalling pathway in synaptic transmission and long-term memory. *Nature* 390: 281–286.

Campeau, S., and Davis, M. (1995). Involvement of subcortical and cortical afferents to the lateral nucleus of the amygdala in fear conditioning measured with fear-potentiated startle in rats trained concurrently with auditory and visual conditioned stimuli. *J. Neurosci.* 15: 2312–2327.

Carew, T.J., and Kandel, E.R. (1973). Acquisition and retention of long-term habituation in Aplysia: Correlation of behavioral and cellular processes. *Science* 182: 1158–1160.

Carew, T.J., Walters, E.T., and Kandel, E.R. (1981). Associative learning in Aplysia: Cellular correlates supporting a conditioned fear hypothesis. *Science* 211: 501–504.

Castellucci, V., Pinsker, H., Kupfermann, I., and Kandel, E.R. (1970). Neuronal mechanisms of habituation and dishabituation of the gill-withdrawal reflex in Aplysia. *Science* 167: 1745–1748.

Chapman, P.F., and Bellavance, L.L. (1992). NMDA receptor-independent LTP in the amygdala. *Synapse* 11: 310–318.

Chapman, P.F., Kairiss, E.W., Keenan, C.L., and Brown, T.H. (1990). Long-term synaptic potentiation in the amygdala. *Synapse* 6: 271–278.

Clugnet, M.C., and LeDoux, J.E. (1990). Synaptic plasticity in fear conditioning circuits: Induction of LTP in the lateral nucleus of the amygdala by stimulation of the medial geniculate body. *J. Neurosci.* 10: 2818–2824.

Clugnet, M.C., LeDoux, J.E., and Morrison, S.F. (1990). Unit responses evoked in the amygdala and striatum by electrical stimulation of the medial geniculate body. *J. Neurosci.* 10: 1055–1061.

Eccles, J.C. (1964). Structural features of chemically transmitting synapses. In J. Eccles (Ed), *The physiology of synapses*, pp. 11–26. Berlin: Springer.

Eichenbaum, H. (1995). The LTP-memory connection. *Nature* 378: 131–132.

Fanselow, M.S., and LeDoux, J.E. (1999). Why we think plasticity underlying Pavlovian fear conditioning occurs in the basolateral amygdala. *Neuron* 23: 229–232.

Gean, P.-W., Chang, F.-C., Huang, C.-C., Lin, J.-H. et al. (1993). Long-term enhancement of EPSP and NMDA receptor-mediated synaptic transmission in the amygdala. *Brain Res. Bull.* 31: 7–11.

Gewirtz, J.C., and Davis, M. (1997). Second-order fear conditioning prevented by blocking NMDA receptors in amygdala. *Nature* 388: 471–473.

Huang, Y.Y., and Kandel, E.R. (1998). Postsynaptic induction and PKA-dependent expression of LTP in the lateral amygdala. *Neuron* 21: 169–178.

Ito, M. (1986). Long-term depression as a memory process in the cerebellum. *Neurosci. Res.* 3: 531–539.

Jarrell, T.W., Gentile, C.G., Romanski, L.M., McCabe, P.M. et al. (1987). Involvement of cortical and thalamic auditory regions in retention of differential bradycardia conditioning to acoustic conditioned stimuli in rabbits. *Brain Res.* 412: 285–294.

Josselyn, S.A., Carlezon Jr., W.A., Shi, C.-J., Neve, R.L. et al. (submitted). Long-term memory is facilitated by CREB overexpression in the amygdala.

Kandel, E.R., and Spencer, W.A. (1968). Cellular neurophysiological approaches to the study of learning. *Physiol. Rev.* 48: 65–134.

Kim, J.J., DeCola, J.P., Landeira-Fernandez, J., and Fanselow, M.S. (1991). N-methy-D-aspartate receptor antagonist APV blocks acquisition but not expression of fear conditioning. *Behav. Neurosci.* 105: 126–133.

Kim, J.J., and Fanselow, M.S. (1992). Modality-specific retrograde amnesia of fear. *Science* 256: 675–677.

Klintsova, A.Y., and Greenough, W.T. (1999). Synaptic plasticity in cortical systems. *Curr. Opin. Neurobiol.* 9: 203–208.

Kupfermann, I., Castellucci, V., Pinsker, H., and Kandel, E. (1970). Neuronal correlates of habituation and dishabituation of the gill-withdrawal reflex in Aplysia. *Science* 167: 1743–1745.

LaBar, K.S., Gatenby, J.C., Gore, J.C., LeDoux, J.E. et al. (1998). Human amygdala activation during conditioned fear acquisition and extinction: A mixed-trial fMRI study. *Neuron* 20: 937–945.

LeDoux, J.E. (2000). Emotion circuits in the brain. *Annu. Rev. Neurosci.* 23: 155–184.

LeDoux, J.E., Cicchetti, P., Xagoraris, A., and Romanski, L.M. (1990a). The lateral amygdaloid nucleus: Sensory interface of the amygdala in fear conditioning. *J. Neurosci.* 10: 1062–1069.

LeDoux, J.E., Farb, C.F., and Ruggiero, D.A. (1990b). Topographic organization of neurons in the acoustic thalamus that project to the amygdala. *J. Neurosci.* 10: 1043–1054.

Lee, H., and Kim, J.J. (1998). Amygdalar NMDA receptors are critical for new fear learning in previously fear-conditioned rats. *J. Neurosci.* 18: 8444–8454.

Li, X., and LeDoux, J.E. (1995). GABA receptors regulate synaptic transmission in the auditory thalamo-amygdala pathway: An *in vivo* microiontophoretic study. *Soc. Neurosci. Abstr.* 21.

Li, X.F., Stutzmann, G.E., and LeDoux, J.L. (1996). Convergent but temporally separated inputs to lateral amygdala neurons from the auditory thalamus and auditory cortex use different postsynaptic receptors: In vivo intracellular and extracellular recordings in fear conditioning pathways. *Learn. Mem.* 3: 229–242.

Mahanty, N.K., and Sah, P. (1998). Calcium-permeable AMPA receptors mediate long-term potentiation in interneurons in the amygdala. *Nature* 394: 683–687.

Maren, S., and Fanselow, M.S. (1996). The amygdala and fear conditioning: Has the nut been cracked? *Neuron* 16: 237–240.

Martin, K.C., Casadio, A., Zhu, H.E.Y., Rose, J.C. et al. (1997). Synapse-specific, long-term facilitation of aplysia sensory to motor synapses: A function for local protein synthesis in memory storage. *Cell* 91: 927–938.

Mascagni, F., McDonald, A.J., and Coleman, J.R. (1993). Corticoamygdaloid and cortico-cortical projections of the rat temporal cortex: A phaseolus vulgaris leucoagglutinin study. *Neuroscience* 57: 697–715.

Mayford, M., Mansuy, I.M., Muller, R.U., and Kandel, E.R. (1997). Memory and behavior: A second generation of genetically modified mice. *Curr. Biol.* 7: R580–589.

McDonald, A.J. (1998). Cortical pathways to the mammalian amygdala. *Progr. Neurobiol.* 55: 257–332.

McKernan, M.G., and Shinnick-Gallagher, P. (1997). Fear conditioning induces a lasting potentiation of synaptic currents in vitro [see comments]. *Nature* 390: 607–611.

Miserendino, M.J.D., Sananes, C.B., Melia, K.R., and Davis, M. (1990). Blocking of acquisition but not expression of conditioned fear-potentiated startle by NMDA antagonists in the amygdala. *Nature* 345: 716–718.

Morris, R.G., and Frey, U. (1997). Hippocampal synaptic plasticity: Role in spatial learning or the automatic recording of attended experience? *Philos. Trans. R. Soc. London B Biol. Sci.* 352: 1489–1503.

Nadel, N.V., Schafe, G.E., Haris, A., Sullivan, G.M. et al. (1999). Immediate posttraining infusion of inhibitors of protein synthesis and PKA activity in the lateral and basal amygdala, but not the hippocampus, interferes with memory consolidation for contextual and auditory fear conditioning. *Soc. Neurosci. Abstr.* 647, 10.

Nicoll, R.A., and Malenka, R.C. (1999). Expression mechanisms underlying NMDA receptor-dependent long-term potentiation. *Ann. N. Y. Acad. Sci.* 868: 515–525.

Phillips, R.G., and LeDoux, J.E. (1992). Differential contribution of amygdala and hippocampus to cued and contextual fear conditioning. *Behav. Neurosci.* 106: 274–285.

Pinsker, H., Kupfermann, I., Castellucci, V., and Kandel, E. (1970). Habituation and dishabituation of the gill-withdrawal reflex in Aplysia. *Science* 167: 1740–1742.

Pitkanen, A., Savander, V., and LeDoux, J.L. (1997). Organization of intra-amygdaloid circuitries: An emerging framework for understanding functions of the amygdala. *Trends Neurosci.* 20: 517–523.

Quirk, G.J., Repa, J.C., and LeDoux, J.E. (1995). Fear conditioning enhances short-latency auditory responses of lateral amygdala neurons: Parallel recordings in the freely behaving rat. *Neuron* 15: 1029–1039.

Quirk, G.J., Armony, J.L., and LeDoux, J.E. (1997). Fear conditioning enhances different temporal components of toned-evoked spike trains in auditory cortex and lateral amygdala. *Neuron* 19: 613–624.

Rogan, M.T., and LeDoux, J.E. (1995a). LTP is accompanied by commensurate enhancement of auditory-evoked responses in a fear conditioning circuit. *Neuron* 15: 127–136.

Rogan, M.T., and LeDoux, J.E. (1995b). Intra-amygdala infusion of APV blocks both auditory evoked potentials in the lateral amygdala and thalamo-amygdala transmission, but spares cortico-amygdala transmission. *Soc. Neurosci. Abstr.* 21: 1930.

Rogan, M.T., and LeDoux, J.E. (1996). Emotion: Systems, cells, synaptic plasticity. *Cell* 85: 469–475.

Rogan, M.T., Staubli, U.V., and LeDoux, J.E. (1997a). AMPA receptor facilitation accelerates fear learning without altering the level of conditioned fear acquired. *J. Neurosci.* 17: 5928–5935.

Rogan, M.T., Stäubli, U.V., and LeDoux, J.E. (1997b). Fear conditioning induces associative long-term potentiation in the amygdala. *Nature* 390: 604–607.

Romanski, L.M., and LeDoux, J.E. (1992). Equipotentiality of thalamo-amygdala and thalamo-cortico-amygdala projections as auditory conditioned sitmulus pathways. *J. Neurosci.* 12: 4501–4509.

Romanski, L.M., and LeDoux, J.E. (1993). Organization of rodent auditory cortex: Anterograde transport of PHA-L from MGv to temporal neocortex. *Cereb. Cortex* 3: 499–514.

Schafe, G.E., Nadel, N.V., Sullivan, G.M., Harris, A. et al. (1999). Memory consolidation for contextual and auditory fear conditioning is dependent on protein synthesis, PKA, and MAP kinase. *Learn. Mem.* 6: 97–110.

Silva, A.J., Giese, K.P., Fedorov, N.B., Frankland, P.W. et al. (1998). Molecular, cellular, and neuroanatomical substrates of place learning. *Neurobiol. Learn. Mem.* 70: 44–61.

Smith, Y., and Pare, D. (1994). Intra-amygdaloid projections of the lateral nucleus in the cat: PHA-L anterograde labeling combined with postembedding GABA and glutamate immunocytochemistry. *J. Comp. Neurol.* 342: 232–248.

Squire, L., and Kandel, E.R. (1999). *Memory: From Mind to Molecules*. New York: Scientific American Books.

Steele, R.J., and Morris, R.G. (1999). Delay-dependent impairment of a matching-to-place task with chronic and intrahippocampal infusion of the NMDA-antagonist D-AP5 [see comments]. *Hippocampus* 9: 118–136.

Thompson, R.F. (1988). The neural basis of basic associative learning of discrete behavioral responses. *Trends Neurosci.* 11: 152–155.

Thompson, R.F., Bao, S., Chen, L., Cipriano, B.D. et al. (1997). Associative learning. *Int. Rev. Neurobiol.* 41: 151–189.

Turner, B., and Herkenham, M. (1991). Thalamoamygdaloid projections in the rat: A test of the amygdala's role in sensory processing. *J. Comp. Neurol.* 313: 295–325.

Walters, E.T., Carew, T.J., and Kandel, E.R. (1979). Classical conditioning in Aplysia californica. *Proc. Natl. Acad. Sci. USA* 76: 6675–6679.

Weinberger, N.M. (1995). Retuning the brain by fear conditioning. In M.S. Gazzaniga (Ed.), *The cognitive neurosciences* (pp. 1071–1090). Cambridge, MA: MIT Press.

Weisskopf, M.G., and LeDoux, J.E. (1999). Distinct populations of NMDA receptors at subcortical and cortical inputs to principal cells of the lateral amygdala. *J. Neurophysiol.* 81: 930–934.

Weisskopf, M., Baner, E., and LeDoux, J.E. (1999). L-type voltage-gated calcium channels mediate NMDA-independent associative LTP at thalamic input synapses to the amygdala. *J. Neurosci.* 19: 10512–10519.

Willenski, A., Schafe, G.E., and LeDoux, J.E. (1998). Immediate post-training infusion of muscimol into the amygdala does not interfere with fear conditioning. *Soc. Neurosci. Abstr.* 24.

CHAPTER THREE

Multiple Roles for Synaptic Plasticity in Pavlovian Fear Conditioning

Stephen Maren

SUMMARY

Long-term potentiation (LTP) is a form of synaptic plasticity that has been proposed to mediate certain forms of learning and memory. In this chapter, it is argued that LTP in the hippocampus and amygdala plays a crucial role in the acquisition of a simple form of emotional learning and memory: Pavlovian fear conditioning. The distinct roles for hippocampal and amygdaloid LTP and the roles for short-term synaptic plasticity mechanisms in the acquisition of learned fear responses are discussed.

Introduction

I would have you imagine, then, that there exists in the mind of man a block of wax, which is of different sizes in different men; harder, moister, and having more or less purity in one than another, and in some an intermediate quality. Let us say that this tablet is a gift of Memory, the mother of the Muses, and that when we wish to remember anything which we have seen, or heard, or thought in our own minds, we hold the wax to the perceptions and thoughts, and in that material receive the impression of them as from the seal of a ring; but when the image is effaced, or cannot be taken, then we forget and do not know.

Plato, ca. 400 B.C.

Throughout history, humans have been fascinated by the nature of memory, the permanent storehouse of the mind's experience. The foregoing passage excerpted from Plato's *Theaetetus* (ca. 400 B.C.) represents an early attempt to describe the process of memory formation in the human brain. In this passage,

This work was supported by a grant from the National Institute of Mental Health (R29MH57865) and the University of Michigan.

Plato envisions that memories are established in the brain when perceptions or thoughts render lasting impressions in the mnemonic wax of the mind. He implies that memories, once impressed in this way, are permanent, unless their trace in the mental "wax" is erased. Despite the figurative nature of Plato's "wax tablet hypothesis," the notion of a pliable or plastic substrate for memory storage continues to be a central tenet of nearly all current neurobiological models of memory formation. Although our comparatively enlightened understanding of brain function has taken the analysis of the neurobiological mechanisms of learning and memory to a molecular level, the question remains: What is the nature of the "waxy" neural substrate for memory and how does it retain a mnemonic "impression"?

Since the beginning of the twentieth century, there has been a general consensus among psychologists, neurobiologists, and even philosophers that memories are represented in the brain as enduring changes in the brain's neuronal circuitry – the "wiring" that interconnects individual nerve cells. In the last 25 years, this view has been extensively elaborated. Indeed, it is now generally believed that synapses, which are the sites for chemical communication between interconnected neurons, are the pliable substrate for memory traces to make their impression.

The involvement of synapses in memory formation has received considerable empirical support from the discovery of a long-lasting change in synaptic function in the mammalian brain. In the early 1970s, a pair of articles was published that described a long-lasting enhancement of synaptic transmission following high-frequency stimulation of excitatory synapses in the brain (Bliss and Gardner-Medwin, 1973; Bliss and Lømo, 1973). This form of synaptic plasticity was discovered in the hippocampus, a seahorse-shaped structure known to be crucial for memory in humans (e.g., Squire and Zola-Morgan, 1991). Bliss, Lømo, and Gardner-Medwin termed the phenomenon long-lasting or long-term potentiation (LTP), because it was considerably more enduring than any previously described form of synaptic enhancement, which typically lasted only minutes. Although it was not evident at the time, the discovery of LTP heralded a new era for the study of the neural mechanisms of learning and memory.

In the years after the discovery of hippocampal LTP, a massive research effort has revealed that it exhibits many properties typical of memory and occurs in brain structures known to be important for learning and memory (Bliss and Collingridge, 1993; Maren and Baudry, 1995). For these and other reasons, there has been great interest in the possibility that LTP serves as a cellular mechanism for learning and memory. Indeed, LTP has served as the primary experimental model for learning and memory in the mammalian brain in the last decade. However, questions have recently been raised concerning the utility of using LTP as an experimental model for the neurobiology of learning and memory (Diamond and Rose, 1994; Shors and Matzel, 1997). For example, the involvement of hippocampal LTP in rodent spatial learning, which has been the preferred behavioral paradigm for examining the LTP-learning connection, has come into question (e.g., Cain, 1997). This confusion may be due, at least in part, to the complicated and multiply determined nature of spatial learning tasks.

To circumvent this problem, a number of laboratories are now exploring the role for LTP in less complicated associative learning paradigms in which the experimenter has exquisite control over the behavioral contingencies. One paradigm that is becoming increasingly popular in this regard is Pavlovian fear conditioning, a robust and rapidly acquired form of emotional learning and memory that is exhibited by mammals throughout the animal kingdom (e.g., Fanselow, 1984). The neurobiological analysis of Pavlovian fear conditioning has revealed exciting insight into the involvement of LTP in learning and memory (Davis et al., 1994; Maren, 1999a; Maren and Fanselow, 1996; Rogan and LeDoux, 1996). This is particularly true insofar as the analysis of LTP has moved beyond the hippocampus into the amygdala, an almond-shaped temporal lobe structure that is crucial for fear conditioning (Davis, 1992; Fanselow, 1994; Maren, 1996; LeDoux, 1998). The aim of this chapter is to describe the considerable progress that has been made in elucidating the roles for hippocampal and amygdaloid LTP in Pavlovian fear conditioning. It will be argued that LTP in the hippocampus and amygdala play complementary, but distinct, roles in mediating different aspects of Pavlovian fear conditioning.

Pavlovian Fear Conditioning in Rodents: A Model System for Exploring the LTP-Learning Connection

After the discovery of LTP in the hippocampus and the realization that it exhibits properties that are expected of a cellular learning mechanism, considerable interest emerged in the role hippocampal LTP might play in behavioral learning and memory. It is not surprising then that the earliest empirical approaches to this issue sought to determine whether forms of learning that were known to require the hippocampus, such as spatial learning in the Morris water maze, also required hippocampal LTP (Morris et al., 1986). As a result of this work, a substantial body of evidence has emerged that implicates hippocampal LTP in spatial learning (Morris et al., 1990; Elgersma and Silva, 1999). However, there are a number of recent studies that have cast doubt on an essential role for LTP in spatial learning (Bannerman et al., 1995; Saucier and Cain, 1995; Cain, 1997). For example, there are several recent reports that genetic mutants that exhibit impaired hippocampal LTP do not exhibit deficits in spatial learning and memory (Meiri et al., 1998; Zamanillo et al., 1999; see also the Introduction of this book). These disparate results may be due to a number of factors, not the least of which is the fact that successful performance in spatial learning tasks involves acquiring several types of information, only some of which involve the hippocampal system.

As an alternative to spatial learning tasks, a number of laboratories have begun to examine the LTP-learning connection in well-characterized and simple associative learning paradigms. The prototypical task of this sort is a Pavlovian (or classical) fear conditioning task, in which rats or mice learn that certain innocuous stimuli (conditional stimuli or CSs), such as tones, lights, or places, are predictive of aversive events (unconditional stimuli or USs), such as electric footshocks. When reexposed to the CSs that were associated with the aversive event, animals exhibit learned or conditional fear responses (CRs), such as freezing (immobility except movement associated with breathing), enhanced acoustic startle, increased heart rate and blood pressure, pupillary dilatation, and defecation. This type of learning is not unique to rodents, but has been described in animals ranging from sea slugs to humans. The ubiquity of fear conditioning is not surprising. It allows animals to encode and remember experiences that are a threat to their survival, and as a result, to engage defensive systems when stimuli predictive of these aversive events are reencountered (Fanselow, 1984).

Pavlovian fear conditioning is an outstanding model system for the study of the neurobiological substrates of learning and memory for a number of reasons. First, the psychological processes underlying Pavlovian fear conditioning have been well characterized. Indeed, it is from this behavioral task that much of the behavioral data forming the core of modern associative learning theory have emerged. Second, Pavlovian fear conditioning is rapidly acquired (with as little training as a single trial) and extremely long-lasting. This makes it an ideal task for studying time-dependent memory processes, such as consolidation. Moreover, because the fear conditioning procedure takes little time to administer, experimental variance can be greatly reduced by running large numbers of animals in parallel. Third, the neural circuitry underlying fear conditioning has been described in some detail. Importantly, the essential locus for CS-US association formation has been identified and many of the sensory pathways that transmit information to this learning center have been mapped (LeDoux, 1998).

Neural Circuitry of Fear Conditioning

It has been recognized for decades that the amygdala is involved in emotional processes, including aversively motivated learning (see Fendt and Fanselow, 1999, for an excellent review). The major amygdaloid nuclei and projections have been well characterized (see Swanson and Petrovich, 1998, for a review of amygdaloid anatomy). Recent anatomic and behavioral evidence indicates that there are at least two distinct subsystems within the amygdala that are important for Pavlovian fear conditioning. The first subsystem of the amygdala consists of the lateral, basolateral, and basomedial nuclei. These nuclei, which are collectively referred to as the basolateral amygdaloid complex (BLA), are the primary sensory interface of the amygdala. Thus, the BLA receives synaptic input from many primary sensory structures, and lesions in these structures yield deficits in Pavlovian fear conditioning. For example, projections from the auditory thalamus and auditory cortex to the BLA are essential for conditioning to auditory CSs (Romanski and LeDoux, 1992; Campeau and Davis, 1995a), projections from the hippocampal formation to the BLA appear to underlie conditioning to contextual CSs (Kim and Fanselow, 1992; Phillips and LeDoux, 1992; Maren and Fanselow, 1997), and projections from the perirhinal cortex transmit visual CS information to the BLA (Rosen et al., 1992; Campeau and Davis, 1995a). Information about the aversive footshock US might reach the BLA via parallel thalamic and cortical pathways (Shi and Davis, 1999). Consistent with this anatomy, single neurons in the BLA respond to auditory, visual, and somatic (shock) stimuli (Romanski et al., 1993), which indicates that the amygdala is a locus of convergence for information about CSs and USs. Thus, the BLA is anatomically situated to integrate information from a variety of sensory domains.

The information processed by the BLA is either relayed back to afferent structures or sent to the second major subsystem of the amygdala, the central nucleus of the amygdala (CEA). The CEA projects to many brain stem targets and is the amygdala's interface with the fear-response systems. For example, the CEA projects to nuclei in the hypothalamus, midbrain, and medulla that control a variety of defensive responses, including freezing and acoustic startle. Electrical stimulation of the CEA produces responses that are similar to those elicited by stimuli paired with shock, and lesions of the CEA also produce profound deficits in both the acquisition and expression of conditional fear (Hitchcock and Davis, 1986; Iwata et al., 1987). Moreover, lesions placed in structures that are efferent to the CEA, such as the lateral hypothalamus or periaqueductal grey, produce selective deficits in either cardiovascular or somatic conditional fear responses, respectively (LeDoux et al., 1988). This suggests that the CEA is the final common pathway for the generation of learned fear responses. Thus, the amygdala contains two distinct subsystems that represent areas of either sensory convergence (BLA) or response divergence (CEA).

Much evidence indicates that the BLA is the crucial neural locus for the formation and storage of fear memories. Selective lesions of the BLA abolish both acquisition and expression of conditional fear in several behavioral paradigms (Helmstetter, 1992; Sananes and Davis, 1992; Campeau and Davis, 1995b; Maren et al., 1996a; Maren, 1998b). In addition, BLA lesions yield deficits in conditional fear when they are made up to 1 month after training (Lee et al., 1996; Maren et al., 1996a; Cousens and Otto, 1998) or after extensive overtraining (Maren, 1998b). Moreover, manipulations that temporarily disable amygdaloid neurons prevent both the acquisition and expression of fear conditioning (Helmstetter and Bellgowan, 1994; Muller et al., 1997). Fear-conditioning deficits are associative in nature, because rats with BLA lesions can perform the freezing response under some conditions (Maren, 1998a; Maren, 1999b).

The view that the BLA is a locus of plasticity during aversive learning is further supported by electrophysiologic studies of neuronal activity in the amygdala during auditory fear conditioning. For example, neurons in the amygdala exhibit short-latency, CS-elicited firing during aversive learning (Maren et al., 1991; Quirk et al., 1995). Associative neuronal firing in the BLA precedes the development of both behavioral CRs and associative firing in other brain structures, including the auditory cortex (Quirk et al., 1997). Moreover, an intact amygdala is required for the acquisition of at least some forms of neuronal plasticity in the auditory cortex (Armony et al., 1998). Because of its essential role in forming and storing fear memories, the BLA serves as an ideal anatomic substrate for analyzing the relationship of synaptic plasticity mechanisms, such as LTP, to behavior.

NMDA Receptor Antagonists and Pavlovian Fear Conditioning

An important breakthrough in understanding the role LTP plays in behavior came with the discovery that some forms of LTP induction require activation of the NMDA subclass of glutamate receptors. Hence, a typical strategy for investigating the role for LTP in learning involves administering NMDA receptor antagonists to animals prior to a learning episode. Methods for delivering NMDA receptor antagonists range from systemic administration of drugs that permeate the blood-brain barrier to discrete intracranial infusion of antagonists into small brain areas. Insofar as some forms of LTP require NMDA receptor activation, the assumption is that learning tasks that are sensitive to NMDA receptor antagonists may also require NMDA receptor-dependent LTP. Of course, NMDA receptors mediate other cellular functions in addition to LTP (Leung and Desborough, 1988; Sah et al., 1989). Therefore, the fact that a learning task is sensitive to NMDA receptor antagonists is a necessary, but not sufficient, condition for involvement of NMDA receptor-dependent LTP in the task.

Studies that have examined the contribution of NMDA receptor antagonists to fear conditioning have used both intracerebroventricular (ICV) infusion of NMDA receptor antagonists into the lateral ventricles and local drug infusions into discrete brain areas. Collectively, the data reveal an important role for NMDA receptors in the acquisition, and, in some cases, the expression of learned fear. For example, Fanselow and colleagues have performed an extensive examination of the effects of ICV administration of the NMDA receptor antagonist, APV, on the acquisition and expression of conditional freezing to contextual stimuli in rats (Kim et al., 1991, 1992; Fanselow et al., 1994). This work indicates that pretraining infusions of APV eliminate the acquisition of conditional freezing to the contextual cues associated with footshock without affecting either footshock sensitivity or the performance of the freezing response (Kim et al., 1991). The disruption of fear conditioning by APV was dose-dependent and stereospecific (i.e., only D-APV blocked conditioning). Moreover, the conditional freezing impairments were not state-dependent, insofar as rats both trained and tested after APV infusion exhibited equally robust deficits in conditional freezing. The impairment in fear acquisition was complete insofar as there was no evidence of savings (learning that is not reflected in performance) following reacquisition training in a drug-free state (Kim et al., 1992). Importantly, APV was only effective in preventing acquisition of conditional freezing if it was present during or before training; immediate posttraining administration of APV did not impair the acquisition of freezing.

In subsequent studies, Fanselow and colleagues examined whether the memory impairments produced by ICV APV were time-limited and/or modality-specific. It was found that rats treated with APV did in fact exhibit conditional freezing immediately following footshock, so-called immediate postshock freezing (Kim et al., 1992). This indicates that APV did not affect the encoding of a short-term memory for the context-shock association. However, APV did interfere with the establishment of a long-term memory for this association. In an effort to determine the extent of fear conditioning deficits after APV infusion, Fanselow and colleagues next examined whether fear conditioning to an auditory CS would be impacted by ICV APV infusion. In these experiments, footshock was always signaled by a tone CS during training. For fear testing, conditional freezing to the contextual CS was assessed in the training chamber, and conditional freezing to the tone CS was assessed in a novel context. These experiments revealed that APV infusion before training only disrupted the acquisition of contextual fear conditioning, and auditory fear conditioning was only minimally affected by APV infusion (Fanselow et al., 1994). Unfortunately, ICV methodology does not allow one to determine the locus upon which the APV was exerting its effects. However, the selective effect of APV on contextual fear conditioning suggests that APV was affecting the hippocampus, because hippocampal lesions typically yield deficits in contextual, but not auditory, fear conditioning (Kim and Fanselow, 1992; Phillips and LeDoux, 1992; but see Maren et al., 1997). Therefore, these studies indicate that NMDA receptor activation is required for contextual fear conditioning, and they implicate NMDA receptor-dependent LTP in the hippocampus in this form of learning.

In addition to the ICV experiments, a number of studies have examined the effects of local administration of APV into discrete brain areas. In the first study of its kind, Davis and colleagues demonstrated that infusion of APV into the basolateral amygdala prevents the acquisition of conditional fear to a visual CS in a fear-potentiated startle paradigm (Miserendino et al., 1990). This effect was dose-dependent and was not due to an APV-induced shift in footshock sensitivity. Importantly, APV infusion into the amygdala before testing did not affect the expression or performance of an already learned CR. Furthermore, APV infusion into the cerebellar interpositus nucleus, a brain structure that is not required for fear conditioning, did not affect acquisition of fear-potentiated startle. Subsequent work has demonstrated that intraamygdala APV also blocks the acquisition, but not expression, of fear-potentiated startle to acoustic CSs (Campeau et al., 1992). The deleterious effect of APV on fear-potentiated startle acquisition has also been demonstrated in second-order conditioning, in which a CS (CS1) that has previously been paired with shock serves as the reinforcer for a novel CS (CS2) in a second phase of training. Under these conditions, conditional fear accrues to CS2 despite the fact that CS2 itself is never paired with the US. APV infusion into the amygdala prior to second-order conditioning does not affect expression of conditional fear to CS1, but does affect the acquisition of the second-order CR to CS2 (Gewirtz and Davis, 1997). This suggests that APV impairs fear conditioning by attenuating an associative mechanism, rather than affecting CS or US processing per se.

In addition to blocking the original acquisition of fear-potentiated startle, intraamygdala APV infusions also prevent the extinction of this conditional fear response (Falls et al., 1992). Lee and Kim (1998) have also demonstrated that intraamygdala APV blocks the extinction of a conditional freezing response (Lee and Kim, 1998). Because extinction appears to represent the acquisition of a new inhibitory CS-"no US" association (as opposed to the erasure of the original CS-

US association), these data extend the role for NMDA receptors in the amygdala to inhibitory forms of learning. It would be of interest to examine whether APV affects the acquisition of other inhibitory associations, such as those acquired during conditioned inhibition training.

In addition to the fear-potentiated startle paradigm, the effects of intraamygdala APV have also been examined in the conditional-freezing paradigm (Maren et al., 1996b). In these experiments, we found that intraamygdala APV administered before training produced a robust impairment in the acquisition of conditional freezing that was not due to a change in footshock sensitivity or motor activity. Intraamygdala APV only blocked conditioning when it was present in the BLA during training; immediate posttraining infusion of APV did not affect conditional freezing (Maren et al., 1996b). The effects of intraamygdala APV did not appear to be time-limited, insofar as immediate postshock freezing was impaired by APV infusion. However, another study has not found impairments in immediate postshock freezing after APV infusion (Lee and Kim, 1998). As with ICV infusions, immediate posttraining administration of NMDA receptor antagonists did not affect the acquisition of conditional freezing. However, unlike the results obtained from the fear-potentiated startle paradigm, we found that the effects of intraamygdala APV were not specific to acquisition; the expression or performance of previously acquired fear CRs was also impaired by intraamygdala APV (Maren et al., 1996b). This pattern of results has recently been replicated (Lee and Kim, 1998) and may be due to the influence of NMDA receptor antagonists on evoked potentials in the amygdala (Li et al., 1995; Maren and Fanselow, 1995). Thus, it appears that NMDA receptor activation is generally involved in the acquisition of fear CRs, but is selectively involved in the expression of the conditional freezing (see Lee and Kim, 1998, for a discussion of this issue). Nonetheless, the evidence implicates NMDA receptor-dependent processes in the amygdala, and possibly amygdaloid LTP, in the acquisition of fear conditioning.

Work in the Morris water maze has revealed that the deficits in learning incurred after administration of NMDA receptor antagonists are often ameliorated by prior familiarization with the task requirements in a drug-free state (Bannerman et al., 1995; Saucier and Cain, 1995). To determine whether this was true for fear conditioning paradigms, Lee and Kim (1998) examined whether the acquisition of a fear CR prior to APV administration affected the subsequent acquisition of a novel CS-US association under the influence of APV. In contrast to the results obtained in the Morris water maze, rats that received aversive "pretraining" still exhibited robust deficits in the acquisition of conditional freezing when subsequently trained on a new CS-US association after intraamygdala APV infusion. These results strongly suggest that intraamygdala APV attenuates the acquisition of conditional fear associations, rather than having a nonassociative effect on task performance.

The amygdala is not the only brain area to have been targeted in APV infusion experiments. The effects of intrahippocampal administration of APV on the acquisition of fear conditioning have also been examined. Fanselow and colleagues found that the acquisition of contextual fear conditioning was impaired by pretraining infusions of APV into the dorsal hippocampus (Young et al., 1994). Unlike the effects of intraamygdala APV infusion, intrahippocampal APV infusion produces a selective effect on contextual fear conditioning (Stiedl et al., 1998). Of great importance, these studies indicate that NMDA receptors in the hippocampus and amygdala play different roles in fear conditioning.

It is well documented that NMDA receptor activation is only the first step in a biochemical cascade that ultimately leads to synaptic modification. Activation of intracellular protein kinases, which are stimulated by NMDA receptor activation, is essential for the induction of LTP. Examinations of the role of protein kinases in fear conditioning have just begun, but there is already evidence that various kinases are required for establishing long-term fear memories. For instance, Kandel and colleagues have shown that posttraining ICV administration of protein kinase A (PKA) inhibitors impairs memory consolidation for contextual fear conditioning (Bourtchouladze et al., 1998). Likewise, LeDoux and colleagues have found that posttraining ICV administration of PKA and mitogen-activated protein kinase (MAPK) inhibitors disrupts the memory for contextual and auditory fear conditioning (Schafe et al., 1999). Furthermore, Davis and colleagues have reported that intraamygdala administration of either PKA or CamKII inhibitors attenuates the acquisition of fear-potentiated startle (Ding et al., 1998). Although these studies are in an early stage, they seem to indicate that many of the kinases that have already been implicated in LTP have a role in Pavlovian fear conditioning.

Less work has been performed on the influence of alpha-amino-3 hydroxy-5-methyl-4-isoaxazoleproprionate (AMPA) receptor ligands on the acquisition of conditional fear. Davis and colleagues have shown that intraamygdala infusion of AMPA receptor antagonists impairs both the acquisition and expression of fear-potentiated startle (Kim et al., 1993; Walker and Davis, 1997). Additionally, LeDoux and colleagues have shown that AMPA receptor agonists infused into the amygdala prior to training enhance the acquisition of conditional freezing (Rogan et al., 1997a).

Collectively, these data reveal an important role for both NMDA and AMPA receptors in the amygdala in the acquisition and expression of Pavlovian fear conditioning. Insofar as these receptors are essential for the induction and expression of LTP, these data also suggest that both hippocampal and amygdaloid LTP are required for the acquisition of learned fear responses. Importantly, however, these results reveal that NMDA receptors in the amygdala and hippocampus play different roles in the acquisition of fear conditioning. Specifically, hippocampal NMDA receptors are only required for the acquisition of long-term conditional fear memories to contextual CSs, whereas amygdaloid NMDA receptors are required for the acquisition and, in some cases, the expression of short- and long-term fear memories to contextual, visual, and auditory CSs. The different involvement of amygdaloid and hippocampal NMDA receptors in the acquisition of fear conditioning suggests that LTP in these structures subserves different roles in this form of learning.

Correlations between LTP and Pavlovian Fear Conditioning

The foregoing studies indicate that both hippocampal and amygdaloid NMDA receptors are involved in the acquisition of Pavlovian fear conditioning in rats. By extension, these results implicate NMDA receptor-dependent LTP in these brain areas in the acquisition of conditional fear. With respect to the involvement of hippocampal LTP in contextual fear conditioning, there are no studies that have attempted to directly measure hippocampal synaptic transmission during the acquisition of contextual fear conditioning. However, a number of studies have used a correlational approach to examine hippocampal LTP, particularly perforant path-dentate granule cell (PP-GC) LTP, in relation to contextual fear conditioning.

In one series of experiments, we attempted to determine whether a behavioral manipulation that was known to enhance acquisition rate in several learning paradigms (e.g., Berry and Swain, 1989) would have facilitatory effects on the induction of hippocampal LTP in anesthetized rats. The behavioral manipulation we chose for this purpose was acute water deprivation, for which access to water was restricted to 1 hour per day for 4 days. In line with the previously reported facilitatory effects of water deprivation on learning, we found that water deprivation reliably enhanced the magnitude of PP-GC LTP induced by high-frequency stimulation (Maren et al., 1994c). This effect was not due to a change in the properties of baseline synaptic transmission at PP-GC synapses. However, water deprivation did increase the proportion of theta-frequency activity in the electroencephalogram, which might have favored greater levels of LTP induction (Huerta and Lisman, 1995).

With this LTP-enhancing manipulation in hand, we next sought to determine whether water deprivation would affect the acquisition of contextual fear conditioning, a hippocampus-dependent task that others had suggested might be mediated by hippocampal LTP (e.g., Kim et al., 1991). We found that water deprivation prior to fear conditioning significantly enhanced the acquisition of contextual fear conditioning (Maren et al., 1994c). The enhancement in conditional freezing to the contextual CSs was only observed with subasymptotic levels of training; therefore, water deprivation increased the rate, but not asymptote, of contextual fear conditioning. This effect was not due to enhanced footshock sensitivity. Interestingly, the enhancement of fear conditioning by water deprivation was specific to contextual fear conditioning; water deprivation did not enhance auditory fear conditioning (Maren et al., 1994b). We have also recently reported that this enhancement of contextual fear conditioning is specific to water deprivation. That is, a comparable period of food deprivation does not affect fear conditioning (Maren and Fanselow, 1998). Collectively, these results reveal that water deprivation has a specific effect on the acquisition rate of contextual fear conditioning, a hippocampus-dependent task, and also augments hippocampal LTP induction.

These experiments suggest a role for hippocampal LTP in contextual fear conditioning. To further explore this relationship, we examined whether individual differences in aversive learning correlated with hippocampal LTP induction, inso-far as we had previously demonstrated a relationship between hippocampal LTP and individual differences in nonassociative fear responses (Maren et al., 1993; 1994d; Mitchell et al., 1993). To this end, we examined whether well-known sex differences in aversive learning correlate with hippocampal LTP. As a first step, we simply assessed the magnitude of PP-GC LTP in adult male and female rats. Somewhat to our surprise, we found a robust sex difference in the magnitude of PP-GC LTP induced *in vivo:* Males exhibited reliably more LTP than females (Maren et al., 1994a; Maren, 1995). Given the sex difference in hippocampal LTP, we hypothesized that male and female rats should exhibit a sex difference in con-textual fear conditioning. To test this hypothesis, we simply examined Pavlovian fear conditioning in male and female rats. Consistent with the sex difference in hippocampal LTP, male rats exhibited greater levels of contextual freezing than female rats (Maren et al., 1994a). There was no sex difference in fear conditioning to an auditory CS, consistent with the specific role for hippocampal LTP in con-textual fear conditioning. The basis for the sex difference in hippocampal LTP and fear conditioning is not known, although a role for circulating testosterone in adult male rats has been ruled out (Anagnostaras et al., 1998). Preliminary results from our laboratory indicate that the ovarian steroid, estrogen, in adult female rats contributes to these sex differences.

The parallel between deprivation-induced enhancements in hippocampal LTP induction and contextual fear conditioning, and the correlation between sex dif-ferences in both hippocampal LTP and contextual fear conditioning, provide fur-ther evidence for a role for hippocampal LTP in the mediation of contextual fear conditioning. Although these correlations do not necessarily implicate causation with regard to the role for LTP in contextual fear conditioning, they are neverthe-less consistent with such a role. Indeed, such correlations are necessary for hypotheses that invoke hippocampal LTP as a mechanism for contextual fear con-ditioning (Fanselow, 1997; Maren, 1997).

In addition to hippocampal LTP, the role of amygdaloid LTP in Pavlovian fear conditioning has received considerable attention (Maren, 1999a). Amygdaloid LTP, which has been studied in thalamic (Clugnet and LeDoux, 1990; Rogan and LeDoux, 1995) and hippocampal (Maren and Fanselow, 1995) projections to the amygdala, exhibits several properties that are similar to those exhibited by hip-pocampal LTP (Maren, 1996). Some forms of amygdaloid LTP are NMDA recep-tor-dependent (Maren and Fanselow, 1995; Huang and Kandel, 1998), although, as in the hippocampus (Grover and Teyler, 1990), there also are NMDA receptor-independent forms of LTP in the amygdala (Chapman and Bellavance, 1992). Amygdaloid LTP also appears to require the activation of protein kinases, such as PKA (Huang and Kandel, 1998), that are also involved in hippocampal LTP. Thus, while differences between the two mechanisms may exist, we will assume for the purpose of this discussion that they are largely similar.

The first nonpharmacologic evidence to link amygdaloid LTP to fear condition-ing has emerged from studies in the LeDoux laboratory examining auditory evoked potentials in the amygdala following either LTP induction or fear conditioning.

Rogan and LeDoux (1995) have shown that induction of LTP at thalamo-amygdaloid synapses *in vivo* potentiates auditory evoked potentials in the amygdala that are transmitted through the thalamus. This suggests that experimental induction of LTP at thalamo-amygdaloid synapses has functional consequences for the processing of acoustic stimuli that use these synapses. In a related study, LeDoux and colleagues have recently demonstrated that auditory evoked potentials in the thalamo-amygdaloid pathway are also augmented during the acquisition of auditory fear conditioning (Rogan et al., 1997b). The increase in the amplitude of auditory evoked potentials in the amygdala was only observed in rats that received paired CS and US presentations. Moreover, the change in the evoked potentials was uncoupled from freezing behavior, insofar as rats receiving unpaired training exhibited similar levels of freezing behavior during training, but did not exhibit an increase in the amplitude of auditory evoked potentials. The similar increases in auditory evoked potentials in the amygdala following both tetanic LTP induction and fear conditioning suggests that LTP-like increases in thalamo-amygdaloid synaptic transmission contribute to the acquisition of auditory fear conditioning.

In a related study, McKernan and Shinnick-Gallagher (1997) have shown that fear-potentiated startle training enhances the amplitude of synaptic currents in amygdaloid neurons *in vitro*. In these experiments, rats were first trained in the fear-potentiated startle task, and then sacrificed for *in vitro* electrophysiologic experiments. Intracellular recordings were obtained from lateral amygdaloid neurons, and currents in these cells were evoked by electrical stimulation of axons presumed to originate from the auditory thalamus. Rats receiving paired CS-US trials, but not those receiving unpaired trials, exhibited a marked increase in stimulus-evoked currents in amygdaloid neurons; this effect appeared to be limited to synaptic currents derived from the AMPA subclass of glutamate receptors. Fear conditioning also reduced paired-pulse facilitation, in which the evoked response to the second stimulus of a pair is larger than that to the first stimulus. This indicates that fear-potentiated startle training had increased neurotransmitter release in the thalamo-amygdaloid pathway. Synaptic transmission in the endopyriform nucleus, which is not believed to play a role in fear conditioning, was not altered by the conditioning procedures. Insofar as tetanus-induced amygdaloid LTP is associated with increased evoked responses and enhanced neurotransmitter release (Maren and Fanselow, 1995; Huang and Kandel, 1998), it would appear that fear-potentiated startle training induced a form of "behavioral" LTP. These results provide strong support for a role for amygdaloid LTP in the acquisition of fear conditioning. Of course, it would be of interest to determine whether these conditioning-related changes in amygdaloid synaptic transmission are blocked by NMDA receptor antagonist administration during training.

Gene Targeting, LTP, and Fear Conditioning

A more direct test of the role for hippocampal LTP in fear conditioning has been provided by several recent studies that have taken advantage of genetically modified mice, which have been engineered with genetic manipulations that either disable or eliminate key proteins in the intracellular biochemical cascades that mediate LTP. Although this technique is clearly a powerful and exciting approach to studying the neural substrates of learning and memory, it must be kept in mind that these studies have several caveats. For instance, the irreversible nature of the mutations, the opportunity for developmental compensation, and the inability to localize the mutations within discrete neural subregions need to be considered when interpreting the results from these studies.

The first study to examine the relationship between hippocampal LTP and Pavlovian fear conditioning involved the use of mice that lacked the gamma isoform of protein kinase C (PKC), an enzyme that has been implicated in both LTP and learning and memory. Mice that lack PKC-gamma exhibited mild deficits in contextual, but not auditory, fear conditioning (Abeliovich et al., 1993b). In contrast, they exhibited normal immediate postshock freezing, suggesting that their short-term memory for contextual fear was intact. The normal level of freezing to the auditory CS indicates that the deficits in contextual freezing were not due to an inability to perform the freezing response. The selective deficit in contextual conditioning is interesting insofar as the mice also exhibited impairments in the induction of hippocampal LTP in area CA1 *in vitro* (Abeliovich et al., 1993a). There were no deficits in either baseline synaptic transmission or paired-pulse facilitation and posttetanic potentiation (PTP), which are measures of presynaptic neurotransmitter release. Interestingly, the deficits in hippocampal LTP induction could be overcome with low-frequency priming stimulation. The fact that some capacity to exhibit LTP was evident in these mice might explain the incomplete nature of the contextual freezing deficits. Unfortunately, amygdaloid LTP was not examined in these animals, although the pattern of behavioral results suggests that it would be normal. Together, these data suggest that hippocampal LTP is involved in establishing memories for long-term contextual fear.

A more recent study has examined the influence of a targeted mutation of the cAMP-responsive element-binding (CREB) protein, which is a transcription factor thought to play an important role in establishing long-term memories, on both fear conditioning and hippocampal LTP. Mice with a disruption of the alpha and delta isoforms of CREB were found to exhibit robust impairments in both contextual and auditory fear conditioning (Bourtchuladze et al., 1994). These impairments were time-dependent insofar as freezing to both contexts and tones was found to be intact when measured within 30 or 60 minutes of training, respectively. However, conditional freezing was nearly absent at long (24-hour) retention intervals. Thus, the sparing of short-term fear memories reveals that the CREB mutants were capable of normal freezing under some conditions. Moreover, the time-dependent loss of conditional freezing over long retention intervals indicates that CREB is essential for consolidating long-term fear memories. Paralleling the time-dependency of fear conditioning, mice that lack CREB also exhibited impairments in hippocampal LTP in area CA1 *in vitro* (Bourtchuladze et al., 1994). While CREB mutants exhibited normal paired-pulse facilitation and PTP, they showed a marked deficit in LTP. This was manifest as a more rapid decay of the potentiation over a 2-hour period. Interestingly, the time period over which LTP decayed appeared to parallel the time period over which fear memories are lost in CREB mutants. A similar pattern of results has been obtained in mice that express an inhibitory form of the regulatory subunit for PKA, an enzyme known to play a role in LTP (Abel et al., 1997). In this case mice also exhibited long-term, but not short-term, impairments in both contextual and auditory fear conditioning. Although neither group of investigators has measured amygdaloid LTP in these mice, the behavioral data would suggest that it should be impaired in CREB mutants. In agreement with the role for CREB in fear conditioning, it has recently been reported that both contextual and auditory fear conditioning rapidly induce CREB in the hippocampus and amygdala (Impey et al., 1998).

In yet another series of studies, Kandel and colleagues have examined mice that overexpress a mutant form of Ca^{2+}-calmodulin-dependent protein kinase II (CamKII) in the amygdala, hippocampus, and striatum (Mayford et al., 1996). In the hippocampus, CamKII is activated by Ca^{2+} influx through the NMDA receptor. It interacts with a number of substrates within neurons, including CREB. Not surprisingly, CamKII has been demonstrated to have a role in LTP induction, and mice that overexpress the transgene for this protein do not exhibit LTP in the hippocampus following theta-frequency stimulation, for example (Mayford et al., 1996). Interestingly, these transgenic mice (Mayford et al., 1996), as well as mice that lack CamKII (Chen et al., 1994), also exhibit impairments in Pavlovian fear conditioning to both contextual and auditory cues. The global impairment in conditional fear to both contextual and auditory cues suggests the existence of amygdala dysfunction in these genetically modified mice. Although the nature of this dysfunction is not yet known, it is tempting to speculate that it will take the form of impaired amygdaloid LTP.

A more direct demonstration of a specific role for amygdaloid LTP in fear conditioning has come from studies of mice that lack Ras-GRF, a neuron-specific guanine nucleotide releasing factor that is activated by both Ca^{2+} and G-protein-coupled messengers. Electrophysiologic recordings from brain slices obtained from mice lacking Ras-GRF have revealed a pronounced deficit in LTP in the basolateral nucleus of the amygdala (Brambilla et al., 1997). Interestingly, these mice also exhibit impairments in consolidating long-term memories for Pavlovian fear conditioning to both contextual and acoustic stimuli. These deficits in LTP and learning were selective for the amygdala and Pavlovian fear conditioning insofar as both hippocampal LTP and spatial learning in Ras-GRF knockouts were normal (Brambilla et al., 1997). Interestingly, Ras-GRF modulates CREB activity through the MAPK pathway. A role for MAPK in fear conditioning has recently been demonstrated (Atkins et al., 1998). Together, these results provide strong support for the view that synaptic LTP in the amygdala is required for the establishment and maintenance of emotional memories.

Differential Roles for Hippocampal and Amygdaloid LTP in Pavlovian Fear Conditioning

Several lines of study converge upon a role for both hippocampal and amygdaloid LTP in the acquisition of Pavlovian fear conditioning. As we have seen, the LTP-learning connection for Pavlovian fear conditioning is supported by behavioral, pharmacologic, electrophysiologic, and molecular experiments. Fear conditioning is (1) prevented by NMDA receptor antagonists, (2) associated with an induction of behavioral LTP, (3) correlated with tetanic LTP, (4) positively modulated by behavioral manipulations that facilitate tetanic LTP, and (5) impaired by manipulations that disrupt or eliminate crucial elements of the biochemical cascade underlying LTP. It is also apparent from the studies discussed to this point that LTP in the amygdala and hippocampus plays different, yet complementary, roles in fear conditioning. This is an important outcome that deserves further attention. It illustrates that even within a simple learning paradigm, such as Pavlovian fear conditioning, synaptic plasticity mechanisms such as LTP play multiple and distinct roles in the learning process.

The roles for amygdaloid and hippocampal LTP in Pavlovian fear conditioning diverge along at least three dimensions: time, sensory modality, and associative function. With respect to the temporal dimension, there is good evidence that LTP is only required for establishing long-term fear memories (i.e., memories that are at least 2 hours old). Short-term fear memories (i.e., memories that last only minutes), such as those evidenced by immediate postshock freezing, do not appear to require LTP. Rather, it is more likely that short-term synaptic plasticity mechanisms, such as PTP, mediate these memories. The requirement for LTP in the establishment of long-term memories might be explained by the important role for protein synthesis in Pavlovian fear conditioning. Indeed, it has recently been demonstrated that infusion of protein synthesis inhibitors into the amygdala prior to fear conditioning prevents the establishment of long-term, but not short-term, fear memories to both contextual and auditory cues (Bailey et al., 1999). However, the role for LTP in conditional fear that is expressed over very long retention intervals (more than 30 days) has not been explored. Recent studies demonstrate a time-limited role for the hippocampus in the expression of contextual fear conditioning (Kim and Fanselow, 1992; Maren et al., 1997; Anagnostaras et al., 1999) and a time-independent role for the amygdala in the expression of contextual and auditory fear conditioning (Kim and Davis, 1993; Lee et al., 1996; Maren et al., 1996a). This suggests that amygdaloid LTP might have a much more temporally enduring role in the consolidation and maintenance of fear memories than hippocampal LTP.

With respect to the sensory dimension, there is strong evidence that hippocampal LTP plays a unique role in fear conditioning to contextual stimuli, whereas amygdaloid LTP has a more general role in fear conditioning to both contextual and discrete CSs, such as tones and lights (see Figure 3.1). This is supported by the fact that manipulations that selectively interfere with hippocampal LTP disrupt only contextual fear conditioning, whereas manipulations that interfere with amygdaloid LTP disrupt both contextual and auditory fear conditioning. The different roles for hippocampal and amygdaloid LTP in conditioning to contextual and discrete CSs is imposed by the anatomy of the fear conditioning circuit. That is, the hippocampus appears to be part of a sensory pathway that conveys contextual CSs to the amygdala for association with footshock. In contrast, as described above, the amygdala appears to be the essential locus for encoding and storing CS-

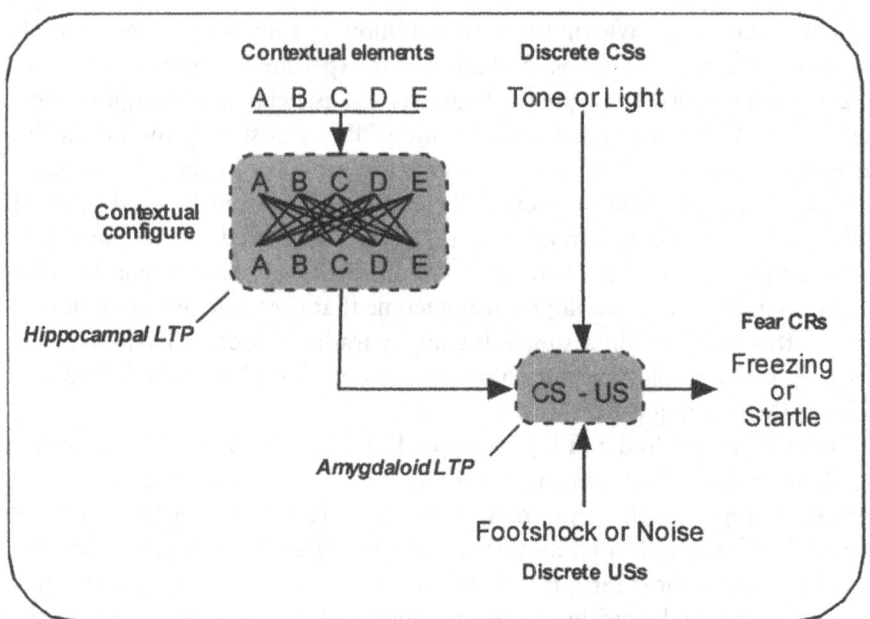

Figure 3.1. Schematic diagram illustrating the role for hippocampal and amygdaloid long-term potentiation (LTP) in different associative processes in Pavlovian fear conditioning. Loci of synaptic plasticity are delineated in the figure by the shaded boxes. Hippocampal LTP is posited to play a role in the formation of contextual representations, which are configural or conjunctive representations formed from individual elemental stimuli (A, B, C, D, E). Amygdaloid LTP, on the other hand, is involved in associating conditional and unconditional stimuli (CSs and USs), such as tones and footshocks. The formation of CS-US associations in the amygdala results in the performance of conditional fear responses (CRs), such as freezing or potentiated acoustic startle. As described in the text, amygdaloid LTP is posited to play a role in establishing long-term fear memories for CSs in all modalities, whereas hippocampal LTP is involved in establishing long-term memories of the contextual CS.

US associations. The different functional roles for the hippocampus and amygdala in fear conditioning provides the foundation for understanding the unique roles LTP plays in these structures in different aspects of Pavlovian fear conditioning.

The role for the hippocampus in processing contextual CSs has been established in a number of studies. From this work, it appears that the hippocampus plays a unique role in forming contextual representations, that is, the process by which the configuration or the conjunction of the contextual cues present during fear conditioning is encoded (Fanselow, 1986; Rudy and Sutherland, 1995). Good and colleagues have suggested that the hippocampus plays an important role in acquiring incidental information about the conditioning context (Good et al., 1998), which might occur during exploration of the conditioning chamber (e.g., Maren et al., 1997). In either case, it does not appear that the hippocampus is important for establishing context-US associations (Young et al., 1994; Maren et al., 1997; Frankland et al., 1998; Cho et al., 1999) – this is the domain of the amygdala (e.g., Maren et al., 1996a). The involvement of the hippocampus in forming contextual representations suggests a unique role for hippocampal LTP in this process (Figure 3.1). There is at least one line of evidence that is consistent with this proposal. It is well established that manipulations that affect CS processing, such as increasing the salience of CSs, affect the rate at which conditional behavior is acquired, but do not affect the level of asymptotic CR performance (Rescorla, 1988). Insofar as hippocampal LTP has a role in representing contextual CSs, manipulations that modulate hippocampal LTP should affect acquisition rate, but not asymptotic CR performance. This selective rate effect might be obscured by LTP impairing manipulations, unless care is taken to train animals to a behavioral asymptote. To avoid this problem, we have examined the effect on contextual fear conditioning of a manipulation that facilitates hippocampal LTP. As predicted, we found that enhancing hippocampal LTP enhanced the rate, but not asymptote, of contextual fear conditioning (Maren et al., 1994c). This reveals that hippocampal LTP has a special role in contextual CS processing during Pavlovian fear conditioning. More specifically, we have suggested that hippocampal LTP represents the conjunction of contextual stimuli experienced at the time of conditioning, and that contextual CS salience is modulated by the strength and/or the inclusiveness of the contextual representation (Maren et al., 1994c). Thus, hippocampal LTP is presumed to regulate phenomena such as the facilitatory effects of context preexposure on the acquisition of contextual fear conditioning (Fanselow, 1990; Rudy, 1996).

In contrast to the hippocampus, the amygdala plays a crucial role in associating CSs and USs during fear conditioning. Thus, the amygdala is also involved in representing stimulus conjunctions, but in this case they are the conjunctions between the CS and the US (Figure 3.1). Therefore, the role for amygdaloid LTP in fear conditioning is quite different from that of hippocampal LTP, insofar as its induction is driven by the US and is expected to occur in CS pathways to the amygdala. The involvement of amygdaloid LTP in CS-US association is demonstrated by the fact that manipulations that impair amygdaloid LTP also disrupt the acquisition of both contextual and auditory fear conditioning. Insofar as amygdaloid LTP is hypothesized to reflect the levels of associative strength that a CS has acquired, it should be highly correlated with CR performance. Unfortunately, studies have not been performed that systematically examine the relationship of amygdaloid LTP to either the rate or asymptote of fear conditioning. One might expect, however, that manipulations that facilitate amygdaloid LTP would enhance both the acquisition rate and asymptotic performance of conditional fear. Further work is required to examine this hypothesis. Nevertheless, the available evidence strongly supports the view that amygdaloid LTP is the crucial plasticity underlying formation and storage of CS-US associations acquired during fear conditioning.

Conclusions

In conclusion, there is now an abundance of data reinforcing the view that there are multiple roles for synaptic plasticity in the acquisition of a simple and adaptive form of associative learning: Pavlovian fear conditioning. It has been established that acquisition of long-term fear memories to the contexts in which shock occurs requires LTP in the hippocampus, whereas the acquisition of conditional fear to both contexts and other discrete cues requires LTP in the amygdala. Hippocampal LTP is proposed to play a special role in the acquisition of contextual CS representations, whereas amygdaloid LTP is proposed to underlie the acquisition of CS-US associations during fear conditioning. Short-lasting forms of synaptic plasticity, such as PTP, may play an important role in encoding short-term fear memories, such as those expressed immediately following an aversive event. Considering all of the available evidence, it is concluded that LTP and related forms of synaptic plasticity are viable mechanisms for memory formation and storage during emotional learning and memory.

REFERENCES

Abel, T., Nguyen, P.V., Barad, M., Deuel, T.A. et al. (1997). Genetic demonstration of a role for PKA in the late phase of LTP and in hippocampus-based long-term memory. *Cell* 88: 615–626.

Abeliovich, A., Chen, C., Goda, Y., Silva, A.J. et al. (1993a). Modified hippocampal long-term potentiation in PKC gamma-mutant mice. *Cell* 75: 1253–1262.

Abeliovich, A., Paylor, R., Chen, C., Kim, J.J. et al. (1993b). PKC gamma mutant mice exhibit mild deficits in spatial and contextual learning. *Cell* 75: 1263–1271.

Anagnostaras, S.G., Maren, S., DeCola, J.P., Lane, N.I. et al. (1998). Testicular hormones do not regulate sexually dimorphic Pavlovian fear conditioning or perforant-path long-term potentiation in adult male rats. *Behav. Brain Res.* 92: 1–9.

Anagnostaras, S.G., Maren, S., and Fanselow, M.S. (1999). Temporally graded retrograde amnesia of contextual fear after hippocampal damage in rats: Within-subjects examination. *J. Neurosci.* 19: 1106–1114.

Armony, J.L., Quirk, G.J., and LeDoux, J.E. (1998). Differential effects of amygdala lesions on early and late plastic components of auditory cortex spike trains during fear conditioning. *J. Neurosci.* 18: 2592–2601.

Atkins, C.M., Selcher, J.C., Petraitis, J.J., Trzaskos, J.M. et al. (1998). The MAPK cascade is required for mammalian associative learning. *Nat. Neurosci.* 1: 602–609.

Bailey, D.J., Kim, J.J., Sun, W., Thompson, R.F. et al. (1999). Acquisition of fear conditioning in rats requires the synthesis of mRNA in the amygdala. *Behav. Neurosci.* 113: 276–282.

Bannerman, D.M., Good, M.A., Butcher, S.P., Ramsay, M. et al. (1995). Distinct components of spatial learning revealed by prior training and NMDA receptor blockade. *Nature (London)* 378: 182–186.

Berry, S.D., and Swain, R.A. (1989). Water deprivation optimizes hippocampal activity and facilitates nictitating membrane conditioning. *Behav. Neurosci.* 103: 71–76.

Bliss, T.V., and Collingridge, G.L. (1993). A synaptic model of memory: Long-term potentiation in the hippocampus. *Nature (London)* 361: 31–39.

Bliss, T.V., and Gardner-Medwin, A.R. (1973). Long-lasting potentiation of synaptic transmission in the dentate area of the unanaesthetized rabbit following stimulation of the perforant path. *J. Physiol. (London)* 232: 357–374.

Bliss, T.V., and Lømo, T. (1973). Long-lasting potentiation of synaptic transmission in the dentate area of the anaesthetized rabbit following stimulation of the perforant path. *J. Physiol. (London)* 232: 331–356.

Bourtchouladze, R., Frenguelli, B., Blendy, J., Cioffi, D. et al. (1994). Deficient long-term memory in mice with a targeted mutation of the cAMP-responsive element-binding protein. *Cell* 79: 59–68.

Bourtchouladze, R., Abel, T., Berman, N., Gordon, R. et al. (1998). Different training procedures recruit either one or two critical periods for contextual memory consolidation, each of which requires protein synthesis and PKA. *Learn. Mem.* 5: 365–374.

Brambilla, R., Gnesutta, N., Minichiello, L., White, G. et al. (1997). A role for the Ras signalling pathway in synaptic transmission and long-term memory. *Nature* 390: 281–286.

Cain, D.P. (1997). LTP, NMDA, genes and learning. *Curr. Opin. Neurobiol.* 7: 235–242.

Campeau, S., and Davis, M. (1995a). Involvement of subcortical and cortical afferents to the lateral nucleus of the amygdala in fear conditioning measured with fear-potentiated startle in rats trained concurrently with auditory and visual conditioned stimuli. *J. Neurosci.* 15: 2312–2327.

Campeau, S., and Davis, M. (1995b). Involvement of the central nucleus and basolateral complex of the amygdala in fear conditioning measured with fear-potentiated startle in rats trained concurrently with auditory and visual conditioned stimuli. *J. Neurosci.* 15: 2301–2311.

Campeau, S., Miserendino, M.J., and Davis, M. (1992). Intra-amygdala infusion of the N-methyl-D-aspartate receptor antagonist AP5 blocks acquisition but not expression of fear-potentiated startle to an auditory conditioned stimulus. *Behav. Neurosci.* 106: 569–574.

Chapman, P.F., and Bellavance, L.L. (1992). Induction of long-term potentiation in the basolateral amygdala does not depend on NMDA receptor activation. *Synapse* 11: 310–318.

Chen, C., Rainnie, D.G., Greene, R.W., and Tonegawa, S. (1994). Abnormal fear response and aggressive behavior in mutant mice deficient for alpha-calcium-calmodulin kinase II [see comments]. *Science* 266: 291–294.

Cho, Y.H., Friedman, E., and Silva, A.J. (1999). Ibotenate lesions of the hippocampus impair spatial learning but not contextual fear conditioning in mice. *Behav. Brain Res.* 98: 77–87.

Clugnet, M.C., and LeDoux, J.E. (1990). Synaptic plasticity in fear conditioning circuits: Induction of LTP in the lateral nucleus of the amygdala by stimulation of the medial geniculate body. *J. Neurosci.* 10: 2818–2824.

Cousens, G., and Otto, T. (1998). Both pre- and posttraining excitotoxic lesions of the basolateral amygdala abolish the expression of olfactory and contextual fear conditioning. *Behav. Neurosci.* 112: 1092–1103.

Davis, M. (1992). The role of the amygdala in fear and anxiety. *Annu. Rev. Neurosci.* 15: 353–375.

Davis, M., Rainnie, D., and Cassell, M. (1994). Neurotransmission in the rat amygdala related to fear and anxiety. *Trends Neurosci.* 17: 208–214.

Diamond, D.M., and Rose, G.M. (1994). Does associative LTP underlie classical conditioning? *Psychobiology* 22: 263–269.

Ding, C., Lee, Y.L., and Davis, M. (1998). Role of PKA and CaM kinases in fear conditioning assessed with fear-potentiated startle using local infusion of Rp-8-Br-cAMP. *Soc. Neurosci. Abstr.* 24: 926.

Elgersma, Y., and Silva, A.J. (1999). Molecular mechanisms of synaptic plasticity and memory. *Curr. Opin. Neurobiol.* 9: 209–213.

Falls, W.A., Miserendino, M.J., and Davis, M. (1992). Extinction of fear-potentiated startle: Blockade by infusion of an NMDA antagonist into the amygdala. *J. Neurosci.* 12: 854–863.

Fanselow, M.S. (1984). What is conditioned fear? *Trends Neursosci.* 7: 460–462.

Fanselow, M.S. (1986). Associative vs topographical accounts of the immediate shock-freezing deficit in rats: Implications for the response selection rules governing species-specific defensive reactions. *Learning Motiv.* 17: 16–39.

Fanselow, M.S. (1990). Factors governing one-trial contextual conditioning. *Anim. Learn. Behav.* 18: 264–270.

Fanselow, M.S. (1994). Neural organization of the defensive behavior system responsible for fear. *Psychon. Bull. Rev.* 1: 429–438.

Fanselow, M.S. (1997). Without LTP the learning circuit is broken. *Behav. Brain Sci.* 20: 616.

Fanselow, M.S., Kim, J.J., Yipp, J., and De Oca, B. (1994). Differential effects of the N-methyl-D-aspartate antagonist DL-2-amino-5-phosphonovalerate on acquisition of fear of auditory and contextual cues. *Behav. Neurosci.* 108: 235–240.

Fendt, M., and Fanselow, M.S. (1999). The neuroanatomical and neurochemical basis of conditioned fear. *Neurosci. Biobehav. Rev.* 23: 743–760.

Frankland, P.W., Cestari, V., Filipkowski, R.K., McDonald, R.J. et al. (1998). The dorsal hippocampus is essential for context discrimination but not for contextual conditioning. *Behav. Neurosci.* 112: 863–874.

Gewirtz, J.C., and Davis, M. (1997). Second-order fear conditioning prevented by blocking NMDA receptors in amygdala. *Nature (London)* 388: 471–474.

Good, M., de Hoz, L., and Morris, R.G. (1998). Contingent versus incidental context processing during conditioning: Dissociation after excitotoxic hippocampal plus dentate gyrus lesions. *Hippocampus* 8: 147–159.

Grover, L.M., and Teyler, T.J. (1990). Two components of long-term potentiation induced by different patterns of afferent activation. *Nature (London)* 347: 477–479.

Helmstetter, F.J. (1992). The amygdala is essential for the expression of conditional hypoalgesia. *Behav. Neurosci.* 106: 518–528.

Helmstetter, F.J., and Bellgowan, P.S. (1994). Effects of muscimol applied to the basolateral amygdala on acquisition and expression of contextual fear conditioning in rats. *Behav. Neurosci.* 108: 1005–1009.

Hitchcock, J., and Davis, M. (1986). Lesions of the amygdala, but not of the cerebellum or red nucleus, block conditioned fear as measured with the potentiated startle paradigm. *Behav. Neurosci.* 100: 11–22.

Huang, Y.Y., and Kandel, E.R. (1998). Postsynaptic induction and PKA-dependent expression of LTP in the lateral amygdala. *Neuron* 21: 169–178.

Huerta, P.T., and Lisman, J.E. (1995). Bidirectional synaptic plasticity induced by a single burst during cholinergic theta oscillation in CA1 in vitro. *Neuron* 15: 1053–1063.

Impey, S., Smith, D.M., Obrietan, K., Donahue, R. et al. (1998). Stimulation of cAMP response element (CRE)-mediated transcription during contextual learning. *Nat. Neurosci.* 1: 595–601.

Iwata, J., Chida, K., and LeDoux, J.E. (1987). Cardiovascular responses elicited by stimulation of neurons in the central amygdaloid nucleus in awake but not anesthetized rats resemble conditioned emotional responses. *Brain Res.* 418: 183–188.

Kim, J.J., and Fanselow, M.S. (1992). Modality-specific retrograde amnesia of fear. *Science* 256: 675–677.

Kim, J.J., DeCola, J.P., Landeira-Fernandez, J., and Fanselow, M.S. (1991). N-methyl-D-aspartate receptor antagonist APV blocks acquisition but not expression of fear conditioning. *Behav. Neurosci.* 105: 126–133.

Kim, J.J., Fanselow, M.S., DeCola, J.P., and Landeira Fernandez, J. (1992). Selective impairment of long-term but not short-term conditional fear by the N-methyl-D-aspartate antagonist APV. *Behav. Neurosci.* 106: 591–596.

Kim, M., and Davis, M. (1993). Lack of a temporal gradient of retrograde amnesia in rats with amygdala lesions assessed with the fear-potentiated startle paradigm. *Behav. Neurosci.* 107: 1088–1092.

Kim, M., Campeau, S., Falls, W.A., and Davis, M. (1993). Infusion of the non-NMDA receptor antagonist CNQX into the amygdala blocks the expression of fear-potentiated startle. *Behav. Neural. Biol.* 59: 5–8.

LeDoux, J. (1998). Fear and the brain: Where have we been, and where are we going? *Biol. Psychiatry* 44: 1229–1238.

LeDoux, J.E., Iwata, J., Cicchetti, P., and Reis, D.J. (1988). Different projections of the central amygdaloid nucleus mediate autonomic and behavioral correlates of conditioned fear. *J. Neurosci.* 8: 2517–2529.

Lee, H., and Kim, J.J. (1998). Amygdalar NMDA receptors are critical for new fear learning in previously fear-conditioned rats. *J. Neurosci.* 18: 8444–8454.

Lee, Y., Walker, D., and Davis, M. (1996). Lack of a temporal gradient of retrograde amnesia following NMDA-induced lesions of the basolateral amygdala assessed with the fear-potentiated startle paradigm. *Behav. Neurosci.* 110: 836–839.

Leung, L.W., and Desborough, K.A. (1988). APV, an N-methyl-D-aspartate receptor antagonist, blocks the hippocampal theta rhythm in behaving rats. *Brain Res.* 463: 148–152.

Li, X.F., Phillips, R., and LeDoux, J.E. (1995). NMDA and non-NMDA receptors contribute to synaptic transmission between the medial geniculate body and the lateral nucleus of the amygdala. *Exp. Brain. Res.* 105: 87–100.

Maren, S. (1995). Sexually dimorphic perforant path long-term potentiation (LTP) in urethane-anesthetized rats. *Neurosci. Lett.* 196: 177–180.

Maren, S. (1996). Synaptic transmission and plasticity in the amygdala. An emerging physiology of fear conditioning circuits. *Mol. Neurobiol.* 13: 1–22.

Maren, S. (1997). Arousing the LTP and learning debate. *Behav. Brain Sci.* 20: 622–623.

Maren, S. (1998a). Neurotoxic basolateral amygdala lesions impair learning but not performance of contextual fear conditioning in rats. *Soc. Neurosci. Abstr.* 24: 1682.

Maren, S. (1999a). Long-term potentiation in the amygdala: A mechanism for emotional learning and memory. *Trends Neurosci.* 22: 561–567.

Maren, S. (1998b). Overtraining does not mitigate contextual fear conditioning deficits produced by neurotoxic lesions of the basolateral amygdala. *J. Neurosci.* 18: 3088–3097.

Maren, S. (1999b). Neurotoxic basolateral amygdala lesions impair learning and memory but not performance of conditional fear in rats. *J. Neurosci.* 19: 8696–8703.

Maren, S., and Baudry, M. (1995). Properties and mechanisms of long-term synaptic plasticity in the mammalian brain: Relationship to learning and memory. *Neurobiol. Learn. Mem.* 63: 1–18.

Maren, S., and Fanselow, M.S. (1995). Synaptic plasticity in the basolateral amygdala induced by hippocampal formation stimulation in vivo. *J. Neurosci.* 15: 7548–7564.

Maren, S., and Fanselow, M.S. (1996). The amygdala and fear conditioning: Has the nut been cracked? *Neuron* 16: 237–240.

Maren, S., and Fanselow, M.S. (1997). Electrolytic lesions of the fimbria/fornix, dorsal hippocampus, or entorhinal cortex produce anterograde deficits in contextual fear conditioning in rats. *Neurobiol. Learn. Mem.* 67: 142–149.

Maren, S., and Fanselow, M.S. (1998). Appetitive motivational states differ in their ability to augment aversive fear conditioning in rats (Rattus norvegicus). *J. Exp. Psychol. Anim. Behav. Process.* 24: 369–373.

Maren, S., Poremba, A., and Gabriel, M. (1991). Basolateral amygdaloid multi-unit neuronal correlates of discriminative avoidance learning in rabbits. *Brain Res.* 549: 311–316.

Maren, S., Patel, K., Thompson, R.F., and Mitchell, D. (1993). Individual differences in emergence neophobia predict magnitude of perforant-path long-term potentiation (LTP) and plasma corticosterone levels in rats. *Psychobiology* 21: 2–10.

Maren, S., De Oca, B., and Fanselow, M.S. (1994a). Sex differences in hippocampal long-term potentiation (LTP) and Pavlovian fear conditioning in rats: Positive correlation between LTP and contextual learning. *Brain Res.* 661: 25–34.

Maren, S., DeCola, J.P., and Fanselow, M.S. (1994b). Water deprivation enhances fear conditioning to contextual, but not discrete, conditional stimuli in rats. *Behav. Neurosci.* 108: 645–649.

Maren, S., DeCola, J.P., Swain, R.A., Fanselow, M.S. et al. (1994c). Parallel augmentation of hippocampal long-term potentiation, theta rhythm, and contextual fear conditioning in water-deprived rats. *Behav. Neurosci.* 108: 44–56.

Maren, S., Tocco, G., Chavanne, F., Baudry, M. et al. (1994d). Emergence neophobia correlates with hippocampal and cortical glutamate receptor binding in rats. *Behav. Neural. Biol.* 62: 68–72.

Maren, S., Aharonov, G., and Fanselow, M.S. (1996a). Retrograde abolition of conditional fear after excitotoxic lesions in the basolateral amygdala of rats: Absence of a temporal gradient. *Behav. Neurosci.* 110: 718–726.

Maren, S., Aharonov, G., Stote, D.L., and Fanselow, M.S. (1996b). N-methyl-D-aspartate receptors in the basolateral amygdala are required for both acquisition and expression of conditional fear in rats. *Behav. Neurosci.* 110: 1365–1374.

Maren, S., Aharonov, G., and Fanselow, M.S. (1997). Neurotoxic lesions of the dorsal hippocampus and Pavlovian fear conditioning in rats. *Behav. Brain Res.* 88: 261–274.

Mayford, M., Bach, M.E., Huang, Y.Y., Wang, L. et al. (1996). Control of memory formation through regulated expression of a CaMKII transgene. *Science* 274: 1678–1683.

McKernan, M.G., and Shinnick-Gallagher, D. (1997). Fear conditioning induces a lasting potentiation of synaptic currents in vitro. *Nature* 340: 607–611.

Meiri, N., Sun, M.K., Segal, Z., Alkon, D.L. (1998). Memory and long-term potentiation (LTP) dissociated: Normal spatial memory despite CA1 LTP elimination with Kv1.4 antisense. *Proc. Natl. Acad. Sci. USA.* 95: 15037–15042.

Miserendino, M.J., Sananes, C.B., Melia, K.R., and Davis, M. (1990). Blocking of acquisition but not expression of conditioned fear-potentiated startle by NMDA antagonists in the amygdala. *Nature (London)* 345: 716–718.

Mitchell, D., Maren, S., and Hwang, R. (1993). The effects of hippocampal lesions on two neotic choice tasks. *Psychobiology* 21: 193–202.

Morris, R.G., Anderson, E., Lynch, G.S., and Baudry, M. (1986). Selective impairment of learning and blockade of long-term potentiation by an N-methyl-D-aspartate receptor antagonist, AP5. *Nature (London)* 319: 774–776.

Morris, R.G., Davis, S., and Butcher, S.P. (1990). Hippocampal synaptic plasticity and NMDA receptors: A role in information storage? *Phil. Trans. R. Soc. London Ser. B.* 329: 187–204.

Muller, J., Corodimas, K.P., Fridel, Z., and LeDoux, J.E. (1997). Functional inactivation of the lateral and basal nuclei of the amygdala by muscimol infusion prevents fear conditioning to an explicit conditioned stimulus and to contextual stimuli. *Behav. Neurosci.* 111: 683–691.

Phillips, R.G., and LeDoux, J.E. (1992). Differential contribution of amygdala and hippocampus to cued and contextual fear conditioning. *Behav. Neurosci.* 106: 274–285.

Quirk, G.J., Repa, C., and LeDoux, J.E. (1995). Fear conditioning enhances short-latency auditory responses of lateral amygdala neurons: Parallel recordings in the freely behaving rat. *Neuron* 15: 1029–1039.

Quirk, G.J., Armony, J.L., and LeDoux, J.E. (1997). Fear conditioning enhances different temporal components of tone-evoked spike trains in auditory cortex and lateral amygdala. *Neuron* 19: 613–624.

Rescorla, R.A. (1988). Behavioral studies of Pavlovian conditioning. *Annu. Rev. Neurosci.* 11: 329–352.

Rogan, M.T., and LeDoux, J.E. (1995). LTP is accompanied by commensurate enhancement of auditory-evoked responses in a fear conditioning circuit. *Neuron* 15: 127–136.

Rogan, M.T., and LeDoux, J.E. (1996). Emotion: Systems, cells, synaptic plasticity. *Cell* 85: 469–475.

Rogan, M.T., Staubli, U.V., and LeDoux, J.E. (1997a). AMPA receptor facilitation accelerates fear learning without altering the level of conditioned fear acquired. *J. Neurosci.* 17: 5928–5935.

Rogan, M.T., Staubli, U.V., and LeDoux, J.E. (1997b). Fear conditioning induces associative long-term potentiation in the amygdala. *Nature (London)* 390: 604–607.

Romanski, L.M., and LeDoux, J.E. (1992). Equipotentiality of thalamo-amygdala and thalamo-cortico-amygdala circuits in auditory fear conditioning. *J. Neurosci.* 12: 4501–4509.

Romanski, L.M., Clugnet, M.C., Bordi, F., and LeDoux, J.E. (1993). Somatosensory and auditory convergence in the lateral nucleus of the amygdala. *Behav. Neurosci.* 107: 444–450.

Rosen, J.B., Hitchcock, J.M., Miserendino, M.J., Falls, W.A. et al. (1992). Lesions of the perirhinal cortex but not of the frontal, medial prefrontal, visual, or insular cortex block fear-potentiated startle using a visual conditioned stimulus. *J. Neurosci.* 12: 4624–4633.

Rudy, J.W. (1996). Postconditioning isolation disrupts contextual conditioning: An experimental analysis. *Behav. Neurosci.* 110: 238–246.

Rudy, J.W., and Sutherland, R.J. (1995). Configural association theory and the hippocampal formation: An appraisal and reconfiguration. *Hippocampus* 5: 375–389.

Sah, P., Hestrin, S., and Nicoll, R.A. (1989). Tonic activation of NMDA receptors by ambient glutamate enhances excitability of neurons. *Science* 246: 815–818.

Sananes, C.B., and Davis, M. (1992). N-methyl-D-aspartate lesions of the lateral and basolateral nuclei of the amygdala block fear-potentiated startle and shock sensitization of startle. *Behav. Neurosci.* 106: 72–80.

Saucier, D., and Cain, D.P. (1995). Spatial learning without NMDA receptor-dependent long-term potentiation [see comments]. *Nature* 378: 186–189.

Schafe, G.E., Nadel, N.V., Sullivan, G.M., Harris, A. et al. (1999). Memory consolidation for contextual and auditory fear conditioning is dependent on protein synthesis, PKA, and MAP kinase. *Learning Memory* 6: 97–110.

Shi, C., and Davis, M. (1999). Pain pathways involved in fear conditioning measured with fear- potentiated startle: Lesion studies. *J. Neurosci.* 19: 420–430.

Shors, T.J., and Matzel, L.D. (1997). Long-term potentiation: What's learning got to do with it? *Behav. Brain Sci.* 20: 597–614; discussion 614–655.

Squire, L.R., and Zola-Morgan, S. (1991). The medial temporal lobe memory system. *Science* 253: 1380–1386.

Stiedl, O., Birkenfeld, K., Palve, M., Heine, C. et al. (1998). APV impairs context- but not tone-dependent fear in mice without discrimination between background and foreground conditioning. *Soc. Neurosci. Abstr.* 24: 1902.

Swanson, L.W., and Petrovich, G.D. (1998). What is the amygdala? *Trends Neurosci.* 21: 323–331.

Walker, D.L., and Davis, M. (1997). Double dissociation between the involvement of the bed nucleus of the stria terminalis and the central nucleus of the amygdala in startle increases produced by conditioned versus unconditioned fear. *J. Neurosci.* 17: 9375–9383.

Young, S.L., Bohenek, D.L., and Fanselow, M.S. (1994). NMDA processes mediate anterograde amnesia of contextual fear conditioning induced by hippocampal damage: Immunization against amnesia by context preexposure. *Behav. Neurosci.* 108: 19–29.

Zamanillo, D., Sprengel, R., Hvalby, O., Jensen, V. et al. (1999). Importance of AMPA receptors for hippocampal synaptic plasticity but not for spatial learning. *Science* 284: 1805–1811.

CHAPTER FOUR

Plasticity of the Hippocampal Cellular Representation of Space

Kathryn J. Jeffery

SUMMARY

If the hippocampus is a site for spatial learning, then it should be possible to see changes occurring in its representation of space following learning. How would we recognize such changes? It is argued in this chapter that if the synaptic plasticity hypothesis of learning is true, then to attribute changes in neuronal activity to memory formation, we need (1) to know what the neurons' inputs were before and after learning, and (2) to show that these changed in a meaningful way. By "meaningful" is meant that they altered the cognitive representation in a manner congruent with the actual experience of the animal. Although it is not yet feasible to record single inputs onto hippocampal cells in awake, behaving animals, it *is* possible to infer the strengths of these inputs by recording the responses of the neurons to environmental stimuli. By showing that the inputs change in an appropriate way following experience, it is possible to derive a simplified model of memory formation that looks at the cognitive representation directly, independent of the animal's behavior. This approach may circumvent some of the difficulties involved in trying to relate very low-level processes, such as synaptic plasticity, with very high-level processes, such as behavior.

Introduction

The hypothesis that a long-term potentiation (LTP)-like process underlies memory formation has the drawback that it is difficult to think of an experimental result

The work described here was carried out in John O'Keefe's laboratory. The author would like to thank John for many illuminating discussions over the past 6 years, and for reviewing this chapter. Colin Lever and Neil Burgess also provided helpful comments. Sean Mathieson conducted the adjacent-box experiment. Stephen Burton, Jim Donnett, Dave Edwards, and Clive Parker gave valuable technical assistance. The work was supported by an MRC programme grant to John O'Keefe.

that could definitively refute it. For every piece of evidence that appears to falsify the hypothesis, there is either another piece of evidence or a hand-waving argument that explains it away. To complicate matters further, even if the hypothesis *were* true, the evidence supporting it to date is so complex and contradictory that it would be difficult ever to convince a true skeptic of the fact. How, then, to arrive at a consensus one way or another?

This situation seems to exist because the memory systems are extremely complex, both anatomically and physiologically, and there are many possible paths of causality linking the very low-level processes of synaptic change (if they exist) with the very high-level processes of behavior. Where we seem to run aground is in not really having a clear picture of what goes on in the middle. The purpose of this chapter is to look at what *does* go on in the middle, to see if it can help us understand whether LTP does or does not mediate learning. The middle ground is the domain of the cognitive representation, the collective activity of neurons that maps the inputs of a structure onto the outputs, and the low-level processes onto the high-level ones. In order to really understand how synaptic processes contribute to behavior, we cannot ignore this representation.

Since the hippocampus has been the target of most studies in both LTP and memory research, the discussion to follow looks at one kind of cognitive representation that the hippocampus seems specialized for, the representation of space. The questions to be asked are these: How is this representation put together, how is it modified by experience, and what are the mechanisms of this modification?

The Hippocampal Cellular Representation of Space

An enormous weight of evidence points to a role for the hippocampus in representing space and/or mediating spatial learning. It is outside the scope of this chapter to examine this evidence in detail, but useful discussions can be found in O'Keefe and Nadel (1978) and Jarrard (1993). We shall also leave aside the contentious issue of whether the hippocampus also has some role in nonspatial cognition. If spatial memory forms at least part of its function, then that is enough for us to begin to tackle the question of how it does this, leaving until later the question of whether it does anything else besides.

One of the most convincing findings to support the spatial cognition hypothesis of hippocampal function came from the discovery by O'Keefe, in the early 1970s, that hippocampal principal cells show spatially localized firing (O'Keefe and Dostrovsky, 1971). O'Keefe was recording single hippocampal cells from rats as they explored an environment, and found that the activity of one class of cell (complex spiking cells, presumed to be the pyramidal cells) showed a very high correlation with the location of the animal. O'Keefe named these cells *place cells* to reflect the high spatial specificity of their activity. An example of the receptive field (the *place field*) of a place cell is shown in Figure 4.1A. In the example shown here, the cell indicated by the black squares was generally silent as the rat wandered over most of the environment (in this case, a square box) foraging for rice grains. However, whenever the rat walked into a particular part of the box (in this

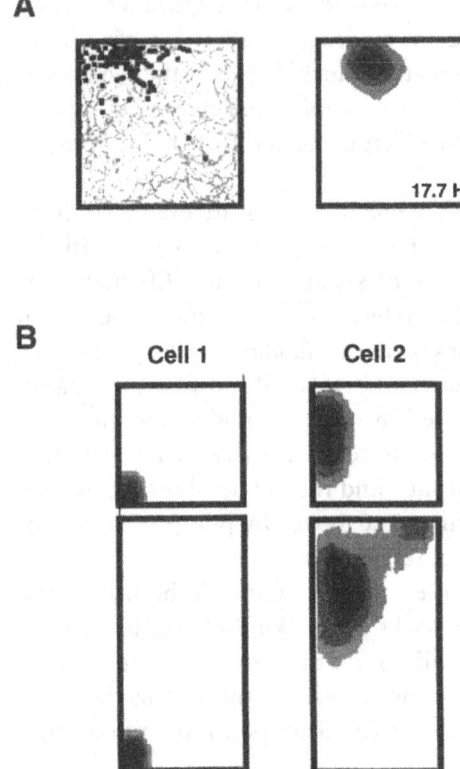

Figure 4.1. (A) Example of a place field recorded in a square box, 60 × 60 cm. **Left:** The gray stippled area shows the places where the rat walked during the 4 minutes of recording. Every time the place cell fired, a small black square was marked on the place where the rat was at the time. This particular cell fired whenever the rat was in the Northwest corner of the box, and was almost silent everywhere else. **Right:** The same data after smoothing and averaging, to show the contour plot representing the field. The peak firing rate of the cell is shown in the bottom right. (B) The behavior of two place cells in the O'Keefe and Burgess moving-walls experiment, showing how different place cells respond to different subsets of the environmental features. Cell 1 maintained its relationship to the South and West walls, while Cell 2 maintained its relationship with the North and West walls. Thus, when the distance between the North and South walls was increased, the fields of the cells were "pulled" apart.

case the Northwest corner) the cell increased its firing rate markedly, reducing it to near zero as the rat walked out of it again.

After ascertaining that these cells were not responding to any particular simple sensory feature in the environment, O'Keefe and Nadel (1978) proposed that they were participating in a maplike representation of space [or what O'Keefe and Nadel called a "cognitive map," an expression coined by Tolman (1948)]. The finding of place cells was supported by emerging evidence from lesion studies that rats with damage to the hippocampus could not solve spatial tasks if these tasks seemed to require the use of some kind of mental map. It seemed, then, that the hippocampus might be some kind of spatial processor within the brain, whose function is to compute where the rat is so that it can navigate to some desirable goal.

If place cells are participating in the hippocampal representation of space, then as the rat learns about its environment, one might expect to see this representation change in some way. Two broad classes of learning could be postulated *a priori*. First, when a rat enters a new environment, it may form an internal representation of the geometry and the salient landmarks, a kind of automatic learning that need not depend on any particular reward (other than the satisfaction of exploratory drive). Second, once it has found a goal (i.e., something in the environment that produces a reward), if the rat is to be able to get back there again it must add the location and nature of that goal into its mental map. These two functions together mean that in the future, when the rat reenters the environment, it (1) recognizes it, and (2) knows where the goal locations are within it. The two processes differ in that the initial mapping may be *latent* (i.e., not visible to an observer) whereas the second process, goal learning, will be manifest as a subsequent tendency for the rat to go straight to the goal whenever it finds itself in that environment again. Most of the discussion in this chapter will be about latent learning, a kind of learning that is much more accessible to physiologists than to psychologists (who have to infer its existence from the way the animal's subsequent behavior changes).

Plasticity

If place cells change their representation to incorporate new spatial knowledge, what kinds of changes would be observed? It is not enough merely to see experience-dependent changes in cellular activity, because such changes might occur during learning for reasons unrelated to memory formation per se. For example, although a neuron in the motor cortex might increase its firing during the course of a session in which a rat is learning to press a lever for food, this does not necessarily mean that the neuron is participating in that memory (although it might be). It may be just a reflection of the fact that the cortex is receiving an increased number of motor commands from somewhere upstream, where the memory *is* being formed. It is important to dissociate changes due to memory itself from changes due to the altered behavioral and emotional state of the animal.

What *is* memory, then, and how could it be observed at a cellular level? To a physiologist, memory is a meaningful change in a cognitive representation following experience, where the changes occur *on the representing cells*. By "meaningful" is meant that the changes are consistent with what might be expected given that we know what the animal experienced, and therefore how the cognitive representation *ought* to have changed. These changes correspond to what Lashley called the *engram*, or the memory trace. We now think, thanks to the insights of Konorski (1948) and Hebb (1949), that the memory trace might consist of changes in connection strength between neurons resulting from their coactivity. As such, it could only be detectable by knowing the state of the neurons (including the strength of each input) before the learning event, and comparing that with what it became afterward.

To understand memory, then, we need to understand

1. What a set of neurons encodes
2. What changes about the representation as a result of experience
3. How these changes occur
4. What the new representation encodes

The hippocampal representation of space is an ideal candidate for this approach to the memory problem, since we now understand much about what its neurons encode. Having established (1), or at least part of (1), how do we go about moving through the remaining steps?

An Associative Approach to Learning by Place Cells

The idea that memories are stored as changes in synaptic strength was first formalized by Hebb (1949), who suggested that the changes should occur as a result of coactivity between the two connected cells, thus providing a mechanism for the association of activity patterns. If Hebb was right, then when a neural representation undergoes learning we would expect to see synaptic changes taking place between coactive neurons involved in this representation. This would have the effect that after learning, a given cell would receive a different pattern of inputs from what it had received before the learning.

To look for associative processes occurring in place cells, it is necessary to know the strengths of the inputs impinging on the cells before and after learning. This is not an easy matter, since it is still not feasible to record from single synapses in awake animals (hence the attractiveness of LTP as an experimental tool). However, one way around this problem is to measure not the physiologic inputs, but the *sensory* inputs. In other words, we can perform what amount to psychological experiments on the place cells by treating each cell as if it were itself a miniature animal, processing incoming stimuli and producing observable responses. Knowing how a place cell responds to a sensory input is not the same as knowing about its synapses. The sensory integration and plasticity may be taking place somewhere upstream from the cell (as we shall see later). However, it enables an assessment of how strongly a given cell is responding to an environmental stimulus, and therefore provides an indirect measure of the strength of a particular pathway between the sensory cortex and the cell. When learning takes place, then if the associativity hypothesis of memory is correct, one would expect to see this pathway change in strength. This is an important first step in localizing the engram, and one that enables the testing of many hypotheses regarding memory formation, without recourse to the recording of synapses themselves.

This, then, is the strategy adopted in the experiments described below. The sequence of steps is as follows:

1. First, identify the sensory inputs to a particular cell.
2. Second, determine which are stronger and which are weaker.
3. Third, change something about the sensory environment in a way that would predictably force learning to occur.
4. Fourth, reassess the relative input strengths. Have they changed? More important, have they changed in a way that accords with what happened in (3)?

Identify the Inputs Onto Place Cells and Assess Their Relative Strengths

What *are* the sensory inputs onto place cells? In other words, how does a place cell know where the rat is?

The most obvious explanation is that perhaps each cell responds to a simple sensory characteristic of the environment, such as a localized odor, and only fires when that sensory stimulus is present. A large body of evidence now exists to show that this is not the case. One of the simplest demonstrations was provided by O'Keefe and Burgess (1996), who recorded place cells in boxes of varying sizes and shapes. The walls of the boxes were constructed out of the same four pieces of wood, clamped together in different ways so that in any given recording session a given wall could be North, South, East, or West and either short or long. The paper covering the floor was also changed periodically. O'Keefe and Burgess found that provided the shape and size of the box were the same, a place cell would always fire in the same place in the box regardless of the arrangement of the walls and floor paper, even if the box were moved around within the room (within certain limits). Thus, the firing of a place cell could only be explained by a combination of sensory features *plus* some kind of spatial information (such as direction and distance; see below).

O'Keefe and Burgess then altered the size and shape of the box by moving some of the walls with respect to the others. They found that somewhat surprisingly, different place cells responded in different ways to this maneuver. Some cells retained their relationship to some walls, and some to others. Other cells stopped firing, or began firing when they had been silent previously. An illustration of such a change is found in Figure 4.1B. This finding has been corroborated by others (e.g., Gothard et al., 1996) and it now appears that when a change is made to an environment, each place cell acts as if it only knows about a subset of the features in the environment, and is oblivious to the remainder. This is an important finding as it suggests that a single place cell cannot code for the location of the rat by itself. Only the combined activity of several or many cells can represent the location of the rat uniquely. O'Keefe and Burgess proposed a model in which each place cell fires maximally when the rat is within a certain distance of a subset of the walls of the box.

The walls that a given place cell responds to will henceforth be referred to as its *proximal* inputs. The proximal inputs to a place cell must be strong, because the box as a whole can usually be moved around over small distances within a room and the fields will follow it around. However, if a box is moved a large enough distance from one part of a room to another, some cells respond to this change by altering or abolishing their fields when the box is in one location, but not when it is in another, as discussed later. This shows that at least some place cells receive information from regions of the environment outside the box. These inputs will henceforth be called the *distal* inputs. The inputs supplied to a place cell by extended surfaces such as walls will be called the cell's *geometric* inputs.

Place cells also seem to make use of nongeometric information. For example, Muller and his colleagues have shown that moving a rat from a cylindrical environment of one color to an identically shaped cylinder of a different color causes place cells to change their fields (Bostock et al., 1991; Kentros et al., 1998). Thus, although the location of a given place field depends on the geometry of the environment, the nongeometric features sometimes seem able to tell the cell whether or not to fire in that location. This leads to the intriguing possibility that the nongeometric inputs *gate* the geometric inputs, telling the place cell which set of inputs to respond to in a given environment. We will return to this possibility later.

What happens in an environment that conveys ambiguous geometric information? For example, in a square environment such as that of O'Keefe and Burgess (1996), where the walls were interchanged, a place cell that is predisposed to fire in a particular geometric location (e.g., 6 cm from one wall and 20 cm from the adjacent wall) has four possible firing locations. How does it know which one to choose, if the walls are all identical? As well as the geometric and nongeometric inputs, a place cell clearly must have some additional information about the location of the rat. One possibility is that the cells can distinguish the walls on the basis of their direction.

We tested this hypothesis in an experiment in which the rat was misled into thinking that North lay in some other direction (East, South, or West; Jeffery, 1998; Jeffery and O'Keefe, 1999). Place cells were recorded as the rat foraged for rice grains in a square box contained within a circular curtained environment. Because of the visual symmetry of both the box and its surround, the only visible directional cue was a large white card, lit by a spotlight and hanging just in front of the curtains, aligned with one of the four walls of the box. Before some trials, the rat was hidden under an opaque cover and then the card moved to a new location behind one of the other box walls. When the rat was released and allowed to forage again, the place fields were consistently found also to have rotated, so that they had the same relationship to the cue card as before.

This control by a cue card over place fields has been previously described by several investigators (O'Keefe and Conway, 1980; Muller et al., 1987; Muller and Kubie, 1987; Knierim et al., 1995; Hetherington and Shapiro, 1997; Rotenberg and Muller, 1997) and is well established. It shows that place cells have *visual directional* inputs. In other words, although the actual location of the fields within the box (the x-y coordinates, so to speak) is governed by the geometric cues supplied by the box walls, the choice of which walls to use (i.e., which is to be "x" and which "y") is governed by the visual cues, either on the walls of the box or outside the box altogether (but not, interestingly, inside it; Cressant et al., 1997), which seem to act like a compass.

What happens when there is no visual directional information available? In the above apparatus, the cue card was removed and place cells recorded again. The results for a typical cell are shown in Figure 4.2A. The first thing to notice is that the field was still localized to a single location within the box, that is, its pattern did not possess fourfold symmetry, even though the environment itself now did. The cell must therefore still have had *some* directional information available. This time, when the rat was enclosed under the opaque cover, the rat itself was rotated (by rotating the piece of box floor that it was standing on) for some multiple of 90 degrees, at a very slow rate that was intended to be undetectable to it. When the rat was released and allowed to forage again, the place field was found to have rotated by the same amount as the rat. This pattern was observed in all four rats tested, and it suggests that the directional information was somehow contained within the rats and carried along with them.

There is now considerable evidence that some kind of directional information can indeed be "contained within" an animal, in the sense of being independent of

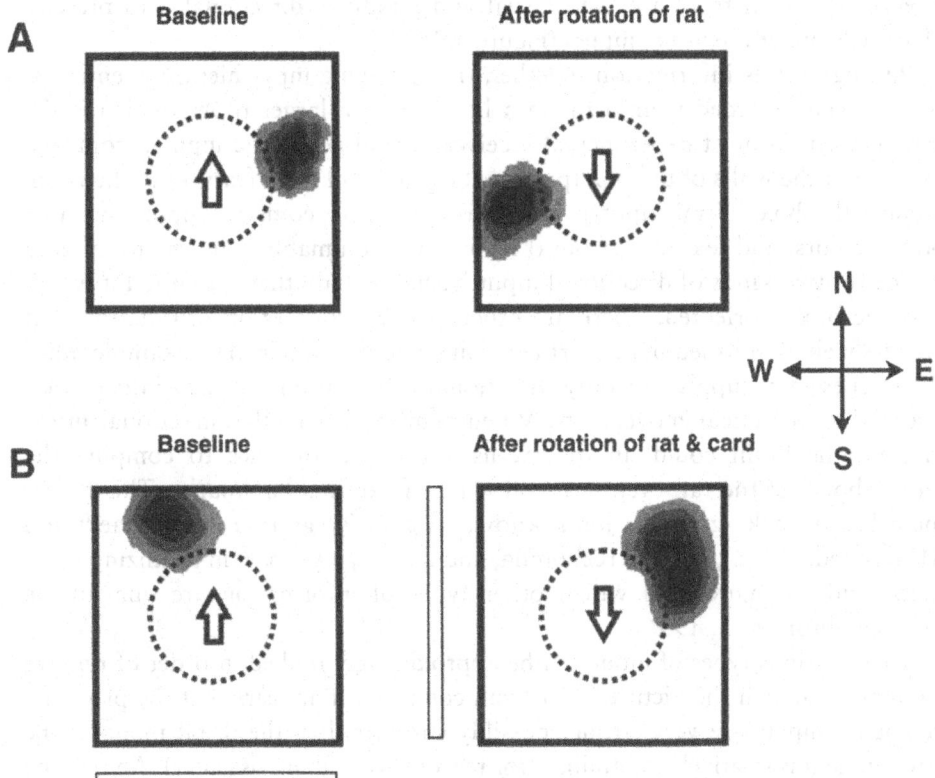

Figure 4.2. (A) The effect of idiothetic cues on the orientation of a place field. **Left box:** Before rotation of the rat, this field lay in the Northeast corner of the box. The rat was then confined under an opaque cover to the circular platter comprising the center of the box floor. This platter was then slowly rotated 180 degrees, and the rat released and allowed to forage again. **Right box:** Now the place field was found in the Southwest corner of the box, suggesting that its orientation with the otherwise symmetrical box was influenced not by external cues, but rather by cues contained within the rat and rotated along with it. (B) When the procedure in A was repeated in the presence of a cue card (shown by the white rectangle), which was rotated by a different amount, the field rotated with the cue card and not with the rat's idiothetic cues. This suggests that the visual directional inputs to this cell were stronger than the idiothetic inputs.

external landmarks (although not independent of external sensory information per se). This *idiothetic* information, which derives from the movements of the animal, is synthesized (Blair and Sharp, 1996) from a mixture of vestibular and proprioceptive information, optic flow (which provides information about movement even if there are no landmarks present), and also probably motor commands (motor efference copy; Taube et al., 1996). The rotation of place fields with rotation of the rat shows that place cells have access to idiothetic directional information when visual directional cues are unavailable. However, recall that when the cue card was present, place fields tended to follow its movements even though these conflicted with the rat's idiothetic cues. It thus appears (at least in this experiment) that when there are both visual and idiothetic directional cues present, place cells prefer the visual inputs (Figure 4.2B).

Putting all this information together, the following input hierarchy emerges. A place cell recorded from a rat in a box within a larger room (which is the arrangement in most experiments) receives several geometric inputs, from two or more of the walls of the box (proximal inputs) and from features in the room outside the box (distal inputs). It also receives nongeometric inputs (such as odors, colors, and textures), from the box and presumably from the room, and it receives two kinds of directional input, visual and idiothetic, that tell it which way the box is oriented. There are other possible sources of information that are less well established but nevertheless likely to play a part. For example, idiothetic cues may supply not only directional information but also information about the rat's linear movements. When combined with the directional information, the brain could, in theory, use these motion cues to compute the whereabouts of the rat, even in the absence of external landmarks. This movement-based tracking of location is known as *path integration* (Mittelstaedt and Mittelstaedt, 1982), or dead reckoning, and it may play a part in localizing place fields under situations in which other types of information are unavailable (McNaughton et al., 1996).

These various types of input can be approximately ranked in order of relative strength, although the picture is far from complete. It appears that the proximal geometric inputs are very strong, possibly stronger than the distal inputs if the environment is relatively unfamiliar (for reasons we will discuss later). Among the proximal inputs, some are stronger than others for a given cell, as evidenced from O'Keefe and Burgess's experiment where the walls were pulled apart. Within the directional inputs, the visual inputs appear to be stronger than the idiothetic inputs, at least in some situations.

The finding that there is a hierarchy of input strengths among the inputs onto place cells opens the door to experiments that attempt to manipulate these inputs, provoking a reordering of the hierarchy, a simple form of learning. The next section describes the results of two such experiments.

Change the Sensory Environment So As to Force Learning, and Reassess the Input Strengths

■ **Experiment 1: The Directional Inputs.** This experiment began with the observation that in our apparatus, visual directional inputs appear to be stronger than the idiothetic ones, as discussed earlier. The intention was to manipulate the inputs so as to make the strong input relatively weaker and the weak one relatively stronger. We reasoned that one situation under which this might occur is if the visual cue were mobile, and therefore unsuitable to act as a spatial landmark. It seems not unreasonable that the spatial system in the hippocampus (or near it) should have evolved a mechanism to rapidly disconnect a mobile object from its representation (Knierim et al., 1995; Biegler and Morris, 1996).

The apparatus was that used in the directional experiments described above: a square box located inside a circular curtained arena in which a white cue card supplied a strong, visual directional signal. The relative strengths of the visual and idiothetic directional inputs onto place cells were tested each day by "conflict" trials in which the rat was enclosed under a cover on the rotating part of the box floor. For each of these trials, the rat was slowly rotated by a multiple of 90 and the card moved by a different multiple of 90, thereby dissociating the visual and idiothetic cues. Place fields were then recorded to see if they had rotated with the card or the rat, thus revealing their preferred directional input.

The learning phase of this experiment took place in the trials preceding these test trials. For some rats, the cue card was visibly moved before each trial. This was achieved by unhooking the card from the curtain rail from which it was suspended, carrying it (in full view of the rat) to a different location behind one of the other walls of the box, and then rehanging it. The rat was therefore able to see that the card was mobile. According to the disconnection hypothesis, these rats should experience a weakening of the influence of the card over their place fields. The remaining four rats, which had been covered during movement of the card, were never given an opportunity to see the card move and should, according to the hypothesis, experience no change in the relative influence of the cue card on the orientation of their fields.

Figure 4.3 shows the results of the test trials, in which the relative strengths of the visual and idiothetic inputs were compared. In rats that had previously seen the card move, the fields gradually stopped following the card and started rotating with the rats' idiothetic cues instead. Place fields in the other rats followed the cue card on all test trials, regardless of the rotation of the rat and its idiothetic cues. Thus, allowing rats to see that a directional indicator was mobile resulted in a weakening of this input and a strengthening of the previously weaker idiothetic inputs.

Two rats from the group that had never seen the card move were subjected to further testing (Jeffery, 1998). First, they underwent several days of recording where, after the test trials, the idiothetic cues were tested in isolation. The results from this phase of testing showed that despite the card's superior control when it was present, the idiothetic cues were still able to influence place fields in the absence of competition. Then the rats underwent 5 days during which, after testing, the card was moved visibly. In these rats, the cue card continued to influence place fields reliably despite the fact that the rats could now see it move. This rather surprising finding seems to indicate that once the cue card had exerted control over place field orientation for some time, the place cells continued to "trust" it even despite its manifest unreliability. This suggests that during the first phases of the experiment, when no learning appeared to be going on, an already strong input was in fact getting even stronger.

How did the place cells "know" that the visual cue was mobile? There seem to be two possibilities. First, perhaps the card activated visual motion-detectors that alerted some part of the brain (such as the object recognition system) to that cue's unreliability. The system could then tag its representation for that object as

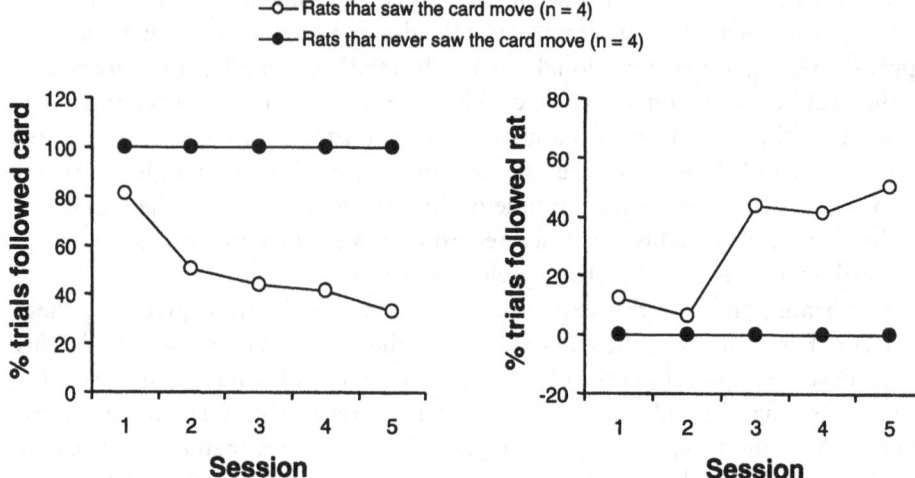

Figure 4.3. Results of trials in which the rat was covered and slowly rotated by one amount, while the card was rotated by a different amount. The left graph shows the percentage of trials in which the fields, after release of the rat, were found to have followed the card. The right graph shows the percentage of trials in which they were found to have followed the rat. The behavior of the fields differed depending on whether the rats had previously seen that the card was mobile. In rats that had seen the card move, the fields stopped following the card and started rotating by the same amount as the rat had been rotated, suggesting an increasing influence of the idiothetic cues with time. In rats that never saw the card move, the fields reliably continued to follow it.

"mobile" or "unreliable" and pass on its tagged output as a weakened input to the spatial system. Note that this is a process that would not necessarily evoke any kind of associative or Hebbian process (in other words, no coactivity need have occurred). On the other hand, Knierim et al. (1995) have suggested that a mobile cue might be recognized as mobile not because of motion detection per se but because the spatial system recognizes that information about its location repeatedly conflicts with idiothetic information. For example, if the idiothetic system tells the rat's hippocampus that the rat is not moving, but the cue changes its location relative to the rat, then the cue itself must be moving. Thus, the idiothetic and the visual systems may compare information to help decide whether an external sensory stimulus is moving or not. This process, if it occurs, could well be associative.

We found that in trials where the rat was rotated by one amount and the card by a different amount, this resulting conflict did not appear to weaken the visual cue at all, provided the rat had never seen the card moving. This seems to suggest that Knierim et al. were wrong in their supposition, and that it was the experience of seeing the card move that caused the place cells to shift their allegiance. However, there is one other important difference between the rats that saw the card move and those that did not, and this is that the latter group was isolated under an opaque cover for between 2 and 4 minutes while the card was being moved. Could it be that this visual (and motor) deprivation weakened the idiothetic cues, causing the fields to continue to follow the card even though it was mobile?

We tested this hypothesis by recording place cells from a third group of four rats that never saw the card move but for which the period of enclosure under the cover was made as brief as possible (30 seconds only, which is the time it took to move the card). If the critical factor was whether the rats perceived the motion of the card visually, then this group, still deprived of such information, should behave no differently from the rats that were enclosed for 2 to 4 minutes. It turned out, however, that this group's behavior was midway between that of the other groups. Fields in two rats behaved like those in rats that had never seen the card move (always following the card) and those in the other two behaved like rats that *had* seen it move (their fields stopped following the card and started following the rat). Since these rats had not seen the card move either, this suggests that perhaps it was not the movement of the card per se that was the crucial factor, but rather the amount of time that the rat was unable to move around and see its environment. Perhaps the isolation of the rat caused the idiothetic cues to weaken. If this were the case, it follows that perhaps if the card could be moved instantaneously, then even if the rats did not actually *see* the card move, their fields might nevertheless stop following the card too.

The above explanation, although complex, is not implausible because it is likely that the idiothetic direction sense needs a constant supply of visual information to keep it updated. If this information is withheld, as it is when the rat is incarcerated under its opaque cover, then perhaps the idiothetic cues get weaker. This might be why the card always "wins" in such competitions. However, if the card is moved when the rat is uncovered, then the full-strength idiothetic system can perhaps compete successfully with the visual cue. It is just a short step from there to positing that such repeated disjunctions could cause the visual cue to be weakened, by a Hebbian (or rather anti-Hebbian) mechanism such as long-term depression (LTD).

In summary, then, the findings of this experiment show that directional inputs onto place cells can be rearranged in strength following a learning experience. The nature of this rearrangement seems consistent with the nature of the information being learned: That is, a strong (visual) input became relatively weaker when it was made an unreliable indicator of direction, a weak (idiothetic) input became stronger, and a strong input seemed to become even stronger when it had been experienced as reliable for some time. Thus, the change in the cognitive representation accords with what one would expect of a memory trace. Does this mean that the place cells *themselves* learned about the spatial cues? Is the engram for directional landmark stability contained within them?

The answer for this particular experiment is probably "no." It was mentioned earlier that to consider a cell to be part of a memory trace, it is necessary to know that the change in its behavior originates from changes in that cell itself. While the place cells in this experiment certainly experienced a change in the strength of environmental inputs, there is reason to think that the inputs did not change on the place cells themselves. This reason is that when learning was occurring (in the rats that were seeing the cue card move around) the place cells always changed their firing patterns together. When one cell stopped rotating with the cue card and started rotating with the rat, all simultaneously recorded cells did so in unison. On no occasion was it ever observed that one cell rotated its field with the cue card while, *at the same time,* another cell rotated with the rat's idiothetic cues. This would be surprising if the input rearrangement was happening on place cell synapses, since one would expect (for purely statistical reasons) that some cells would learn faster than others. Instead, this observation strongly suggests that the learning was taking place elsewhere and that an integrated, coherent signal was being passed onto the place cells. There are several brain regions, such as the postsubiculum (Taube et al., 1990a, 1990b), thalamus (Taube, 1995), and other structures (Chen et al., 1994a, 1994b) that process directional information directly and express their computation in the form of the activity of *head direction cells.* The firing of these cells is highly correlated with the direction that the rat's head is pointing at a given moment, and we also know that brain regions containing head direction cells do communicate with the hippocampus (albeit indirectly). It thus seems likely that the learning revealed in this experiment was taking place in one of the head direction areas. A discussion of how and where this integration may be achieved can be found in Taube et al. (1996).

Two conclusions about learning can be drawn from this experiment. First, learning can be observed at a cellular level by exposing an animal to a change in its environment and recording a change in the way the cells behave subsequently. If this change makes sense in the context of what we know the cells are representing (and in this case it does) then it seems likely that what is observed is learning itself, and not a by-product of it even though it was never expressed as a change in the overt behavior of the animal. "Likely" does not mean "proven," however. Second, it is not enough merely to observe such a change. It is also necessary to know that the change was localized to those cells themselves. In this case, there are strong grounds for thinking this is not the case.

■ **Experiment 2: The Geometric Inputs.** The second experiment examined another pair of place cell inputs in which there appears to be a difference in input strengths: the proximal and distal inputs. Recall that the proximal inputs generally seem to be very much stronger, as evidenced by the observation that moving a box around within a room causes fields to shift along with the box, rather than remaining attached to the room. We tested whether these relative strengths could be varied by creating a conflict between them (that is, by moving the proximal cues with respect to the distal cues). In other words, could a place cell be forced to learn over time that the proximal and distal cues did not always coincide, and modify their representation accordingly?

Three rats participated in this experiment. The apparatus used was a 72 cm square box, which lacked a floor so that the rat walked around on paper taped to the floor of the room. Since this paper was fixed throughout all the trials on each day (although changed each day), the floor effectively constituted one of the "static" cues. The box, which was 25 cm high, was located inside the curtained-off arena described in the previous experiment, so that the rat, if it looked up, could see only the curtains and the ceiling. This was done so as to minimize the salience of the distal cues and slow down learning enough for it to be measured on a day-by-day basis. To provide a weak directional cue, a spotlight was shone on the North side of the curtains so that there was a gradient of illumination across the environment from North to South. For one rat, a cue card was also present, to enable rotation of the direction sense (by the covering procedure described above) and therefore disconnection from the static olfactory cues in the arena. The lighting, in conjunction with the rat's idiothetic direction sense, was intended to keep the rat directionally oriented while the nondirectional aspects of the environment changed.

Place cells were recorded as the proximal and distal cues were dissociated by moving the box back and forth between two locations that overlapped slightly. The rat remained within the box enclosure during the moving of the box so that no disruption to its path integration system was introduced. The question asked in this experiment was, Did the box-moving procedure cause place cells to alter the relative pattern of inputs from the two sources of information? Each session consisted of four pairs of trials, alternating between the two locations, so that any changes seen could be checked for stability.

Fifty-four cells were analyzed in detail, of which six had variable fields and were therefore excluded. At first, moving the box back and forth between the two locations did not appear to affect the place cell representation much, if at all. The majority of cells shifted their fields along with the box and did not appear to "notice" that the pattern of distal cues was different in the two locations. Over time, however, more and more cells began to differentiate the two locations, behaving differently in one box location than the other. Cells that showed different behavior in the two box locations were called *discriminating* cells and those that had the same field in both places were called *nondiscriminating*. In total, twenty cells were discriminating and twenty-eight were nondiscriminating. Figure 4.4A shows an example of three cells, one of which did not discriminate (cell 1) and two that fired only when the box was in the Northwest location (cell 2) or the Southeast location (cell 3).

The proportions of discriminating and nondiscriminating cells did not, however, remain constant over time. Figure 4.4B shows that over the course of several sessions, the proportion of nondiscriminating cells decreased and the proportion of discriminating cells increased. A chi-square analysis comparing the first two sessions with the last two sessions showed a significant change in the proportions of discriminating versus nondiscriminating cells ($\chi^2 = 6.30$, $df = 1$, $p < .05$). Usually a discriminating cell possessed a field only in one or another location, but occasionally a cell demonstrated a different field in one of the two locations. On one occasion, a cell was observed to change from nondiscriminating to discriminating behavior, suggesting that individual cells might be able to change their behavior.

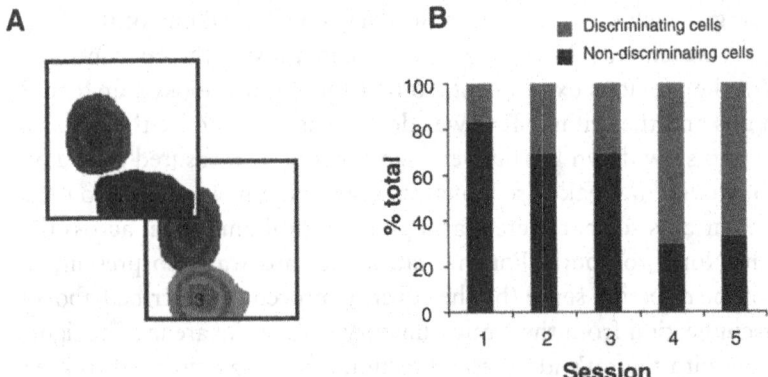

Figure 4.4. Discrimination of geometrically identical environments by place cells. When a box was moved from its Northwest location in the curtained arena to its Southeast location, most cells maintained their fields in the usual position within the box. However, over time, cells appeared that showed discriminatory behavior, firing differently in the two locations. (A) Cell 1 was nondiscriminating, having the same field in both the Northwest and Southeast box locations, while cells 2 and 3 discriminated the two locations, firing only when the box was in one of them. (B) Histogram showing the relative proportions of discriminating versus nondiscriminating cells over time.

How did the cells discriminate the two locations? One possibility is that they were able to use information generated by the movement of the rat (path integration) as it walked from location Northwest to location Southeast when the box was moved. The other possibility is that they were able to use information from distal cues as the primary discriminative stimulus. We attempted to discriminate these two possibilities in a fourth animal. For this rat, the visually identical environments were adjacent, both constructed out of pieces of gray laminated wood, 60 cm square, that were rearranged between trials or between sessions. The pieces were arranged so as to form adjacent rectangular enclosures, a West box and an East box, that were 120 cm long × 60 cm wide and that shared one of the long walls. The floor was covered with white paper that was rotated, inverted, or changed completely at the start of each day. When the rat was required to move under its own volition from one box to the other, one of the pieces of wood forming the dividing wall was pulled back to open up a gap in the center of the wall. After the rat had passed through, this gap was closed up again. Because the outside walls of the box also had a join in the center, closure of the gap meant that the East and West boxes became visually identical.

The electrodes remained stable in the CA1 cell layer for several weeks, and ninety-four complex spiking cells were isolated, of which forty-six had stable place fields and proceeded to further analysis. Of these, twenty-six discriminated the two environments and twenty did not. Of the cells that discriminated the environments, fourteen lost a field in one or another box and twelve developed a different field. As in the previous experiment, however, the relative proportions of discriminating and nondiscriminating cells did not remain constant over time.

In the first block of six sessions, only one of the six cells had discriminated the two boxes, and this was only observed on the final day of the block. At the end of this block, the partition between the boxes was opened up to let the rat walk through from the East box to the West. It was predicted that there would be a sudden change in the place cell representation as the rat discovered that there were, in reality, two boxes. This, however, did not happen; there was no change in the pattern of fields in the two boxes (not shown).

For the remainder of the experiment, the rat passed from one box to the other by walking through the gap in the partition, when this was made available. As the days progressed, the proportion of cells showing discriminating behavior changed so that eventually more cells became discriminating than not (Figure 4.5A). Thus, as before, there appeared to be an effect of time on the proportion of cells that fell into each category. A chi-square analysis comparing the first two blocks with the last two blocks showed a significant change in the proportions of discriminating versus nondiscriminating cells ($\chi^2 = 11.31$, $df = 1$, $p < .001$).

What information did the discriminating cells use to know what firing pattern to adopt? Three possibilities seemed likely candidates. First, perhaps the cells used path integration information; in other words, because the rat had the opportunity to walk from one box to the other, perhaps the cells were able to combine this motion information along with sensory information to determine which box was which. Second, perhaps the East box possessed different sensory characteristics (such as odor) from the West box. Third, perhaps the cells could use the slightly

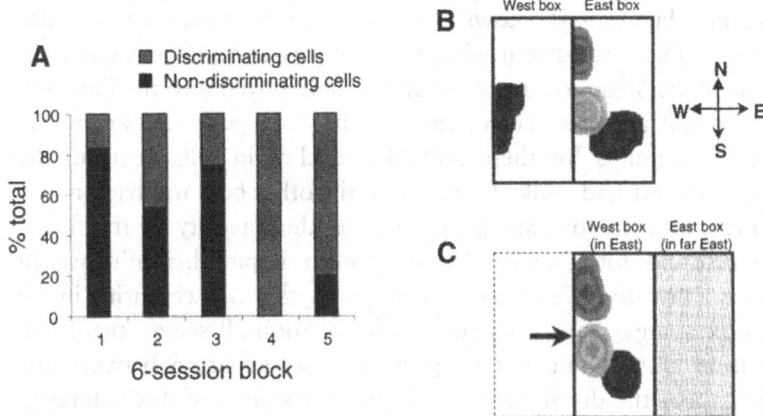

Figure 4.5. (A) Histogram showing the increasing proportion of discriminating cells over time in a rat that walked between two adjacent identical boxes. (B) Fields from three place cells in this apparatus, showing that one cell did not discriminate (fired in the same relative place in both boxes) and two discriminated, firing only in the East box. (C) When the box ensemble (including the floor paper) was moved Eastward, so that the West box lay in the place within the room previously occupied by the East box, the cells adopted the "East" firing pattern, even though the rat had just walked there from the East box (now in a "Far-East" location). This suggests that it was the location of the box within the room, and not either a sensory characteristic of the box or the relative locations of the East and West boxes, that told the cells which firing pattern to exhibit.

different view of the room from the two boxes to distinguish the two, for example, the computer was nearer to the East box, and the door nearer to the West box.

These possibilities were tested by means of probe trials. First, the rat was removed from the environment while the whole box ensemble (the two boxes and the floor paper) was shifted East so that the West box now lay in the position (with respect to the room) formerly occupied by the East box. The rat was then replaced in the West box, and a trial of place cell recording conducted. Then the rat was allowed to walk through to the East box (now in a Far East position). Recording of place fields was not possible from this box as it lay outside the camera viewing area; however, the rat was encouraged to explore this box as usual, and then allowed back into the West box. It was predicted that if path integration were the major determinant in these cells, then at least after the rat's return (if not before) they should fire in the West pattern in the West box, regardless of its location in the room. Similarly, if olfactory information emanating from the box and the floor paper were the determining factors then the cells should also fire in their "West pattern." However, if cues outside the box were the determining factors, then the cells should fire in the "East pattern," even though the rat was in the West half of the box ensemble.

The results of this procedure were examined for fourteen discriminating cells. For the first trial, before the rat had passed into the East box (in the Far East location), ten of the cells fired in the "East" pattern and only one cell fired in the "West" pattern, seeming to rule out olfaction as an important discriminative stimulus. For the second trial, after the rat had passed into the East box and returned to the West box again, seven of the cells fired in the "East" pattern and none fired in the "West" pattern. Figure 4.5B shows a typical result from such a manipulation: the cells fired in the East pattern when the box was shifted eastward, even though the rat was in the West box and even after it had moved into the East box and back again. Thus, it appears that for this rat, the distal room cues were the major discriminative stimulus for these cells. The decline in cells firing in the "East" pattern after the rat had walked through to the other box and back might suggest a disruptive influence of path integration on the integrity of the fields. Nevertheless, the cells did not assume a "West" pattern despite this influence. In fact, at no time was a "relative West" cell ever observed, that is, a cell firing in the West of the two boxes, regardless of its position in the room. It seems, therefore, that path integration alone could not support the discrimination between the boxes, and suggests that the distal cues were a primary source of discriminative information.

The development of a new pattern of place cell activity in an environment is usually called *remapping,* to reflect the belief that it constitutes development of a new representation (map) of the environment. The remapping seen in the identical-box experiments discussed here is unusual because it is an example of what might be called *piecemeal remapping;* in other words, the change happened one cell at a time.

The existence of piecemeal (as contrasted with all-or-nothing) remapping casts some light on how place cells construct and modify their representations. Since the two box locations differed only with respect to their location in the outside room, cells that discriminated the locations seem to have done so by using information from these cues. Assuming that the discrimination was acquired by individual cells (although this was only actually observed directly on one occasion), it seems that the effective input from the distal cues must have become stronger over time. Furthermore, the proximal inputs must have become effectively weaker at the same time. If they had not, then they would still have been able to drive the cells to firing threshold in both box locations, just as they had done previously. That the discriminating cells usually stopped firing in one or the other box location shows that for these cells, the correct configuration of proximal cues was no longer enough to make them fire. Now, the cells appeared to need a conjunction of both the correct proximal *and* the correct distal cues. Figure 4.6 depicts a scheme showing the apparent change in inputs onto these cells over time.

These changes might reflect an associative redistribution of input strengths. Because the proximal cues and distal cues were paired, the distal inputs might have become strengthened because of the coactivity with the firing cell, as it was being driven by the (initially strong) proximal inputs. However, there are alternative, nonassociative explanations for the changes in input strength. Perhaps the distal inputs increased in strength because as time passed, the rat began to pay more "attention" to its surroundings, this attention being manifest neurophysiologically as an increase in activity along this pathway (the synaptic weights them-

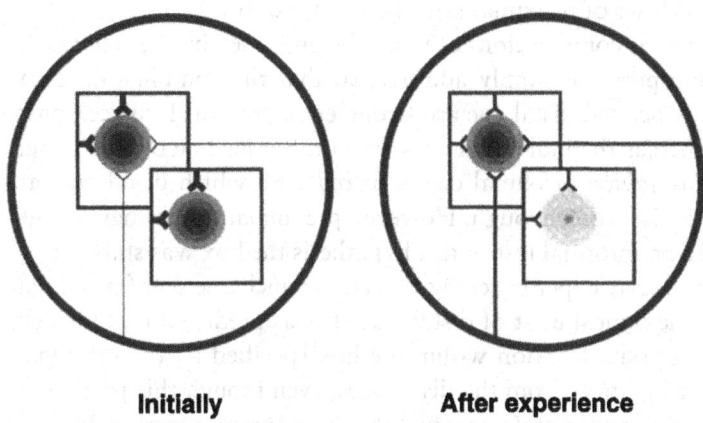

Initially   **After experience**

Figure 4.6. Change in inputs strengths onto place cells after experience in a cue conflict situation. The floorless box was moved diagonally between the two locations shown. **Left:** Initially, this cell had the same fields in both location, showing that it must have been driven strongly from the proximal cues (the box walls, shown by the thick lines). However, this model postulates that there is also a weak input onto some of the cells from the distal cues (the curtains, shown by the thin lines). **Right:** After time, the cell stopped firing in the Southeast box location. This shows that the proximal cues must have become relatively weaker, otherwise they should still be able to drive the cell to its firing threshold in either location. However, the distal cues became stronger, so that the cell can only fire when it receives a conjunction of both distal *and* proximal inputs. Therefore, it has become able to discriminate the two locations.

selves perhaps remaining unchanged). Place cells receiving a relatively larger percentage of their inputs from the distal cues would tend to reflect this increase first, explaining the piecemeal nature of the change. Perhaps the proximal inputs became relatively weaker because the cell raised its firing threshold to compensate for the increased drive it was receiving. Perhaps the distal inputs were able to inhibit the proximal ones by some feedforward process.

Whether the mechanism is associative or not, it seems clear that the pattern of inputs onto these cells was able to change in a meaningful way as a result of the rat's experience. In other words, the development of discriminatory ability by place cells seems to reflect the acquisition by the spatial map of useful knowledge about the environment, and might reasonably correspond to or even underlie the ability of the rat as a whole to make such discriminations.

As well as shedding light on the processes of memory formation, the finding that subclasses of inputs can be dissociated by changing parts of the environment opens up the possibility of experiments that determine how place cells integrate the various sources of information impinging on them. For example, the observation that a small proportion of cells, rather than losing a field, developed a *different* field in one or the other of the boxes shows that at any one time, a given cell might have two or even more simultaneous sets of inputs, of which it only selects one at a given moment. It must have the proximal inputs to know where in the box to fire (and a control experiment, not shown here, found that moving the box a small amount caused the fields to follow along with it, so there must have been *some* proximal drive onto the cell). Similarly, it must have the distal inputs, or else it would not know which set of proximal inputs to respond to.

How might these various combinations of inputs be processed by the cells? One possibility is that the inputs are simply additive, so that the combination of a proximal cue and its associated distal cue are strong enough to push the cell past its firing threshold, whereas the individual cues are not. By this line of reasoning, the cell should not care *which* proximal cue is paired with which distal cue, as long as the combination is strong enough. However, preliminary data suggest this may not be the case. In an informal test of this hypothesis the box was shifted to a novel location, not previously experienced by the rat, in which one set of proximal cues was paired with the opposite set of distal cues. It was predicted that the cell should fire in the appropriate location within the box specified by the proximal cues because of supporting drive from the distal cues, even though this particular combination of proximal and distal cues had never occurred together before. Somewhat surprisingly, no such thing happened; instead, the pattern of fields was the same as that in one of the previously experienced locations (as it happens, the one most recently experienced by the rat, which may or may not be significant). In other words, it seems as though, at least in this example, the cell did not respond to a simple combination of inputs; rather, it seemed to know which sets of inputs belonged together.

How could this be achieved? There are various possibilities, but perhaps the most interesting is that the distal cues might *gate* the proximal cues, that is, enable the cell to select, from among its various sets of proximal inputs, which ones to respond to and which to ignore at a given time. In this scenario, the strength of the proximal input would be modulated by whether or not its corresponding distal input is active. If it is, then the proximal input will be strong enough to drive the cell; if not, then it will not. In other words, the pattern of inputs onto a place cell is arranged in such a way that certain combinations belong together and that the presence of only parts of a given combination will not affect the cell.

Such a gating arrangement is not entirely implausible. As mentioned earlier, it has been known for some time that the presence of nonspatial inputs (such as the color of the environment) can determine which set of spatial inputs is selected by the cell. The possibility that a subclass of spatial input might act in the same way is intriguing. It might explain, for example, why rats that have learned a given proximal environment (such as a water maze) might be able subsequently to learn a spatial goal the whereabouts of which is signaled by the distal cues, even under conditions such as NMDA blockade, where spatial learning had been presumed impossible (Bannerman et al., 1995). It also suggests that the ability of the hippocampus to learn about context (corresponding in our example to the distal environment) might be experimentally dissociable from its spatial learning capability.

The main conclusion from the shifting-box experiment is that spatial inputs can be manipulated independently, so as to investigate the relative influences on the place cell. Furthermore, it appears that the pattern of input strengths can be modulated by experience, just as with the directional inputs. This rearrangement is consistent with what we know about what the rat as a whole should be learning; in other words, the place cells are "learning" to discriminate the two locations, just as the rat might be (although this was not tested explicitly).

Does this constitute true learning? Much more experimentation is needed to determine if this is the case. To begin with, it is far from clear where in the brain these changes are taking place. Maybe the increase in distal input strength is due to an increase of the synaptic strength onto place cells; however, it could equally well be due to increased activity on the input pathway as a result of increased attention by the rat to the distal cues. Although such an attentional change arguably constitutes a kind of memory (because it comes about as a result of experience), it is nonassociative and likely to be extrahippocampal. Until the exact anatomic nature and location of changes such as these have been identified, it will not be possible to conclude firmly that the site of the engram has been localized. Nevertheless, the results suggest that the study of latent learning by cognitive representations provides a worthwhile ground for future research.

Conclusion

One of the findings that is gradually emerging from both current and past research is that "memory" is in reality a multitude of processes, perhaps a different process in every brain system. For example, is the attentional change that we speculated about above a type of memory? What about path integration ("memory" for recent movements)? What about the downregulation of AMPA receptors as a result of overactivity in a pathway? Or a change in a cell's firing threshold?

Rather than "memory," it is perhaps preferable to be more explicit about one's meaning and to talk, for example, about cognitive representations and how they are constructed, how they change as a result of experience, and whether the changed representation overwrites the original, or is somehow stored alongside it. To this end, the spatial cognitive system is one of the most interesting and useful areas for study, as so much is known both about its anatomic organization and physiology.

The theme of this book is LTP, and whether it is a mechanism for "memory." The purpose of the present chapter was to show that what goes on within the spatial cognitive representation when an animal is exposed to a new environment (and so learns about it) is multifarious and complex. It is likely that there are many processes, some that are obviously manifest as a change in the output of the rat (its behavior) and some, such as latent learning of directional or distal cues, that may change the cognitive representation inside the rat even if never observed by an experimenter. To understand spatial learning, then, and to explore its physiologic basis, we need to know much more about what actually goes on in the cells themselves as they acquire new information about the world. It seems likely that by the time we have isolated these changes to our satisfaction, the question of whether the processes are LTP, or even something vaguely like it, will have evolved to become the far more interesting question of how each system modifies its own particular representation. There are probably many different processes, occurring in different parts of the brain both within and without the hippocampal formation, and some of them probably resemble LTP to a greater or lesser degree (with, for example, dependence on the NMDA receptor) while others probably do not.

Should we give up studying LTP altogether then? The answer is obviously "no," since the LTP model of synaptic change has been enormously useful in unraveling the machinery of the synapses, and likely will be for some time to come. However, it is worth remembering that LTP is simply an artificial way of persuading synapses to alter their strengths. Whether and to what extent the changes that mediate LTP also play a part in spatial learning is in some senses a naïve question, given the tangled web of complexity behind what looks deceptively like a simple behavioral function. Rather than speculate too long about the extent to which nature imitates "art" (if LTP induction can be considered an art, which is often the case), it surely makes more sense to look at nature herself, and ask her directly how she does what she does.

REFERENCES

Bannerman, D.M., Good, M.A., Butcher, S.P., Ramsay, M. et al. (1995). Distinct components of spatial learning revealed by prior training and NMDA receptor blockade [see comments]. *Nature* 378: 182–186.

Biegler, R., and Morris, R.G. (1996). Landmark stability: Further studies pointing to a role in spatial learning. *Q. J. Exp. Psychol. B.* 49: 307–345.

Blair, H.T., and Sharp, P.E. (1996). Visual and vestibular influences on head-direction cells in the anterior thalamus of the rat. *Behav. Neurosci.* 110: 643–660.

Bostock, E., Muller, R.U., and Kubie, J.L. (1991). Experience-dependent modifications of hippocampal place cell firing. *Hippocampus* 1: 193–205.

Chen, L.L., Lin, L.H., Barnes, C.A., and McNaughton, B.L. (1994a). Head-direction cells in the rat posterior cortex. II. Contributions of visual and ideothetic information to the directional firing. *Exp. Brain Res.* 101: 24–34.

Chen, L.L., Lin, L.H., Green, E.J., Barnes, C.A. et al. (1994b). Head-direction cells in the rat posterior cortex. I. Anatomical distribution and behavioral modulation. *Exp. Brain Res.* 101: 8–23.

Cressant, A., Muller, R.U., and Poucet, B. (1997). Failure of centrally placed objects to control the firing fields of hippocampal place cells. *J. Neurosci.* 17: 2531–2542.

Gothard, K.M., Skaggs, W.E., Moore, K.M., and McNaughton, B.L. (1996). Binding of hippocampal CA1 neural activity to multiple reference frames in a landmark-based navigation task. *J. Neurosci.* 16: 823–835.

Hebb, D.O. (1949). *The Organization of Behavior.* New York: Wiley.

Hetherington, P.A., and Shapiro, M.L. (1997). Hippocampal place fields are altered by the removal of single visual cues in a distance-dependent manner. *Behav. Neurosci.* 111: 20–34.

Jarrard, L.E. (1993). On the role of the hippocampus in learning and memory in the rat. *Behav. Neural Biol.* 60: 9–26.

Jeffery, K.J. (1998). Learning of landmark stability and instability by hippocampal place cells. *Neuropharmacology* 37: 677–687.

Jeffery, K.J., and O'Keefe, J. (1999). Learned interaction of visual and idiothetic cues in the control of place field orientation. *Exp. Brain Res.* 127: 151–161.

Kentros, C., Hargreaves, E., Hawkins, R.D., Kandel, E.R. et al. (1998). Abolition of long-term stability of new hippocampal place cell maps by NMDA receptor blockade. *Science* 280: 2121–2126.

Knierim, J.J., Kudrimoti, H.S., and McNaughton, B.L. (1995). Place cells, head direction cells, and the learning of landmark stability. *J. Neurosci.* 15: 1648–1659.

Konorski, J. (1948). *Conditioned Reflexes and Neuron Organization.* Cambridge: Cambridge University Press.

McNaughton, B.L., Barnes, C.A., Gerrard, J.L., Gothard, K. et al. (1996). Deciphering the hippocampal polyglot: The hippocampus as a path integration system. *J. Exp. Biol.* 199: 173–185.

Mittelstaedt, H., and Mittelstaedt, M.-L. (1982). Homing by path integration. In F. Papi and H.G. Wallraff (Eds.), *Avian navigation* (p. 290). Berlin, Heidelberg: Springer-Verlag.

Muller, R.U., and Kubie, J.L. (1987). The effects of changes in the environment on the spatial firing of hippocampal complex-spike cells. *J. Neurosci.* 7: 1951–1968.

Muller, R.U., Kubie, J.L., and Ranck, J.B., Jr. (1987). Spatial firing patterns of hippocampal complex-spike cells in a fixed environment. *J. Neurosci.* 7: 1935–1950.

O'Keefe, J., and Burgess, N. (1996). Geometric determinants of the place fields of hippocampal neurons [see comments]. *Nature* 381: 425–428.

O'Keefe, J., and Conway, D.H. (1980). On the trail of the hippocampal engram. *Physiol. Psychol.* 8: 229–238.

O'Keefe, J., and Dostrovsky, J. (1971). The hippocampus as a spatial map. Preliminary evidence from unit activity in the freely-moving rat. *Brain Res.* 34: 171–175.

O'Keefe, J., and Nadel, L. (1978). *The Hippocampus as a Cognitive Map.* Oxford: Clarendon Press.

Rotenberg, A., and Muller, R.U. (1997). Variable place-cell coupling to a continuously viewed stimulus: Evidence that the hippocampus acts as a perceptual system. *Philos. Trans. R. Soc. London B. Biol. Sci.* 352: 1505–1513.

Shapiro, M.L., Tanila, H., and Eichenbaum, H. (1997). Cues that hippocampal place cells encode: Dynamic and hierarchical representation of local and distal stimuli. *Hippocampus* 7: 624–642.

Taube, J.S. (1995). Head direction cells recorded in the anterior thalamic nuclei of freely moving rats. *J. Neurosci.* 15: 70–86.

Taube, J.S., Muller, R.U., and Ranck, J.B., Jr. (1990a). Head-direction cells recorded from the postsubiculum in freely moving rats. II. Effects of environmental manipulations. *J. Neurosci.* 10: 436–447.

Taube, J.S., Muller, R.U., and Ranck, J.B., Jr. (1990b). Head-direction cells recorded from the postsubiculum in freely moving rats. I. Description and quantitative analysis. *J. Neurosci.* 10: 420–435.

Taube, J.S., Goodridge, J.P., Golob, E.J., Dudchenko, P.A. et al. (1996). Processing the head direction cell signal: A review and commentary. *Brain Res. Bull.* 40: 477–484.

Tolman, E.C. (1948). Cognitive maps in rats and men. *Psychol. Rev.* 40: 40–60.

There Is More to the Picture Than Long-Term Potentiation

Theta or Gamma Oscillations in the Brain and the Facilitation of Synaptic Plasticity

CHAPTER FIVE

Synaptic Potentiation by Natural Patterns of Activity in the Hippocampus

Implications for Memory Formation

Fenella Pike, Sturla Molden, Ole Paulsen, and Edvard I. Moser

SUMMARY

Although our understanding of the relationship between hippocampal long-term potentiation (LTP) and learning is limited, a fresh approach presented here bears promise for resolving this important issue. Blockade of LTP frequently leads to blockade of hippocampus-dependent learning, but there are examples of intact learning in the absence of LTP, and the function of LTP during learning is poorly understood. This lack of understanding may partly stem from the preoccupation with tetanus-induced LTP in experimental designs, since such long-lasting high-frequency activity has never been demonstrated to occur *in vivo*. A closer understanding of memory-related plasticity in the brain requires detailed study of the neuronal activity patterns occurring when an animal learns. Replication of natural patterns of activity in an *in vitro* preparation suggests that bursting activity in hippocampal pyramidal neurons may play a specific role during encoding of new memories. These data have led to the development of a novel model for information processing in cortical networks, in which separate processing modes may coexist.

Introduction

The question of whether long-term potentiation (LTP) is the basis for learning and memory is one of the most exciting and controversial issues in cognitive neuroscience. Previous attempts to link LTP and memory seem to have gone up the wrong path since, in several respects, we are as confused about this important question today as we were 30 years ago. One reason why we went astray might be that in our enthusiasm to use novel cellular and molecular techniques to explore the mechanisms underlying LTP, we forgot what we were actually trying to understand,

Christian Hölscher, editor, *Neuronal Mechanisms of Memory Formation*. © 2001 Cambridge University Press. Printed in the United States of America. All rights reserved.

namely the mechanism of memory. In this chapter we will discuss a fresh approach
to this problem, which we believe will lead to a more definitive outcome.

The Link between LTP and Learning: A Jungle of Inconsistencies

Long-term potentiation (Bliss and Lømo, 1973; Bliss and Collingridge, 1993) is
thought to be an experimentally induced overexpression of a physiologic process
involved in the regulation of synaptic weights during certain types of memory formation. Under natural conditions in the behaving animal, LTP-like synaptic modifications have been suggested to form distributed patterns, which may be
organized according to a correlational or Hebbian rule (McNaughton and Morris,
1987). Hebb's rule postulates that synaptic potentiation will occur when presynaptic and postsynaptic neurons are simultaneously active. Long-term potentiation in several synapses of the hippocampus supports the Hebb rule because it is
dependent on the N-methyl-D-aspartate (NMDA) receptor, which requires both
presynaptic release of transmitter and postsynaptic depolarization for its activation (Mayer et al., 1984; Nowak et al., 1984).

Much of the validity of the LTP model of memory formation rests on the apparently overlapping mechanisms of hippocampal LTP and hippocampus-dependent
spatial learning. In particular, blockade of NMDA receptor function impairs both
hippocampal LTP and hippocampus-dependent spatial learning (Morris et al.,
1986; Sakimura et al., 1995; Tsien et al., 1996). NMDA receptors are necessary
for induction but not for expression or maintenance of LTP (Collingridge et al.,
1983). Similarly, the NMDA receptor seems to be essential for successful encoding
of spatial memory but is not required for retrieval of a previously acquired spatial
task (Morris, 1989; Steele and Morris, 1999). However, the technique of NMDA
receptor blockade leads to an interpretational problem, since it is difficult to identify exactly which physiologic deficit accounts for the behavioral effects.

Similar results are seen following interference with the putative molecular
mechanisms downstream of the NMDA receptor. For example, mice with targeted
mutations of the α-calcium/calmodulin dependent protein kinase II, *fyn* tyrosine
kinase, Ca^{2+}-stimulated adenylyl cyclase, or cAMP-responsive element binding
(CREB) have been reported to demonstrate parallel impairments of hippocampus-
dependent learning and hippocampal LTP (Grant et al., 1992; Silva et al., 1992a,
1992b; Bourtchuladze et al., 1994; Wu et al., 1995). However, these studies also
suffer from several interpretational problems. Mutant strains frequently have a
broad profile of behavioral and physiologic abnormalities, including changes in
activity, vigilance, fear responses, aggression, pain sensitivity, or susceptibility to
seizures (Silva et al., 1992b; Chen et al., 1994; Miyakawa et al., 1996), and these
probably account for a significant proportion of the range of behavioral impairment in mutant mice (Lipp and Wolfer, 1998). For example, fearfulness and ataxia
may account for the deficit in water maze learning observed in *fyn* knock-out
mice. If *fyn* knock-outs are given mechanical stimulation through their hind feet,
swimming is enhanced and they display robust reference memory in the water
maze (Huerta et al., 1996). Several other reports also indicate a dissociation

between LTP and spatial memory following genetic interventions with the molecular machinery involved in LTP (Huang et al., 1995; Nosten-Bertrand et al., 1996; Schurmans et al., 1997; Meiri et al., 1998; Zamanillo et al., 1999). These problems have led some researchers to question the usefulness of the genetic approach in studying the role of LTP until the knock-out can be restricted spatially to certain cell types and the expression of the gene temporally controlled.

A different approach is to occlude the LTP process physiologically. LTP does not grow indefinitely but will saturate upon repeated stimulation (Bliss and Lømo, 1973). If memories are encoded as distributed patterns of potentiated synapses, it follows that network saturation should disrupt encoding and retrieval (McNaughton and Morris, 1987). Spatial learning is blocked by mere repetition of the LTP induction procedure, but only if a sufficient proportion of the perforant-path synapses to the dentate gyrus and the hippocampus are stimulated (McNaughton et al., 1986; Castro et al., 1989; Moser et al., 1998) (Figure 5.1). The validity of this approach rests on the assumption that the saturation procedure is not accompanied by nonspecific damage to the hippocampal network (Moser and Moser, 1999). Preliminary observations suggest that the impairment is reversible and specific to memory at long intervals (2 hours, but not 15 seconds) (Molden et al., 1999). This is what would be expected if long-term memory is disrupted specifically and the disruption is caused by occlusion of further LTP rather than a systemic lesion of the hippocampus.

However, a problem with all of these studies is the extraction of the specific LTP-related behavioral impairment. Spatial or nonspatial pretraining in a different water maze fully protects against an impairment of spatial learning in rats with LTP blocked either by NMDA receptor antagonists (Bannerman et al., 1995; Saucier and Cain, 1995) or by a saturation protocol (Otnæss et al., 1999). This effect of pretraining does not require NMDA receptors during pretraining (Hoh et al., 1999). Thus, it is clear that NMDA receptors are required neither for learning general strategies nor for spatial mapping per se in the water maze, if these components are acquired one after another. A deficit develops only when the capacity for LTP formation is blocked during simultaneous acquisition of procedural and mapping components of the task. These observations clearly indicate that our knowledge of the specific function of LTP during memory formation is limited.

We Need to Study Natural Activity Patterns

Why, despite all this effort, does the specific function of LTP during memory processes remain elusive? Perhaps the failure to establish the cellular mechanisms underlying memory stems from the preoccupation with tetanus-induced LTP in experimental designs. It is noticeable that the type of activity used experimentally to induce LTP has never been demonstrated to occur *in vivo*. In fact, the highly synchronous ensemble activity commonly used to induce LTP is very different from the neuronal activity observed in animals during learning behaviors. Therefore, if we are to come closer to an understanding of memory-related plasticity in the brain, we might need to study in more detail the neuronal activity

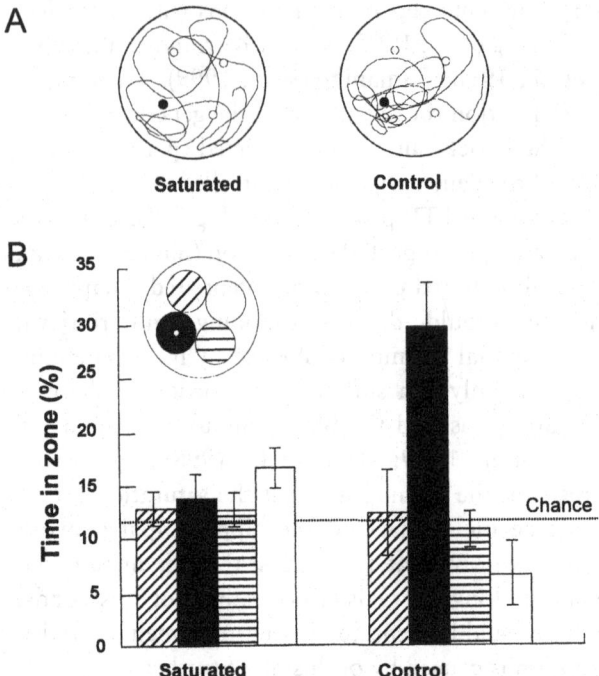

Figure 5.1. Blockade of spatial learning in a water maze in animals in which LTP was satu-rated in the perforant-path synapses of the dentate gyrus. Rates received either high-fre-quency stimulation ("Saturation") or low-frequency stimulation ("Control") through multiple electrodes in the angular bundle. This stimulation occluded further LTP in the high-frequency stimulated group, whereas LTP could be induced in the control group. (A) Search pattern of representative animals on a probe test in which the platform was unavailable. Only the control animals searched more around the location of the platform (**black**) than elsewhere in the pool. (B) Mean time (± SEM) spent in a zone around the platform position and in cor-responding, equally large zones in the three other quadrants of the pool on the final spatial probe test (platform unavailable). The inset indicates location and size of the four zones. The animals were trained with the platform in the center of the black zone. The stippled line indi-cates the chance level. (Adapted from Moser et al., 1998, with permission.)

occurring when an animal learns. For this purpose, there is no substitute for direct recording of hippocampal activity during performance of memory tasks. Although the postulated distributed nature of LTP makes it difficult to detect lasting changes in just those synapses that are modified during a specific learning episode, a lot can be achieved by closer inspection of firing patterns of hippocampal neurons during encoding and retrieval of memory. Such firing patterns can in turn be sim-ulated in *in vitro* preparations that allow a detailed investigation of their effects on synaptic transmission between identified types of neurons.

Network Activity and Memory

During exploration in rats, the hippocampal network is engaged in rhythmic oscil-latory activity at "theta" (4 to 12 Hz) frequencies, as seen in electroencephalographic (EEG) recordings *in vivo* (Vanderwolf, 1969; Buzsáki et al., 1983; Wiener et al., 1989). It is often assumed that such theta oscillations are necessary for hippocampus-dependent learning to take place. A recent study reports that theta activity is present in the brains of epileptic patients during encoding or retrieval of spatial memory in a computer-animated T-maze (Kahana et al., 1999), but the specific conditions during which theta activity does and does not occur are not clear from this study. In animals, theta rhythm and spatial learning are disrupted in parallel by lesions of the medial septum (Winson, 1978; Mitchell et al., 1982), which is consistent with, but does not prove, the idea that theta rhythm is necessary for memory formation. Finally, theta activity is not exclusively associated with memory formation but can be observed during more stereotypic locomotor movement as well. Clearly, more direct evidence relating theta oscillations to memory functions is required.

Single-Cell Activity and Memory

More information about the cellular conditions during learning can be gleaned from studies of individual neurons within a network. Based on their firing patterns in freely moving rats, hippocampal neurons are frequently divided into two classes: complex-spike cells and theta cells (Ranck, 1973). Complex-spike cells, which are likely to be pyramidal cells (Fox and Ranck, 1975, 1981), fire at low rates, but often in bursts. These bursts typically consist of two to seven spikes at 150 to 200 Hz. A major proportion of the complex-spike cells have spatial correlates (O'Keefe and Dostrovsky, 1971). During exploratory behavior, each of these "place cells" fires in a specific location, the "place field" of the cell, but is virtually silent in other positions. As an animal traverses the place field, the activity of a place cell advances progressively relative to the EEG theta ("phase precession"; O'Keefe and Recce, 1993). Collectively, adjacent place cells appear to cover the entire experimental environment (Wilson and McNaughton, 1993).

Exploratory behavior and theta activity are also associated with characteristic rhythmic discharges in "theta cells" (Ranck, 1973; Buzsáki et al., 1983). These cells have higher spontaneous firing rates than complex-spike cells, and spatial correlates are less apparent (McNaughton et al., 1983). Theta cells are particularly active during movement, when the hippocampal EEG is dominated by theta rhythm (Vanderwolf, 1969; Buzsáki et al., 1983). Many theta cells are likely to be local-circuit interneurons (Fox and Ranck, 1975, 1981). At least some of these presumed interneurons appear to be basket cells, because thetalike activity in intact, but anesthetized, animals is associated with rhythmic discharges of interneurons that have been identified as basket cells (Ylinen et al., 1995). These discharges occur at theta frequencies and are phase-related to the ongoing extracellular theta oscillation.

An important challenge for memory research is to relate activity in either of these types of cell directly to memory processing. A step in this direction was taken by Wood et al. (1999), who observed that a class of hippocampal complex spike cells apparently fired specifically during nonmatches in a delayed-non-matching-to-sample odor memory task. However, the hippocampus is not required for memory in this task (Dudchenko et al., 2000), and it has not been ruled out that differences in EEG state or behaviour contribute to the different activity during matches and nonmatches. More recently, it has been demonstrated that a subset of hippocampal pyramidal cells exhibit activity related to the hidden platform in an adapted, hippocampus-dependent version of the Morris watermaze memory task, regardless of the position of the platform (Moser et al., 1999a, 1999b). This retrieval-related activity, observed on probe tests in the absence of the platform, appeared despite maintained hippocampal theta oscillations. Finally, there is evidence that memory is expressed in activity patterns of complex spike cells comes from investigations of firing patterns during sleep episodes subsequent to presumed learning events. It was found that complex spike cells that were active during a preceding exploration episode maintained their increased or correlated firing patterns during slow-wave sleep several hours subsequently (Pavlides and Winson, 1989; Wilson and McNaughton, 1994; Kudrimoti et al., 1999). Together, these recent data suggest that we may learn a lot about mechanisms of memory by studing natural activity patterns of hippocampal neurones in animals that perform memory tasks.

How Can We Use These Insights in the Study of Synaptic Plasticity?

Although substantial progress has been made in uncovering some of the behavioral correlates of hippocampal complex-spike cell activity, we know little about their role during encoding and retrieval of memory. The questions we need to ask are, first, what occurs at the individual synaptic level during memory encoding, and, second, how these changes collectively encode new information. We are technically limited in the study of individual synapses *in vivo*. Therefore, at present, in order to answer our questions, we need to transfer the experimental observations *in vivo* to an *in vitro* preparation. LTP has primarily been studied in excitatory synapses between pyramidal cells of the hippocampus. Previous attempts at using behaviorally relevant activity to induce LTP in hippocampal slices have used field recordings and mimicked the theta bursting pattern in the afferent input. It was demonstrated that a theta burst pattern presynaptically could indeed induce LTP (Larson et al., 1986; Stäubli and Lynch, 1987; Huerta and Lisman, 1993). However, single action potentials at theta frequency can also produce synaptic potentiation under such conditions (Mayford et al., 1995). It was later found that this potentiation required postsynaptic bursting (Thomas et al., 1998).

We set out to investigate whether bursting at theta frequency had any special role in the induction of synaptic plasticity, compared to single spikes (Pike et al., 1999). We found that bursting was indeed essential for induction of potentiation, and by controlling both presynaptic and postsynaptic activity we were able to show that it was postsynaptic bursting paired with presynaptic activity that was vital for synaptic potentiation (Figure 5.2). Whereas it has been commonly assumed that presynaptic bursting was essential to provide sufficient postsynaptic depolarization, our data demonstrate that it is rather postsynaptic bursting that may be the critical factor. This learning rule comes close to a literal interpretation

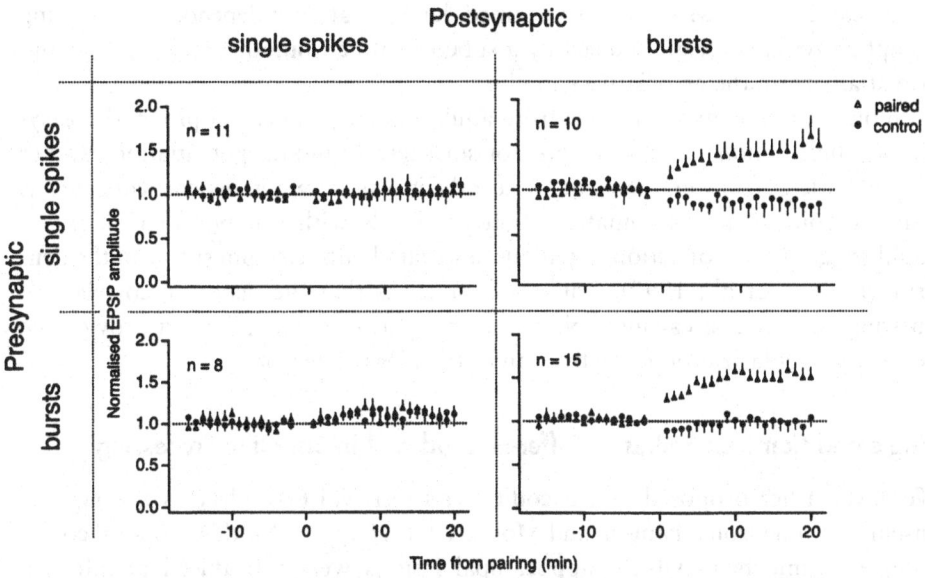

Figure 5.2. Experiments to investigate the pre- and postsynaptic requirements for synaptic potentiation. Synaptic efficacy was monitored in two separate afferent pathways among the Schaffer collaterals during intracellular recording of single CA1 pyramidal neurons *in vitro*. Four pairing paradigms were compared, pairing either single or triple ("burst") presynaptic activity with either single spikes or bursts postsynaptically. Each pairing was repeated ten times at 5 Hz, and each set repeated four times at 10-second intervals. Only paradigms with postsynaptic bursting resulted in input-specific potentiation. Error bars represent SEM. (Modified from Figure 2 of Pike et al., 1999, with permission.)

of Hebb's postulate, that coincidence of presynaptic and postsynaptic activity leads to strengthening of the synapse between the active neurons.

How Can Postsynaptic Bursts Enable Synaptic Potentiation?

The conventional view of induction of LTP has been that a local depolarization induced by synaptic high-frequency activity provides the necessary postsynaptic requirement for NMDA receptor-mediated synaptic change (Bliss and Collingridge, 1993). However, since then an alternative mechanism of signaling postsynaptic activity has been discovered. It was shown that action potentials can actively backpropagate into the dendrites (Stuart and Sakmann, 1994). This provides an efficient mechanism whereby the postsynaptic neuron can signal a copy of the output of the neuron to input synapses. Thus, this provides a substrate for the Hebb rule (Linden, 1999). Rather than the local dendritic learning rules that have been promoted following the discovery of tetanus-induced LTP, our data suggest that the postsynaptic neuron serves as a single compartment during associative learning, such that any input active at the time of postsynaptic bursting will be potentiated. If backpropagating action potentials can provide the local depolarization requirement, widely separated synapses can associated also. For example, a synapse located in the basal dendrites may be associated with an activity in the apical dendrite. Moreover, a sustained depolarization independent of ongoing synaptic excitation (e.g., induced by a subcortical neuromodulatory input) could potentially form the associative stimulus.

In our experiments with tissue from adult animals, coincident pre- and postsynaptic single action potentials were not sufficient to induce potentiation. Rather postsynaptic bursts were necessary. Recently, it was shown in neocortical neurons that the coincidence of somatic action potentials with synaptic depolarization could trigger bursts of action potentials associated with calcium spikes in the dendrite (Larkum et al., 1999). This result suggests that the dendritic correlate of bursting activity is a calcium spike, and that this calcium spike can provide the necessary depolarization for activation of the NMDA receptor.

Single and Complex Spikes as Different Modes of Information Processing

We have earlier proposed that encoding and retrieval take place in overlapping ensembles of neurons (Paulsen and Moser, 1998). Support for this proposal comes from experiments in which hippocampal lesions were introduced at different stages of memory processing, which demonstrated that the amount and location of hippocampal tissue required for retrieval of a water maze task directly reflected the amount and location of the tissue used for encoding (Moser and Moser, 1998).

Specifically, it was proposed in the model that hippocampal pyramidal cells alternate between a burst mode, in which information is encoded and synaptic weights modified in their dendrites ("read-in" mode), and a single-spike mode, in which the information stored in the network is retrieved from the network ("read-out" mode) (Figure 5.3). Encoding and retrieval processes may take place at the

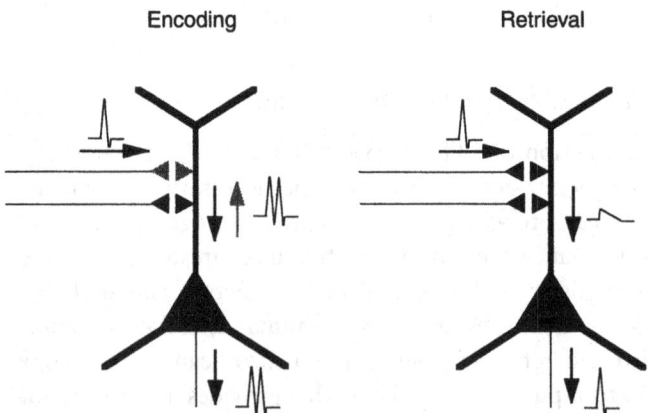

Figure 5.3. Model for encoding and retrieval of memory in the hippocampus. During encoding (**left**) bursts of action potentials backpropagate into dendritic compartments (**gray arrow**). When backpropagating bursts coincide with synaptic input, the active synapses (**gray triangles**) are strengthened by a process similar to LTP. During retrieval (**right**), backpropagation and synaptic plasticity are minimal, whereas information stored in the synapses is transferred to downstream regions of the network via axonal conduction of single action potentials. (Adapted from Paulsen and Moser, 1998, with permission.)

same time, with some principal cells performing read-in functions (bursts) and others performing read-out functions (Single spikes). The differential threshold for read-in and read-out functions may be mediated by selective changes in the activity of inhibitory circuits (Paulsen and Moser, 1998).

Conclusion

Replication of natural patterns of activity occurring during learning can lead to new insight into the network and synaptic mechanisms responsible for memory encoding in the hippocampus. We have summarized here evidence from *in vivo* and *in vitro* data that bursting activity in hippocampal pyramidal neurons may play a specific role during encoding of new memories. These data also suggest a novel model for information processing in cortical networks, in which separate processing modes can coexist. This adds another level of sophistication to the understanding of brain mechanisms involved in memory. A future challenge is to understand the information content of hippocampal single cell and network activity, both during encoding and retrieval of memories.

REFERENCES

Bannerman, D., Good, M.A., Butcher, S.P., Ramsay, M. et al. (1995). Distinct components of spatial learning revealed by prior training and NMDA receptor blockade. *Nature* 378: 182–186.

Bliss, T.V.P., and Collingridge, G.L. (1993). A synaptic model of memory—long-term potentiation in the hippocampus. *Nature* 361: 31–39.

Bliss, T.V.P., and Lømo, T. (1973). Long-lasting potentiation of synaptic transmission in the dentate area of the anaesthetized rabbit following stimulation of the perforant path. *J. Physiol.* 232: 331–356.

Bourtchuladze, R., Frenguelli, B., Blendy, J., Cioffi, D. et al. (1994). Deficient long-term memory in mice with a targeted mutation of the cAMP-responsive element-binding protein. *Cell* 79: 59–68.

Buzsáki, G., Leung, L., and Vanderwolf, C.H. (1983). Cellular bases of hippocampal EEG in the behaving rat. *Brain Res. Rev.* 6: 139–171.

Castro, C.A., Silbert, L.H., McNaughton, B.L., and Barnes, C.A. (1989). Recovery of spatial learning deficits after decay of electrically induced synaptic enhancement in the hippocampus. *Nature* 342: 545–548.

Chen, C., Rainnie, D.G., Greene, R.W., and Tonegawa, S. (1994). Abnormal fear response and aggressive behavior in mutant mice deficient for α-calcium-calmodulin kinase II. *Science* 266: 291–294.

Collingridge, G.L., Kehl, S.J., and McLennan, H. (1983). Excitatory amino acids in synaptic transmission in the Schaffer collateral-commissural pathway of the rat hippocampus. *J. Physiol.* 34: 33–46.

Dudchenko, P.A., Wood, E.R., and Eichenbaum, H. (2000). Neurotoxic hippocampal lesions have no effect on odor span and little effect on odor recognition memory but produce significant impairments on spatial span, recognition, and alternation. *J. Neurosci.* 20: 2964–2977.

Fox, S.E., and Ranck, J.B. Jr. (1975). Localization and anatomical identification of theta and complex spike cells in dorsal hippocampal formation of rats. *Exp. Neurol.* 49: 299–313.

Fox, S.E., and Ranck, J.B. Jr. (1981). Electrophysiological characteristics of hippocampal complex-spike cells and theta cells. *Exp. Brain. Res.* 41: 399–410.

Grant, S.G.N., O'Dell, J., Karl, K.A., Stein, P.L. et al. (1992). Impaired long-term potentiation, spatial learning, and hippocampal development in fyn mutant mice. *Science* 258: 1903–1910.

Hoh, T., Beiko, J., Boon, F., Weiss, S. et al. (1999). Complex behavioral strategy and reversal learning in the water maze without NMDA receptor-dependent long-term potentiation. *J. Neurosci.* 19: RC2 (1–5).

Huang, Y.Y., Kandel, E.R., Varshavsky, L., Brandon, E.P. et al. (1995). A genetic test of the effects of mutations in PKA on mossy fiber LTP and its relation to spatial and contextual learning. *Cell* 83: 1211–1222.

Huerta, P.T., and Lisman, J.E. (1993). Heightened synaptic plasticity of hippocampal CA1 neurons during a cholinergically induced rhythmic state. *Nature* 364: 723–725.

Huerta, P.T., Scearce, K.A., Farris, S.M., Empson, R.M. et al. (1996). Preservation of spatial learning in fyn tyrosine kinase knockout mice. *Neuroreport* 7: 1685–1689.

Kahana, M.J., Sekuler, R., Caplan, J.B., Kirschen, M. et al. (1999). Human theta oscillations exhibit task dependence during virtual maze navigation. *Nature* 399: 781–784.

Kudrimoti, H.S., Barnes, C.A., and McNaughton, B.L. (1999). Reactivation of hippocampal cell assemblies: Effects of behavioral state, experience, and EEG dynamics. *J. Neurosci.* 19: 4090–4101.

Larkum, M.E., Zhu, J.J., and Sakmann, B. (1999). A new cellular mechanism for coupling inputs arriving at different cortical layers. *Nature* 398: 338–341.

Larson, J., Wong, D., and Lynch, G. (1986). Patterned stimulation at the theta frequency is optimal for the induction of hippocampal long-term potentiation. *Brain Res.* 368: 347–350.

Lipp, H.-P., and Wolfer, D.P. (1998). Genetically modified mice and cognition. *Curr. Opin. Neurobiol.* 8: 272–280.

Linden, D.J. (1999). The return of the spike: Postsynaptic action potentials and the induction of LTP and LTD. *Neuron* 22: 661–666.

Mayer, M.L., Westbrook, G.L., and Guthrie, P.B. (1984). Voltage-dependent block by Mg2+ of NMDA responses in spinal cord neurones. *Nature* 309: 261–263.

Mayford, M., Wang, J., Kandel, E.R., and O'Dell, T.J. (1995). CaMKII regulates the frequency-response function of hippocampal synapses for the production of both LTD and LTP. *Cell* 81: 891–904.

McNaughton, B.L., and Morris, R.G.M. (1987). Hippocampal synaptic enhancement and information storage within a distributed memory system. *Trends Neurosci.* 10: 408–415.

McNaughton, B.L., Barnes, C.A., and O'Keefe, J. (1983). The contribution of position, direction, and velocity to single unit activity in the hippocampus of freely-moving rats. *Exp. Brain Res.* 52: 41–49.

McNaughton, B.L., Barnes, C.A., Rao, G., Baldwin, J. et al. (1986). Long-term enhancement and the acquisition of spatial information. *J. Neurosci.* 6: 563–571.

Meiri, N., Sun, M.K., Segal, Z., and Alkon, D.L. (1998). Memory and long-term potentiation (LTP) dissociated: Normal spatial memory despite CA1 LTP elimination with Kv1.4 antisense. *Proc. Natl. Acad. Sci. USA* 95: 15037–15042.

Mitchell, S.J., Rawlins, J.N.P., Steward, O., and Olton, D.S. (1982). Medial septal area lesions disrupt theta rhythm and cholinergic staining in medial entorhinal cortex and produce impaired radial arm maze behavior in rats. *J. Neurosci.* 2: 292–302.

Miyakawa, T., Yagi, T., Tateishi, K., and Niki, H. (1996). Susceptibility to drug-induced seizures of Fyn tyrosine kinase-deficient mice. *Neuroreport* 7: 2723–2726.

Molden, S., Morris, R.G.M., Moser, M.-B., and Moser, E.I. (1999). Preservation of short-term working memory after massive tetanization of the perforant path. *Soc. Neurosci. Abstr.* 25: 649.10.

Morris, R.G.M. (1989). Synaptic plasticity and learning: Selective impairment of learning in rats and blockade of long-term potentiation in vivo by the N-methyl-D-aspartate receptor antagonist D-AP5. *J. Neurosci.* 9: 3040–3057.

Morris, R.G.M., Anderson, E., Lynch, G.S., and Baudry, M. (1986). Selective impairment of learning and blockade of long-term potentiation by an N-methyl-D-aspartate receptor antagonist, AP5. *Nature* 319: 774–776.

Moser, E.I., Krobert, K.A., Moser, M.-B., and Morris, R.G.M. (1998). Impaired spatial learning after saturation of long-term potentiation. *Science* 281: 2038–2042.

Moser, E.I., and Moser, M.-B. (1999). Is learning blocked by saturation of synaptic weights in the hippocampus? *Neurosci. Biobehav. Rev.* 23: 661–672.

Moser, M.-B., and Moser, E.I. (1998). Distributed encoding and retrieval of spatial memory in the hippocampus. *J. Neurosci.* 18: 7535–7542.

Moser, E.I., Hollup, S.A., Donnett, J.G., and Moser, M.-B. (1999a). Dissociation of place and goal in CA1 pyramidal cells in a water-maze reversal task. *Soc. Neurosci. Abstr.* 25: 649.6.

Moser, M.-B., Hollup, S.A., Donnett, J.G., and Moser, E.I. (1999b). Skewed distribution of place fields in a water-maze retrieval task. *Soc. Neurosci. Abstr.* 25: 649.5

Nosten-Bertrand, M., Errington, M.L., Murphy, K.P., Tokugawa, Y. et al. (1996). Normal spatial learning despite regional inhibition of LTP in mice lacking Thy-1. *Nature* 379: 826–829.

Nowak, L., Bregestovski, P., Ascher, P., Herbet, A. et al. (1984). Magnesium gates glutamate-activated channels in mouse central neurones. *Nature* 307(5950): 462–465.

O'Keefe, J., and Dostrovsky, J. (1971). The hippocampus as a spatial map. Preliminary evidence from unit activity in the freely-moving rat. *Brain Res.* 34: 171–175.

O'Keefe, J., and Recce, M. (1993). Phase relationship between hippocampal place units and the EEG theta rhythm. *Hippocampus* 3: 317–330.

Otnæss, M.K., Moser, M.-B., and Moser, E.I. (1999). Pretraining prevents spatial learning impairment following saturation of LTP. *Soc. Neurosci. Abstr.* 25: 649.8.

Paulsen, O., and Moser, E.I. (1998). A model of hippocampal memory formation and retrieval: GABAergic control of synaptic plasticity. *Trends Neurosci.* 21: 273–278.

Pavlides, C., and Winson, J. (1989). Influences of hippocampal place cell firing in the awake state on the activity of these cells during subsequent sleep episodes. *J. Neurosci.* 9: 2907–2918.

Pike, F.G., Meredith, R.M., Olding, A.W., and Paulsen, O. (1999). Postsynaptic bursting is essential for 'Hebbian' induction of associative long-term potentiation at excitatory synapses in rat hippocampus. *J. Physiol.* 518: 571–576.

Ranck, J.B. Jr. (1973). Studies on single neurons in dorsal hippocampal formation and septum in unrestrained rats. I. Behavioral correlates and firing repertoires. *Exp. Neurol.* 41: 461–535.

Sakimura, K., Kutsuwada, T., Ito, I., Manabe, T. et al. (1995). Reduced hippocampal LTP and spatial learning in mice lacking NMDA receptor epsilon 1 subunit. *Nature* 373: 151–155.

Saucier, D., and Cain, D.P. (1995). Spatial learning without NMDA receptor-dependent long-term potentiation. *Nature* 378: 186–189.

Schurmans, S., Schiffmann, S.N., Gurden, H., Lemaire, M. et al. (1997). Impaired long-term potentiation induction in dentate gyrus of calretinin-deficient mice. *Proc. Natl. Acad. Sci. USA* 94: 10415–10420.

Silva, A.J., Paylor, R., Wehner, J.M., and Tonegawa, S. (1992a). Impaired spatial learning in alpha-calcium-calmodulin kinase II mutant mice. *Science* 257: 206–211.

Silva, A.J., Stevens, C.F., Tonegawa, S., and Wang, Y. (1992b). Deficient hippocampal long-term potentiation in alpha-calcium-calmodulin kinase II mutant mice. *Science* 257: 201–206.

Staubli, U., and Lynch, G. (1987). Stable hippocampal long-term potentiation elicited by 'theta' pattern stimulation. *Brain Res.* 435: 227–234.

Steele, R.J., and Morris, R.G.M. (1999). Delay-dependent impairment of a matching-to-place task with chronic and intrahippocampal infusion of the NMDA-antagonist D-AP5. *Hippocampus* 9: 118–136.

Stuart, G.J., and Sakmann, B. (1994). Active propagation of somatic action potentials into neocortical pyramidal cell dendrites. *Nature* 367: 69–72.

Thomas, M.J., Watabe, A.M., Moody, T.D., Makhinson, M. et al. (1998). Postsynaptic complex spike bursting enables the induction of LTP by theta frequency synaptic stimulation. *J. Neurosci.* 18: 7118–7126.

Tsien, J.Z., Huerta, P.T., and Tonegawa, S. (1996). The essential role of hippocampal CA1 NMDA receptor-dependent synaptic plasticity in spatial memory. *Cell* 87: 1327–1338.

Vanderwolf, C.H. (1969). Hippocampal electrical activity and voluntary movement in the rat. *Electroencephalogr. Clin. Neurophysiol.* 26: 407–418.

Wiener, S.I., Paul, C.A., and Eichenbaum, H. (1989). Spatial and behavioral correlates of hippocampal neuronal activity. *J. Neurosci.* 9: 2737–2763.

Wilson, M.A., and McNaughton, B.L. (1993). Dynamics of the hippocampal ensemble code for space. *Science* 261: 1055–1058.

Wilson, M.A., and McNaughton, B.L. (1994). Reactivation of hippocampal ensemble memories during sleep. *Science* 265: 676–679.

Winson, J. (1978). Loss of hippocampal theta rhythm results in spatial memory deficit in the rat. *Science* 201: 160–163.

Wood, E.R., Dudchenko, P.A., and Eichenbaum, H. (1999). The global record of memory in hippocampal neuronal activity. *Nature* 397: 613–616.

Wu, Z.-L., Thomas, S.A., Villacres, E.C., Xia, Z. et al. (1995). Altered behavior and long-term potentiation in type I adenylyl cyclase mutant mice. *Proc. Natl. Acad. Sci. USA.* 92: 220–224.

Ylinen, A., Soltesz, I., Bragin, A., Penttonen, M. et al. (1995). Intracellular correlates of hippocampal theta rhythm in identified pyramidal cells, granule cells, and basket cells. *Hippocampus* 5: 78–90.

Zamanillo, D., Sprengel, R., Hvalby, O., Jensen, V. et al. (1999). Importance of AMPA receptors for hippocampal synaptic plasticity but not for spatial learning. *Science* 284: 1805–1811.

CHAPTER SIX

Plasticity in Local Neuronal Circuits

In Vivo Evidence from Rat Hippocampus and Amygdala

Mouna Maroun, Dan Yaniv, and Gal Richter-Levin

SUMMARY

At present, long-term potentiation (LTP) of synaptic transmission is the leading neurophysiologic model for learning and memory processes, despite controversial results regarding its behavioral correlates. The evidence we present in this chapter demonstrates lasting plasticity at the level of local neuronal assemblies in both hippocampus and amygdala. Local circuit plasticity (LCP) is induced by tetanic stimulation of afferent fibers and is mediated, in the hippocampus, by a reduction in GABA release. Different interneuronal populations are suggested to be involved in the LCP and LTP and at least one type of LCP correlates with age-related spatial memory abilities while the levels of LTP that can be induced initially were found unchanged in this respect. The results suggest that GABAergic interneurons play a major role in LCP and that the involved molecular/cellular modifications do not necessarily occur at the synaptic level. Overall, these data support the conception of LCP as a candidate mnemonic device that may be involved in more than one type of memory.

Introduction

A general principle of biology is that any given behavior of an organism depends on a hierarchy of levels of organization. As applied to the brain, it means that one needs to identify the main levels of organization in order to provide a framework for understanding the principles underlying its construction and function. The study of brain and mind has led to the recognition of several important levels of analysis from large information processing blocks down to the finest details of molecular structure and subcellular biophysics.

Within this conceptual framework, the study of learning and memory (as well as other cognitive processes) has grown rapidly over the past four decades and

Christian Hölscher, editor, *Neuronal Mechanisms of Memory Formation.* © 2001 Cambridge University Press. Printed in the United States of America. All rights reserved.

allowed some fascinating insights into the biological machine underlying these capacities. One of the first widely known theories to propose a mechanism for storing and retrieving information in the brain was Hebb's theory of cell assemblies (1949). Hebb's work (1949), accompanied by papers from McCulloch and Pitts (McCulloch and Pitts, 1943; McCulloch, 1947; Pitts and McCulloch, 1947), launched a generation of neuroscientists on a course of studying the dynamic properties of assemblies of interconnected neurons (e.g., Rapoport, 1952; White, 1961; Ashby et al., 1962; Smith and Davidson, 1962). According to this view, coactive and potentially interconnected neurons would, after repeated coactivity, become more strongly connected. This change in connection strength implemented learning, its persistence comprised memory, and the reactivation of *assemblies* of such neurons was memory retrieval. Hebb's theory provided one way in which learning and memory could occur in the brain, *through* an activity-dependent, associative *synaptic* plasticity. Long-term potentiation (LTP), an electrophysiologic phenomenon that resembled Hebb's idea of an activity-dependent, modifiable synapse, was first observed in the hippocampus only 26 years later (Bliss and Lomo, 1973) and in other brain areas as well later on (see the introduction to this book).

"Assembling" the three italic words in the last paragraph reflects two different hierarchical levels – the synapse and neural assemble – and emphasizes what we consider to be a cornerstone in the work we present in this chapter. We differentiate, experimentally, between two assertions recently reviewed by Martinez and Derrick (1996). One is that memory is stored in networks of neurons, and the second is that such ensembles require dynamic interactions among neurons and an ability to modify these interactions. In other words, because neurons communicate with each other only at synapses, the activity of the assembly or network is most easily altered by changes in synaptic function. LTP reflects such a synaptic change, one that is a mechanism by which memory can occur (or at least one that is likely to enable it). Yet, we are interested in exploring memory at the higher level, that of the operation of local neuronal circuits that, analogously, reflects the first assertion (i.e., memory itself). In fact, as will be described, changes in local circuitry can occur independently of LTP occurrence, a fact that supports the search for synaptic processes other than those focused on isolated excitatory synapses.

This chapter focuses on distinct cellular processes that may be responsible for the activation of local circuit plasticity, for example, interneuronal activity. We present experimental evidence of the activation of local circuitry as well as its modifiability following different procedures, some of which do and some of which do not affect LTP. As we are interested in different types of memory, the circuits investigated are located in two brain areas – the hippocampus and the amygdala – which represent, for that matter, cognitive and emotional memory systems.

Local Circuit Plasticity in Hippocampal Dentate Gyrus

Local circuit activity is defined as interactions between neurons of similar or different properties. Its functional meaning is that under given conditions local circuits function as an independent integrative unit (Rakic, 1976). In this sense, the general design of the hippocampus (as well as that of the cerebellum and neocortex) is compatible: an input stage of granule cells equipped with feedforward and/or feedback inhibition that outputs to many principal (pyramidal) cells that have inhibitory interactions. Lately it became evident that one cannot overemphasize the role of GABAergic interneurons in modifying information processing in hippocampal circuits (for a recent consideration, see Paulsen and Moser, 1998).

One way of activating local circuit activity within the dentate gyrus (DG) is by increasing perforant path stimulus frequency from 0.1 Hz to 1.0 Hz for a short interval (a few seconds). This results in a transient reduction of the population spike of the field potential response (Sloviter, 1991; Richter-Levin et al., 1994), and therefore is called frequency-dependent inhibition (FDI). FDI is GABA-mediated and reflects mainly feedforward inhibition by perforant path-activated interneurons on DG granule cells (Sloviter, 1991). We have recently revealed that FDI in the DG is NMDA-dependent (Rosenblum et al., 1999). This means that N-methyl-D-aspartate receptor (NMDAR)-mediated currents contribute to the basal level responses of inhibitory interneurons. In addition, by applying different doses of MK-801 (a noncompetitive NMDA receptor antagonist) we have found dissociation between FDI and LTP in relation to NMDAR activation. At an intermediate dosage, MK-801 had yet no significant effect on LTP but markedly reduced FDI while, at a higher dose, MK-801 had effect on both phenomena. These results are in agreement with other studies that suggest that NMDARs on interneurons may have different properties from those located on granule cells (for an in-depth discussion, see McBain et al., 1999). In fact, our results hint that different interneuronal populations are involved in FDI and LTP.

In another study (Maroun and Richter-Levin, 2000) we have examined the modifiability of FDI and its relation to aging-associated impairments in spatial learning abilities. Comparing the effects of theta burst stimulation (TBS) on LTP induction and FDI in young and old rats, we found that although the two groups showed similar levels of LTP, the tetanic stimulation also gave rise to a lasting reduction in FDI in young but not aged rats. Furthermore, this age-associated reduction in local circuit plasticity was correlated with an age-associated impairment of performance in a reversal spatial memory task in the Morris water maze. This set of results indicates that, in the hippocampus, TBS induces a form of local circuit plasticity independently of its known capacity to induce synaptic plasticity. The fact that this additional capacity is compromised in aged animals, an impairment that was correlated with spatial memory capabilities, supports the conception of local circuitry as an attractive candidate mnemonic device.

By which mechanisms TBS attenuate FDI? Based on the GABAergic role in the basic phenomenon, a plausible possibility is a reduction in GABA function. So we next examined the effects of bicuculline (a GABAA receptor blocker) on FDI in the dentate gyrus (Maroun and Richter-Levin, 2000). Indeed, FDI was attenuated by the application of bicuculline, similar to the effects of TBS. These results indicate that TBS-induced reduction in FDI is mediated, at least in part, by a reduction in GABA release. This may result from decreased efficacy of both inhibitory synapses from interneurons onto pyramidal cells and excitatory synapses from pyramidal cells onto interneurons (see Nakajima et al., 1991; McMahon and Kauer, 1997). The hippocampal circuitry furthermore exhibits a different type of local circuit activity apart from FDI. The inner third of the molecular layer of the dentate gyrus receives a projection that originates exclusively from the cells in the polymorphic layer (Blackstad, 1956; Laurberg and Sorensen, 1981). Since this projection originates both on the ipsilateral and contralateral sides, it has been called *ipsilateral associational/commissural projection*. Both projections appear to originate as collaterals from axons of the mossy cells of the hillus (Laurberg and Sorensen, 1981). Since the mossy cells are immunoreactive for glutamate (Soriano and Frotscher, 1993), it is likely that they release this excitatory transmitter substance at their terminals within the ipsilateral associational/commissural zone of the molecular layer.

Stimulation of the commissural projection at different intervals prior to stimulation of the perforant path has been shown to induce a biphasic inhibitory/excitatory effect on granule cells' responsiveness to the perforant path stimulation (Richter-Levin and Segal, 1991). We found that TBS, in addition to inducing LTP, also lastingly reduces both the commissure-induced inhibition (at 25 msec ISI) and facilitation (at 85 msec ISI) (Maroun and Richter-Levin, 2000).

In a similar fashion to FDI, we examined the role of GABA in mediating this type of plasticity (Maroun and Richter-Levin, unpublished observation). The application of bicuculline reduced the commisural-induced inhibition, similarly to TBS, while enhancing the commissure-induced facilitation. Thus, commissural-dependent inhibition of granule cells' responsiveness to perforant path stimulation is GABAergic and may lastingly change in response to TBS, probably through a reduction in GABA release. It is not clear whether commissure-induced facilitation is interneuronal or principal cells modulated. In any case, as was suggested before (Kanda et al., 1989), because the commissural facilitation at longer intervals is observed as a result of the counteraction between the GABAergic inhibition and commissural facilitatory influence, any procedure reducing the GABAergic transmission should result in the potentiation of commissural-dependent facilitation.

LTP and Local Circuit Plasticity in the Amygdala

The amygdalar complex is a medial temporal lobe structure in the brain that is widely considered to be involved in the neural substrates of emotional memory processes (reviewed by Davis, 1994; LeDoux, 1995; Gallagher and Chiba, 1996; LaBar and LeDoux, 1997; Phelps and Andersen, 1997). In particular, it appears that the basolateral complex of the amygdala (BLA), which includes the lateral and basal nuclei, is a site of plasticity that may be crucial for fear conditioning (Davis et al., 1994; Rogan and LeDoux, 1996; Maren and Fanselow, 1996). Like other forms of classical conditioning, fear conditioning is believed to involve physiologic changes in the pathways processing the CS, as a result of the convergence with inputs from the unconditioned pathway (Pavlov, 1927; Hebb, 1949; Konorski, 1967; Kandel and Spencer, 1968).

In an elegant series of studies, LeDoux and colleagues have shown that the lateral amygdala is a crucial site of plasticity for auditory fear conditioning (reviewed by LeDoux, 1998). This group showed that the processing of sound by the amygdala was amplified by the induction of LTP through thalamic tetanization (Rogan and LeDoux, 1995) and that fear conditioning did the same thing to sound processing as LTP induction (Rogan et al., 1997). In fact, this latter study and another one published at the same time (McKernan and Shinnick-Gallagher, 1997) constitute the best evidence to date that LTP has anything to do with learning (Malenka and Nicoll, 1997; Stevens, 1998).

In addition to its sensory input from the thalamus, the amygdala receives massive projections from the overlying visual, auditory, and multimodal temporal lobe cortex (for a recent comprehensive review, see McDonald, 1998). Consistent with this position, behavioral reports have demonstrated that posttraining but not pretraining lesions of the perirhinal cortex (PRC) interfere with the expression of conditioned fear responses to visual (Rosen et al., 1992), auditory (Campeau and Davis, 1995; Corodimas and LeDoux, 1995), and contextual stimuli (Corodimas and LeDoux, 1995) (but see Herzog and Otto, 1997, 1998). Pretraining lesions of the anterior PRC have also been reported to disrupt olfactory fear conditioning (Herzog and Otto, 1997, 1998). This is consistent with studies in the monkey, which suggest that the primate PRC plays a role in memory consolidation (Squire and Alvarez, 1995; Higuchi and Miyashita, 1996). Although the PRC [together with the hippocampal formation (Squire and Zola-Morgan, 1991)] has typically been associated with the declarative or explicit memory system, these behavioral data suggest that this area may also be involved in the storage, consolidation, or retrieval of emotional memory along with the amygdala (Suzuki, 1996). Recent anatomic data support this assumption by showing that the basal amygdaloid nucleus (BN) receives inputs from both the fundus and ventral bank (area 35) of the rhinal sulcus, while projections from the more dorsal bank (area 36) are distributed fairly evenly across the lateral nucleus (Shi and Cassell, 1999). We therefore set out to examine whether we could reliably evoke field responses in the BN by stimulating the vPRC and, if so, to examine their long-term modifiability (Yaniv and Richter-Levin, unpublished results). Indeed we have observed and characterized field potentials within the BN. Moreover we found that delivering TBS to the PRC produced an enduring LTP of the evoked potentials.

In this pathway, preliminary results also suggest the existence of local circuit activity and plasticity. We employed a paired-pulse stimulation protocol and measured the effects of the first stimulus on the slope and amplitude of the second response. In addition to paired-pulse facilitation at short intervals (15 to 120 msec), we observed paired-pulse inhibition at 240 msec ISI. Recent studies done in cats (Lang and Pare, 1997, 1998; Smith et al., 1998) indicate that BN interneurons play a critical role in regulating the activity of projection cells. Interneurons receive direct input from cortical afferents (Pare et al., 1997) as well as feedback excitation from lateral projection axon collaterals (Lang and Pare, 1998). Both these mechanisms could induce the local inhibitory effect reported here. Following the delivery of TBS we remeasured the effects of paired-pulse stimulation to the

PRC. Although no significant change occurred in paired-pulse facilitation, a lasting and significant reduction in inhibition occurred at 240 msec ISI.

Conclusion

Out data demonstrate the modifiability of different types of local circuit activity, that is, LCP. Hippocampal LCP may be relevant to spatial memory and its absence may be connected with aging-associated impairments in this ability. As to the mechanisms, our data suggest that oscillations at the theta frequency, by activating GABAergic interneurons, may induce LCP. We think that this capacity is separated from LTP and that distinct interneuronal populations are involved in both phenomena. The presence of LCP in the basolateral amygdala, although preliminary, hints that this mechanism may also participate in different forms of memory (e.g. emotional memory). While it seemed to be related to the theta frequency – recently shown to exist in the BLA (Pare and Gaudreau, 1996; Pape et al., 1998) – the responsible mechanisms are less clear at present.

Our work stresses that different processes may participate in information storage and that these processes may be separate. Although working within the Hebb's rule frame, lasting changes in local circuit activity may result from changes other than synaptic (e.g., changes in membrane conductance, ionic channels, formation of new synapses, or elimination of existing ones). In other words, although changes in synaptic weights may accompany LCP they may as well not and thus reflect separate molecular and cellular modifications. In this case, LCP may be considered a distinct mnemonic device.

This stance is supported by the participation of interneurons in LCP, stemming from their documented role in the basic activity of local circuits. Abundant differences exist between hippocampal "principal" neurons and GABAergic interneurons in their anatomic and neurochemical features (reviewed by McBain et al., 1999), which affect short- and long-term synaptic plasticity. The simplest example is the lack of conventional forms of LTP and LTD in most interneurons. We consider this fact favorable to our assumption and evidence of LCP independence of LTP-like mechanisms.

In conclusion, our observations strengthen current views regarding the prominent role of GABAergic interneurons, of distinct classes, in memory processes, and demonstrate the importance of widening one's observations of plastic processes beyond those occurring at the synapse, that is, those expressed at the local circuit level.

REFERENCES

Ashby, W.R., von Foerster, H., and Walker, C.C. (1962). Instability of pulse activity in a net with a threshold. *Nature* 196: 561–562.

Blackstad, T.W. (1956). Commissural connections of the hippocampal region in the rat, with special reference to their mode of termination. *J. Comp. Neurol.* 105: 417–537.

Bliss, T.V.P., and Lomo, T. (1973). Long-lasting potentiation of synaptic transmission in the dentate area of an anesthetized rabbit following stimulation of the perforant path. *J. Physiol.* (London), 232: 331–356.

Campeau, S., and Davis, M. (1995). Involvement of subcortical and cortical afferents to the lateral nucleus of the amygdala in fear conditioning measured with fear potentiated startle in rats trained concurrently with auditory and visual conditioned stimuli. *J. Neurosci.* 15: 2312–2327.

Corodimas, K.P., and LeDoux, J.E. (1995). Disruptive effects of posttraining perirhinal lesions on conditioned fear: Contributions of contextual cues. *Behav. Neurosci.* 109: 613–619.

Davis, M. (1994). The role of the amygdala in emotional learning. *Int. Rev. Neurobiol.* 36: 225–266.

Davis, M., Rainnie, D., and Cassell, M. (1994). Neurotransmission in the raet amygdala related to fear and anxiety. *TINS* 17: 208–214.

Gallagher, M., and Chiba, A.A. (1996). The amygdala and emotion. *Curr. Opin. Neurobiol.* 6: 221–227.

Hebb, D.O. (1949). *The Organization of Behavior.* New York: Wiley.

Herzog, C., and Otto, T. (1997). Odor-guided fear conditioning in rats: 2. Lesions of the anterior perirhinal cortex disrupt fear conditioned to the explicit conditioned stimulus but not the training context. *Behav. Neurosci.* 111: 1265–1272.

Herzog, C., and Otto, T. (1998). Contributions of anterior perirhinal cortex to olfactory and contextual fear conditioning. *Neuroreport* 9: 1855–1859.

Higuchi, S.-I., and Miyashita, Y. (1996). Formation of mnemonic neural responses to visual paired associates in inferotemporal cortex is impaired by perirhinal and entorhinal lesions. *Proc. Natl. Acad. Sci. USA* 93: 739–743.

Kanda, M., Maru, E., Ashida, H., Tatsuno, J., and Takatani, O. (1989). Effects of LTP-inducing tetanic stimulations of the perforant path on the commissural inhibition and facilitation of dentate granule cell discharge. *Brain Res.* 484: 325–332.

Kandel, E.R., and Spencer, W.A. (1968). Cellular neurophysiological approaches to the study of learning. *Physiol. Rev.* 48: 65–134.

Konorski, J. (1967). *Integrative Activity of the Brain.* Chicago: University of Chicago Press.

LaBar, K.S., and LeDoux, J.E. (1997). Emotion and the brain: An overview. In T.E., Feinberg and M.J. Farah (Eds.), *Behavioral neurology and neuropsychology* (pp. 675–689). New York: McGraw-Hill.

Lang, E.J., and Pare, D. (1997). Similar inhibitory processes dominate the responses of cat lateral amygdaloid projection neurons to their various afferents. *J. Neurophysiol.* 77: 341–352.

Lang, E.J., and Pare, D. (1998). Synaptic responsiveness of interneurons of the cat lateral amygdaloid nucleus. *Neuroscience* 83: 877–889.

Laurberg, S., and Sorensen, K.E. (1981). Associational and commissural collaterals of neurons in the hippocampal formation (hilus fasciae dentete and subfield CA3). *Brain Res.* 212: 287–300.

LeDoux, J.E. (1995). Emotion: Clues from the brain. *Annu. Rev. Psychol.* 46: 209–235.

LeDoux, J.E. (1998). Fear and the brain: Where have we been, and where are we going? *Biol. Psychiatr.* 44: 1229–1238.

Malenka, R.C., and Nicoll, R.A. (1997). Learning and memory: Never fear, LTP is here. *Nature* 390: 552.

Maren, S., and Fanselow, M.S. (1996). The amygdala and fear conditioning: Has the nut been cracked? *Neuron* 16: 237–240.

Martinez, J.L., and Derrick, B.E. (1996). Long-term potentiation and learning. *Annu. Rev. Psychol.* 47: 173–203.

McBain, C.J., Freund, T.F., and Mody, I. (1999). Glutamatergic synapses onto hippocampal interneurons: Precision timing without lasting plasticity. *TINS* 22: 228–235.

McCulloch, W.S. (1947). Modes of functional organization of the cerebral cortex. *Fed. Proc.* 6: 448–452.

McCulloch, W.S., and Pitts, W.H. (1943). A logical calculus of the ideas immanent in nervous activity. *Bull. Math. Biophys.* 5: 115–133.

McDonald, A.J. (1998). Cortical pathways to the mammalian amygdala. *Prog. Neurobiol.* 55: 257–332.

McKernan, M.G., and Shinnick-Gallagher, P. (1997). Fear conditioning induces a lasting potentiation of synaptic currents in vitro. *Nature* 390: 607–611.

McMahon, L.L., and Kauer, J.A. (1997). Hippocampal interneurons express a novel form of synaptic plasticity. *Neuron* 18: 295–305.

Nakajima, S., Franck, J.E., Bilkey, D., and Schwartzkroin, P.A. (1991). Local circuit synaptic plasticity interactions between CA1 pyramidal cells and interneurons in the kainate-lesioned hyperexcitable hippocampus. *Hippocampus* 1: 67–78.

Pape H.C., Pare D., and Driesang R.B. (1998). Two types of intrinsic oscillations in neurons of the lateral and basolateral nuclei of the amygdala. *J. Neurophysiol.* 79: 205–16.

Pare D., and Gaudreau H. (1996). Projection cells and interneurons of the lateral and basolateral amygdala: Distinct firing patterns and differential relation to theta and delta rhythms in conscious cats. *J. Neurosci.* 16: 3334–3350.

Pare, J.-F., Smith, Y., Pare, D., and Fillion, M. (1997). Cortical inputs to inhibitory interneurons of the basolateral amygdaloid complex. *Soc. Neurosci. Abstr.* 23: 817.7.

Paulsen, O., and Moser, E.I. (1998). A model of hippocampal memory encoding and retrieval: GABAergic control of synaptic plasticity. *TINS* 21: 273–278.

Pavlov, I.P (1927). *Conditioned Reflexes.* New York: Dover.

Phelps, E.A., and Andersen, A.K. (1997). What does the amygdala do? *Curr. Biol.* 7: R311–R314.

Pitts, W.H., and McCulloch, W.S. (1947). How we know universals: The perception of auditory and visual form. *Bull. Math. Biophys.* 9: 127–147.

Rakic, P. (1976). *Local Circuit Neurons.* Cambridge, MA: MIT Press.

Rapoport, A. (1952) "Ignition" phenomena in randon nets. *Bull. Math. Biophys.* 14: 35–44.

Richter-Levin, G., and Segal, M. (1991). The effects of serotonin depletion and raphe grafts on hippocampal electrophysiology and behavior. *J. Neurosci.* 11: 1585–1596.

Richter-Levin, G., Greenberger, V., and Segal, M. (1994). The effects of general and restricted lesions on hippocampal electrophysiology and behavior. *Brain Res.* 642: 111–116.

Rogan, M., and LeDoux, J.E. (1995). LTP is accompanied by commensurate enhancement of auditory-evoked responses in a fear conditioning circuit. *Neuron* 15: 127–136.

Rogan, M.T., and LeDoux, J.E. (1996). Emotion: Systems, cells, synaptic plasticity. *Cell* 85: 469–475.

Rogan, M.T., Staubli, U.V., and LeDoux, J.E. (1997). Fear conditioning induces associative long-term potentiation in the amygdala. *Nature* 390: 604–607.

Rosen J.B., Hitchcock J.M., Miserendino M.J.D., Falls W.A. et al. (1992). Lesions of the perirhinal cortex but not of the frontal, medial prefrontal, visual, or insular cortex block fear-potentiated startle using a visual conditioned stimulus. *J. Neurosci.* 12: 4624–4633.

Rosenblum, K., Maroun, M., and Richter-Levin, G. (1999). Frequency-dependent inhibition in the dentate gyrus is attenuated by the NMDA receptor blocker MK-801 at doses which do not yet affect long-term potentiation. *Hippocampus* 9: 491–494.

Shi C.-J., and Cassell M.D. (1999). Perirhinal cortex projections to the amygdaloid complex and hippocampal formation in the rat. *J. Comp. Neurol.* 406: 299–328.

Sloviter, R.S. (1991). Feedforward and feedback inhibition of hippocampal principal cell activity evoked by perforant path stimulation: GABA-mediated mechanisms that regulate excitability. *Hippocampus* 1: 31–40.

Smith, D.R., and Davidson, C.H. (1962). Maintained activity in neural nets. *J. Assoc. Comp. Mach.* 9: 268–279.

Smith, Y., Pare, J.-F., and Pare, D. (1998). Cat intraamygdaloid inhibitory network: Ultrastructural organization of parvalbumin-immunoreactive elements. *J. Comp. Neurol.* 391: 164–179.

Soriano, E., and Frotscher, M. (1993). Spiny nonpyramidal neurons in the CA3 region of the rat hippocampus are glutamate-like immunoreactive and receive convergent mossy fiber input. *J. Comp. Neurol.* 333: 435–448.

Squire, L., and Alvarez, P. (1995). Retrograde amnesia and memory consolidation: A neuro-biological perspective. *Curr. Opin. Neurobiol.* 5: 169–177.

Squire, L., and Zola-Morgan, S. (1991). The medial temporal lobe memory system. *Science* 253: 1380–1386.

Stevens, C.F. (1998). A million dollar question: Does LTP = memory? *Neuron* 20: 1–2.

Suzuki, W.A. (1996). The anatomy, physiology and functions of the perirhinal cortex. *Curr. Opin. Neurobiol.* 6: 179–186.

White, H. (1961). The formation of cell assemblies. *Bull. Math. Biophys.* 23: 43–53.

Yaniv, D., and Richter-Levin, G., (2000). LTP in the basal amygdala induced by perirhinal cortex stimulation, in vivo. *Neuroreport* 11(3): 525–530.

CHAPTER SEVEN

Theta-Facilitated Induction of Long-Term Potentiation

A Better Model for Memory Formation?

Christian Hölscher

SUMMARY

As described in the introduction of this book, the induction of long-term potentiation (LTP) of synaptic transmission in the hippocampus using high-frequency stimulation (HFS) cannot be seen as a physiologic method that models synaptic plasticity that might occur during learning. Several other stimulation protocols have been developed that emulate natural neuronal firing patterns more closely, and LTP obtained with such a technique may therefore provide a better model of learning-related plasticity. The novel stimulation protocol presented here makes use of the reduction of local inhibition during theta rhythm. This stimulation technique (five pulses at 200 Hz phase-locked with peaks of theta oscillations *in vivo*) is able to induce stable LTP with as few as fifteen stimuli. Such bursts of stimuli are comparable to natural activity that can be recorded in the living brain. This type of stimulation protocol appears to induce LTP in a different way than HFS does. The metabotropic glutamate receptor agonist 1S,3S-ACPD blocks HFS-induced LTP, but does not affect the ability of rats to learn spatial tasks. However, LTP induced by a stimulation protocol of short bursts that are given phase-locked with theta rhythm was not blocked by 1S,3S-ACPD. Hence, the novel stimulation protocol appears to induce LTP in a more physiologic way that correlates with learning abilities of rats. It is suggested that this protocol, which not only resembles natural firing patterns found in the hippocampus in a living brain, but also models changes in synaptic transmission that are linked to memory formation more closely than HFS-induced LTP, has the potential to be a better model for putative synaptic changes that occur during learning. Although this novel stimulation protocol is still very unphysiologic in the way large areas in the brain are simultaneously activated, it can be seen as a step in the right direction by making use of endogenous facilitating mechanisms that might play a role in alteration of synaptic transmission during learning.

Introduction

As discussed in the introduction to this book, we cannot automatically assume that all types of long-term potentiation (LTP), induced by high-frequency stimulation (HFS) or otherwise, are a model for synaptic processes that might occur during learning. When LTP was first described, it was an exciting new model that offered great promise (Bliss and Lømo, 1973). However, we have learned a lot since. We now know that different areas (CA1/CA3, dentate, cortex, superior cervical ganglion, and others) express different types of LTP that show different pharmacologic profiles and are induced by activation of different receptor types (Lanthorn et al., 1984; Johnston et al., 1992; Luján et al., 1996; Alkadhi and Altememi, 1997; Lu et al., 1997). We also know a lot more about neuronal activity in the brain in behaving animals. This chapter will describe attempts to make use of this knowledge and to employ stimulation techniques that are closer to naturally occurring neuronal activity patterns, and also to take advantage of intrinsic mechanisms that modulate local inhibition and can greatly facilitate synaptic plasticity.

Theta Rhythm

Theta rhythm is defined as electroencephalogram (EEG) field potential oscillations in the 3 to 12 Hz range (Winson, 1972; Vanderwolf, 1975; Fox et al., 1983; Vanderwolf and Leung, 1983; Buzsáki, 1986). Theta in the hippocampal formation is generated by two main inputs: a cholinergic/GABAergic afferent projection from rhythmically discharging cells of the medial septum and diagonal band (Petsche et al., 1962) and a glutamatergic projection from stellate cells in layer II of the entorhinal cortex (Steward, 1976; Vanderwolf and Leung, 1983; Alonso and Ilinás, 1989). Axons of pyramidal cells of layer II of both the medial and the lateral entorhinal cortex terminate on the CA1 pyramidal cell dendrites. In the dentate gyrus, entorhinal stellate cells from layer II project to granule cells (Steward, 1976; Buzsáki, 1986). Septal neurons terminate on inhibitory interneurons in the dentate and CA1 and on granule cells (Buzsáki et al., 1983). In addition, subtypes of hippocampal interneurons in the stratum moleculare may also exhibit low-threshold membrane oscillations (Buhl and Buzsáki, 1998). The intracellular mechanism that produces neuronal oscillations is dependent on the activation of a low-threshold sodium current and the deactivation of hyperpolarization-activated currents (I_H). These currents have properties indistinguishable from previously described pacemaker currents termed I_H, I_Q, or I_F (Gauss et al., 1998; Ludwig et al., 1998). These currents are mediated by hyperpolarization-activated cyclic nucleotide sensitive nonselective cation channels. In thalamic neurons, I_H causes membrane potential resonance in response to inputs of around 6 Hz (Strohmann et al., 1994). In the entorhinal cortex, I_H interacts with a noninactivating sodium current to generate theta oscillations (Alonso and Ilinás, 1989). CA1 pyramidal neurons also express such channels and have membrane currents with properties characteristic of I_H, which could amplify oscillating pacemaker input from the septum (Gauss et al., 1998; Ludwig et al., 1998).

However, theta rhythm is not simply the product of pacemaker activity but is also dependent on and amplified by local neuronal networks of the hippocampus. For example, somatostatin-containing interneurons receive their main excitatory input from local collaterals of pyramidal neurons and preferentially synapse with distal dendrites of pyramidal cells (Buhl and Buzsáki, 1998). Such a local circuit is capable of oscillating if either the excitatory or the inhibitory neurons are activated by afferent inputs. If the pyramidal neurons fire, they will activate the inhibitory interneurons, which in turn inhibit pyramidal neurons by negative feedback loops, thereby reducing firing probability in the pyramidal neurons. Once inhibition drops again, the firing probability of the pyramidal neurons increases (Leung, 1980).

Hence, theta rhythm depends on the network architecture and is the result of overall network activity and not just on passive resonance induced by oscillating input of pacemakers. These properties of local networks in the hippocampus can be shown in paired-pulse facilitation *in vivo*. In area CA1 of the hippocampus, giving a second stimulus ca. 50 msec after a first will produce a stronger excitatory postsynaptic potential (EPSP) response. One of several reasons for this potentiation is the fact that all local inhibitory interneurons have been activated simultaneously during the first stimulation. A short time afterward, all local inhibitory interneurons will reduce their activity due to the lack of excitatory input coming from the negative feedback loops described earlier, since they inhibited pyramidal cell firing. Local inhibition will be reduced simultaneously during a defined time window after the first stimulus, and the second EPSPs will be larger if a stimulus is given within this time window (Schulz et al., 1995; Son and Carpenter, 1996; Hölscher et al., 1997b).

What has interested researchers for many decades is that the onset of theta rhythm is dependent on motor activity or arousal (e.g., by presentation of a novel object, or during paradoxical sleep; Leung, 1980; Fox et al., 1983; Vanderwolf and Leung, 1983). Initial suggestions that theta itself encoded or transmitted information had to be abandoned, since regular oscillation cannot contain information in itself. However, it was clear from lesion and pharmacologic studies that theta rhythm was necessary for proper information processing and learning (Winson, 1978; Sinz, 1979; Bland, 1986). Hence, the correlation between theta and exploring/learning intrigued many researchers as it suggested that theta rhythm is a crucial aspect of proper neuronal network functions and could hold the key to the answer of how information is actually processed by the brain.

Gamma Activity

Apart from field potential oscillations in the theta range, high-frequency oscillations can be observed (40 to 100 Hz) in the awake, exploring rat (Vanderwolf, 1969; Buzsáki et al., 1983). These oscillations are not the product of activation by pacemaker nuclei but by inhibitory interneurons (Freund and Buzsáki, 1996; Penttonen et al., 1998; Csicsvari et al., 1999). Active neurons within the cortex or the hippocampus have been shown to be synchronized in the gamma frequency if the neurons have been activated by the same stimulus (and therefore presumably process the same information) but are desynchronized if they are activated by the different stimuli (and therefore might not process the same information) (Singer, 1994; Neuenschwander and Singer, 1996; Fries et al., 1997; Singer, 1999). As described in different chapters in this book, this synchronization of neuronal activity could functionally "bind" neurons in their activity to produce a coherent representation within a neuronal network. This difference is crucial, as a gamma pacemaker could not discriminate between neurons that collaborate on processing of the same stimuli and nearby neurons that are not involved in it. If synchronization does bind neurons in such a way, gamma oscillation has to be produced in a decentralized and highly localized way according to local requirements.

Gamma oscillations occur at higher frequency than theta activity. This enables a higher time resolution of information relay. However, the disadvantage is that high-frequency synchronization has a much lower "time tolerance"; a delay of only a few milliseconds could prevent phase-locking of oscillation with the firing of other cells. Since action potentials take a certain time to travel, the area that can be synchronized by gamma oscillation is much smaller than that by theta oscillations. Gamma activity therefore is ideal for synchronizing cortical areas that together process a subdetail of information input, while the lower frequency theta oscillation is more suitable for synchronization of neuronal activities over the whole length of the entorhinal cortex-hippocampal formation system. Nevertheless, the brain seems to be able to synchronize gamma oscillation over large areas that are involved in the same task. In cats that were trained to respond to visual stimuli by lever presses it was observed that neuronal activity in the parietal association cortex (area 7) was synchronized with activity in area 17, the primary visual cortex, with zero time-lag (Roelfsema et al., 1997). Such high-precision synchrony over long distances requires finely tuned feedback loop projections (see also Castelo-Branco et al., 1998, and Chapter 8 in this book).

Complex Spike Activity

Other types of neuronal activity can be measured in the living brain. Since theta does not contain any information per se but is of importance for information processing and learning, the question is of what theta actually modulates and how information is encoded by neurons. Endogenous neuronal firing patterns are observed in CA1 as high-frequency bursts of about two to seven spikes ("complex spikes"; Ranck, 1973; Buzsáki, 1986; Muller and Kubie, 1989; Otto et al., 1991). Single spikes are also observed. However, since neurons are "noisy" and the single spikes could be noise, it appears that the network architecture of the nervous system is designed to prevent single spikes from being conducted very far through the neuronal networks. Bursts of spikes, however, are conducted more reliably as the first spikes reduce local inhibition and facilitate the relay of following spikes. Bursts can perhaps encode and relay information in a more reliable manner (see Lisman, 1997, for a review, and Chapter 9 in this book).

How Does Theta Rhythm Control Hippocampal Activity?

From the available data one could postulate what role theta rhythm might play in the central nervous system (CNS) and why theta would be of importance for synchronizing excitatory neuronal activity and to increase the signal-to-noise ratio. When theta activity is strongest, activity of inhibitory neurons would be highest and excitatory neurons "clamped." While pyramidal neurons still receive dendritic input they could not fire. Spontaneous activity (noise) would be minimal at this stage. When theta activity ceases, firing of inhibitory neurons would be much reduced and pyramidal neurons free to discharge if the threshold was reached after "computation" of the inhibitory and excitatory input. Firing of pyramidal cells would activate inhibitory interneurons, and together with the next phase of theta activity local inhibition would be raised again. The advantage of such a negative feedback system is that it is very stable since it keeps itself in check. Furthermore, it is a "high-tolerance" and safe way to activate neuronal networks. When brain areas are not in use they tend to be under high inhibition to prevent spontaneous activity (see below). Therefore, in order to shift brain areas into an activated state, inhibition has to be reduced toward a level in which neuronal activity and information processing is possible. Reducing inhibition too much would result in uncontrolled discharge of neurons. If a system existed that reduced inhibition for longer periods of time, the fine-tuning of this system would be crucial. Neurons, however, are difficult to calibrate (especially during development and over long time), and an oscillating negative feedback system is ideal to do such a task without the need of finely tuned neurons. Theta pacemaker cells simply start to activate local oscillations and increase them until sufficient excitatory neurons fire at the low phase of local inhibition. The firing then reduces local inhibition and feedback to pacemaker cells in a negative way. This way, large networks can be maintained at the fragile threshold between too much and too little inhibition over a long time without any risk or the need for precisely turned specialized neurons.

In the anesthetized animal this model fits the observed phenomena well. Spike and complex burst activity is highest when the theta cycle is at the lowest inhibition phase (Vanderwolf and Leung, 1983; Kamondi et al., 1998). In the awake rat, however, spike activity can precede the theta phase of lowest inhibition (Muller and Kubie, 1989; O'Keefe and Recce, 1993; Jensen and Lisman, 1996; Skaggs and McNaughton, 1996; Tsodyks et al., 1996; Csicsvari et al., 1999). It is feasible that stronger input to pyramidal cells enable them to overcome interneuronal inhibition earlier. Some authors constructed theories of how information could be encoded in the shifts of firing times such that pyramidal cell firing precedes theta wave troughs of lowest network inhibition (Muller and Kubie, 1989; O'Keefe and Recce, 1993; Buzsáki and Chrobak, 1995; Muller et al., 1996; Samsonovich and McNaughton, 1997; Lisman, 1999).

Induction of LTP by Theta-Patterned Stimulation

As described earlier, due to the nature of the network architecture and dynamics it is possible to produce paired-pulse facilitation by stimulating once (which activates excitatory and inhibitory neurons indiscriminantly) and then stimulating again in the right time window when the activity of inhibitory neurons has gone down. One strategy to induce LTP by making use of this intrinsic disinhibitory mechanism is to give short bursts of stimuli with an interburst interval of around 200 msec. Such high-frequency bursts of around five pulses resemble complex spike activity that occurs predominantly on the positive or negative phase of theta rhythm (Buzsáki, 1986; Otto et al., 1991; Stewart et al., 1992; Jeffery et al., 1996). The interburst interval of around 200 msec during theta-patterned stimulation mimics theta-type activity. A 200-msec interburst interval therefore mimics theta-type activity, and interneuron inhibition is greatly altered at that time, facilitating the induction of LTP by theta-patterned burst stimulation (Larson et al., 1986; Stäubli and Lynch, 1987; Diamond et al., 1988). However, such patterned stimulation only imitates theta rhythm and does not make use of naturally occurring theta activity. Furthermore, LTP induced by theta-patterned stimulation does not always correlate with learning abilities of animals and therefore is probably not a good model for learning-related synaptic changes. *Icv* injection of the metabotropic glutamate receptor group II agonist 1S,3S-1-amino-cyclo-pentyl-1,3-dicarboxylic acid (1S,3S-ACPD) blocked induction of LTP by high-frequency stimulation (Hölscher et al., 1997a, 1997d) or by theta-patterned stimulation in area CA1 *in vivo* (Figures 7.1 and 7.2; Hölscher et al., 1997c). However, icv injection of the same dose did not impair learning of spatial tasks in a water maze or a radial arm maze (Figure 7.1).

Induction of LTP by Stimulation Phase-Locked with Theta Rhythm

A more physiologic stimulation protocol than long trains of standard HFS or theta-patterned stimulation is the technique of stimulating neurons during actual theta rhythm. Such a technique has been reported to facilitate the induction of LTP both *in vitro* (Huerta and Lisman, 1995) and *in vivo* (Pavlides et al., 1988). Thetalike field oscillations can be induced *in vitro* using cholinergic agonists. In one study LTP was obtained by a single burst of four pulses at 100 Hz if given on the phase of theta rhythm in the hippocampal slice that represents the time window of lowest inhibition. The same burst on the opposite phase of theta (during the state of highest inhibition) induced depotentiation of previously potentiated EPSPs (Huerta and Lisman, 1995). It is possible to elicit theta activity in anesthetized animals (dependent on the type of anesthetizing agent). For example, electrical stimulation of septal nuclei can elicit theta activity (Pavlides et al., 1988; Kocsis and Vertes, 1996; Sik et al., 1997). A different technique is to induce theta in urethane-anesthetized rats by sensory stimulation such as tail-pinch (Green et al., 1990; Dickson et al., 1994; Hölscher et al., 1997b). Studies in anesthetized rats showed a similar result: stimulation with ten bursts of five pulses at 400 Hz on the positive phase of theta rhythm (during the state of lowest inhibition) induced LTP of 8 percent of the slope of field EPSPs in the dentate gyrus, while stimulation on the negative phase of theta with ten bursts reversed this (comparatively small) LTP (Pavlides et al., 1988).

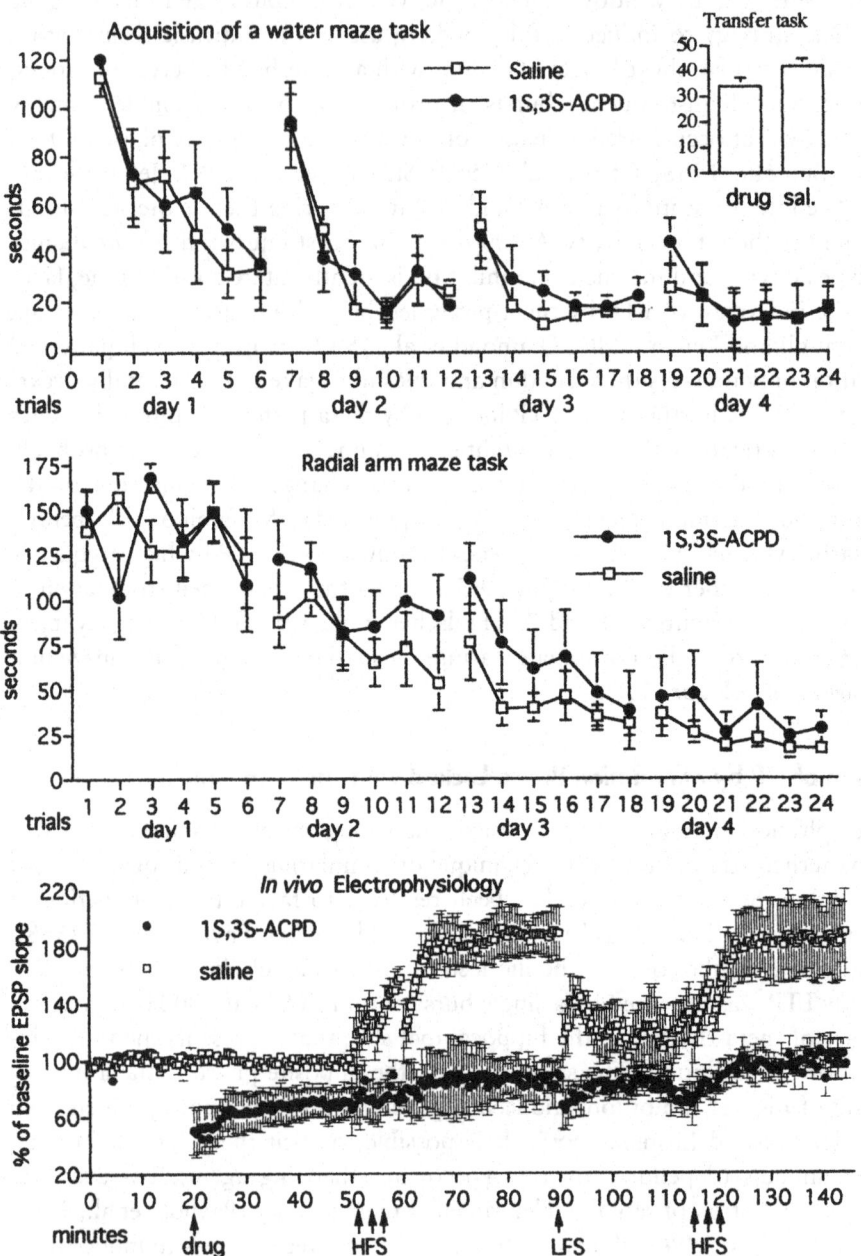

The drug 1S,3S-ACPD blocks LTP but does not affect learning in rats

In a similar study in area CA1 in urethane-anesthetized rats, single pulses given phase-locked with the positive phase of sensory stimuli-evoked theta rhythm did not change the slopes of field EPSPs. However, a train of five pulses at 200 Hz increased the slope of field EPSPs to around 115 percent of the baseline slope (Figure 7.3). Stimulating with three such trains increased slopes of field EPSPs to

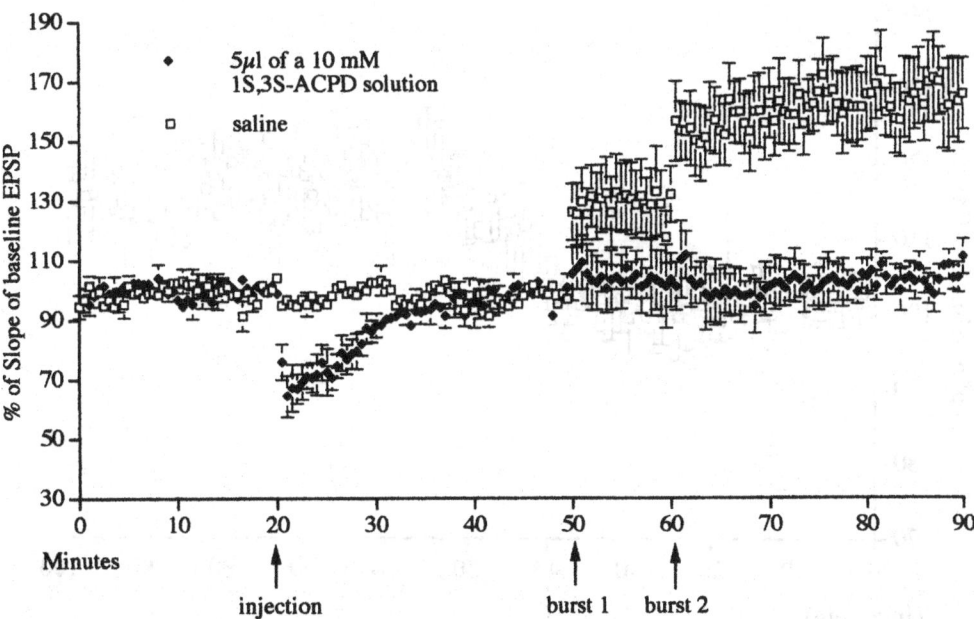

Figure 7.2. Two sets of "theta-patterned" stimulation (each consisting of four trains of five pulses at 75 Hz, 200 msec inter-train interval) induced stable LTP of field EPSPs in area CA1 in urethane anesthetized control animals. This LTP induction was blocked in animals injected with the mGluR agonist 1S,3S-ACPD (5 μL of a 10 mM solution icv). For details see Hölscher et al. (1997).

approximately 160 percent of baseline values (Figure 7.4). Stimulation on the negative phase or on the neutral phase or the absence of theta using one to ten trains did not change EPSPs in any way. Stimulating with three trains phase-locked with the negative phase of theta activity did not affect previously potentiated field EPSPs. However, stimulation on the negative phase (during the state of highest

Figure 7.1. Effect of the metabotropic glutamate receptor agonist 1S,3S-ACPD on high-frequency stimulation-induced LTP in area CA1 and on spatial learning in rats. Groups of rats ($n = 7$ to 8 per group) were trained in a spatial task involving a submerged platform in a water tank that the animal has to find. The top graph shows the effect of injecting 5 μL of a 20 mM solution of 1S,3S-ACPD icv on learning performance (time required by rats to find the platform). The insert graph shows the result of a transfer task in which the platform had been removed and rats were allowed to swim for 60 seconds. The distance swum in the quadrant that contained the platform previously was measured. There was no difference between drug and control groups. A second spatial task in a radial arm maze showed a similar result: There was no difference between groups in the time needed to find three baited arms (middle graph). Measuring the slope of field EPSP in area CA1 after injection of the same dose showed an effect on baseline and a block of LTP after HFS (lower graph). A lower dose (5 μL of a 10 mM solution of 1S,3S-ACPD icv) that did not affect baseline still blocked LTP in a separate experiment. Depotentiation was also blocked. Values are the mean ± SEM percentage of baseline EPSP slope. (Adapted from Hölscher et al., 1997, with permission.)

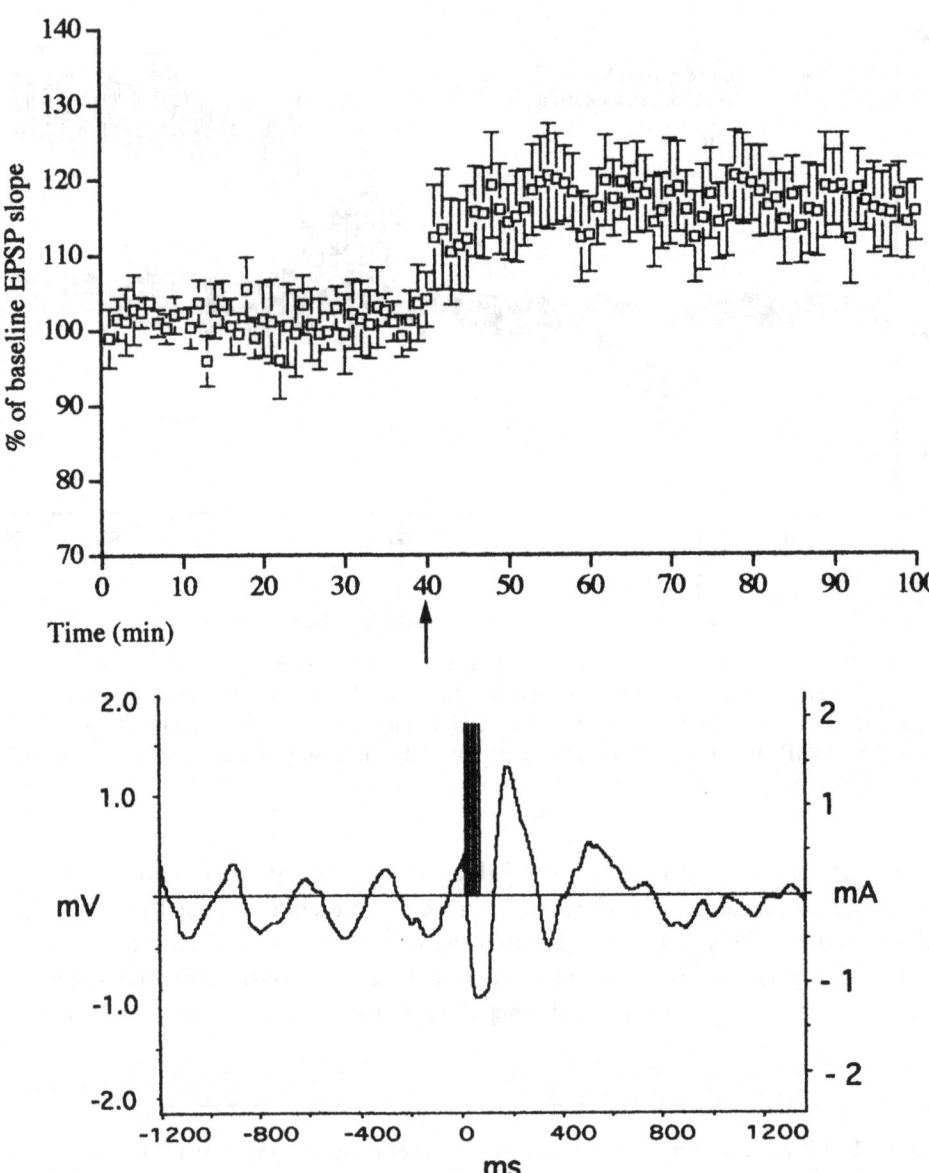

Figure 7.3. Effect of stimulation on the positive phase of theta rhythm in area CA1 in ure-thane anesthetized rats. One burst of five pulses at 200 Hz on the peak of theta (**arrow**) induced LTP of field EPSPs over 60 minutes of recording. The insert below shows a sample trace of stimulation on the positive phase of theta rhythm. The left scale shows the theta wave amplitude, and the right scale shows stimulus amplitude as measured on a different channel. Theta rhythm was induced by tail pinch, and a burst of five pulses at 200 Hz was triggered on a preset amplitude level of theta rhythm. For details see Hölscher et al. (1997).

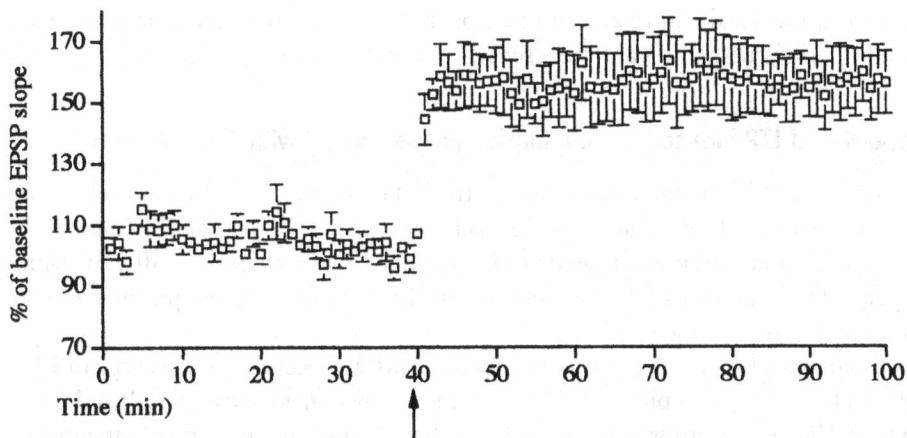

Figure 7.4. Stimulation with 3 bursts (5 pulses at 200 Hz per burst; see arrow) on the positive phase of theta rhythm induced larger LTP in area CA1. This stimulation protocol appeared to saturate LTP as additional stimulation did not increase LTP any further (see Hölscher et al., 1997).

inhibition) with ten trains did reduce previously potentiated field EPSPs (Hölscher et al., 1997b). Why such stimulation at the time of highest inhibition of local networks depotentiates EPSPs is not quite understood, especially since the same stimulation in the absence of theta did not change the slopes of previously potentiated EPSPs.

Making use of the modulation of local inhibition by theta oscillation greatly reduces the required number of stimuli to induce synaptic plasticity. In comparison, in the same setup, a minimum of 200 to 600 pulses is required to induce LTP of the same magnitude (Doyle et al., 1996; Hölscher et al., 1997d). Stimulating with high-frequency trains has the drawback of not only stimulating excitatory neurons (or axons) but also inhibitory neurons. Depending on the circumstances it is possible that such stimulation actually inhibits the system more than excites it, which explains why sometimes HFS does not produce LTP at all. In *in vitro* studies of the dentate gyrus, GABA antagonists are added to the artificial cerebrospinal fluid (CSF) to reduce the strong inhibition in this area and to make LTP induction possible (Brown and Reymann, 1995; Bushell et al., 1995; O'Mara et al., 1995; Nosten-Bertrand et al., 1996). In one investigation, it was shown that mice that do not express the cell adhesion molecule Thy-1 did not express LTP in the dentate gyrus when recorded *in vivo* in anesthetized animals. In the slice preparation, however, LTP was inducible in the presence of GABA antagonists. Injecting GABA antagonists locally into the hippocampus rescued LTP induction in the dentate *in vivo* in these mice (Nosten-Bertrand et al., 1996). In a follow-up study recording in awake mice, it was shown that a small increase of about 10 percent of the EPSP slope was achieved with HFS (Errington et al., 1997). Since Thy-1 deficient mice were able to learn spatial tasks and appeared not much different from control mice in their general behavior, one can assume that the extraordinarily high inhibition in the dentate gyrus in the anesthetized mouse is reduced in the awake animal and most probably is greatly reduced in the active dentate during theta and gamma activity.

Properties of LTP Induced by Stimulation Phase-Locked with Theta Activity

One question that emerged from the fact that LTP can be induced by as few as five stimuli is whether LTP induced by this technique is identical to HFS-induced LTP. It is possible that the novel type of LTP is induced by mechanisms different from standard HFS-induced LTP. One way to test this is to identify the pharmacologic profile of the novel type of LTP.

It is not possible to test the involvement of NMDA receptors in this type of LTP induced by stimulation phase-locked with theta, since theta activity itself is dependent on NMDA receptor activity and is reduced after application of antagonists (Leung and Desborough, 1988). A block of LTP induced by theta phase-locked stimulation after application of such antagonists could be an indirect effect by reducing theta activity. The same argument holds true for drugs that act on the cholinergic system. Investigations of the pharmacology of the type of LTP induced by stimulation phase-locked with theta is therefore limited to pharmaceutical manipulations that do not interfere with theta activity.

Theta activity is dependent on cholinergic, serotonergic, GABAergic, and NMDA-receptor dependent neurotransmission (Fox et al., 1983; Green and Greenough, 1986; Leung and Desborough, 1988; Dickson et al., 1994; Marrosu et al., 1996; Natsume and Kometani, 1997). As described previously the mGluR agonist 1S,3S-ACPD blocked LTP but did not impair spatial learning in rats. Therefore, it is of interest to test what effect this drug has on LTP induced by stimulation phase-locked with theta activity. A dose that was previously seen to block HFS-induced LTP or theta-patterned stimulation induced LTP (Hölscher et al., 1997a–d; Figures 7.1 and 7.2) did not affect LTP induced by stimulation phase-locked with theta activity. Also, theta rhythm was not affected by the drug. The selective mGluR group I and II antagonist (±)alpha-methyl-4-carboxyphenyl-glycine (MCPG) also had no effect on the induction of LTP (Figure 7.5). These results are surprising and suggest that the novel type of LTP is induced in a different way than HFS-induced LTP. There has been some debate as to what degree mGluRs play a role in the induction process of LTP. It was reported that the mGluR antagonist MCPG was found to block LTP (Bashir et al., 1993), or that MCPG blocked LTP only under certain conditions, when mGluRs have not been activated previously (which would activate a "molecular switch") (Bortolotto et al., 1994), or not to block LTP at all (Bordi and Ugolini, 1995; Selig et al., 1995; Thomas and O'Dell, 1995) (see Hölscher et al., 1999, for a review). Since some mGluR subtypes have a relatively low affinity to glutamate and can be located at the periphery of synapses (Luján et al., 1996; Shigemoto et al., 1997), one could speculate that mGluRs are activated primarily during strong stimulation (Petrozzino and Connor, 1994). The efficacy of the brief burst stimulation during positive phase theta activity in eliciting LTP in the CA1 area is comparable to HFS. The magnitude of LTP following 15 pulses was equivalent to that observed

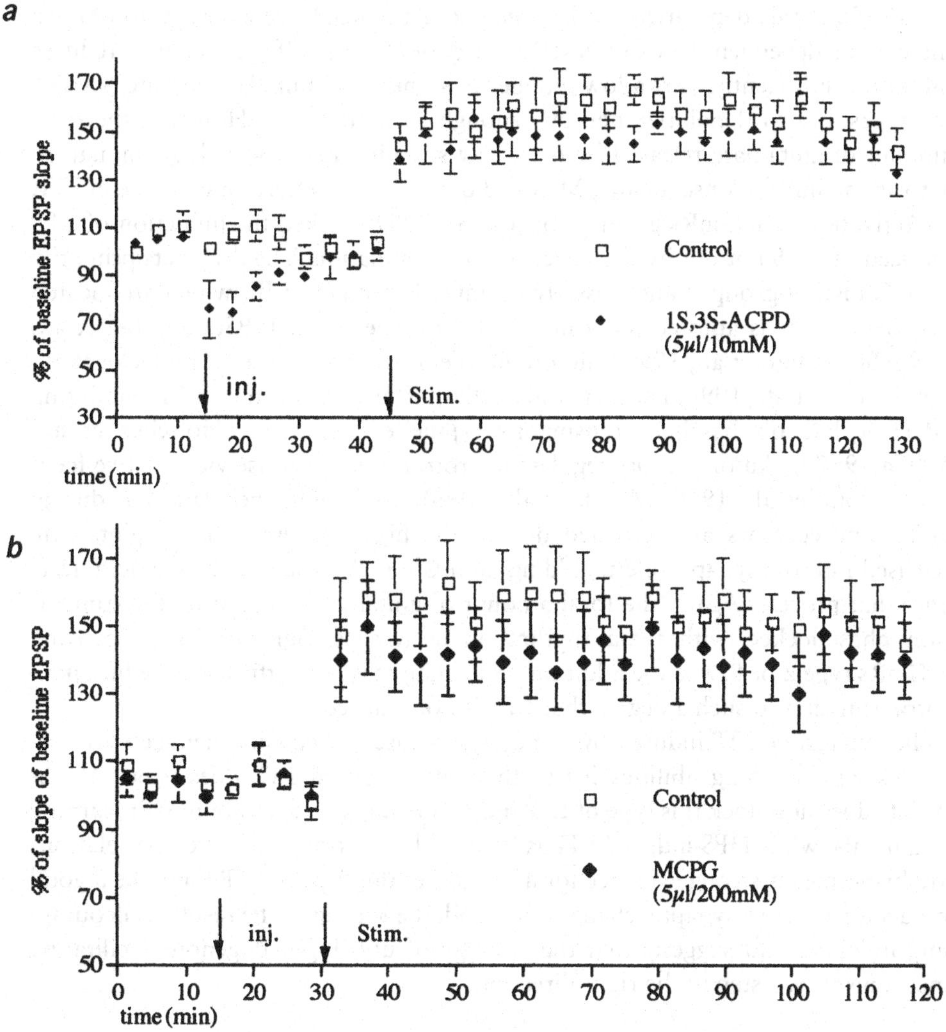

Figure 7.5. Effect of the mGluR agonist 1S,3S-ACPD and the antagonist MCPG on LTP induced by stimulation phase-locked with theta rhythm. (a) The effect of 5 µL/10 mM icv on LTP induced by stimulation phase-locked with theta rhythm is shown in the top graph. This dose of 1S,3S-ACPD transiently reduced baseline transmission but the effect had reversed at the time of conditioning stimulation. LTP was not affected by 1S,3S-ACPD. Values are the mean ± SEM percentage baseline EPSP slope. *n* = 6 per group. (b) The mGluR antagonist MCPG (5 µL/200 mM icv) did not significantly affect the magnitude of LTP induced by stimulation phase-locked with theta rhythm. *n* = 6 per group. Theta activity was not impaired by the drugs.

after 600 pulses using the standard HFS protocol (Hölscher et al., 1997a, 1997d). The threshold for eliciting LTP with this protocol was a single burst of three to five pulses (Huerta and Lisman, 1995; Hölscher et al., 1997b). During the positive phase of theta it is thought that synchronous depolarization across large sections of the hippocampus occurs due to a reduction in GABAergic inhibition (Ylinen et al., 1995). If this depolarization is large enough it would be expected to remove the voltage-dependent block of NMDA receptor channels. If theta-activity reduces inhibition sufficiently, only a low number of stimuli is required to activate NMDA receptors and to depolarize neurons enough to induce LTP. However, the total amount of glutamate released by these few stimuli might not be high enough to activate mGluRs. Consequently, MCPG did not have an effect on this type of LTP.

Activation of mGluRs group II by 1S,3S-ACPD blocked the induction of LTP induced by HFS but not by the novel type of stimulation. The drug acts primarily on mGluR2 of group II and possibly on mGluR8 of group III, which are located presynaptically as autoreceptors in area CA1 (Jane et al., 1995; Saugstad et al., 1996; Shigemoto et al., 1997) and on interneurons and glial cells (Blümcke et al., 1996; Neki et al., 1996; Petralia et al., 1996). This explains the strong inhibiting effect it has on baseline transmission (Jane et al., 1996; Hölscher et al., 1997a,1997d). Autoreceptors regulate neurotransmitter release via negative feedback (Conn et al., 1996; Macek et al., 1996). One could speculate that during HFS, autoreceptors are activated due to the high concentration of glutamate released into the synaptic cleft. Adding an mGluR2/8 agonist clearly would acerbate that process. Again, the total amount of glutamate released by the stimulation phase-locked with theta rhythm might not be high enough to activate mGluRs type 2 or 8, and the addition of an agonist is not sufficient to reduce neurotransmission to such a degree that LTP is not induced.

In conclusion, LTP induced by stimulation phase-locked with theta activity correlates with learning abilities better than HFS-induced LTP does, since 1S,3S-ACPD does not block this type of LTP induction and also does not impair learning in animals, while HFS-induced LTP is blocked by the drug. However, correlations are by no means strong evidence for a claim that this type of LTP might be a good model for putative synaptic changes that underlie learning. The result is encouraging, however, and suggests that the strategy of utilizing endogenous facilitating mechanisms is a step in the right direction.

Prospects for the Future

The results show that making use of facilitating mechanisms that are intrinsic to neuronal networks of the hippocampus can greatly reduce the threshold for induction of synaptic plasticity. This suggests that perhaps similar processes of modulation of synaptic transmission are induced during learning. However, one has to concede that this novel stimulation protocol still is very unphysiologic. Stimulations are evoked artificially, using comparatively strong shocks that depolarize large areas in the brain simultaneously, indiscriminantly of cell type (excitatory or inhibitory, projection neuron or interneuron, spontaneously active or silent neurons, etc.). Hence, this protocol can only be a step toward more realistic and physiologic experimental conditions and models for memory processes.

Ideally, one would stimulate a single neuron and record from a neuron that receives input from this stimulated neuron. If the response evoked in the recorded neuron changed during a learning situation, one possibility is that the learning process altered synaptic transmission (O'Mara, 1995). Unfortunately, such an experiment is almost impossible with currently available techniques, and furthermore, there is no guarantee that one happens to record from neurons that are actually involved in a learning process. Also, single neurons can be spontaneously active, and such noise might affect synaptic transmission to some extent. Additionally, there are numerous confounding variables and learning-independent influences. For example, stress can reduce EPSPs and impair LTP development (Diamond et al., 1990, 1994; Pavlides et al., 1996; Joëls, 1997). A downregulation or upregulation of a single synaptic contact would not necessarily prove the point.

A more pragmatic approach is the simultaneous recording of a number of single neurons during learning. Using a multirecording electrode array it is possible to monitor a large number of neurons of which some will be active in synchronization. This will not measure synaptic activity directly, but can give a fairly accurate account of which neurons are active during specific activities. One would assume that information is encoded in active neuronal assemblies that are involved in processing information. Observing a group of so-called place cells that fire predominantly when the animal is in a defined location (O'Keefe and Dostrovsky, 1971; O'Keefe, 1979) in a spatial task, for example, can show emerging firing patterns of neuronal ensembles that correlate with learning and familiarization of the animal with the environment. This new pattern then is consistently observed when placing the animal in the same environment (Wilson and McNaughton, 1993; Burgess et al., 1996; Barnes et al., 1997; Jeffery, 1997; Mehta et al., 1997; Wilson and Tonegawa, 1997; see also chapters on single cell recording in this book). These emerging patterns are not static and can adapt after alteration of the environment (Bostock et al., 1991; Wilson and McNaughton, 1993). Such network dynamics shows that these are indeed plastic changes in neuronal responses that correlate with experience. The working hypothesis is that the changes are of a synaptic nature, but the technique does not allow one to test directly that conjecture since firing probability of neurons is dependent on many factors, not just on synaptic input. However, it is possible to measure neuronal connections indirectly by cross-correlating the activity of one neuron with the activity of a second. If the second neuron consistently fires shortly after the first, it is probable that the first neuron participates in driving the second. Such connected pairs can be monitored during exploration and could suggest changes in the efficacy of neurons driving other neurons after learning (Jeffery, 1997).

What the physiologic basis for these changes is will have to be investigated in further detail. Since such activity patterns do not involve all neurons within a given brain area it will be difficult to record from many neurons simultaneously that are part of the same ensemble. Also, it is obvious that such an ensemble is very different from a full-scale activation of all synapses using HFS. When utilizing gamma or theta rhythm activity, the neuronal network can reduce the noise or irrelevant neuronal activity that is not involved in the particular information of interest. Ideally, one should be able to isolate the neuronal assemblies that are synchronized in their activity by gamma rhythm. Using hundreds of electrodes that record from single neurons it could be possible to observe the emergence of synchronized neuronal assemblies that process the information of a learning task. Recall should also reactivate the same neuronal assembly.

Once a reliable recording technique and a suitable learning task have been developed and established, it could be possible to identify which types of receptors are activated during the process or the emergence of neuronal assemblies, and which enzymes, second messengers, and immediate early genes play a role. Furthermore, we could compare these data with experimental findings in aged animals, perhaps even in models for stroke or Alzheimer's disease.

In other words, we would not use a "model" for putative synaptic changes during learning (such as HFS-induced LTP) but we would use the endogenous, intrinsic changes themselves. Such natural synaptic changes would most probably be quite different from those observed after HFS. Since many biophysical and biochemical processes (ion channel activation, enzyme activation, receptor modification, etc.) in neurons are threshold dependent, it would not be a surprise to see that a number of processes that have been described to be activated by HFS are not activated during learning at all. For example, the amount of calcium influx into neurons is dependent on the strength and duration of membrane depolarization. Strong HFS produces different results than weak HFS. In some studies, the effect of blocking nitric oxide synthase was visible using weak HFS but was overridden by strong HFS (Haley et al., 1993). In a patch clamp experiment in the cerebellar slice it was found that strong stimulation not only induced LTD in the stimulated synapses but also in neighboring synapses. Interestingly, the LTD induced by direct stimulation was not susceptible to nitric oxide synthase inhibitors, while the "indirect" LTD was blocked by these inhibitors (Hartell, 1996). These are just a few examples to show that stimulation strength and technique determine the outcome to a large degree, and how important it is to stimulate neurons in a "realistic" way to prevent artifactual results. Using artificial stimulation makes it is virtually impossible to estimate how realistic the stimulation was. Without a goalpost nobody can decide which of the many possible result is the "correct" one.

Another point is that we do not know to what extent synapses might be changed in their response during learning. In *in vitro* studies, large LTP is good LTP, and small LTP is considered to be bordering on failure. However, as described in the opening chapter of this book, there is evidence that animals can learn a spatial task if their (artificially induced) LTP in the hippocampus is at least 10 percent (Errington et al., 1997; Moser et al., 1998). This indicates that perhaps a very small change of synaptic efficacy is sufficient to encode information. One would not assume that synaptic transmission is always upregulated to maximal values during learning. In fact, making use of the full spectrum of synaptic modulation from zero to full potentiation would give the neuronal system an analogue gradient that could, for example, resemble the strength of memory formation. This would also imply that some weak synaptic modulation would not activate all those biochemical cascades that have been identified using the *in vitro* LTP technique (Bliss and Lynch, 1988; Crepel and Jaillard, 1990; Coffey et al., 1994; Thomas et al., 1994). It has been suggested that memory formation is dependent on the successful activation of several biochemical cascades that are gradually activated in time. Any failure or interruption of activation of these chains of cascades would then result in loss of memory storage (McGaugh, 1968; Rose, 1991; Rosenzweig et al., 1992; Hölscher, 1995). It would be of great interest to analyze the biochemical changes induced by plastic changes during learning and compare them with those induced by HFS.

In conclusion, our goal should be to develop reliable recording techniques that observe emerging neuronal ensembles during and after learning, and to identify where and how (and if) synaptic plasticity develops. This is our task for the new millennium.

REFERENCES

Alkadhi, K.A., and Altememi, G.F. (1997). Nitric oxide mediates long-term potentiation in rat superior cervical ganglion. *Brain Res* 753: 315–317.

Alonso, A., and Ilinás R.R. (1989). Subthreshold Na$^+$-dependent theta-like rhythmicity in stellate cells of entorhinal cortex layer II. *Nature* 342: 175–177.

Barnes, C.A., Suster, M.S., Shen, J., and McNaughton, B.L. (1997). Multistability of cognitive maps in the hippocampus of old rats. *Nature* 388: 272–275.

Bashir, Z.I., Bortolotto, Z.A., Davies, C.H., Berretta, N. et al. (1993). Induction of LTP in the hippocampus needs synaptic activation of glutamate metabotropic receptors. *Nature* 363: 347–350.

Bland, B.H. (1986). The physiology and pharmacology of hippocampal formation theta rhythms. *Prog. Neurobiol.* 26: 1–54.

Bliss, T., and Lømo, T. (1973). Long-lasting potentiation of synaptic transmission in the dentate area of the anaesthesised rabbit following stimulation of the perforant path. *J. Physiol. London* 232: 331–356.

Bliss, T.V.P., and Lynch, M.A. (1988). Long-term potentiation of synaptic transmission in the hippocampus: Properties and mechanisms. In *Long-term potentiation: From biophysics to behavior* (pp. 3–72). New York: Alan R. Liss.

Blümcke, I., Behle, K., Malitschek, B., Kuhn, R. et al. (1996). Immunohistochemical distribution of metabotropic glutamate receptor subtypes mGluR1b, mGluR2/3, mGluR4a and mGluR5 in human hippocampus. *Brain Res.* 736: 217–226.

Bordi, F., and Ugolini, A. (1995). Antagonists of the metabotropic glutamate receptor do not prevent induction of long-term potentiation in the dentate gyrus of rats. *Eur. J. Pharmacol.* 273: 291–294.

Bortolotto, Z.A., Bashir, Z.I., Davies, C.H., and Collingridge, G.L. (1994). A molecular switch activated by metabotropic glutamate receptors regulates induction of long-term potentiation. *Nature* 368: 740–743.

Bostock, E., Muller, R., and Kubie, J. (1991). Experience-dependent modifications of hippocampal cell firing. *Hippocampus* 1: 193–206.

Brown, R.E., and Reymann, K.G. (1995). Class I metabotropic glutamate receptor agonists do not facilitate the induction of long-term potentiation in the dentate gyrus of the rat *in vitro*. *Neurosci. Lett.* 202: 73–76.

Buhl, E.H., and Buzsáki, G. (1998). Remembering the Caribbean: The spring hippocampal research conference. *Neuron* 21: 27–35.

Burgess, N., Recce, M., and O'Keefe, J. (1996). A model of hippocampal function. *Neuronal Networks* 7: 1065–1081.

Bushell, T.J., Jane, D.E., Tse, H.-W., Watkins, J.C. et al. (1995). Antagonism of the synaptic depressant actions of L-AP4 in the lateral perforant path by MAP4. *Neuropharmacology* 34: 239–241.

Buzsáki, G. (1986). Generation of hippocampal EEG patterns. In R. Isaacson and K. Pibram (Eds.), *The hippocampus* (pp. 137–167). New York: Plenum Press.

Buzsáki, G., and Chrobak, J.J. (1995). Temporal structure in spatially organized neuronal ensembles: A role for interneuronal networks. *Curr. Opin. Neurobiol.* 5: 504–510.

Buzsáki, G., Leung, L., and Vanderwolf C. (1983). Cellular bases of hippocampal EEG in the behaving rat. *Brain Res.* 225: 235–247.

Castelo-Branco, M., Neuenschwander, S., and Singer W. (1998). Synchronization of visual responses between the cortex, lateral geniculate nucleus, and retina in the anesthetized cat. *J. Neurosci.* 18: 6395–6410.

Coffey, E.T., Herrero, I., Sihra, T.S., Sánchez-Prieto, J. et al. (1994). Glutamate exocytosis and MARCKS phosphorylation are enhanced by a metabotropic glutamate receptor coupled to a protein kinase C synergistically activated by diacylglycerol and arachidonic acid. *J. Neurochem.* 63: 1303–1310.

Conn, P.J., Macek, T.A., and Gereau, R.W. (1996). Physiological roles of multiple mGluR subtypes in rat hippocampus. *Neuropharmacology* 35: A9.

Crepel, F., and Jaillard, D. (1990). Protein kinases, nitric oxide and long-term depression of synapses in the cerebellum. *Neuroreport* 1: 133–136.

Csicsvari, J., Hirase, H., Czurko, A., Mamiya, A. et al. (1999). Oscillatory coupling of hippocampal pyramidal cells and interneurons in the behaving rat. *J. Neurosci.* 19: 274–287.

Diamond, D., Bennett, M., Fleshner, M., and Rose, G. (1994). Stress impairs LTP and hippocampal-dependent memory. In *Brain corticosteroid receptors* (pp. 411–414). New York: New York Academy of Science.

Diamond, D.M., Dunwiddie, T.V., and Rose, G.M. (1988). Characteristics of hippocampal primed burst potentiation *in vitro* and in the awake rat. *J. Neurosci.* 8: 4079–4088.

Diamond, D.M., Bennett, M.C., Stevens, K.E., Wilson, R.L. et al. (1990). Exposure to a novel environment interferes with the induction of hippocampal primed burst potentiation in the behaving rat. *Psychobiology* 18: 273–281.

Dickson, C.T., Trepel, C., and Bland, B.H. (1994). Extrinsic modulation of theta field activity in the entorhinal cortex of the anesthetized rat. *Hippocampus* 4: 37–51.

Doyle, C., Hölscher, C., Rowan, M.J., and Anwyl, R. (1996). The selective neuronal NO synthase inhibitor 7-nitro-indazole blocks both long-term potentiation and depotentiation of field EPSPs in rat hippocampal CA1 *in vivo*. *J. Neurosci.* 16: 418–426.

Errington, M.L., Bliss, T.V.P., Morris, R.J., Laroche, S. et al. (1997). Long-term potentiation in awake mutant mice. *Nature* 387: 666–667.

Fox, S.E., Wolfson, S., and Ranck, J.B. (1983). Investigating the mechanisms of hippocampal theta rhythms: Approaches and progress. In W. Seifert (Ed.), *Neurobiology of the hippocampus* (pp. 303–319). London: Academic Press.

Freund T., and Buzsáki G. (1996). Interneurons of the hippocampus. *Hippocampus* 6: 347–470.

Fries, P., Roelfsema, P., Engel, A., König, P. et al. (1997). Synchronization of oscillatory responses in visual cortex correlates with perception in interocular rivalry. *Proc. Natl. Acad. Sci. USA* 94: 12699–12704.

Gauss, R., Seifert, R., and Kaupp, U. (1998). Molecular identification of a hyperpolarisation-activated channel in sea urchin sperm. *Nature* 393: 583–587.

Green, E.J., and Greenough, W.T. (1986). Altered synaptic transmission in dentate gyrus of rats reared in complex environments: Evidence from hippocampal slices maintained *in vitro*. *J. Neurophysiol.* 55: 739–750.

Green, E.J., McNaughton, B.L., and Barnes, C.A. (1990). Role of the medial septum and hippocampal theta rhythm in exploration-related synaptic efficacy changes in rat fascia dentata. *Brain Res.* 537: 102–108.

Haley, J.E., Malen, P.L., and Chapman, P.F. (1993). Nitric oxide synthase inhibitors block long-term potentiation induced by weak but not strong tetanic stimulation at physiological brain temperatures in rat hippocampal slices. *Neurosci. Lett.* 160: 85–88.

Hartell, N.A. (1996). Strong activation of parallel fibers produces localized calcium transients and a form of LTP that spreads to distant synapses. *Neuron* 16: 601–610.

Hölscher, C. (1995). Release of prostaglandins during memory consolidation in the chick. *Eur. J. Pharmacol.* 294: 253–259.

Hölscher, C., Anwyl, R., and Rowan, M. (1997a). Block of HFS-induced LTP in the dentate gyrus by 1S,3S-ACPD: Further evidence against LTP as a model for learning. *Neuroreport* 8: 451–454.

Hölscher, C., Anwyl, R., and Rowan, M. (1997b). Stimulation on the positive phase of hippocampal theta rhythm induces long-term potentiation which can be depotentiated by stimulation on the negative phase in area CA1 *in vivo. J. Neurosci.* 17: 6470–6477.

Hölscher, C., Anwyl, R., and Rowan, M.J. (1997c). Block of theta-burst induced LTP by 1S,3S-ACPD: Further evidence against LTP as a model for learning. *Neuroscience* 81: 17–22.

Hölscher, C., McGlinchey, L., Anwyl, R., and Rowan, M.J. (1997d). HFS-induced long-term potentiation and depotentiation in area CA1 of the hippocampus are not good models for learning. *Psychopharmacology* 130: 174–182.

Hölscher, C., Gigg, J., and O'Mara, S. (1999). Metabotropic glutamate receptor activation and blockade. Consequences for long-term potentiation, learning and neurotoxicity. *Neurosci. Biobeh. Rev.* 23: 399–410.

Huerta, P.T., and Lisman, J.E. (1995). Bidirectional synaptic plasticity induced by a single burst during cholinergic theta oscillation in CA1 in vitro. *Neuron* 15: 1053–1063.

Jane, D.E., Pittaway, K., Sunter, D.C., Thomas, N.K. et al. (1995). New phenylglycine derivatives with potent and selective antagonist activity at presynaptic glutamate receptors in neonatal rat spinal cord. *Neuropharmacology* 34: 851–856.

Jane, D.E., Thomas, N.K., Tse, H.W., and Watkins, J.C. (1996). Potent antagonists at the L-AP4- and (1S,3S)-ACPD-sensitive presynaptic metabotropic glutamate receptors in the neonatal rat spinal cord. *Neuropharmacology* 35: 1029–1035.

Jeffery, K.J. (1997). LTP and spatial learning—Where to next? *Hippocampus* 7: 95–110.

Jeffery, K.J., Donnett, J.G., and O'Keefe, J. (1996). Medial septal control of theta-correlated unit firing in the entorhinal cortex of awake rats. *Neuroreport* 6: 2166–2170.

Jensen, O., and Lisman, J. (1996). Hippocampal CA3 region predicts memory sequences: Accounting for the phase precession of place cells. *Learning Memory* 3: 279–287.

Joëls, M. (1997). Steroid hormones and excitability in the mammalian brain. *Frontiers Neuroendocrinol.* 18: 2–48.

Johnston, D., Williams, S., Jaffe, D., and Gray, R. (1992). NMDA-independent long-term potentiation. *Annu. Rev. Physiol.* 54: 489–505.

Kamondi, A., Acsady, L., Wang, X.J., and Buzsaki, G. (1998). Theta oscillations in somata and dendrites of hippocampal pyramidal cells in vivo: Activity-dependent phase-precession of action potentials. *Hippocampus* 8: 244–261.

Kocsis, B., and Vertes, R.P. (1996). Midbrain raphe cell firing and hippocampal theta rhythm in urethane-anaesthetized rats. *Neuroreport* 7: 2867–2872.

Lanthorn, T.H., Ganong, A.H., and Cotman, C.W. (1984). 2-amino-4-phosphonobutyric acid selectively blocks mossy fiber CA3 responses in guinea pig but not rat hippocampus. *Brain Res.* 290: 174–178.

Larson, J., Wong, D., and Lynch, G. (1986). Patterned stimulation at the theta frequency is optimal for the induction of hippocampal long-term potentiation. *Brain Res.* 368: 347–350.

Leung, L.-W.S. (1980). Behavior-dependent evoked potentials in the hippocampal CA1 region of the rat. 1. Correlation with behavior and EEG. *Brain Res.* 198: 95–117.

Leung, L.W.S., and Desborough, K.A. (1988). APV, an N-methyl-D-aspartate receptor antagonist, blocks the hippocampal theta rhythm in behaving rats. *Brain Res.* 463: 148–152.

Lisman, J. (1999). Relating hippocampal circuitry to function: Recall of memory sequences by reciprocal dentate-CA3 interactions. *Neuron* 22: 233–242.

Lisman, J.E. (1997). Bursts as a unit of neural information: Making unreliable synapses reliable. *Trends Neurosci.* 20: 38–43.

Lu, Y., Jia, Z., Janus, C., Henderson, J. et al. (1997). Mice lacking metabotropic glutamate receptor 5 show impaired learning and reduced CA1 long-term potentiation (LTP) but normal CA3 LTP. *J. Neurosci.* 17: 5196–5205.

Ludwig, A., Zong, X., Jeglitsch, M., Homann, F. et al. (1998). A family of hyperpolarisation-activated mammalian cation channels. *Nature* 393: 587–591.

Luján, R., Nusser, Z., Roberts, J.D.B., Shigemoto, R. et al. (1996). Perisynaptic location of metabotropic glutamate receptors mGluR1 and mGluR5 on dendrites and dendritic spines in the rat hippocampus. *Eur. J. Neurosci.* 8: 1488–1500.

Macek, T.A., Winder, D.G., Gereau, R.W., Ladd, C.O. et al. (1996). Differential involvement of group II and group III mGluRs as autoreceptors at lateral and medial perforant path synapses. *J. Neurophysiol.* 76: 3798–3806.

Marrosu, F., Fornal, C.A., Metzler, C.W., and Jacobs, B.L. (1996). 5-HT$_{1A}$ agonists induce hippocampal theta activity in freely moving cats: Role of presynaptic 5-HT$_{1A}$ receptors. *Brain Res.* 739: 192–200.

McGaugh, J.L. (1968). A multi-trace view of memory storage processes. In R. Bovert (Ed.), *Attuali orentamenti della ricerca sull'apprendimento e la memoria* (pp. 13–24). Rome: Academia Nazional dei Lincei, Quaderno.

Mehta, M.R., Barnes, C.A., and McNaughton, B.L. (1997). Experience-dependent, asymmetric expansion of hippocampal place fields. *Proc. Natl. Acad. Sci. USA* 94: 8918–8921.

Moser, E., Krobert, K., Moser, M.-B., and Morris, R. (1998). Impaired spatial learning after saturation of long-term potentiation. *Science* 281: 2038–2042.

Muller, R.U., and Kubie, J.L. (1989). The firing of hippocampal place cells predicts the future position of freely moving rats. *J. Neurosci.* 9: 4101–4110.

Muller, R.U., Stead, M., and Pach, J. (1996). The hippocampus as a cognitive graph. *J. Gen. Physiol.* 107: 663–694.

Natsume, K., and Kometani, K. (1997). Theta-activity-dependent and -independent muscarinic facilitation of long-term potentiation in guinea pig hippocampal slices. *Neurosci. Res.* 27: 335–341.

Neki, A., Ohishi, H., Kaneko, T., Shigemoto, R. et al. (1996). Pre- and postsynaptic localization of a metabotropic glutamate receptor, mGluR2, in the rat brain. *Neurosci. Lett.* 202: 197–200.

Neuenschwander, S., and Singer, W. (1996). Long-range synchronization of oscillatory light reponses in the cat retina and lateral geniculate nucleus. *Nature* 379: 728–733.

Nosten-Bertrand, M., Errington, M.L., Murphy, K.P.S.J., Tokugawa, Y. et al. (1996). Normal spatial learning despite regional inhibition of LTP in mice lacking Thy-1. *Nature* 379: 826–829.

O'Keefe, J. (1979). A review of the hippocampal place cells. *Prog. Neurobiol.* 13: 419–439.

O'Keefe, J., and Dostrovsky, J. (1971). The hippocampus as a spatial map: Preliminary evidence from unit activity in the freely-moving rat. *Brain Res.* 34: 171–175.

O'Keefe, J., and Recce, M.L. (1993). Phase relationship between hippocampal place units and the EEG theta rhythm. *Hippocampus* 3: 317–330.

O'Mara, S., Rowan, M.J., and Anwyl, R. (1995). Metabotropic glutamate receptor-induced homosynaptic long-term depression and depotentiation in the dentate gyrus of the rat hippocampus *in vitro*. *Neuropharmacology* 34: 983–989.

O'Mara, S.M. (1995). A review of the hippocampal place cells. *Prog. Neurobiol.* 13: 419–439.

Otto, T., Eichenbaum, H., Wiener, S., and Wible, C. (1991). Learning-related patterns of CA1 spike trains parallel stimulation parameters optimal for inducing hippocampal long-term potentiation. *Hippocampus* 1: 181–192.

Pavlides, C., Greenstein, Y.J., Grudman, M., and Winson, J. (1988). Long-term potentiation in the dentate gyrus is induced preferentially on the positive phase of θ-rhythm. *Brain Res.* 439: 383–387.

Pavlides, C., Kimura, A., Magariños, A.M., and McEwen, B.S. (1996). Hippocampal homosynaptic long-term depression/depotentiation induced by adrenal steroids. *Neuroscience* 68: 379–385.

Penttonen, M., Kamondi, A., Acsady, L., and Buzsaki, G. (1998). Gamma frequency oscillation in the hippocampus of the rat: Intracellular analysis in vivo. *Eur. J. Neurosci.* 10: 718–728.

Petralia, R.S., Wang, Y.X., Niedzielski, A.S., and Wenthold, R.J. (1996). The metabotropic glutamate receptors, mGluR2 and mGluR3, show unique postsynaptic, presynaptic and glial localizations. *Neuroscience* 71: 949–976.

Petrozzino, J.J., and Connor, J.A. (1994). Dendritic Ca^{2+} accumulations and metabotropic glutamate receptor activation associated with an N-methyl-D-aspartate receptor-independent long-term potentiation in hippocampal CA1 neurons. *Hippocampus* 4: 546–558.

Petsche, H., Stumpf, C., and Gogolar, G. (1962). The significance of the rabbit's septum as a relay station between the midbrain and the hippocampus: The control of hippocampus arousal activity by septum cells. *Electroencephalogr. Clin. Neurophysiol.* 14: 202–211.

Ranck, J.B.J. (1973). Studies on single neurons in dorsal hippo-campal formation and septum in unrestrained rats. I. Behavioral correlates and firing repertoires. *Exp. Neurol.* 41: 461–531.

Roelfsema, P., Engel, A., König, P., and Singer, W. (1997). Visuomotor integration is associated with zero time-lag synchronization among cortical areas. *Nature* 385: 157–161.

Rose, S.P.R. (1991). How chicks make memories: The cellular cascade from c-fos to dendritic remodelling. *Trends Neurosci.* 14: 390–397.

Rosenzweig, M.R., Bennett, E.L., Martinez, J.L., Colombo, P.J. et al. (1992). Studying stages of memory formation with chicks. In S. Butters (Ed.), *Neuropsychology of memory* (pp. 533–546). New York: Guilford Press.

Samsonovich, A., and McNaughton, B.L. (1997). Path integration and cognitive mapping in a continuous attractor neural network model. *J. Neurosci.* 17: 5900–5920.

Saugstad, J.A., Kinzie, J.M., Segerson, T.P., and Westbrook, G.L. (1996). Agonist profile of recombinant rat mGluR8. *Neuropharmacology* 35: A27.

Schulz, P.E., Cook, E.P., and Johnston, D. (1995). Using paired-pulse facilitation to probe the mechanisms for long-term potentiation. *J. Physiol. (Paris)* 89: 3–9.

Selig, D.K., Lee, H.K., Bear, M.F., and Malenka, R.C. (1995). Re-examination of the effects of MCPG on hippocampal LTP, LTD, and depotentiation. *J. Neurophysiol.* 74: 1075–1082.

Shigemoto, R., Kinoshita, A., Wada, E., Nomura, S. et al. (1997). Differential presynaptic localization of metabotropic glutamate receptor subtypes in the rat hippocampus. *J. Neurosci.* 17: 7503–7522.

Sik, A., Penttonen, M., and Buzsaki, G. (1997). Interneurons in the hippocampal dentate gyrus: An in vivo intracellular study. *Eur. J. Neurosci.* 9: 573–588.

Singer, W. (1994). Time as coding space in neocortical processing: A hypothesis. In G. Buszáki (Ed.), *Temporal coding in the brain* (pp. 51–79). Berlin: Springer Verlag.

Singer, W. (1999). Striving for coherence. *Nature* 397: 391–436.

Sinz, R. (1979). *Neurobiology und Gedächtnis*. Stuffgart: Gustav Fischer Verlag.

Skaggs, W.E., and McNaughton, B.L. (1996). Replay of neuronal firing sequences in rat hippocampus during sleep following spatial experience. *Science* 271: 1870–1873.

Son, H., and Carpenter, D.O. (1996). Interactions among paired-pulse facilitation and post-tetanic and long-term potentiation in the mossy fiber CA3 pathway in rat hippocampus. *Synapse* 23: 302–311.

Stäubli, U., and Lynch, G. (1987). Stable hippocampal long-term potentiation elicited by 'theta' pattern stimulation. *Brain Res.* 435: 227–234.

Steward, O. (1976). Topographic organization of the projections from the entorhinal area to the hippocampal formation of the rat. *J. Comp. Neur.* 167: 285–314.

Stewart, M., Luo, Y., and Fox, S.E. (1992). Effects of atropine on hippocampal theta cells and complex-spike cells. *Brain Res.* 591: 122–128.

Strohmann, B., Schwarz, D., and Puil, E. (1994). Subthreshold frequency selectivity in avian auditory thalamus. *J. Neurophysiol.* 71: 1361–1372.

Thomas, K.L., Laroche, S., Errington, M.L., Bliss, T.V.P. et al. (1994). Spatial and temporal changes in signal transduction pathways during LTP. *Neuron* 13: 737–746.

Thomas, M.J., and O'Dell, T.J. (1995). The molecular switch hypothesis fails to explain the inconsistent effects of the metabotropic glutamate receptor antagonist MCPG on LTP. *Brain Res.* 695: 45–52.

Tsodyks, M.V., Skaggs, W.E., Sejnowski, T.J., and McNaughton, B.L. (1996). Population dynamics and theta rhythm phase precession of hippocampal place cell firing: A spiking neuron model. *Hippocampus* 6: 271–280.

Vanderwolf, C.H. (1969). Hippocampal electrical activity and voluntary movement in the rat. *Electroencephologr. Clin. Neurophysiol.* 26: 407–418.

Vanderwolf, C.H. (1975). Neocortical and hippocampal activation in relation to behavior: Effects of atropine, eserine, phenothiazines and amphetamin. *J. Comp. Physiol. Psychol.* 88: 300–323.

Vanderwolf, C.H., and Leung, L.-W.S. (1983). *Hippocampal Rhythmical Slow Activity: A Brief History and the Effects of Entorhinal Lesions and Phencyclidine.* London: Academic Press.

Wilson, M., and McNaughton, B. (1993). Dynamics of the hippocampal ensemble code for space. *Science* 261: 1055–1058.

Wilson, M.A., and Tonegawa, S. (1997). Synaptic plasticity, place cells and spatial memory: Study with second generation knockouts. *Trends Neurosci.* 20: 102–105.

Winson, J. (1972). Interspecies differences in the occurrence of theta. *Behav. Biol.* 7: 479–487.

Winson, J. (1978). Loss of hippocampal theta rhythm results in spatial memory defects of the rat. *Science* 201: 160–163.

Ylinen, A., Soltesz, I., Bragin, A., Penttonen, M. et al. (1995). Intracellular correlates of hippocampal theta rhythm in identified pyramidal cells, granule cells, and basket cells. *Hippocampus* 5: 78–90.

CHAPTER EIGHT

Role of Gamma Oscillations for Information Processing and Memory Formation in the Neocortex

Matthias H. J. Munk

SUMMARY

The neuronal code that is used by the brain to represent complex information is not yet identified. Two complementary representational strategies, smart neurons and neuronal assemblies, have been proposed as solutions to the coding problem. Neurons that respond selectively to particular feature combinations are called "smart." Neuronal assemblies are large populations of neurons that represent information in distributed form by their correlated discharge. These different strategies seem to be optimized for different functional aspects of the neuronal processes underlying perception and sensorimotor integration. Smart neurons could serve the fast processing of familiar information by operating as coincidence detectors for converging inputs arriving on feed-forward connections. In contrast, neuronal assemblies appear to provide a flexible coding mechanism that can cope with the combinatorial complexity of new material during creation and reorganization of representations. Synchronized neuronal responses have been proposed as constituting functional assemblies that could code for the relations among individual features of an input pattern in the case of perceptual processes, or sensory information and motor activity in the case of sensorimotor integration. Neuronal oscillations in the gamma-frequency range are often observed to accompany precisely synchronized responses. Oscillatory modulation of neuronal discharge may therefore serve as a mechanism to synchronize responses even over large distances. Oscillatory discharge is induced by activation of the same modulatory systems like the reticular formation that control vigilance and improve sensorimotor performance of the awake performing brain. As the two described representa-

I am grateful to Suzana Herculano-Houzel for her enduring effort to make difficult experiments work, Hanka Klon-Lipok and Michaela Klinkmann for excellent technical help, Sergio Neuenschwander for his innovative analysis software, Renate Ruhl and Selina Völsing for help with the figures, David E.J. Linden and Sonja Grün for valuable comments on an earlier version of this manuscript, and Wolf Singer for his constant support.

tional strategies function in rather different ways, the mechanisms by which they can be modified during learning and memory formation may also differ considerably. The functional connectivity that can support information processing based on smart neurons consists of feed-forward connections that converge on individual neurons. In contrast, the organization of synchronously firing assemblies requires mutual interactions among reciprocally linked neuronal populations. Mutual interactions can be supported by the corticocortical tangential and feedback connections. These connections have been shown to mediate and modulate cortical synchronization. Millisecond-precise coincidences of pre- and postsynaptic activation can determine the direction and strength of synaptic gain changes. Such gain changes have been shown to directly change response properties of individual neurons and their functional connectivity. In the presence of neuromodulatory substances such as acetylcholine and norepinephrine, synaptic gain changes can be modulated both *in vitro* and *in vivo*. The temporal contingency of synchronized neuronal firing with behavioral training or the activation of modulatory systems such as the basal forebrain has been shown to enable changes of single unit response properties as well as the layout of cortical maps in response to sensory stimulation. In the case of assembly-coded information, learning-induced changes of neuronal representations are expected to be expressed in altered synchronization patterns, and leave the response properties of the synchronously firing neurons unaffected. As synchronous oscillatory discharge is facilitated by the same modulators that facilitate synaptic gain changes and support massive reorganization of cortical representations, synchronous oscillatory activity may constitute the link between the activation of the cholinergic system and learning-induced changes of synaptic transmission in the cortical network. Synchronization of oscillatory neuronal firing would then serve as a mechanism that supports both the ad hoc formation of assemblies and at the same time facilitates synaptic modifications that stabilize the newly formed assemblies. As recent evidence shows, malfunction of the cholinergic system does not directly lead to memory deficits but impairs attention. Hence, oscillatory activity may be a constituent of the neuronal mechanisms controlling attention, both in processing and learning.

Introduction

The high speed of neuronal processing and the ability of the brain to process complex information require neuronal coding strategies that are optimized for very different parameters. The speed with which complex sensory information can be processed is impressively high. For example, faces and other complex objects can be recognized within less than a tenth of a second. The brain and in particular the neocortex, therefore, have to have developed a neuronal processing strategy that allows them to decompose a visual scene very rapidly and detect those constituents that are of behavioral relevance. The high degree of complexity that arises from the practically unlimited number of combinations of elementary features constituting sensory and sensorimotor information has to be encoded in a neuronal representation that allows the brain to process the information with sufficient detail and speed and store the important constituents in memory. Because of the infinite number of possible feature constellations, a coding strategy is required that allows the representation of feature combinations by a dynamic recombination of subsets of combinations or simpler components (primitives). If the nervous system would dedicate individual cells for the representation of individual feature combinations, coding capacity (i.e., the number of possible combinations that can be represented) would be limited at best to the number of cells in the cortex (Singer, 1993). New feature combinations could not be identified and processed successfully. If instead of individual cells, large numbers of cells constitute the representation of related information, a mechanism to coordinate and distinguish their activity is required.

Neuronal activity in the neocortex that is evoked by a sensory stimulus or is involved in the processing of sensorimotor information is always distributed among numerous different areas. In sensory systems, different areas represent and process different aspects of the same input pattern in parallel. Early processing stages such as the primary sensory areas serve the purpose of extracting and representing very detailed information about the most basic parameters of the input. High spatial resolution (e.g., in the visual system) is achieved by distributing afferent activity over a large cortical surface. This kind of representation appears to be suitable to detect fine detail in the input patterns. However, the perception of structures in the entire pattern requires that the distributed information is integrated and related to the context in space and time. Integration of information from a complex input pattern can only be achieved if the relations among individual features of the input are identified and made available to subsequent processing stages. Further processing involves neuronal operations in numerous other cortical areas that receive afferent activity through feed-forward connections. With further processing, information needs to be selected with respect to its behavioral relevance. The selection of inputs to subsequent processing stages can either depend on the relative saliency of the arriving signals (bottom-up) or attentional processes (top-down). As attentional modulation of sensory activity can be traced back into the primary sensory areas of the neocortex (Roelfsema et al., 1998), attentional mechanisms are very likely to influence the distribution of neuronal activity to higher areas. The subsequently occurring simultaneous processing in multiple areas needs to be organized in a way that permits the local and intra-areal neuronal operations to interact in order to generate a coherent percept and to organize adequate behavior. Both at the level of primary representations as well as at later stages of processing, a general mechanism is required that can structure and select neuronal activity so that related information can be identified and used to generate new representations.

Our environment keeps changing so that the sensory input and the behavioral context are never the same. The mechanisms of perception and sensorimotor integration, therefore, have to adapt constantly. Representations of sensory and sensorimotor information need to be highly flexible and have to have direct access to the stored information in memory. To enable the system to improve performance, information about previous experience needs to be available during the processes underlying perception and sensorimotor integration. If in turn the information about recent experience is to influence subsequent instances of perception and behavior, those preceding processes should be able to immediately alter the content of relevant memories. This implies that the substrate of processing of new information and storage of information about previous experience should be identical or very closely related. Direct interaction of ongoing perceptual and sensorimotor processing and memory operations such as read-out (recall) and updates (encoding and consolidation) is of particular relevance for the optimization and fine-tuning of perceptual and sensorimotor operations through training. The neuronal representation used by the brain and in particular by the neocortex needs to be stable and robust in some situations to allow for efficient and fast processing. At other times, representations have to be highly flexible in order to adapt the functional structure to new computational requirements.

Representational Strategies of the Neocortex

Two complementary representational strategies have been identified in the brain: smart neurons and synchronized neuronal assemblies. The term *smart neurons* refers to cells that respond selectively to a particular set of elementary stimulus features and are typically found in higher areas of the cortex. For example, cells in higher visual areas such as in the inferotemporal region respond selectively to complex stimuli such as faces. Concepts of cortical function that rely exclusively on smart neurons assume that for each unique constellation of features, a few dedicated cells signal the presence of a particular feature conjunction. Smart neurons are an efficient strategy for representing complex information that frequently occurs with a fixed combination of individual features. Smart neurons can be generated by the selection of converging feed-forward connections by which the response profiles of each layer of afferent cells is combined in a way that the respective postsynaptic cell will only respond if the appropriate input pattern has occurred. They operate as coincidence detectors for sets of component features. Smart neurons are optimized to detect frequently recurring feature combinations and thus provide a mechanism for very fast sensorimotor processing.

A radically different but complementary coding strategy consists of synchronized neuronal assemblies. Neuronal assemblies are based on large groups of cells that are coactivated by a given input pattern. Each of the neurons that may become a member of an assembly responds to individual features or a subset of features of the input pattern. The mere coactivation that is evaluated for population codes is only a prerequisite for the formation of assemblies. Assemblies require that upon activation by a given set of features some of the coactivated neurons respond in a coordinated way to signal the presence of a unique set of features. It has been proposed that this coordination could be instantiated by millisecond precise synchronization of the neuronal responses (Singer et al., 1997). Synchronized firing facilitates the integration of synaptic activity at subsequent neurons that receive converging inputs from different members of the same assembly. Assemblies are most suitable to represent information that occurs with frequently changing feature combinations of individual objects or if contextual information has to be immediately integrated. Assemblies are thought to constitute themselves without prior selection of a particular set of connections, provided that a substrate for mutual neuronal communication exists.

Mutual interactions that result in either synchronized or desynchronized firing would allow simultaneously active cells in the cortex to determine the members of an assembly by means of a self-organizing process. The substrate required for this kind of operation are the long-range tangential corticocortical connections, which are known to be mostly reciprocal (Salin and Bullier, 1995). Mutual operations across these connections are certainly more time consuming than the transmission of activity through converging feed-forward connections; however, self-organizing ensemble activity can operate with higher flexibility and can cope with a higher degree of complexity. Rapid changes of the representation of relations can be achieved by the dynamic recombination of the members of synchronized assemblies. If different levels of complexity, such as the processing of local features and a context, are involved, top-down influences from higher areas may be required to structure or bias the organization of assemblies. Attentional mechanisms responsible for spatially selective attention could be modulating the information processing in topographically restricted sections of lower areas by sending synchronizing signals through feedback connections.

The Substrate of Neuronal Interactions in the Neocortex

Three major types of corticocortical connections have been isolated and characterized functionally. Based on the pattern of their origin and termination, corticocortical connections have been classified as feed-forward, lateral, or feedback connections (Felleman and Van Essen, 1991). Feed-forward connections serve the transmission and distribution of afferent activity that causes neurons to respond to a stimulus and determine the basic properties of their receptive fields. The information they convey exhibits topologic or in the case of the visual system retinotopic selectivity. This topologic selectivity has been shown to correspond between the source and target cells of corticocortical projections (Salin et al., 1989). For example in the visual system, feed-forward connections that arise from neurons in V1 transmit information from the same sector of the visual field to neurons in V2 that is actually represented by the responses of the target neurons of this projection in V2 (Salin and Bullier, 1995). This is not the case for lateral and feedback connections. They violate topographic correspondence, which clearly indicates that they serve functions other than generating primary response properties or receptive fields. Lateral and feedback connections appear to be involved in the organization of correlated firing (Munk et al., 1995) (see also Figure 8.1A and B) and feedback connections may play a role in the modulation of receptive field surround (Hupe et al., 1998). The topographic aspect of neuronal interactions suggests that lateral and feedback connections primarily serve to mediate contextual information (Phillips and Singer, 1997).

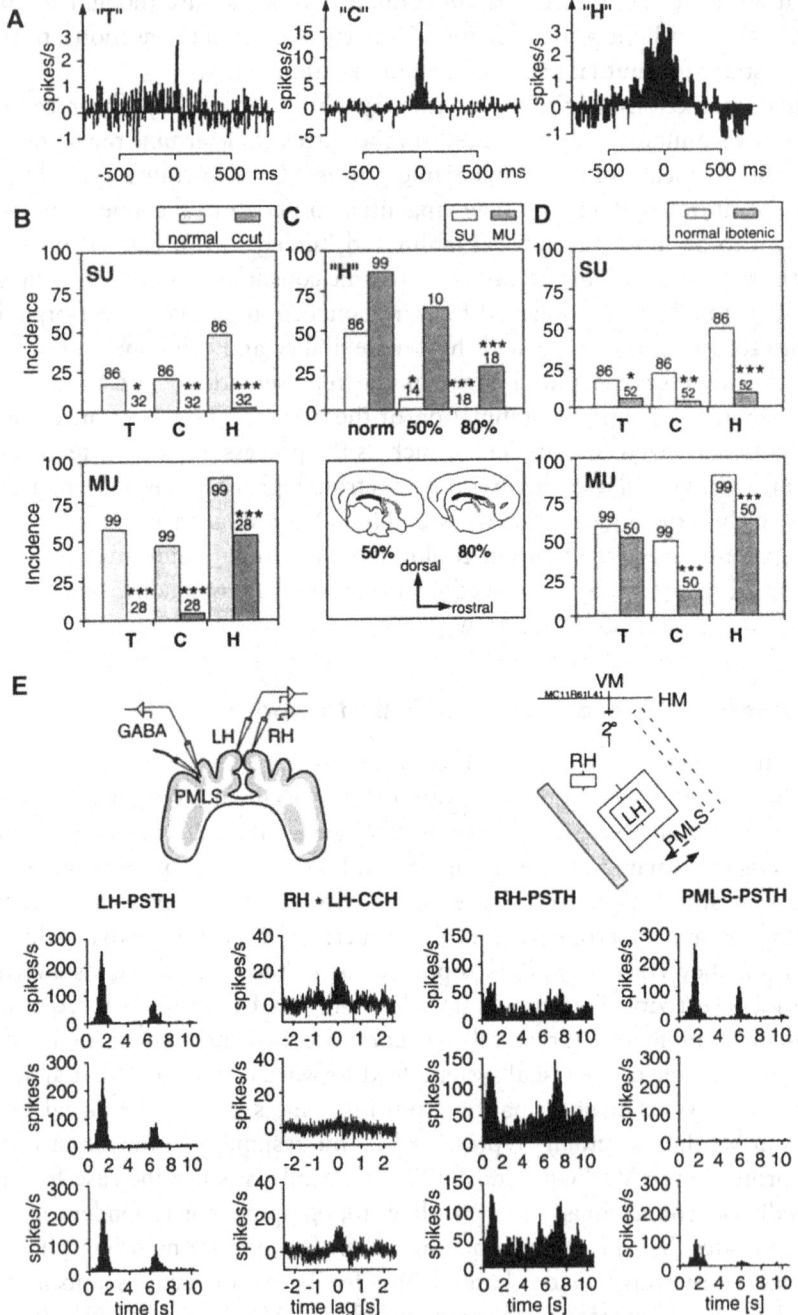

In addition to their different functional topography, corticocortical connections differ in their susceptibility to modification during different developmental stages (see Singer, 1995, for review). Feed-forward connections in the visual system are largely determined by genetic information and retain only very limited susceptibility to induction of long-term plasticity. Changes of receptive field properties have only been achieved experimentally with invasive conditioning procedures or extensive training. In contrast, lateral and feedback connections seem to preserve considerable capacity to change in later developmental stages. These observations also suggest that feed-forward on the one hand and lateral and feedback connections on the other hand serve quite distinct functions.

The majority of corticocortical connections is reciprocal. A connection is considered to be reciprocal if the neurons that send their axons to a different population of cells either in the same or another cortical area will also receive projections from their targets. What does this mean in functional terms? In a feed-forward/feedback system, given that this projection is topographically organized, the cells in the higher area can control the cells in the lower area that provide their excitatory drive. In a horizontal direction (i.e., through intrinsic long-range or lateral inter-areal connections) interactions may support the generation and fine-tuning of response selectivity. However, it has been shown that these connections are also necessary to mediate synchronized firing (Engel et al., 1991a; Munk et al., 1995). The temporal precision of neuronal interactions seems to reflect the type of mediating connections. Horizontal and lateral connections are necessary to main-

---

Figure 8.1. Functional connectivity in the visual cortex of the cat as revealed by cross-correlation of spike firing: normal pattern, mediating connections, supporting neuronal populations, and remote modulation of functional connectivity in the visual cortex. (A) The normal pattern of functional connectivity consists of millisecond-precise correlations ("T"), several tens ("C") and hundreds ("H") of milliseconds dispersed correlations, as determined by cross-correlation analysis of single unit responses to a moving visual stimulus. The three different examples shown represent discrete classes of peaks that can be related to the interaction of different cortical circuits. (B) Cutting the posterior part of the corpus callosum ("ccut") destroys precise synchronization, whereas temporally dispersed correlations persist, even if only the most anterior part is left intact. (C) The incidence of H-peaks gradually decreases with the number of callosal fibers severed. Note, however, that with only the most anterior portion of the corpus callosum intact, the firing of neurons in the visual cortex is still coordinated through polysynaptic pathways. (D) The neuron populations supporting temporally dispersed correlations could be localized in widespread regions of extrastriate cortex. After destroying the majority of areas with monosynaptic connections to A17 by cytotoxic lesions ("ibotenic" acid), the incidence of temporally precise correlations ("T") was much less affected than that of temporally dispersed correlations ("C" and "H") as compared to normal animals. However, the coupling strength of precise correlations was strongly reduced (not shown here) which points toward a modulatory role of those areas responsible for the generation of temporally dispersed correlations. (E) Reversible inactivation of neuron populations in an extrastriate cortical area (PMLS) leads to reversible suppression of correlated firing in primary cortex. Pressure injection of GABA into the visuotopically corresponding region of PMLS silences these neurons (**rightmost column**). In the meantime, the temporally dispersed correlation that occurred in responses (LH-PSTH and RH-PSTH) that synchronize across the hemispheres is reversibly suppressed (column labeled "RH*LH-CCH").

tain temporally precise synchronization as its incidence is most affected by destroying the direct connectivity (Figure 8.1B), whereas the experimental manipulation of those cell populations from which feedback connections arise has a greater effect on temporally disperse correlations (Fig. 8.1C and D). This means that horizontal (intra-areal) and lateral (inter-areal) connections sustain mutual neuronal interactions with high temporal precision as can be observed during the synchronization of gamma oscillations, whereas the reciprocal connections based on feed-forward and feedback projections may not only control the excitatory drive from afferents, but may also modulate interactions within and between lower order areas (Nelson et al., 1992a) (Figure 8.1E).

Why is the reciprocity of corticocortical connections an important property for the organization of information processing? In the case of the horizontal connections, structure and function of the reciprocal connections is symmetrical, which means they have in principle the same impact on the respective target cells. This provides a neuronal substrate for simultaneous multilateral interactions. Mutual interactions in a diverging and reciprocally converging structure of connections allow that a large number of local processes initiated by feed-forward activation determine their relatedness without supervision. Several different kinds of interactions between any two sites in such a multilateral network can be imagined to occur. The most interesting case for dynamic grouping operations is if the cells at both sites are already activated through feed-forward input and then start to mutually exchange signals. In this situation, the exact timing of the exchanged signals will determine the result of the interaction. If the exchanged signals arrive precisely at the same time, they will stabilize synchronized firing and may even lead to reverberations. If the signals arrive with very different delays, no interaction may occur. Local processes that exhibit oscillatory firing patterns as is often the case if the cortex is activated [e.g., by stimulation of the

---

→

Figure 8.2. Immediate and delayed onset of response synchronization in primary visual cortex. Receptive fields, visual stimuli (A, a), and stimulus timing relative to neuronal responses (B, a), are identical for both data sets recorded from the same cells 50 minutes apart in time. Each data set consists of the responses to ten identical stimulus presentations. Four histograms labeled (b) show the responses of neurons in two sites of A17 to the moving visual stimuli. The label "MRF" denotes the stimulation artifact. Average cross-coincidence histograms (d) show different types of synchronized oscillations. (c) The decomposition of correlations in peri-stimulus time allows the determination of when correlations appear or disappear with respect to the response. This analysis is a modified form of the JPSTH and represents the time difference of correlated events on the ordinate and peri-stimulus time on the abscissa. The strength of correlation is coded by different levels of gray. The insets on the upper right represent the average correlations in shorter time intervals. Synchronous high-frequency (80 to 120 Hz) oscillations (A), which are transmitted from the retina to the cortex, appear early in the visual response of the cortical neurons and cease after a few hundred milliseconds. Response synchronization based on gamma-frequency oscillations (B) is generated in the cortex (here after MRF stimulation) and therefore need time to organize themselves. The latency of synchronous gamma oscillations in spike responses is several hundred milliseconds as can be seen in the example in (B, c). Note that frequency and phase of the oscillations change during the responses.

mesencephalic reticular formation (MRF, see Figures 8.2 and 8.3)], small phase shifts due to different conduction velocities and synaptic integration times on the reciprocal connections may result in dynamic adaptation of the spike firing times. Then, either the phase at one site is advanced toward the phase at the majority of its inputs so that firing is synchronized, or the phase will be further delayed so

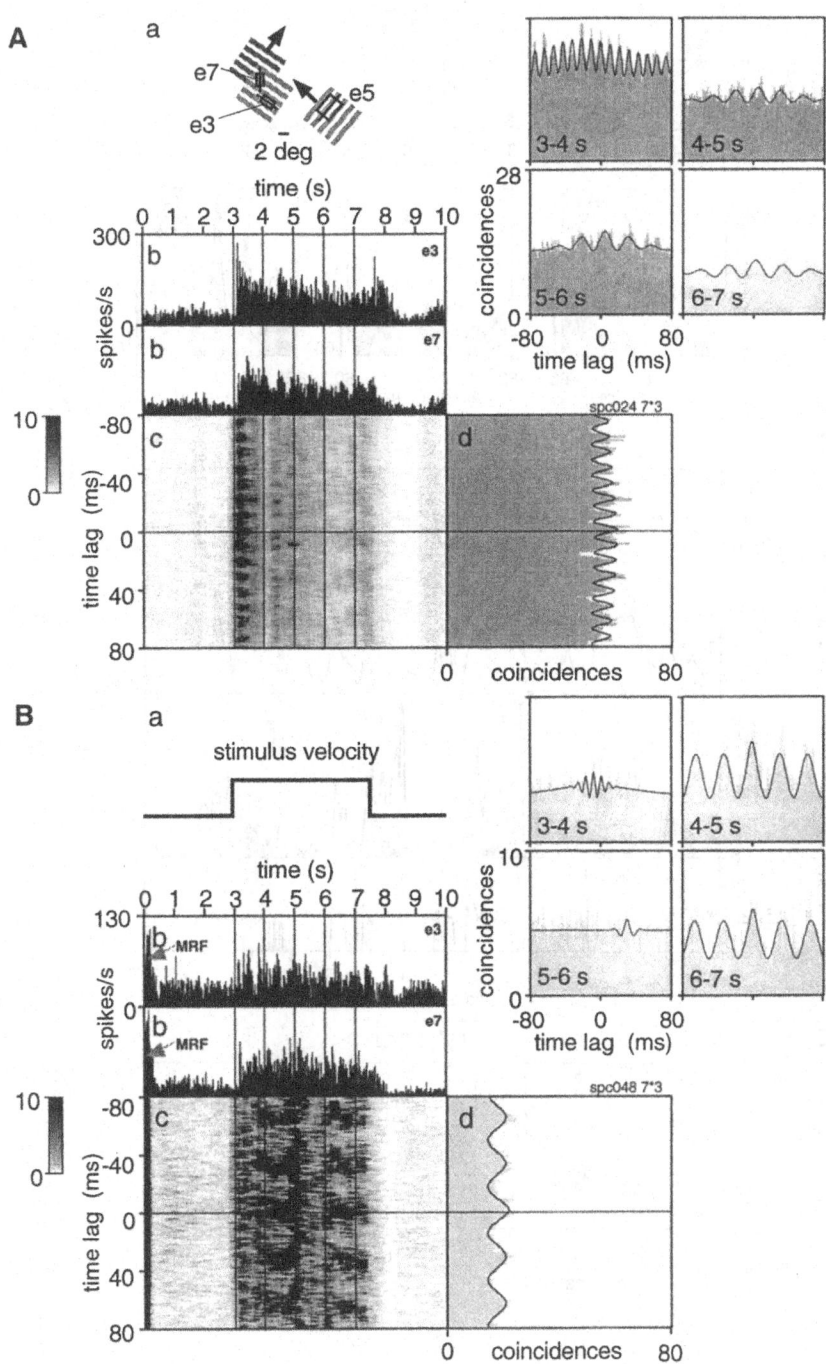

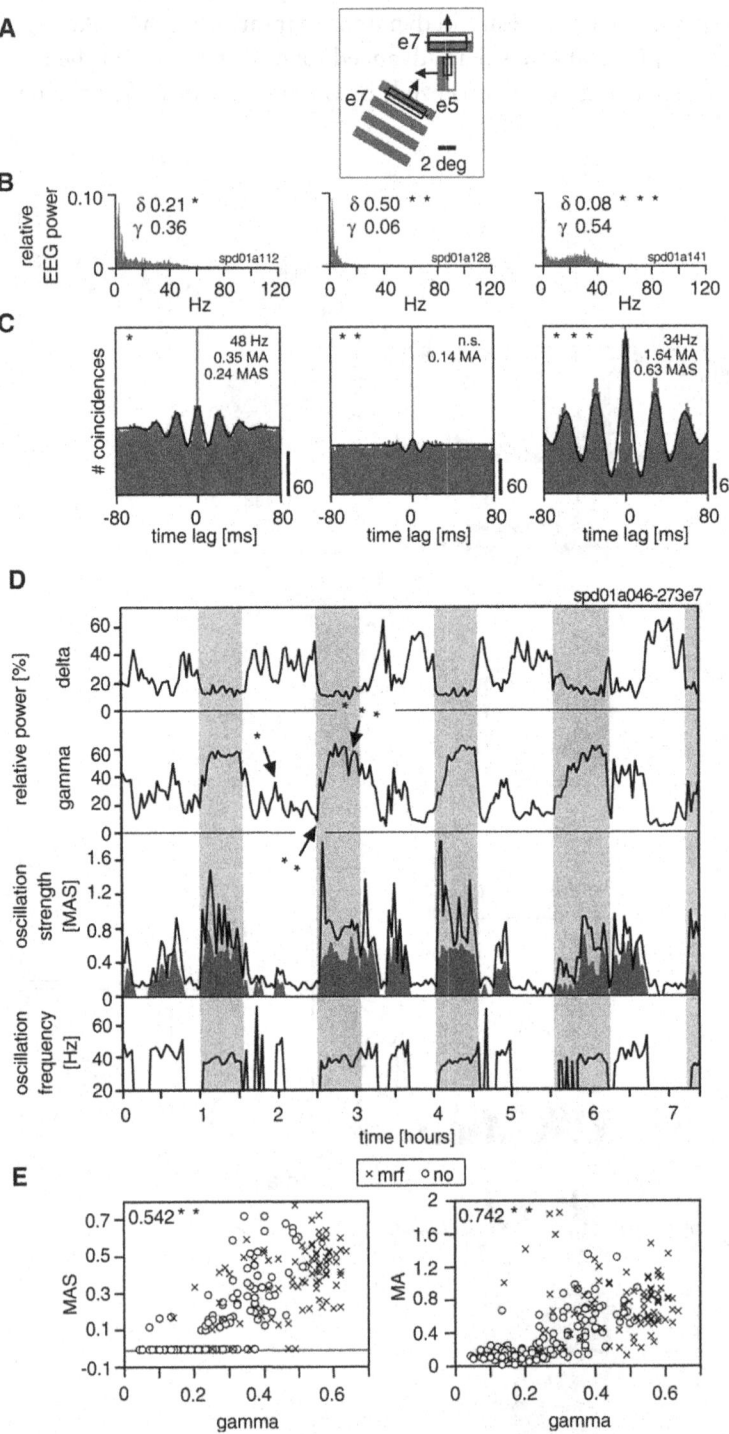

that firing is finally desynchronized. The direction of phase changes will depend on the average timing of all active inputs to the respective cells. If two or more input populations of synchronously firing cells exist that fire at different delays relative to each other, the target cell will follow the rhythm of those inputs that are most efficient in driving its own spike generator. This way, mutual interactions can serve to initiate assemblies of synchronously firing neurons or modify their composition by recruiting new members or separating previously synchronized neurons. As this process of mutual interactions can operate without instructive or biasing signals it represents some kind of self-organization. This kind of organization differs fundamentally from the conception of brain function based on serial chains of neurons. Learning-induced changes of this process will require that the temporal properties of signal transmission of the reciprocal connections are modified.

Representations Based on Synchronized Responses

Individual neurons in sensory areas of the cortex each respond to a whole range of stimulus parameters, which is referred to as *coarse coding*. Cells, for example, in V1 of the monkey respond to a range of orientations and may in addition be sensitive to color or prefer a certain range of directions of moving stimuli. Any visual stimulus will therefore evoke simultaneous responses in huge populations of neurons. The mere coactivation of neurons with similar response properties does not by itself reflect a representation of the relations among the individual features being present in the input pattern. If the simultaneous activation of large groups of neurons is considered as a population code, different but not too dissimilar features in the input pattern would be represented in the same or at least largely overlapping neuronal populations and therefore run the risk to be confounded. Based on the experience and the expectation of the system, an active grouping process

Figure 8.3. Oscillatory modulation of multiunit responses covaries with EEG activation. (A) Receptive fields and pattern of visual stimuli. (B) Normalized power spectra from epicortically recorded EEG show different proportions of power in the delta-frequency band (1 to 3 Hz) and in the gamma-frequency band (20 to 70 Hz) as indicated by numbers. The different stars denote positions in the time series shown in (D). (C) Autocoincidence histograms computed from multiunit responses to visual stimulation in A17 of anesthetized paralyzed cats. Note that with decreasing power in the delta band and increasing power in the gamma band the strength of the oscillation increases. (D) Time course of relative power in delta (1 to 3 Hz) and gamma (20 to 70 Hz) bands (**upper traces**) of the EEG and oscillation strength (gray histogram), strength of local synchronization (**thin line**), and oscillation frequency (**last trace**) of units at electrode 7. The strength of oscillations is quantified by the modulation amplitude of the satellite peak (Mastronarde, 1983), which is defined as the ratio of the height of the first satellite peak divided by the offset of the correlogram. The gray columns mark those epochs during the experiment during which the MRF was electrically stimulated just prior to each presentation of the visual stimulus. Note how reliably oscillation and synchronization are enhanced during epochs of MRF conditioning and that they have a tendency to persist after MRF stimulation is discontinued. (E) Scattergrams for oscillation (**left**) and synchronization strength (**right**) in the unit responses as a function of gamma activation in the EEG. Spearman correlation coefficients are given in the upper left corner.

has to occur that will extract the relevant feature combinations and make them available to subsequent processing stages. Experience is stored in the connectivity pattern and the weights of the involved synapses and the weights of the synapses involved in the mutual interactions underlying the formation and reorganization of synchronized assemblies. If the system can generate expectations about the results of a grouping process, they could be mediated by feedback signals from higher areas, which may directly bias the grouping operation or be compared to the results of the self-organizing dynamic grouping process and the error signal may be used to optimize the latter. During the grouping operation, each individual cell starts communicating to the large number of postsynaptic target cells through their reciprocal connections, with the result that part of the circuits will arrive at a cooperative state (e.g., engage in a synchronous gamma oscillation) whereas other circuits will not find a stable state of interaction or may even actively disengage. Synchronization of spike firing appears to be a suitable candidate mechanism for dynamic grouping operations because the readout of such a temporal code at subsequent processing stages can take advantage of spatial summation of converging inputs. As spatial summation of simultaneously arriving action potentials is much less time consuming than the summation of temporally dispersed input, neuronal signal integration based on synchronized inputs can be achieved without further delay and therefore constitutes a highly efficient mechanism to detect related responses.

The following observations suggest that synchronization of distributed neuronal responses could serve as a mechanism for dynamic grouping. (1) Response synchronization involves widespread neuronal populations distributed both within (König et al., 1995; Maldonado et al., 2000) and across cortical areas (Nelson et al., 1992b; Frien et al., 1994; Nowak et al., 1999) and hemispheres (Engel et al., 1991a; Nowak et al., 1995; Murthy and Fetz, 1996). (2) Millisecond-precise response synchronization is stimulus-dependent (i.e., it is strong if the participating neurons are activated by stimuli that have certain features in common and it is weak or absent between neurons responding to unrelated stimuli) (Engel et al., 1991b; Kreiter and Singer, 1996). (3) Millisecond precise synchronization of visual responses has been shown to be stronger during lower levels of anesthesia (Herculano-Houzel et al., 1999) and can be strengthened by experimental activation of the cortex by stimulation of the MRF (Munk et al., 1996; Herculano-Houzel et al., 1999). Synchronization can be expected to be stronger among responses that represent related features during more aroused states if response synchronization is relevant for information processing. (4) In awake behaving cats, the synchronization of oscillations in visual (A17,18,21) and parietal (A7,5) as well as parietal and motor (A4) areas was strengthened during periods of attentional demand (Roelfsema et al., 1997). The frequency of these oscillations changed systematically during the task, being high during periods of increased attention and dropping significantly during reward. (5) Rapid changes in correlated firing of neurons in the frontal cortex of awake monkeys have been shown to be closely related to changes in their behavior (Aertsen et al., 1989; Vaadia et al., 1995). In awake squinting cats stimulated dichoptically (separate stimuli for each eye) with rivaling

moving stimuli, millisecond-precise synchronization of gamma-frequency oscillations in area 17 allows the prediction of the direction of the optokinetic nystagmus
(Fries et al., 1997). (6) Synchronized oscillations in the gamma-frequency range
occur during visual responses (Gray and Singer, 1989; Nowak et al., 1995) and the
pattern of change in time during visual responses is highly suggestive of the unfolding of a dynamic process (see Castelo-Branco et al., 1998; Herculano-Houzel et al.,
1999, and Figure 8.2).

Oscillations in the Gamma-Frequency Range and Their Role for Synchronized Firing

Since their discovery 70 years ago (Berger, 1929), electroencephalographic (EEG)
signals have been described as containing oscillatory waves that have been classified into numerous different frequency bands (Niedermeyer, 1987). From the very
beginning, changes in the frequency distribution of the EEG have been related to
changes of the functional state of the brain. The concept of synchronized and
desynchronized EEG activity was based on the following ideas. If huge populations of neurons engage in the same rhythm, their synaptic potentials summate
and therefore generate a signal strong enough to be measured on the surface of the
brain or skull. Conversely, if input from sensory organs arrived or the subject
became mentally involved, then many neurons operate in different modes and at
different times and therefore would cause a low-amplitude signal of higher frequencies on the surface. This classical observation of a reproducible shift of the
dominant frequency was first described for the occipital alpha rhythm (8 to 13
Hz) that was replaced by the faster and smaller beta (14 to 30 Hz) waves (Berger,
1929). The term *gamma-frequency band* was introduced to designate frequencies
above 30 Hz (Jasper and Andrews, 1938) and that were originally described as
being superimposed on the occipital alpha rhythm.

Not long after the discovery of brain potentials and their state dependency, the
mechanisms responsible for the dramatic changes in the EEG were investigated.
Electrical stimulation of the MRF was shown to cause an arousal reaction accompanied by a reliable increase of the dominant frequency of the EEG in cats
(Moruzzi and Magoun, 1949). An important observation was that the modulatory systems in the brain stem not only regulate wakefulness but also modulate
brain performance in the alert state. Stimulating the MRF in awake behaving
monkeys that performed a haptic discrimination task resulted in improved sensorimotor processing as reaction times shortened and error rates decreased (Fuster,
1958, 1962).

Combined studies of EEG and single unit activity in the olfactory system
revealed for the first time that defined neuronal circuits involved in sensory processing are responsible for the generation of gamma oscillations (Freeman and
Skarda, 1985). In the neocortex, gamma oscillations were discovered in the local
field potential of visual areas in anesthetized cats (Gray and Singer, 1987). During
light anesthesia, responses of the neurons to a moving visual stimulus were accompanied by a strong periodic modulation of the local field potential (Eckhorn et al.,

1988; Gray and Singer, 1989). These oscillations could be readily detected in multiunit responses, whereas single unit responses would only participate in about a third of the investigated cells (Eckhorn and Obermueller, 1993; Gray and McCormick, 1996). Oscillations in the gamma-frequency range synchronise across large and remote populations of neurones that respond to the same or a related stimuli (Eckhorn et al., 1988; Gray and Singer, 1989; Engel et al., 1991b) and can be quickly attenuated if the continuity of stimulus motion is reduced by superposition of a random motion (Kruse and Eckhorn, 1996). In the awake cat the incidence of gamma-frequency oscillations during visual responses is higher (26 percent) than during anesthesia (17 percent) (Gray and Viana, 1997).

In the awake macaque monkey, response-related oscillations have originally been described to occur either in extrastriate areas (Kreiter and Singer, 1996), or with higher frequencies (Eckhorn et al., 1993; Frien et al., 1994) than described for the cat or in V1 of squirrel monkeys (Livingstone, 1996). It has been shown only recently that gamma oscillations occur in a large proportion (46 percent) of single cells in V1 of the awake macaque (Friedman-Hill et al., 2000) and structure the responses in many other areas of the neocortex, in the inferotemporal cortex during passive viewing of complex visual objects (Freiwald et al., 1998), in parietal cortex during the preparatory period of a visually guided reaching movement (MacKay and Mendonca, 1995), and in sensorimotor (Murthy and Fetz, 1996) and motor cortex (Sanes and Donoghue, 1993).

One factor that may explain the different incidences of gamma oscillations in different studies is the level of anesthesia maintained during recording (Friedman-Hill et al., 2000). A direct demonstration that the vigilance level determines the incidence and strength of gamma oscillations could be provided by manipulating the MRF while recording cortical responses to visual stimulation. Already spontaneous state fluctuations under anesthesia showed a tight positive correlation of the incidence and strength of gamma oscillations in multiunit responses and the dominant frequency of the EEG (Herculano-Houzel et al., 1999). Most important, through activation of the MRF, the occurrence of gamma oscillations was stabilized and with prolonged repetition of sensory activation accompanied with MRF stimulation significantly increased their strength and synchronicity (see Figure 8.3).

One of the reasons why gamma oscillations are an attractive mechanism for the dynamic reorganization of large neuronal circuits is their ability to synchronize the spike discharge of neurons with millisecond precision, although the driving input may lack any relevant time structure (Volgushev et al., 1998). Before this direct demonstration was provided, this idea had inspired a computer simulation study in which disinhibitory feedback loops from inhibitory interneurons with diverging connections to large populations of pyramidal cells were responsible for the ability of the neuronal network to synchronize with millisecond precision (Bush and Douglas, 1991). Along these lines, it was proposed that oscillatory discharge of neurons in the visual cortex may serve synchronization because the incidence of oscillations dominating the correlation pattern increased with distance (König et al., 1995). Based on single trial analysis, there is some first evidence that oscillatory modulation often precedes the onset of synchrony in successive stimulus responses (Herculano-Houzel et al., 1998). Although a causal relation between gamma oscillations and synchronization is not yet established, there is evidence that they are tightly linked. Inducing gamma oscillations in visual responses by activating the MRF reliably increased the probability of observing synchronization even across large distances (Munk et al., 1996; Herculano-Houzel et al., 1999). It is therefore necessary to understand which mechanisms are responsible for the generation of oscillatory activity.

Numerous proposals have been made of how gamma oscillations may be generated (Traub et al., 1996; Ritz and Sejnowski, 1997). In many visual cortical neurons, oscillatory modulation of membrane potentials seems to originate from synaptic inputs (Bringuier et al., 1992). This finding is compatible with the observation that some pacemaker cells generate the rhythm by intrinsic properties and entrain the network transsynaptically. In the visual cortex of anesthetized cats, about one-third (25:73) of the neurons have been shown to generate oscillations upon progressive depolarization and visual stimulation. These cells were later identified as superficial pyramidal neurons called "chattering cells" (Gray and McCormick, 1996). There is accumulating evidence that acetylcholine can induce rhythmic firing in neocortical neurons (McCormick, 1993; Wang and McCormick, 1993; Lukatch and MacIver, 1997) that may be able to entrain the entire network or at least parts of it. Studies of the temporal structure of neuronal activity in the hippocampus (Buzsaki and Chrobak, 1995) and more recently *in vitro* and simulation studies of the neocortex (Whittington et al., 1995) suggest that apart from pacemaker cells, networks of connected inhibitory interneurons may also be able to generate oscillations in the gamma-frequency range. It is, however, not yet clear which of the numerous candidate mechanisms is relevant under realistic conditions of brain function. However, the behavioral and cognitive conditions under which gamma activity occurs have recently been investigated.

Gamma activity has been observed to occur in human EEG recordings either in a fixed phase relation to external events ("phase-locked") or only initiated by external events, but with variable phase from trial to trial, the so-called induced gamma. Early reports described gamma activity as part of the event-related potentials (Galambos et al., 1981; Ribary et al., 1991). In animals, most of the observed gamma oscillations recorded intracortically did not occur with a fixed phase relation to, for example, sensory stimulation, which raised the question whether induced gamma activity would also exist in human brain activity. By means of a new analysis method it has been made possible to distinguish "evoked" (phase-locked) and "induced" (non–phase-locked) gamma activity even in single trials (Tallon-Baudry and Bertrand, 1999). Initially, induced gamma activity was shown to depend on the processing demands during visual pattern detection (Tallon-Baudry et al., 1996). In the meantime, a number of elegant studies have confirmed that induced gamma activity can be observed during visual search (Tallon-Baudry et al., 1997), visual short-term memory (Tallon-Baudry et al., 1998), and auditory tone discrimination (Yvert et al., 1998), that is, when an active internal representation or reorganization of sensory information (Keil et al., 1999) is needed to perform a task successfully. The fact that gamma oscillations are detectable in surface signals drawing from huge populations of neurons suggests that the underlying oscillatory neuronal firings are synchronized to some degree. More recent experiments suggest that phase synchronization and active desynchronization of activity in the gamma-frequency range characterize different processes during perceptual and sensorimotor integration and provide more information about the underlying neuronal operations than the mere up- and down-modulation of gamma activity (Rodriguez et al., 1999).

Oscillations in the gamma-frequency range become particularly prominent in behavioral conditions in which attention and active representations of sensory information are required. During epochs of synchronized oscillatory activity, synaptic inputs to individual cells are synchronized with postsynaptic discharge. Therefore gamma oscillations are directly involved in the generation of very large numbers of coincidences in synaptically connected neurons. Millisecond-precise coincidences of pre- and postsynaptic activation have been shown to induce changes in synaptic transmission and determine the direction of change depending on the exact temporal relation (Markram et al., 1997). Small phase shifts between synchronized oscillations could therefore be a very efficient mechanism to control synaptic change. Therefore, the conditions under which oscillations can influence the modulation of synaptic plasticity will be more closely reviewed.

Cortical Mechanisms of Plasticity for Feed-Forward and Assembly-Forming Connections

It is now well established that the connections between neocortical neurones express long-term potentiation (LTP) and long-term depression (LTD). Although coincident activation of pre- and postsynaptic membranes has long been postulated to be the relevant signal to initiate synaptic modification (Hebb, 1949; Bienenstock et al., 1982; Sejnowski, 1977), it has only recently been demonstrated for neocortical connections. The temporal contingency of presynaptic activation with postsynaptic depolarization or hyperpolarization can cause lasting changes of synaptic efficacy in opposite directions, whereas random temporal delays between pre- and postsynaptic events have no effect (Frégnac et al., 1994). Synaptic efficacy is regulated by millisecond precise ($<<100$ msec) timing of excitatory postsynaptic potentials (EPSPs) and postsynaptic action potentials (Markram et al., 1997), which had been interpreted as an effect of interactions of the backpropagating action potentials (Stuart et al., 1997) and synaptic input in the dendrite. Direct evidence for such a mechanism was provided recently by simultaneous recordings from dendrite and soma of the same cell. Single action potentials backpropagated from the axon that coincided with dendritic EPSPs led to dendritic calcium action potentials that in turn elicited high-frequency bursts of axonal action potentials (Larkum et al., 1999). This is a mechanism for increasing the intracellular calcium concentration, which is the prerequisite for the induction of synaptic plasticity and for integrating information arriving from different inputs by converting coincidence-encoded inputs into a rate-coded output.

In feed-forward architectures, changes in synaptic gain can be expected to result in modified response strength, if the same set of afferent connections is modified, and in modified response specificity if previously weak connections are strengthened and/or previously strong inputs are weakened. The synaptic changes depend on the degree of postsynaptic depolarization, which determines the intracellular calcium concentration. As described above, the latter can be boosted by coincident pre- and postsynaptic activation. These mechanisms have mostly been studied by testing postsynaptic responses to single presynaptic test stimuli. However, under *in vivo* conditions, neurons often fire trains and bursts of action potentials. It has recently been demonstrated that the time course of a postsynaptic response to a regular 20-Hz burst of presynaptic action potentials can be modified without changing the net efficacy of the involved synapses after the connection was exposed to repeated synchronous activation of the pre- and postsynaptic cell (Markram and Tsodyks, 1996). This redistribution of response amplitude is due to a modification of the frequency attenuation of the postsynaptic response. If synchronous activation of the pre- and postsynaptic cells can cause a systematic shift of the response maximum in time without changing the average level of activation in a broader time window, the exact latency of a neuron's response can be modified so that the time at which a cell participates in an assembly can be adapted by neuronal mechanisms. If the timing of synaptic responses can change independently of their strength, two different algorithms for synaptic modifications can be conceived. Changing the strength of postsynaptic responses may be the mechanism by which the cortex can select the cells that respond to a certain input pattern, whereas the modification of the response timing could determine or at least bias the participation of a given cell in neuronal assemblies.

What is the evidence that response properties change under experimental conditions? Only in very few studies could *in vivo* response properties of individual neurons be changed without the additional presence of neuromodulators or appropriate learning behavior. Invasive conditioning procedures with direct postsynaptic depolarization (Frégnac et al., 1992) or very prolonged synchronous sensory conditioning (Eysel et al., 1998) have been effective in inducing lasting changes. As the *in vitro* facilitation of synaptic change by cholinergic or adrenergic stimulation (Bröcher et al., 1992) suggests, numerous *in vivo* studies in which neuromodulators were either directly applied or released after activation of modulatory systems such as the basal forebrain could demonstrate strong and robust effects. In the visual cortex of kittens, pairing the presentation of a nonoptimal light stimulus with the application of acetylcholine (ACh), noradrenaline (NE), or excitatory amino acids (NMDA, L-Glu) were effective in changing ocular dominance, orientation, and direction selectivities after a few hundred pairings in about half of the cells tested (Greuel et al., 1988). In the auditory cortex of adult cats, pairing single tones with application of ACh induced modification of frequency-specific responses. In subsequent studies, similar changes of auditory receptive fields could be induced by conditioning with electrical stimulation of the basal forebrain (Bakin and Weinberger, 1996) or by classical conditioning during anesthesia, which caused changes that were evident up to 8 weeks after induction

(Weinberger, 1993). Conditioning of auditory responses to single tones in awake rats with electrical stimulation of their nucleus basalis (the origin of the major cholinergic projection to the cortex) led to dramatic changes of the cortical map as determined by the tuning of unit responses in favor of the conditioned frequency (Kilgard and Merzenich, 1998a). This modulatory influence was not only effective in the spatial reorganization, but was shown to enable the generation of new response properties in the temporal domain that did not exist prior to conditioning (Kilgard and Merzenich, 1998b). Surprisingly similar are the changes of cortical response properties if instead of basal forebrain stimulation the mesencephalic reticular cholinergic system is used to condition visual responses to a particular orientation of the stimulus, suggesting that similar mechanisms could be involved. In a study of the adult visual cortex in anesthetized cats, the orientation tuning of multiunit responses could be altered reversibly upon MRF conditioning with different orientations of the visual stimulus (Galuske et al., 1997).

The validity of experiments that have substituted the naturally occurring effects of modulatory systems by electrical stimulation or local application of drugs is confirmed by the results of studies of behaviorally induced changes of neuronal response properties. Training monkeys to perform a haptic discrimination task induced massive changes in the size and location of receptive fields in area 3B of somatosensory cortex representing the contralateral hand (Wang et al., 1995), whereas no such extension was found for the ipsilateral hand in the same animals. Training-induced expansions of frequency representations in the somatosensory (Recanzone et al., 1992) and auditory cortex (Recanzone et al., 1993) have been shown to correlate with behavioral performance.

A first direct demonstration that the behavioral context is not only effective in modifying response properties but can also facilitate modifications of functional connectivity in the cortex was provided by studying temporal contingencies in the auditory cortex (Ahissar et al., 1992). Cellular conditioning was applied by inducing temporal contingency between the response of one auditory neuron with the response of another simultaneously recorded neuron that responded to sensory activation triggered by the first neuron's spikes. In some of the conditioning periods the monkeys performed an auditory discrimination task, whereas in other periods contingencies were generated without the monkey having to attend. Although cellular contingency without behavioral training was able to induce weak but significant changes ($r = 0.4$ for the correlation between induced and retained changes), a highly significant effect was observed for cellular contingency during training ($r = 0.8$), which was extinguished when contingency was decreased. No correlation was found with changes in the firing rates of the neurons. The results of this study imply that changes of synaptic interactions in the neocortex can be induced much more efficiently if the modulatory systems that are implicated in controlling attention are activated.

In the case of learning that requires the storage of assembly-coded information, changes of the neuronal representation are expected in the form of modified response synchronization and not in the response strength of those neurons that constitute the assemblies. Elements of a visual scene that belong to the features defining the same perceptual object are expected to evoke synchronized responses with higher probability than unrelated features. This has been shown to be the case for line segments of identical orientation that move either in the same direction (related) or in opposite directions (unrelated) (Engel et al., 1991b; Munk et al., 1996). With repeated presentation of related stimuli or the frequent recurrence of related features in behaviorally significant situations, the probability and strength of synchronized firing are expected to increase, and, vice versa, to decrease for the frequent recurrence of unrelated features. To test whether the neuronal representation of spatially segregated visual stimuli changes in accordance with this prediction, we devised an experiment in which the repeated presentation of visual stimuli was conditioned with electrical stimulation of the MRF. As can be seen in Figure 8.4, during the conditioning periods the strength of response synchronization was reliably increased. Such changes in response synchronization are often accompanied by enhanced oscillatory patterning of the responses (see Figure 8.3). If response synchronization is abolished or reduced due to changes of the sensory stimuli during conditioning, synchronization will be weakened or absent during the next test period. Desynchronization was reversible as subsequent conditioning of synchronous firing was successful (last pairing period in Figure 8.4). These changes in synchronization strength could be due to fluctuations of cortical activation or the depth of anesthesia. However, this is not the case as can be judged from the time course and the distributions of fractional power in the gamma-frequency band of the simultaneously recorded EEG. In the case shown in Figure 8.4, power in the gamma-frequency band even reaches its maximum during the period of conditioning decorrelated firing (third pairing period). The high gamma during this period most likely reflects the stimulus-induced oscillatory activity of those circuits that respond to the new set of visual stimuli (see Figure 8.4A). The fact that the degree of EEG activation is almost identical during all the test conditions allows us to conclude that the synaptic substrate underlying correlated firing of the neurons has been modified.

Oscillatory modulation of neuronal firing patterns are reliably induced by reticular activation of the cortex, which is at least in part mediated through cholinergic projections from the basal forebrain (Jones, 1995). Oscillatory patterning of responses can synchronize groups of neurons that receive the same oscillatory signals. If different groups of neurons that each have established their own oscillatory firing pattern start to interact via their horizontal reciprocal connections, a synchronization pattern will emerge that at the beginning of the interactions reflects the phase relations of all the local oscillatory processes. With the unfolding of dynamic lateral interactions, the synchronization pattern will be more and more determined by the temporal transmission properties of the effective horizontal connectivity. As the temporal transmission properties determine which neurons can engage in synchronized firing, learning-induced changes of these properties can cause the reorganization of assembly-coded information. In the presence of neuromodulatory substances such as ACh, the sensitivity of synapses to change their properties is enhanced. If under these circumstances the same modulators cause stronger oscillatory patterning, more precisely coincident EPSPs impinge on

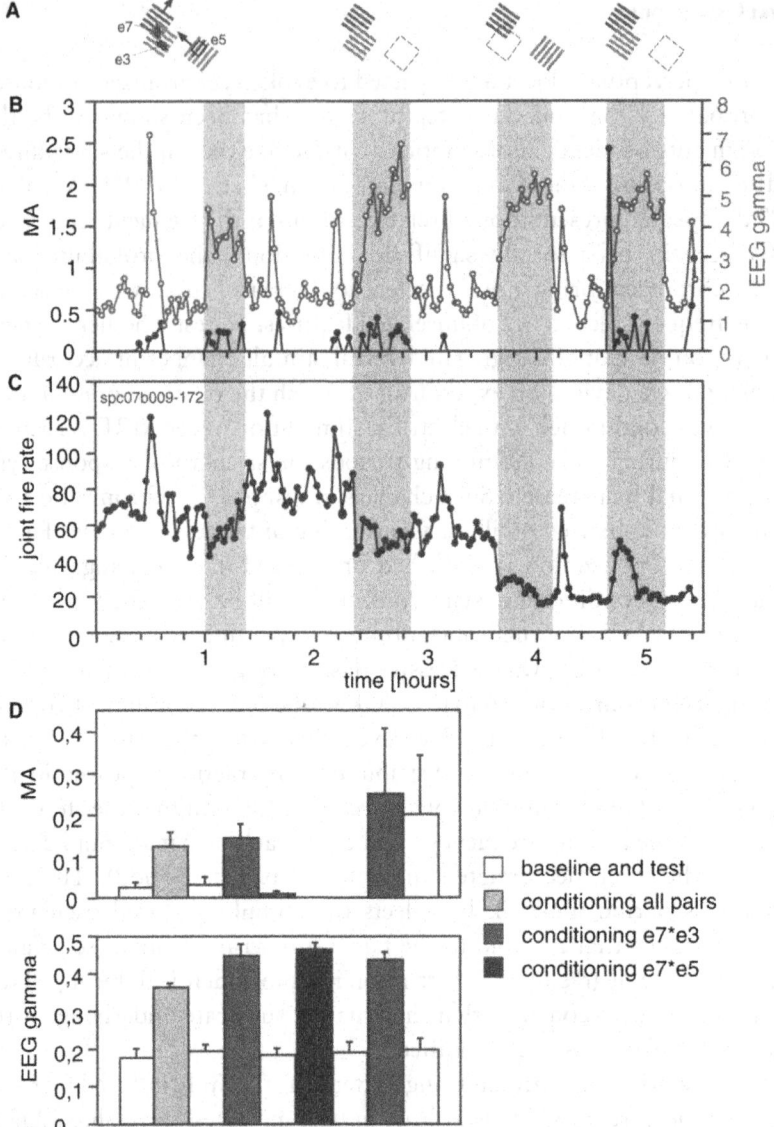

Figure 8.4. MRF conditioning of synchronised and decorrelated visual responses leads to lasting changes in the correlation pattern that depends on the pattern of sensory stimulation. (**A**) Stimulus pattern superimposed on the receptive fields. Stimuli were small patches of gratings moving in the preferred direction of the cells. (**B**) Time course of synchronization strength (black line with filled symbols) as quantified by the modulation amplitude (MA) in multi-unit cross-correlation histograms (see Figure 8.2). The MA is computed by taking the ratio of the height of the center peak of a fitted Gabor function divided by the offset of the correlogram. Note that synchronization is high during and after MRF conditioning, is abolished if a different pair of cells (e5 and e7) is conditioned, but comes back after a further period of conditioning pair e3*e7. The time course of fractional power in the gamma-frequency band (20 to 70 Hz, grey line with open symbols) reflects the level of cortical activation. (**C**) Joint firing rate of the multi-unit responses at e3 and e7. Note that the changes in firing rate do not account for the changes in synchronization strength. (**D**) Mean values for synchronization strength in the unit responses (**upper row**) and gamma activation in the EEG (**lower row**) demonstrate that the difference in correlation strength cannot be explained by a difference in global excitability as revealed by the gamma fraction in the EEG.

synoptically connected (pre- and postsynaptic) neurons. The direct effects of ACh on intracellular signaling and the effects on oscillatory firing patterns may act synergistically to change synaptic transmission characteristics and as a consequence the spatiotemporal patterns of synchronized activity. Under conditions of increased cortical activation as they characterize attentional states, the probability of altering the composition of neuronal assemblies could therefore be increased.

Originally, evidence came from lesion studies and human pathology (Alzheimer's disease) that an intact cholinergic system is required for normal learning. A critical review (Everitt and Robbins, 1997) of the studies that tested the effect of manipulating the cholinergic forebrain system revealed that this system facilitates learning by enhancing attention rather than by interacting directly with mechanisms of synaptic plasticity. A behavioral study in macaque monkeys had demonstrated that lesions of the basal forebrain did not interfere with a number of mnemonic tasks, but disrupted attentional focusing (Voytko et al., 1994). It is well established that attention is required for successful learning and therefore the effects of the cholinergic modulators may influence learning processes through the intermediate step of controlling attention. As synchronous oscillatory discharge is elicited by the same modulators that facilitate synaptic changes and support massive reorganization of cortical representations, synchronous oscillatory activity may constitute the link between the activation of the cholinergic system and learning-induced changes of synaptic transmission in the cortical network. Synchronization of oscillatory neuronal firing would then serve as a representational mechanism that constitutes assemblies and at the same time controls synaptic modification.

Learning-induced changes of feed-forward and assembly-forming connections are based on different neuronal mechanisms. This is the consequence of the rather distinct modes of operation in which the two types of connections are involved. Feed-forward transmission is fast and quickly invades many processing levels of the cortex. It relies on coincidence detection of converging inputs that is entirely dependent on the previously set synaptic gains. Assembly-based transmission is slower because the processes underlying synchronization take time to unfold; however, synchronization can rapidly adapt its spatiotemporal structure in order to represent new content. Assemblies represent an active self-organizing process that groups large populations of active neurons by synchronization and desynchronization and thus determines the composition of different assemblies. The output of assemblies is synchronized activity that also converges on cells at subsequent processing stages. Assemblies, therefore, contribute to feed-forward transmission, but only after some delay. However, the synchronized activity of assemblies could be an instructive signal that guides the change of feed-forward connectivity in order to modify response properties at subsequent processing stages.

In conclusion, precise timing of spike discharge during neuronal responses in the neocortex may serve the representation and processing of complex information and at the same time constitute a mechanism to select behaviorally relevant information to be stored in memory by modifying synaptic transmission. There is growing evidence that oscillatory modulation of neuronal firing patterns could be a mechanism for synchronizing large distributed neuronal populations and thus for organizing neuronal assemblies. As millisecond-precise synchronous oscillations are facilitated by the same neuromodulators that facilitate changes of synaptic transmission and support massive reorganization of cortical representations, synchronous gamma oscillations may constitute the link between the activation of the cholinergic system and learning-induced changes of cortical function.

REFERENCES

Aertsen, A.M., Gerstein, G.L., Habib, M.K., and Palm, G. (1989). Dynamics of neuronal firing correlation: Modulation of "effective connectivity." *J. Neurophysiol.* 61: 900–917.

Ahissar, E., Vaadia, E., Ahissar, M., Bergman, H. et al. (1992). Dependence of cortical plasticity on correlated activity of single neurons and on behavioral context. *Science* 257: 1412–1415.

Bakin, J.S., and Weinberger, N.M. (1996). Induction of a physiological memory in the cerebral cortex by stimulation of the nucleus basalis. *Proc. Natl. Acad. Sci. USA* 93: 10546–10547.

Berger, H. (1929). Über das Elektrencephalogramm des Menschen. *Arch. Psychiat. Nervenkr.* 87: 527–570.

Bienenstock, E.L., Cooper, L.N., and Munro, P.W. (1982). Theory for the development of neuron selectivity: Orientation specificity and binocular interaction in visual cortex. *J. Neurosci.* 2: 32–48.

Bringuier, V., Frégnac, Y., Debanne, D., Shulz, D. et al. (1992). Synaptic origin of rhythmic visually evoked activity in kitten area 17 neurones. *Neuroreport* 3: 1065–1068.

Bröcher, S., Artola, A., and Singer, W. (1992). Agonists of cholinergic and noradrenergic receptors facilitate synergistically the induction of long-term potentiation in slices of rat visual cortex. *Brain Res.* 573: 27–36.

Bush, P.C., and Douglas, R.J. (1991). Synchronization of bursting action potential discharge in a model network of neocortical neurons. *Neural Comp.* 3: 19–30.

Buzsaki, G., and Chrobak, J.J. (1995). Temporal structure in spatially organized neuronal ensembles: A role for interneuronal networks. *Curr. Opin. Neurobiol.* 5: 504–510.

Castelo-Branco, M., Neuenschwander, S., and Singer, W. (1998). Synchronization of visual responses between the cortex, lateral geniculate nucleus, and retina in the anesthetized cat. *J. Neurosc.* 18: 6395–6410.

Eckhorn, R., and Obermueller, A. (1993). Single neurons are differently involved in stimulus-specific oscillations in cat visual cortex. *Exp. Brain Res.* 95: 177–182.

Eckhorn, R., Bauer, R., Jordan, W., Brosch, M. et al. (1988). Coherent oscillations: A mechanism of feature linking in the visual cortex? Multiple electrode and correlation analyses in the cat. *Biol. Cybern.* 60: 121–130.

Eckhorn, R., Frien, A., Bauer, R., Woelbern, T. et al. (1993). High frequency (60–90 Hz) oscillations in primary visual cortex of awake monkey. *Neuroreport* 4: 243–246.

Engel, A.K., König, P., Kreiter, A.K., and Singer, W. (1991a). Interhemispheric synchronization of oscillatory neuronal responses in cat visual cortex. *Science* 252: 1177–1179.

Engel, A.K., Kreiter, A.K., König, P., and Singer, W. (1991b). Synchronization of oscillatory neuronal responses between striate and extrastriate visual cortical areas of the cat. *Proc. Natl. Acad. Sci. USA* 88: 6048–6052.

Everitt, B.J., and Robbins, T.W. (1997). Central cholinergic systems and cognition. *Ann. Rev. Neurosci.* 48: 649–684.

Eysel, U.T., Eyding, D., and Schweigart, G. (1998). Repetitive optical stimulation elicits fast receptive field changes in mature visual cortex. *Neuroreport* 9: 949–954.

Felleman, D.J., and Van Essen, D. (1991). Distributed hierarchical processing in the primate cerebral cortex. *Cereb. Cortex* 1: 1–47.

Freeman, W.J., and Skarda, C.A. (1985). Spatial EEG patterns, non-linear dynamics and perception: The neo-Sherringtonian view. *Brain Res.* 357: 147–175.

Frégnac, Y., Shulz, D., Thorpe, S., and Bienenstock, E. (1992). Cellular analogs of visual cortical epigenesis. I. Plasticity of orientation selectivity. *J. Neurosci.* 12: 1280–1300.

Frégnac, Y., Burke, J.P., Smith, D., and Friedlander, M.J. (1994). Temporal covariance of pre- and postsynaptic activity regulates functional connectivity in the visual cortex. *J. Neurophysiol.* 71: 1403–1421.

Freiwald, W.A., Kreiter, A.K., and Singer, W. (1998). Oscillatory and synchronous activity states in the macaque inferotemporal cortex. *Soc. Neurosci. Abstr.* 24: 355.15.

Friedman-Hill, S., Maldonado, P.E., and Gray, C.M. (2000). Temporal dynamics of neuronal activity in the striate cortex of alert macaque: I. Incidence and stimulus-dependence of oscillations. *J. Cerebral Cortex* (in press).

Frien, A., Eckhorn, R., Bauer R., Woelbern, T. et al. (1994). Stimulus-specific fast oscillations at zero phase between visual areas V1 and V2 of awake monkey. *Neuroreport* 5: 2273–2277.

Fries, P., Roelfsema, P.R., Engel, A.K., König, P. et al. (1997). Synchronization of oscillatory responses in visual cortex correlates with perception in interocular rivalry. *Proc. Natl. Acad. Sci. USA* 94: 12699–12704.

Fuster, J.M. (1958). Effects of stimulation of brain stem on tachistoscopic perception. *Science.* 127: 150.

Fuster, J.M. (1962). Facilitation of tachistoscopic performance by stimulation of midbrain tegmental points in the monkey. *Exper. Neurol.* 6: 384–406.

Galambos, R., Makeig, S., and Talmachoff, P.J. (1981). A 40-Hz auditory potential recorded from the human scalp. *Proc. Natl. Acad. Sci. USA* 78: 2643–2647.

Galuske, R.A.W., Singer, W., and Munk, M.H.J. (1997). Reticular activation facilitates use-dependent plasticity of orientation preference maps in the cat visual cortex. *Soc. Neurosci. Abstr.* 23: 801.8.

Gray, C.M., and McCormick, D.A. (1996). Chattering cells: Superficial pyramidal neurons contributing to the generation of synchronous oscillations in the visual cortex. *Science* 274: 109–113.

Gray, C.M., and Singer, W. (1987). Stimulus-specific neuronal oscillations in the cat visual cortex: A cortical functional unit. *Soc. Neurosci. Abstr.* 13: 404.3.

Gray, C.M., and Singer, W. (1989). Stimulus-specific neuronal oscillations in orientation columns of cat visual cortex. *Proc. Natl. Acad. Sci. USA* 86: 1698–1702.

Gray, C.M., and Viana, D.P. (1997). Stimulus-dependent neuronal oscillations and local synchronization in striate cortex of the alert cat. *J. Neurosci.* 17: 3239–3253.

Greuel, J.M., Luhmann, H.J., and Singer, W. (1988). Pharmacological induction of use-dependent receptive field modifications in the visual cortex. *Science* 242: 74–77.

Hebb, D.O. (1949). *The Organization of Behavior.* New York: Wiley.

Herculano-Houzel, S., Munk, M.H.J., and Singer, W. (1998). Relation between response synchronisation and oscillatory modulation in cat visual cortex. *Eur. J. Neurosci.* 10: 93–32.

Herculano-Houzel, S., Munk, M.H., Neuenschwander, S., and Singer, W. (1999). Precisely synchronized oscillatory firing patterns require electroencephalographic activation. *J. Neurosci.* 19: 3992–4010.

Hupe, J.M., James, A.C., Payne, B.R., Lomber, S.G. et al. (1998). Cortical feedback improves discrimination between figure and background by V1, V2 and V3 neurons. *Nature* 394: 784–787.

Jasper, H.H., and Andrews, H.L. (1938). Electroencephalography. III. Normal differentiation of occipital and precentral regions in man. *Arch. Neurol. Psychiat. (Chicago)* 39: 96–115.

Jones, B.E. (1995). Reticular formation. Cytoarchitecture, transmitters and projections. In G. Paxmos (Ed.), *The rat nervous system* (pp. 155–171). New South Wales: Academic Press Australia.

Keil, A., Müller, M.M., Ray, W.J., Gruber, T. et al. (1999). Human gamma band activity and perception of a gestalt. *J. Neurosci.* 19: 7152–7161.

Kilgard, M.P., and Merzenich, M.M. (1998a). Cortical map reorganization enabled by nucleus basalis activity. *Science* 279: 1714–1718.

Kilgard, M.P., and Merzenich, M.M. (1998b). Plasticity of temporal information processing in the primary auditory cortex. *Nat. Neurosci.* 1: 727–731.

König, P, Engel, A.K., and Singer, W. (1995). Relation between oscillatory activity and long-range synchronization in cat visual cortex. *Proc. Natl. Acad. Sci. USA* 92: 290–294.

Kreiter, A.K., and Singer, W. (1996). Stimulus-dependent synchronization of neuronal responses in the visual cortex of the awake macaque monkey. *J. Neurosci.* 16: 2381–2396.

Kruse, W., and Eckhorn, R. (1996). Inhibition of sustained gamma oscillations (35–80 Hz) by fast transient responses in cat visual cortex. *Proc. Natl. Acad. Sci. USA* 93: 6112–6117.

Larkum, M.E., Zhu, J.J., and Sakmann, B. (1999). A new cellular mechanism for coupling inputs arriving at different cortical layers. *Nature* 398: 338–341.

Livingstone, M.S. (1996). Oscillatory firing and interneuronal correlations in squirrel monkey striate cortex. *J. Neurophysiol.* 75: 2467–2485.

Lukatch, H.S., and MacIver, M.B. (1997). Physiology, pharmacology, and topography of cholinergic neocortical oscillations in vitro. *J. Neurophysiol.* 77: 2427–2445.

MacKay, W.A., and Mendonca, A.J. (1995). Field potential oscillatory bursts in parietal cortex before and during reach. *Brain Res.* 704: 167–174.

Maldonado, PE, Friedman-Hill, S., and Gray, C.M. (2000). Temporal dynamics of neuronal activity in the striate cortex of alert macaque: II. Short and long-range temporally correlated activity. *J. Cerebral Cortex* (in press).

Markram, H., Lübke, J, Frotscher, M., and Sakmann, B. (1997). Regulation of synaptic efficacy by coincidence of postsynaptic APs and EPSPs. *Science* 275: 213–215.

Markram, H., and Tsodyks, M. (1996). Redistribution of synaptic efficacy between neocortical pyramidal neurons. *Nature* 382: 807–810.

Mastronarde, D.N. (1983). Interactions between ganglion cells in cat retina. *J. Neurophysiol.* 49/2: 350–365.

McCormick, D.A. (1993). Actions of acetylcholine in the cerebral cortex and thalamus and implications for function. *Prog. Brain Res.* 98: 303–308.

Moruzzi, G., and Magoun, H.W. (1949). Brain stem reticular formation and activation of the EEG. *Electroencephalog. Clin. Neurophysiol.* 1: 455–473.

Munk, M.H., Nowak, L.G., Nelson, J.I., and Bullier, J. (1995). Structural basis of cortical synchronization. II. Effects of cortical lesions. *J. Neurophysiol.* 74: 2401–2414.

Munk, M.H., Roelfsema, P.R., König, P., Engel, A.K. et al. (1996). Role of reticular activation in the modulation of intracortical synchronization. *Science* 272: 271–274.

Murthy, V.N., and Fetz, E.E. (1996). Oscillatory activity in sensorimotor cortex of awake monkeys: Synchronization of local field potentials and relation to behavior. *J. Neurophysiol.* 76: 3949–3967.

Nelson, J.I., Nowak, L.G., Chouvet, G., Munk, M.H.J. et al. (1992a). Synchronization between cortical neurons depends on activity in remote areas. *Soc. Neurosci. Abstr.* 18: 11.8.

Nelson, J.I., Salin, P.A., Munk, M.H., Arzi, M. et al. (1992b). Spatial and temporal coherence in cortico-cortical connections: A cross-correlation study in areas 17 and 18 in the cat. *Vis. Neurosci.* 9: 21–37.

Niedermeyer, E. (1987). The normal EEG of the waking adult. In E. Niedermeyer, and F. Lopes da Silva (Eds.), *Elektroencephalography* (pp. 97–117). Baltimore, Munich: Urban & Schwarzenberg.

Nowak, L.G., Munk, M.H., James, A.C., Girard, P. et al. (1999). Cross-correlation study of the temporal interactions between areas V1 and V2 of the macaque monkey. *J. Neurophysiol.* 81: 1057–1074.

Nowak, L.G., Munk, M.H., Nelson, J.I., James. A.C. et al. (1995). Structural basis of cortical synchronization. I. Three types of interhemispheric coupling. *J. Neurophysiol.* 74: 2379–2400.

Phillips, W.A., and Singer, W. (1997). In search of common foundations for cortical computation. *Behav. Brain Sci.* 20: 657–683.

Recanzone, G.H., Merzenich, M.M., Jenkins, W.M., Grajski, K.A. et al. (1992). Topographic reorganization of the hand representation in cortical area 3b owl monkeys trained in a frequency-discrimination task. *J. Neurophysiol.* 67: 1031–1056.

Recanzone, G.H., Schreiner, C.E., and Merzenich, M.M. (1993). Plasticity in the frequency representation of primary auditory cortex following discrimination training in adult owl monkeys. *J. Neurosci.* 13: 87–103.

Ribary, U., Ioannides, A.A., Singh, K.D., Hasson. R. et al. (1991). Magnetic field tomography of coherent thalamocortical 40-Hz oscillations in humans. *Proc. Natl. Acad. Sci. USA* 88: 11037–11041.

Ritz, R., and Sejnowski, T.J. (1997). Synchronous oscillatory activity in sensory systems: New vistas on mechanisms. *Curr. Opin. Neurobiol.* 7: 536–546.

Rodriguez, E, George, N., Lachaux, J.P., Martinerie, J. et al. (1999). Perception's shadow: Long-distance synchronization of human brain activity. *Nature* 397: 430–433.

Roelfsema, P.R., Engel, A.K., König, P., and Singer, W. (1997). Visuomotor integration is associated with zero time-lag synchronization among cortical areas. *Nature* 385: 157–161.

Roelfsema, P.R., Lamme, V.A., and Spekreijse, H. (1998). Object-based attention in the primary visual cortex of the macaque monkey. *Nature* 395: 376–381.

Salin, P.A., and Bullier, J. (1995). Corticocortical connections in the visual system: Structure and function. *Physiol. Rev.* 75: 107–154.

Salin, P.A., Bullier, J, and Kennedy, H. (1989). Convergence and divergence in the afferent projections to cat area. 17. *J. Comp. Neurol.* 283: 486–512.

Sanes, J.N., and Donoghue, J.P. (1993). Oscillations in local field potentials of the primate motor cortex during voluntary movement. *Proc. Natl. Acad. Sci. USA* 90: 4470–4474.

Sejnowski, T.J. (1977). Statistical constraints on synaptic plasticity. *J. Theoret. Biol.* 69: 385–389.

Singer, W. (1993). Synchronization of cortical activity and its putative role in information processing and learning. *Ann. Rev. Physiol.* 55: 349–374.

Singer, W. (1995). Development and plasticity of cortical processing architectures. *Science* 270: 758–764.

Singer, W., Engel, A.K., Kreiter, A.K., Munk, M.H. et al. (1997). Neuronal assemblies: Necessity, signature and detectability. *Trends Cogn. Sci.* 1: 252–261.

Stuart, G., Schiller, J., and Sakmann, B. (1997). Action potential initiation and propagation in rat neocortical pyramidal neurons. *J. Physiol.* 505: 617–632.

Tallon-Baudry, C., and Bertrand, O. (1999). Oscillatory gamma activity in humans and its role in object representation. *Trends Cogn. Sci.* 3: 151–162.

Tallon-Baudry, C., Bertrand, O., Delpuech, C., and Permier, J. (1997). Oscillatory gamma-band (30–70 Hz) activity induced by a visual search task in humans. *J. Neurosci.* 17: 722–734.

Tallon-Baudry, C., Bertrand, O., Delpuech, C., and Pernier, J. (1996). Stimulus specificity of phase-locked and non-phase-locked 40 Hz visual responses in human. *J. Neurosci.* 16: 4240–4249.

Tallon-Baudry, C., Bertrand, O., Peronnet, F., and Pernier, J. (1998). Induced gamma-band activity during the delay of a visual short-term memory task in humans. *J. Neurosci.* 18: 4244–4254.

Traub, R.D., Whittington, M.A., Stanford, I.M., and Jefferys, J.G. (1996). A mechanism for generation of long-range synchronous fast oscillations in the cortex. *Nature* 383: 621–624.

Vaadia, E., Haalman, I., Abeles, M., Bergman, H. et al. (1995). Dynamics of neuronal interactions in monkey cortex in relation to behavioural events. *Nature* 373: 515–518.

Volgushev, M., Chistiakova, M., and Singer, W. (1998). Modification of discharge patterns of neocortical neurons by induced oscillations of the membrane potential. *Neuroscience* 83: 15–25.

Voytko, M.L., Olton, D.S., Richardson, R.T., Gorman, L.K. et al., (1994). Basal forebrain lesions in monkeys disrupt attention but not learning and memory. *J. Neurosci.* 14: 167–186.

Wang, X., Merzenich, M.M., Sameshima, K., and Jenkins, W.M. (1995). Remodelling of hand representation in adult cortex determined by timing of tactile stimulation. *Nature* 378: 71–75.

Wang, Z., and McCormick, D.A. (1993). Control of firing mode of corticotectal and cortico-pontine layer V burst-generating neurons by norepinephrine, acetylcholine, and IS,3R-ACPD. *J. Neurosci.* 13: 2199–2216.

Weinberger, N.M. (1993). Learning-induced changes of auditory receptive fields. *Curr. Opin. Neurobiol.* 3: 570–577.

Whittington, M.A., Traub, R.D., and Jefferys, J.G. (1995). Synchronized oscillations in interneuron networks driven by metabotropic glutamate receptor activation. *Nature* 373: 612–615.

Yvert, B., Bertrand, O., Pernier, J., and Ilmoniemi, R.J. (1998). Human cortical responses evoked by dichotically presented tones of different frequencies. *Neuroreport* 9: 1115–1119.

Making Models from Empirical Data of Synaptic Plasticity

CHAPTER NINE

Toward a Physiologic Explanation of Behavioral Data on Human Memory

The Role of Theta-Gamma Oscillations and NMDAR-Dependent LTP

John Lisman, Ole Jensen, and Michael Kahana

SUMMARY

Psychological studies of list learning provide a quantitative behavioral description of human episodic memory. Our goal here is to describe this literature and to attempt, insofar as possible, to relate these finding to underlying physiologic processes. One prominent hypothesis to emerge from psychological studies is that of a short-term memory (STM) buffer (e.g., Atkinson and Shiffrin, 1968). It is thought that this buffer stores a small number of items (e.g., 7 ± 2 digits) using maintained neural activity. The repetitive firing produced by the STM buffer is important for the transfer to long-term memory (LTM). The rapid formation of LTM is revealed by the pre-recency part of the serial position curve in free-recall experiments. The information stored in LTM include intraitem associations, asymmetric interitem heteroassociations, and associations of items to context. Despite the success of buffer models, some observations, particularly long-term recency, argue against two-store models and alternative models have been developed. Additional information relevant to this controversy comes from neuropsychological, pharmacologic, physiologic, and computational studies. In free-recall studies, hippocampal lesions selectively reduce the recall of early list items consistent with a selective effect on LTM. Furthermore, the rapid formation of LTM (within seconds) and the selective inhibition of this process by cholinergic antagonists is consistent with what is known about the induction of long-term potentiation (LTP) and further supports the distinction between LTM and STM.

A second hypothesis to emerge from behavioral studies (the Sternberg task) is the idea of rapid serial search of the STM buffer. A model has been developed that relates these findings to brain oscillations. According to this model, a memory is encoded by the subset of neurons that fire during an individual gamma cycle; different memories in STM are serially activated in the ~7 gamma subcycles of slower theta oscillations. Initial experiments

---

using subdural electrode arrays provide strong evidence for human theta and the tight linkage of this oscillation to STM tasks. Computational studies also give insight into the consequences of the theta/gamma buffer for LTM formation by LTP. One conclusion is that the time window of LTP determines whether autoassociation or heteroassociation occurs. A second conclusion is that the buffer allows heteroassociative interitem linkages to form, even when the items occurred with a temporal separation much larger than the window. Because so much information is available about the hippocampus, it is possible to generate a working hypothesis about which synapses store particular types of information. It is proposed that autoassociation occurs in the dentate, heteroassociation in the recurrent connections of CA3, and linkages to context in the perforant path connections to CA3 and hilar cells. It is thus beginning to be possible to relate human memory performance to specific brain processes. With the rapidly developing methods for studying humans during memory tasks, it should be possible to distinguish between models and gain insight into the underlying mechanisms.

Introduction

The effort to understand memory will require both a behavioral description of the process and a mechanistic explanation of the underlying neural events. The experimental study of human memory, and in particular verbal learning, already goes a long way toward providing the needed behavioral description. Human learning is easy to study and much is known about it. Despite this success, the field of human learning has not yet had much impact on the physiologists working to understand the mechanisms of memory. This situation is beginning to change, as methods for studying physiologic events during human behavioral learning paradigms are being expanded. These include electroencephalography (EEG), magnetoencephalography (MEG), functional magnetic resonance imaging (fMRI), and intracranial recording methods. Furthermore, based on insight into neural mechanisms derived from lower animals, insight is being gained into how the key behavioral findings in human learning might be explained in mechanistic terms.

In the first section of this chapter we review some of the behavioral data on list learning that led to the idea of the distinction between short-term memory (STM) and long-term memory (LTM). One popular hypothesis is that STM acts as a limited-capacity buffer, capable of storing a small number of memory items for several seconds. It is generally assumed that STM is stored by patterns of maintained neural activity. LTM is a very high-capacity network in which synaptic modifications encode intraitem autoassociation, interitem heteroassociations, and links between items and context. It should be stressed that we follow the behavioral literature in defining LTM formation as a rapid process, which is then slowly consolidated. Other fields in neuroscience have used the term LTM to describe the stable form of memory that occurs after consolidation.

Despite the success of buffer models in accounting for a broad range of data, certain phenomena present serious challenges to these models. In the next section we will discuss some of these challenges and alternative models that do not posit a distinct STM buffer. The following section reviews neuropsychological, physiologic, and pharmacologic data relevant to this issue. The data suggesting that LTM and STM can be differentially affected are consistent with the hypothesis that the formation of LTM occurs by the NMDA-dependent form of long-term potentiation (LTP), the best studied form of activity-dependent synaptic plasticity. These data strengthen the case for the distinction between STM and LTM. The next section reviews the data on the Sternberg task, which describes the retrieval time from STM. These data suggest that memory items are rapidly, serially, and exhaustively activated during a search through STM. These data can be accounted for by the Lisman-Idiart-Jensen model, according to which the STM buffer is clocked by known theta/gamma oscillations. Some of the evidence for such a model will be discussed, including recent work that directly demonstrates the presence of theta oscillations during the Sternberg task. In the final section, we consider how NMDA-mediated LTP could transfer information from the theta/gamma STM buffer into the hippocampal LTM network.

It should be emphasized at the outset that the attempt to provide a physiologic explanation for behavioral findings on human learning are in their infancy, and that no definite conclusions can yet be reached. We hope the reader will appreciate, however, that there are interesting points of contact between the physiologic and behavioral results and that a common language is being developed that will help to integrate the behavioral and physiologic approaches.

Behavioral Data That Led to the Formulation of the Two-Store (STM-LTM) Memory Model

■ **Serial Recall and the Limits on Immediate Memory Span.** Serial recall is one of the oldest tasks used in the experimental study of human memory and provides the clearest evidence for capacity limits. In this task, subjects are presented a short list of items and asked to recall them in order immediately. The length of a series of items that can be recalled without error is termed *memory span*. For most subjects memory span is approximately seven for digits, six for letters, and five for words (Crannell and Parish, 1957). It is the small size of span, compared to the huge number of items that a person can learn with greater practice, that provides one argument for a limited-capacity STM buffer.

■ **The Effect of Serial Position in Free Recall (Recency and Primacy).** Additional arguments for an STM buffer are based on results of the free-recall task. In this task, a list of words is presented to a subject who is asked for immediate recall of those items in any order. These lists typically contain fifteen to thirty words and are thus much longer than memory span. Practiced subjects tend to recall about eight items, beginning by recalling the last few list items in forward order, and then jumping around among list items from earlier serial positions. The probability of recalling an item having a given serial position is shown in Figure 9.1A. Subjects

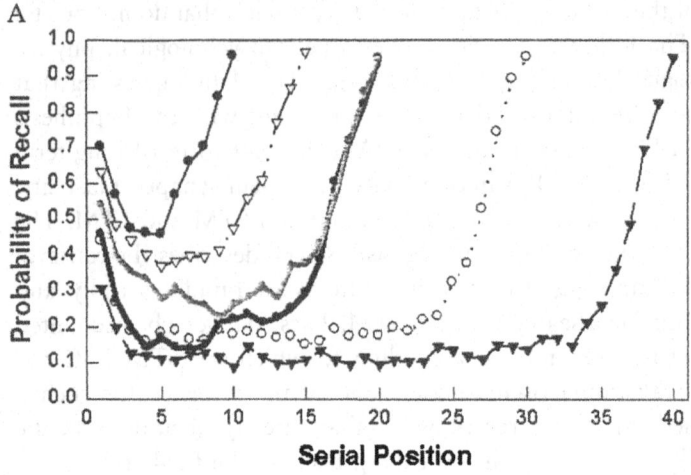

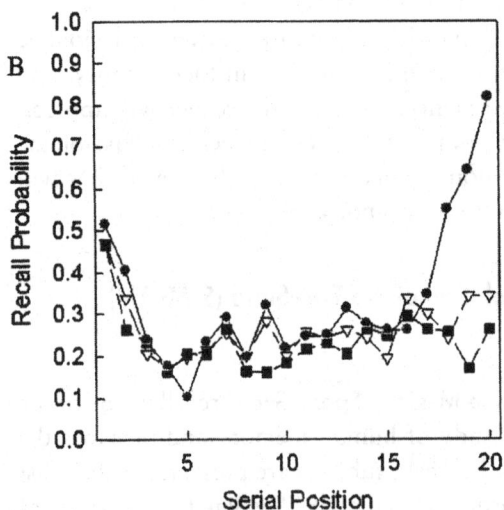

Figure 9.1. Psychological evidence for forms of memory (STM, LTM). (A) In free-recall experiments, the probability of recall varies as a function of the item's serial position in the list. Data are shown for various list lengths (indicated by rightmost point). Presentation rate is 2 s/item expect for lower 20-item list and 1 s/item for 30-item list. (Data from Murdock, 1962.) (B) A distractor given for 15 or 30 seconds at the end of the list affects free recall by selectively reducing the recency part of the curve. Circles are without distractor. (Data from Postman and Phillips, 1965.)

show the highest probability of recalling items near the end of the list, a phenomenon termed the *recency effect*. There is also a fairly high probability of recalling items near the beginning of the list, a phenomenon termed the *primacy effect*. The items in between have a lower constant probability of recall; this is termed the *asymptotic region* of the serial position curve.

The idea of a separate STM and LTM store emerged from the finding that the pre-recency (the primacy and asymptote regions) and recency parts of the curve can be differentially affected. As seen in Figure 9.1A, list length has a large effect on recall probability in the primacy and asymptotic portion of the serial position curve, but the recency effects in the six experimental conditions are virtually identical. Other experimental variables that have different effects on these two parts of the curve include semantic similarity (Watkins et al., 1974), incidental learning (Marshall and Werder, 1972), presentation rate (Murdock, 1962), and modality of presentation (Murdock and Walker, 1969). Most dramatically (Figure 9.1B), the recency effect can be made to disappear altogether if a brief (~15 seconds) arithmetic task (a "distractor") is given between the end of list presentation and the beginning of recall (Howard and Kahana, 1999; Postman and Phillips, 1965). These dissociations provide the basis for attributing the recency and pre-recency regions to different kinds of memory stores, as described below.

Experiments on serial recall suggest that the representation of information in STM is phonologic (with confusions based on sound), whereas the LTM representation is based on semantic coding (with confusions based on meaning). These findings explain why memory span depends on word length and strengthens the case for separate STM and LTM stores (Baddeley, 1996).

■ **The Atkinson-Shiffrin "Buffer" Model.** To account for these findings, models have been developed that assume three distinct stages of processing. First, sensory input due to individual items is temporarily maintained in modality-specific sensory buffers. Next, recognition systems act to identify known patterns in these buffers. These patterns, now translated into symbols, are then maintained in a modality-nonspecific, multi-item STM buffer through a process called rehearsal (it remains unclear whether this is unconscious or literally involves subvocal articulation). The amount of time that information remains in STM determines how well it is transferred to LTM. Although many models have this basic flavor, the most comprehensive is the Atkinson-Shiffrin buffer model (Atkinson and Shiffrin, 1968).

The Atkinson-Shiffrin model explains the recency and primacy data as follows. It is assumed that STM has a limited capacity approximately equal to memory span. Each new item is added to the first position in the buffer, pushing previously presented items to a later position. When the buffer is full, each new item is still added to the first position of the buffer, thereby preserving order, but one existing item drops out (older items have a higher probability of dropping out). As a result of these rules, early items spend a longer time in the buffer than other items. When subjects begin the recall process, they start by emptying the contents of the buffer. Because the buffer necessarily contains the last, and with high probability the previous few items, the probability of recalling items near the end of the list is highest. It is this that accounts for the recency effect. After all items in the buffer have been recalled, the subject turns to LTM and recalls items with a probability proportional to the associative strength of the synaptic encoding. Since this strength depends on the time the item spent in the buffer and since early items spend the most time in the buffer, early items will be recalled with higher probability than items in the asymptotic region. This accounts for the primacy effect. If the content of the buffer is *emptied* by a distractor task immediately after presentation of the last list item, then the subsequent ability to recall should be based solely on LTM. Since the last items have been in the buffer the least amount of time, their transfer to LTM should be minimal; this explains why the recency effect should be selectively eliminated by disrupting the buffer (Figure 9.1B). Indeed, Rundus predicted that if the buffer is optimally disrupted after presentation of the last item, recall of the last items should fall below the asymptotic region. This surprising prediction was confirmed by Craik (1970; see also Craik et al., 1970). The idea of separate STM and LTM storage thus nicely explains the experimental findings of Figure 9.1A and B.

■ **The SAM Model: The Role of Item Autoassociation, Heteroassociation, and Linkage to Context.** What makes it so favorable to study human memory is that it is possible to make subtle variations in the content of list items and to study, in detail, how this affects recall. This has made it possible to learn about the kind of information that is stored in LTM. The search of associative memory (SAM) model, a detailed mathematical implementation of the classic buffer model (e.g., Raaijmakers and Shiffrin, 1981; Kahana, 1996) provides an account of these findings. In principle, learning could involve nonassociative modifications (Figure 9.2A); cells representing a given memory might become more excitable or all their synapses onto all targets might become stronger. This kind of nonassociative process could potentially be used by the brain to determine whether an item was recently presented. Alternatively, associative synaptic modification might strengthen the connection between the cells that encode a given item (Figure 9.2C). This "Hebbian" process is the basis of most attractor network models of associative memory and is termed *autoassociation*. Autoassociation could also occur between cells representing a list item and the current "context." The term *context* has various definitions, but can best be thought of as a complex combination of the general conditions under which the list was learned, including place

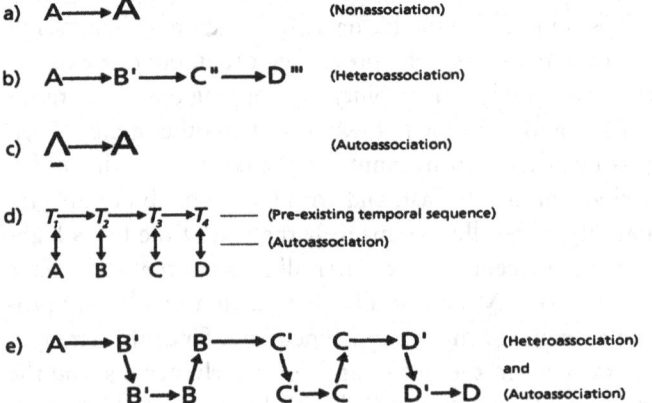

Figure 9.2. Types of nonassociative or associative modifications that could be involved in list learning.

and time. There is general agreement that item-context associations must be important in providing a way to distinguish which of the many lists learned during an experimental session should be recalled (Howard and Kahana, 1999). Furthermore, if context changes in an ordered way from moment to moment, association of items to context could become a basis of storing the order of list items by using only autoassociative modification (Figure 9.2D). Finally, a second class of associative synaptic modification links different list items across time. This is called *heteroassociation* and is the most direct way of encoding item order information (Figure 9.2B).

Is order information in fact preserved in LTM? The data of free recall, a task in which the subject is not specifically asked to recall list order, show that there is nevertheless a strong tendency to preserve order information. After recalling a given list item, the probability of recalling one of its neighbors is much higher than more distant items (Figure 9.3). This graph, which is called the *conditional response probability curve* (CRP), is asymmetric (higher recall for the next item than the previous one). According to the SAM model, this order information is stored in LTM by asymmetric *heteroassociative* interitem weights (Figure 9.2B). A physiologic model of how interitem heteroassociation might occur is presented later. However, as we will see in the next section, the idea that heteroassociations

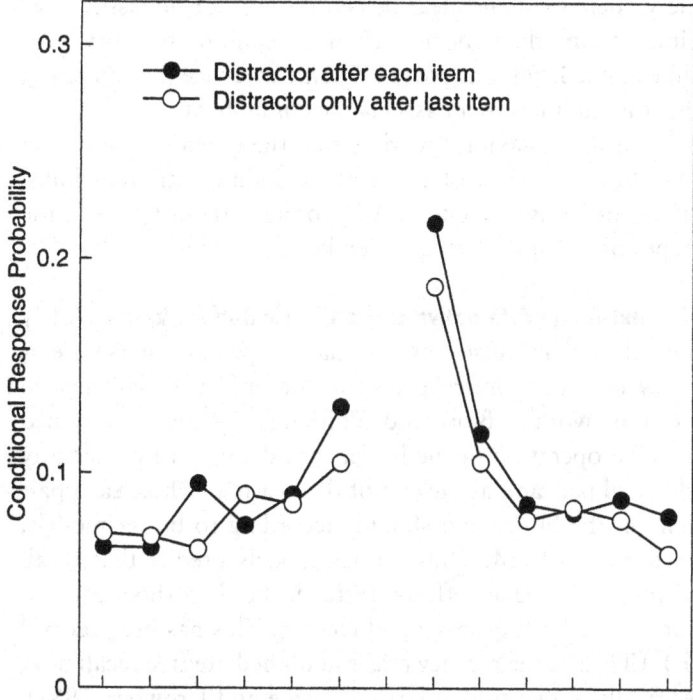

Figure 9.3. The conditional response probability curve (CRP) is not strongly affected by a procedure thought to disrupt the buffer (a distractor is given after each item and at the end of the list). The curve is similar to that measured when a distractor is given only at the end (delayed condition). (Data from Howard and Kahana, 1999.)

actually occur is controversial and altogether different models using autoassociations of items to an ordered context sequence can also explain how order is stored (Figure 9.2D).

To provide a coherent framework for explaining recall, recognition, and priming tasks, SAM also posits that item-specific (i.e., not interitem) information is strengthened during list presentation (e.g., Gillund and Shiffrin, 1984). The storage of item-specific information enables SAM, for instance, to explain how subjects can rapidly recognize individual items from a long list after a long delay. If subjects had to do recognition by first re-creating the whole list using interitem links, reaction time would increase linearly with list length at the same increment/item for short and long lists, contrary to what is observed (Burrows and Okada, 1973).

The stored item-specific information could be either nonassociative (e.g., Murdock, 1982, 1997) or associative (e.g., Metcalfe, 1991; Chappel and Humphreys, 1994), or both (e.g., Mandler et al., 1981). Clear evidence for associative changes comes from experiments on fragment or stem completion. In these tests, it is found that prior exposure to an item enhances the ability to recall the item from a component of the item.

A question of particular relevance to physiologists is whether memories could be stored, at least in part, by nonassociative cellular or synaptic modifications. For example, mossy fiber synapses onto hippocampal CA3 cells can undergo nonassociative LTP. Unfortunately, there exists no clear behavioral test for nonassociative learning. Recent experimental and theoretical work on recognition memory (e.g., Yonelinas, 1997; McElree et al., 1999) has provided some evidence that there is a nonassociative component in addition to an associative component.

The general conclusion of the behavioral work is that the type of information stored in LTM involves different types of linkages, including intraitem links, interitem links, and linkage of items to context. A hypothesis about where in the brain these particular types of linkages occur is given later.

■ **Retrieved Temporal Context As an Alternative to the Classic Buffer Models.** A key assumption of buffer models is that recency and primacy depend on which items are in the buffer and how long they are rehearsed in the buffer. A challenge to buffer models comes from the work of Bjork and Whitten (1974), who examined free recall of item pairs. The operation of the buffer was disrupted by a lengthy distractor between each word pair and at the end of the last pair. Thus, each pair spent the same brief time in the buffer and should, according to buffer models, have been equally transferred to LTM. Thus, buffer models predict that recall should show neither primacy or recency effects. Instead, the data show a traditional serial position curve with both primacy and recency. This has been termed *long-term recency* (LTR). LTR and the recency effect in immediate free recall have similar properties. Specifically, semantic similarity (Greene and Crowder, 1984), incidental instructions (Glenberg et al., 1980), and list length (Greene, 1986) all have a significant effect on the retrieval of pre-recency items and little or no impact on recency items.

A second assumed property of multi-item buffers is that interitem heteroassociations will form between two items only while they are both active in the buffer. If this is the case, preventing multiple items from being active by disrupting the buffer after each item presentation should prevent multiple items from being in the buffer at the same time. Thus, interitem heteroassociations should not be formed. Figure 9.3 shows, however, that the CRP function is unaltered by such disruption.

One possible explanation for LTR is simply that efforts to disrupt the buffer may not have been successful. Subjects may somehow accommodate to the distractor and rehearse list items while performing the distractor. This view was put forward by Koppenaal and Glanzer (1990), who found that switching distractors at the very end of the list disrupted LTR; this was subsequently challenged by Thapar and Greene (1993), who found significant LTR even when subjects were given different kinds of distractor tasks after every list item. In addition, a robust LTR effect is found even when the distractor task is extremely taxing, making it unlikely that subjects are surreptitiously rehearsing items during the distractor interval (Watkins et al., 1989). Nevertheless, there remains some uncertainty about the implications of LTR because there is no independent way of verifying that buffer disruption has been achieved.

If there was no buffer, what could account for recency? An alternative to buffer models has been put forward by Howard and Kahana (1999). They propose that as each item is presented, there is an immediate (within <500 msec) transfer to LTM by autoassociation of the item with context (this is physiologically plausible given how fast LTP can be induced, as shown in Figure 9.11). When the next item arrives, the activity of the previous item ceases (i.e., there is thus no multi-item buffer). Kahana and Howard assume that context is a slowly changing pattern of activity and is thus an ordered sequence. Therefore, item information will be stored in an ordered way if each item is autoassociated to a given moment in the context sequence (see also Levy et al., 1995). At the time of testing, the subject uses the current context to retrieve items. The current context is most similar to that of the context associated with the last few list items, and it is this similarity that produces the recency effect. Once an item is recalled, the context that was associated with it cues the recall of the most similar context, which will be that of a nearby time. This, in turn, aids the recall of the item with which that context is associated. Because order information is based on associations to context, it can occur in the absence of direct interitem heteroassociation. This explains why buffer disruption after each item presentation has little effect on the CRP curve (Figure 9.3). Our model does handle asymmetry effects in a much more elegant way than the buffer model. Primacy effects can be explained by either model.

In summary, the behavioral evidence about human memory has revealed some striking findings and has led to interesting models of the underlying processes. However, the concept of a buffer remains controversial as does the concept of serial search of STM, a concept that will be described later. It is perhaps not surprising that multiple explanations should emerge for the same behavioral data given the limited questions one can ask by purely behavioral means and the limitless imagination of modelers. In the next sections we turn to insights into these questions provided by physiologic methods.

Physiologic Evidence for a Multi-item STM Buffer

■ **The Load Dependence of Signals Provides Evidence for a Multi-Item STM Buffer.** If multiple items are actively maintained in an STM buffer, the overall level of activity would be expected to vary with the number of items being held. Thus, the existence of a multi-item buffer is supported by a number of positron emission tomography (PET) and fMRI studies of STM in which activity in certain brain regions is shown to increase with memory load. In these studies variants of the Sternberg task (Manoach et al., 1997; Rypma and D'Esposito, 1999; Rypma et al., 1999) and the n-back task (Paulesu et al., 1993; Braver et al., 1997; Cohen et al., 1997a, 1997b; Smith and Jonides, 1998) have been applied. Activity in prefrontal, temporal, and parietal cortex increases with load of STM. Thus the collaboration of multiple brain areas appears to form the basis of STM. An fMRI study by Cohen et al. (1997b) nicely demonstrates load dependence (Figure 9.4). A variant of the n-back task was used, where a list of numbers is presented visually, one item every 10 seconds. The subject must indicate if the last presented item matches the digit n items back. The larger the value of n, the larger the

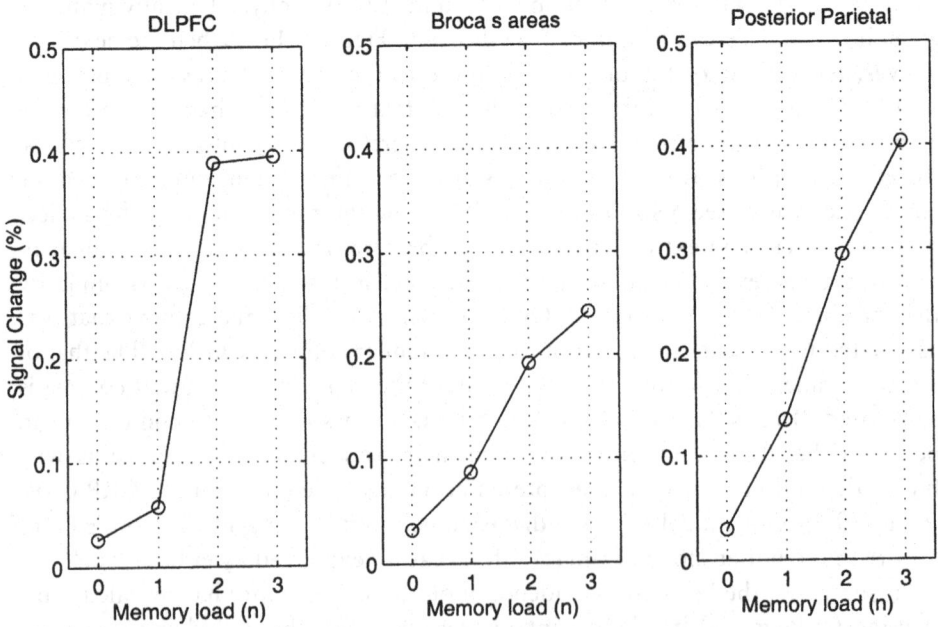

Figure 9.4. Load dependence—the averaged fMRI signal between item presentations in the n-back task for dorsolateral prefrontal cortex (DLPFC), Broca's areas, and posterior parietal cortex. In all regions the signal increases systematically with memory load ($n = 1, 2, 3,$ and 4). An element is presented every 10 seconds, thus allowing four scans. (Adapted from Cohen et al., 1997b.)

memory load. Figure 9.4 shows the averaged activity as a function of time during the retention interval for Broca's area, dorsolateral prefrontal, and parietal cortex. The increase in activity with load is present during the full retention interval (scan 2, 3, and 4). Hence the elevated activity cannot be explained by recall or encoding mechanisms that usually are over within a second after item presentation. One could argue that the increased signal simply reflects higher demands on attention. This question was addressed in a study where both task difficulty and memory load were manipulated. It was established that the activity of the dorsolateral prefrontal cortex correlated with memory load rather than attention (Barch et al., 1997). The activity in other regions, such as the anterior cingulate, seemed to be controlled by attention. These results favor the hypothesis that items in STM are maintained by activity and that activity depends on the number of items stored. Additional evidence for load-dependent signals come from EEG measurements (Mecklinger et al., 1992; Mecklinger and Pfeifer, 1996; Gevins et al., 1997).

■ **STM and LTM Formation Are Differentially Affected by Temporal Lobe Damage and by Cholinergic Antagonists.** Further support for the distinction between STM and LTM derives from pharmacologic and neuropsychological work. If STM and LTM are physiologically different processes, it should be possible to find drugs or lesions that differentially affect the two processes. In terms of the Atkinson and Schiffrin model, this would mean that one should be able to differentially affect the recency part of the curve, which reflects the STM buffer, and the other parts of the curve, collectively termed the *pre-recency region*, which reflect LTM. Furthermore, agents that selectively affect the pre-recency part of the curve should not affect digit span, which is a pure measure of STM. In the following paragraphs we review evidence that supports these predictions.

As illustrated in Figure 9.5A damage to the hippocampal region selectively affects the pre-recency part of the curve (Drachman and Arbit, 1966; Baddeley and Warrington, 1970; Cave and Squire, 1992). This is consistent with the idea that the hippocampal region is required for LTM storage, but not STM. A similar picture emerges from the study of Alzheimer's patients (Burkart et al., 1998; Linn et al., 1995). Particularly relevant to the issue of the mechanism of LTM is the finding that the NMDA antagonist ketamine interferes with free recall (Ghoneim et al., 1985; Krystal et al., 1994; Malhotra et al., 1996; Rockstroh et al., 1996; Newcomer et al., 1999). These findings are of interest because the only associative form of LTP known is dependent on NMDA channel function. Unfortunately, the published behavioral work does not show whether the pre-recency items were selectively affected, so it is difficult to determine the relative contributions of LTM and STM to the memory deficits. Data are available showing that a cholinergic antagonist, scopolamine (Drachman, 1978; Frith et al., 1984), affects pre-recency more strongly than recency (Figure 9.5B) and has only minor effects on digit span (Ostfeld and Aruguete, 1962; Drachman, 1978). Importantly, the effect of scopolamine is counteracted by a cholinesterase inhibitor (Drachman, 1978), indicating a specificity of action of cholinergic

A

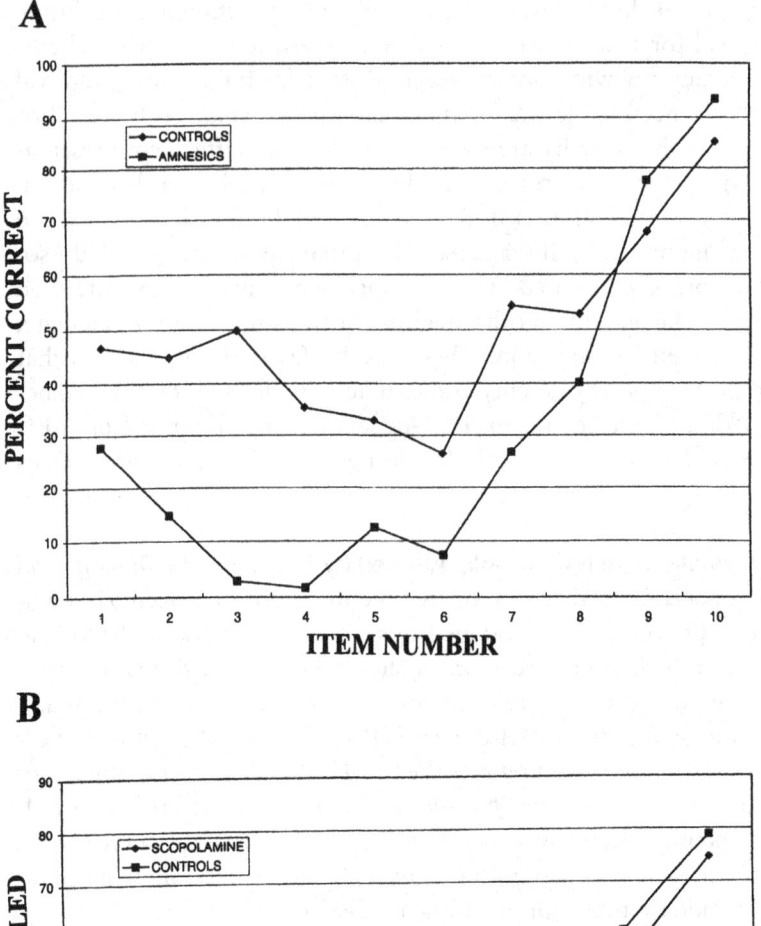

B

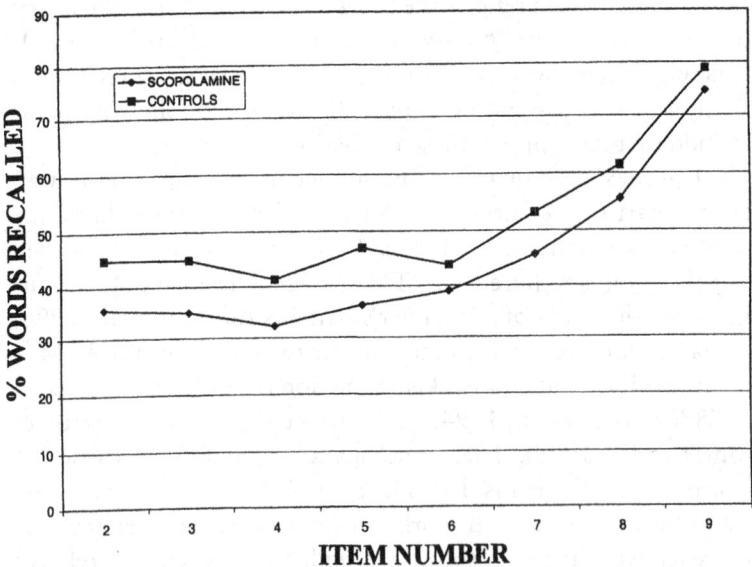

Figure 9.5. Pre-recency parts of the serial position curve are selectively reduced by (**A**) damage to the hippocampal region (data replotted from Baddeley and Warrington, 1970); (**B**) the cholinergic antagonist scopolamine (data replotted from Crow and Grove-White, 1973).

receptors. The vulnerability of LTM formation to cholinergic antagonists is consistent with the finding that cholinergic modulation greatly enhances LTP in the hippocampal slice (see later).

An opposite type of dissociation between STM and LTM comes from the observations of Shallice and Warrington (1970) and Vallar and Shallice (1990). They described a patient with very low digit span (2 to 3). The surprising finding is that these patients have fairly normal LTM.

In summary, the neuropsychological literature and the pharmacologic literature provide support for the idea that there are separate locations and mechanisms involved in STM and LTM. Furthermore, the existence of load-dependent signals suggests that the STM buffer can store more than one item.

A Physiologic Model of a Multi-item STM Buffer: A Role of Theta and Gamma Oscillations

By what mechanism could a buffer keep multiple items active at the same time? The Atkinson-Shiffrin model used the computer metaphor of separate "registers," as if multiple brain networks existed, one for each item. An alternative idea is that multiple items are held in the *same* network, which uses a multiplexing scheme to serially cycle through different items. The results of the Sternberg memory task suggest that a serial process may indeed be involved. We will first review the main findings of the Sternberg task and then describe how the Lisman/Idiart/Jensen (LIJ) model accounts for these data in physiologic terms.

■ **The Sternberg Probe-Recognition Task.** In the Sternberg task (Sternberg, 1966), a short list of items is presented (list lengths are generally varied between two and seven elements) and then a single probe item is presented. A probe is termed *positive* if it was on the list or *negative* if it was not. Subjects are asked to indicate as quickly and accurately as possible whether the probe was positive or negative. Because the list is subspan, there are very few errors (typically less than 5 percent). The variable of interest is the reaction time (RT).

The key finding in the Sternberg test is that the mean RT increases linearly with list length (Figure 9.6A). The slopes of the RT-list length functions for positive and negative probes are both approximately 40 msec item. Sternberg (1966) proposed a serial exhaustive scanning (SES) model to account for these data. According to this model, list items are held in some type of buffer. When the probe item appears, it is compared with each list item in a serial fashion (i.e., a new comparison does not begin until the previous comparison has been completed). As a result of the serial comparison process, mean RT increases linearly with list length. To explain the equivalent slopes for positive and negative probes, Sternberg proposed that a response is not made until all comparisons have been completed (if a response could be made as soon as a match were found, one would expect that the slope for positive probes would be half of the slope for negative probes, which is not the case). This is what is meant by "exhaustive" search.

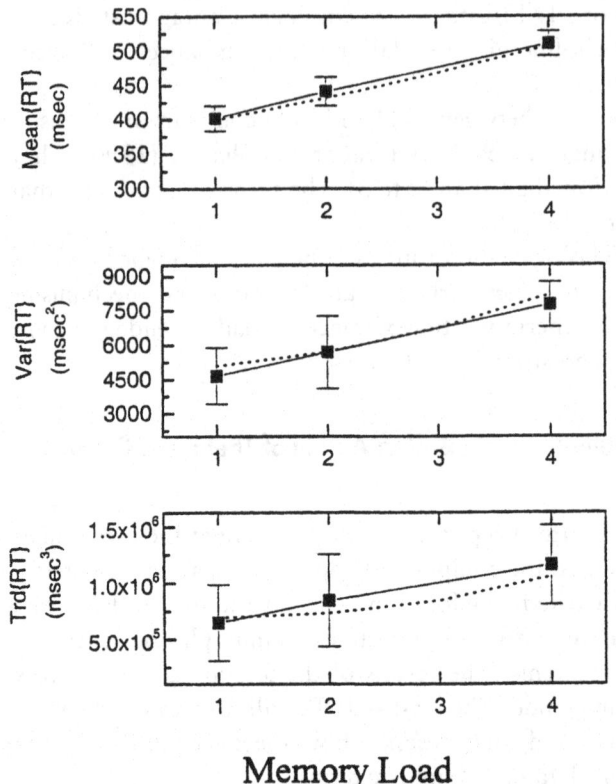

Memory Load

Figure 9.6. Data from the Sternberg item recognition task (**solid**) and the fit of these data by the LIJ theory (**dashed**). The mean reaction time (RT) increases with memory load (slope = 37 msec/item). The variance and third moment also increase with memory load (S) (10 subjects; data courtesy of S. Sternberg). The fit is using the "Reset" model of Jensen and Lisman (1998). The derived period of a gamma cycle is 20 to 25 msec (40–46 Hz).

■ **The Lisman/Idiart/Jensen Model of an Oscillating Multi-Item Buffer.** The LIJ model addresses the question of the physiologic mechanisms that might underlie a multiplexing multi-item buffer (Lisman and Idiart, 1995; Jensen et al., 1996; Jensen and Lisman, 1996a). A central assumption is that a memory item is represented by the synchronous firing of a subset of cells that encode the item. Different items are represented by different subsets that fire at different times.

But what is the time separation of different memories? In a different context (perceptual grouping) it has been suggested that the gamma-frequency field oscillations observed in the brain reflect the synchronous firing of many neurons and that gamma itself can be subdivided into different phases; one group of cells representing one item would fire at one phase of a gamma cycle while another group representing a different item would fire at a different phase of the same gamma cycle. The LIJ uses the value of the slope in the Sternberg task to argue for a very different view. The interitem temporal separation suggested by the slope is ~40 msec. This is about equal to the period of gamma cycle. It is therefore posited in the LIJ model that different memories fire in *different* gamma cycles. Gamma-frequency oscillations often occur together with a slower oscillation (4 to 10 Hz) termed *theta* (Bragin et al., 1995). Since the number of gamma cycles that can fit within a theta cycle is around 7, this could be the related to the span of STM, which is also ~7; thus the buffer would operate on the principle that the entire group of memories held in STM, each in a different gamma cycle, would repeat each theta cycle, as shown in Figure 9.7.

One way of testing the idea that oscillations underlie STM is to see if oscillatory models can account for the detailed results on the Sternberg task, specifically the full distribution of RTs and the way these distributions depend on load. These distributions show some very long RTs that could not be accounted for by scanning through a single theta cycle. Therefore, to fit the distributions it was proposed (Jensen and Lisman, 1998) that with some probability, scanning of a second or

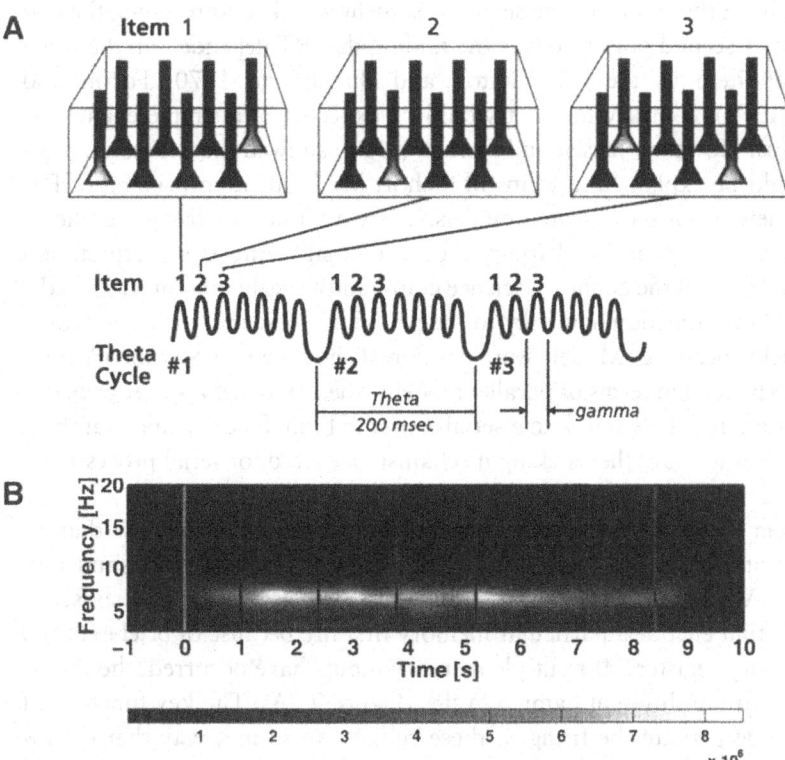

Figure 9.7. The role of theta and gamma in STM. **(A)** Scheme showing a neural code in which different memory items are active in different gamma subcycles of a theta cycle. Memories repeat each theta cycle. **(B)** Evidence for theta oscillations during the Sternberg task, as measured by subdural electrodes. The time-frequency energy averaged over multiple trials of the Sternberg task for four items shows enhanced activity in the theta band time locked to the onset of the list and the arrival of the probe. An orienting cue is given (green bar), followed by list items (narrow black bar) followed by the probe (thick black bar) and the response (red bar).

third theta cycle could occur. An additional question that arises in trying to develop a model is whether the theta frequency is reset by presentation of the probe or simply goes on unperturbed. Finally, there is the question of whether theta frequency is constant or varies with memory load (if there are only two memory items, does it make sense to have five empty slots)? Jensen and Lisman (1998) tried to fit the RT distribution with various assumptions and several variants were found that could fit the entire RT distribution. One of those is shown in Figure 9.6. An important conclusion of this work is that the increment in RT/memory item (~40 msec) is not exactly equal to the period of the underlying oscillation, but needs to be corrected. When this correction is done, the temporal separation of memories is estimated to be about 20 to 25 msec, close to the period of gamma oscillations in the 40-Hz range.

There have been several objections to the idea of exhaustive serial search, as proposed by Sternberg. One objection was that exhaustive search seemed unlikely. Oscillatory models provide a plausible explanation for this feature; it need only be assumed that giving the results of the search is somehow linked to reaching the end of a theta cycle. A second objection was the finding that RT depended on the serial position of the item in the list (Clifton and Birenbaum, 1970; Forrin and Cunningham, 1973), contrary to what would be expected of a simple exhaustive scanning process. However, Jensen and Lisman (1998) showed that the serial position effects could be explained in terms of a short-lived repetition priming of RT, within the framework of serial search models. There are thus no strong arguments against Sternberg's interpretation. Perhaps the reason that Sternberg's interpretation fell into such disfavor in the cognitive science community was because it suggested a serial aspect to brain function, contrary to the prevailing view that the brain works through parallel processing. Models were developed showing that Sternberg's findings could be explained in terms of parallel models. The LIJ model now reopens this debate by positing that there is indeed a serial aspect to brain function and that theta and gamma oscillations are the clocking mechanism required for serial processing.

■ **Is a Multi-Item Buffer Physiologically Feasible?** Simulation studies show that an oscillatory multiplexing buffer can be implemented by known cellular and network processes. We briefly review these studies here. It is assumed that a subset of pyramidal cells that encode a particular memory first fire because of brief external input from sensory registers. If multiple memory inputs have occurred, the different subsets will fire in different gamma cycles (Figure 9.7A). The key function of the buffer is to perpetuate the firing of these cells to do so in a way that retains order. In the LIJ model (Figure 9.8) this occurs because firing affects intrinsic conductances of the cell by (1) resetting the membrane potential to near resting potential and (2) producing a depolarizing ramp termed the *afterdepolarization* (ADP) (Lisman and Idiart, 1995; Jensen et al., 1996). Thus, cells that fire in an order will have ramps that are temporally offset and that will bring the cells to threshold again in the same order as their initial firing. The repeat time is determined by theta oscillations, which are due to an external input. Within a theta cycle, the separate firing of different memories is organized by gamma oscillations, which

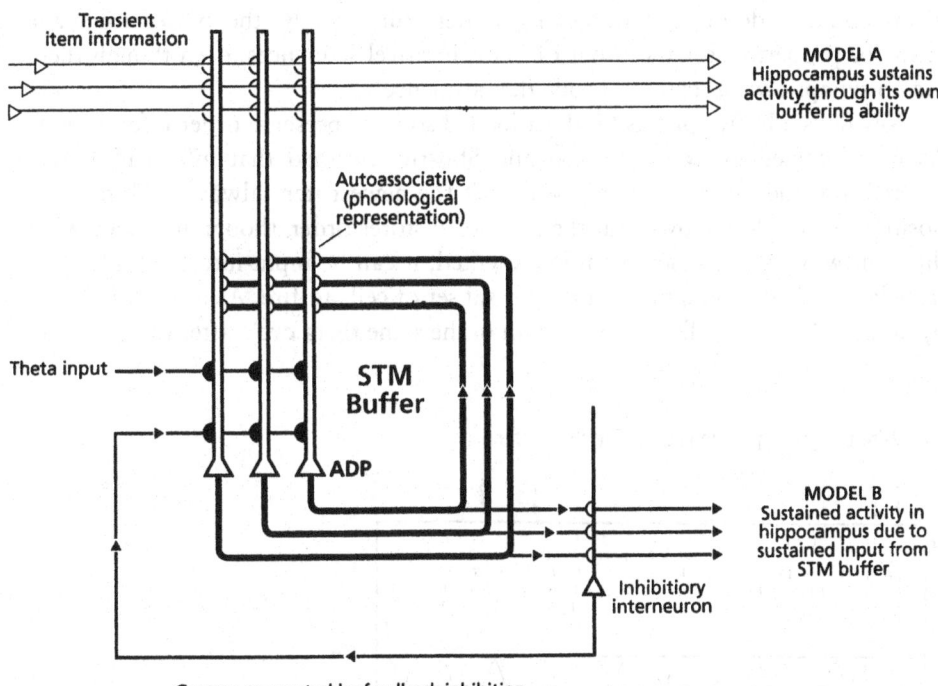

Transient
item information

MODEL A
Hippocampus sustains
activity through its own
buffering ability

Autoassociative
(phonological
representation)

Theta input

STM
Buffer

ADP

MODEL B
Sustained activity in
hippocampus due to
sustained input from
STM buffer

Inhibitiory
interneuron

Gamma generated by feedback inhibition

Figure 9.8. Properties of a network that functions as a multi-item STM buffer. An afterdepolarization (ADP) is triggered after a cell fires and creates a depolarizing ramp that serves to trigger the same cell to fire again after a delay. These ramps are temporally offset for different memories, an offset that causes the different memories to fire in different gamma cycles. For references regarding the biological basis of the ADP, see Lisman and Idiart (1995). According to Model B, the multi-item STM buffer produces the repetitive firing that drives the formation of LTM in the hippocampus. According to model B, the sustained activity required for LTM formation is due to buffering ability of the hippocampal network itself.

arises from global feedback inhibition. Thus, after one memory is active, it rapidly inhibits all others; as this inhibition wears off, the cell group with the most depolarized ramp will fire, thus reactivating the next memory in the sequence. This triggers another cycle of inhibition. This alternating excitation and inhibition creates gamma oscillations. Jenson et al. (1996) showed that these mechanisms alone were sufficient to generate a buffer, but that the buffer will gradually fail as cells encoding each item become desynchronized. Jensen and Lisman (1996a) showed, however, that this desynchronization could be avoided if the recurrent synapses store autoassociative information about items. The use of autoassociative information is reasonable since in many learning situations and almost all list learning experiments, the items are familiar (e.g., digits). As shown in Figure 9.9 (top), a buffer containing autoassociative LTM about digits can retain the novel sequence of digits presented to the network. Order is preserved despite noise; cells that fire in the wrong gamma cycle will subsequently fire in the correct gamma cycle because of the cooperative properties of the autoassociative network. The conclusion of this line of theoretical work is that known cellular and network mechanisms could underlie a multiplexing buffer. Surprisingly, the buffer can have attractor properties for the order of items in novel sequences, even though there are no synaptic weights that encode that sequence.

How does a buffer of this kind get loaded so as to preserve order information? As we discussed before, Atkinson and Shiffrin assumed that information was entered into the buffer in such a way that the newest item always took the first position. Figure 9.9 shows that the LIJ model stores order, though in a somewhat different way. When a new item is presented, it can be input into the buffer at a trough of a theta oscillation, causing a subset of cells to fire. As a result of ramp dynamics, the same cells then fire again in the same theta cycle after the end of all

A   7-item digit sequence is stored in the buffer

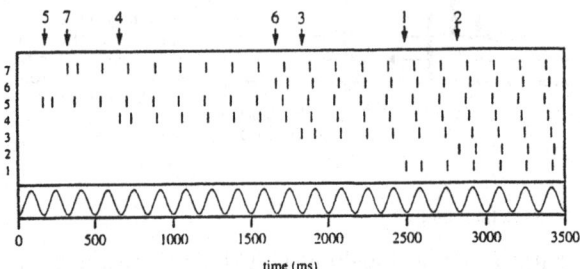

The synaptic weight matrix shows the information transferred to LTM

Recall of the sequence from LTM evoked by a two item cue

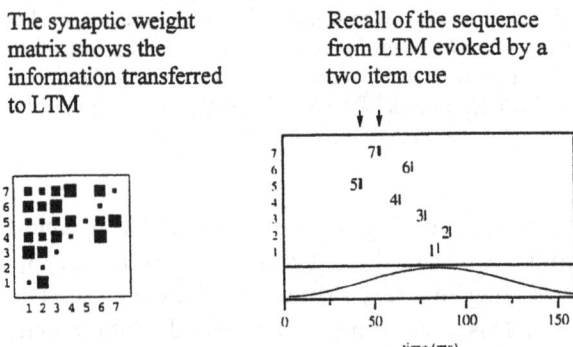

Figure 9.9. Simulation of the storage of seven digits in STM, the storage of the sequence in LTM, and the recall of the sequence from LTM. (Top) Digits are presented over a 3-second period, causing a particular cell to fire near the trough of the theta cycle in the STM network. This cell then fires in every subsequent theta cycle with a fixed phase. The phase preserves the order of item presentation (e.g., during last theta cycle at far right). (Bottom left) Synaptic weight matrix shows heteroassociative memory formed by activity in an LTM network driven by output from an STM network. It is assumed that LTM forms by an NMDA-mediated LTP-type process and that the strength of LTM formed between an item that fires (x-axis) and an item that fires in another gamma cycle (y-axis) is proportional to the magnitude of the remaining NMDA conductance in the second cell (the conductance decays with tau = 50 msec). (Bottom right) The ability of the network to recall is illustrated by presenting the network with the first two digits in the sequence; the network then recalls the remaining digits during the remainder of the theta cycle.

previously incorporated items. This order-preserving pattern then repeats on each subsequent theta cycle. This illustrates that there are simple ways of loading the buffer in a way that preserves order.

■ **Evidence for Buffering in the LTM Store.** One of the key reason for postulating the existence of a buffer is that activity will outlive the sensory stimulus, a persistence that can be important for the formation of LTM. Recordings from the hippocampus during presentation of sensory stimuli provide evidence that activity in the hippocampus can persist for many seconds and long outlive the stimulus itself (Berger et al., 1983; Givens, 1996; Colombo and Gross, 1994; Hampson et al., 1993; Vinogradova, 1984). This either means that the hippocampus is being driven by a buffer or that the hippocampus itself has buffer properties. Since STM can occur after removal of the hippocampal region, the STM buffer must be elsewhere, and it is tempting to suppose that the hippocampus is driven by the STM buffer. However, as mentioned previously, there are patients that have very weak STM but fairly normal LTM, raising the possibility that the hippocampus may itself be a buffer (Figure 9.8).

■ **Evidence for Theta/Gamma Coding.** The idea that information about different items is contained in different gamma cycles of a theta cycle is a fundamentally new idea about neural coding (Jensen and Lisman, submitted). The idea has not yet been tested in the context of STM function. The strongest evidence that the timing of firing in a theta cycle carries information comes from work on place cells in the hippocampus (O'Keefe and Recce, 1993). This work shows that when the animal enters a place field, the cell fires with late phase (thus presumably in a late gamma cycle); as the animal progresses through the place field, cells fire with progressively earlier phase (thus presumably in earlier gamma cycles). This process is thought to be the readout of known place sequences from LTM and so is not directly relevant to STM (Jensen and Lisman, 1996b; Lisman, 1999). However, it seems reasonable to suppose that the brain uses a similar timing structure based on oscillations both to deal with the storage of multiple items in STM and to read out multiple items from LTM.

■ **Evidence for Theta in the Human Temporal Lobe.** For many years there have been reports that theta oscillations, although easily seen in rats and cats, were not easily detected in primates, including humans. For this reason there was serious concern that extrapolation from lower animals to humans was inappropriate. However, in the last few years, several groups have obtained evidence for theta-band activity in humans. An EEG method called *event-related synchronization* (ERS) provides evidence of the enhanced synchronization in the theta band during encoding of new memories (Klimesch et al., 1996, 1997; Burgess and Guzelier, 1997). Gevins used EEG localization methods to detect theta-bound actions coming from the cingulate cortex, while Tesche (Tesche and Karhu, 1999) used MEG localization to identify a theta source near the hippocampus. These results, however, did not reveal the large amplitude theta that can be seen in single traces in the rat. Recently, very clear evidence for large amplitude theta has been obtained from humans using subdural electrode arrays that recorded the local brain surface activity from the temporal lobes of epileptic patients. Recordings during a maze navigation task reveal dramatic theta oscillations in single traces and the power spectrum of such traces has a peak in the 4 to 8 Hz range (Kahana et al., 1999). In this report, theta oscillations were not always present, but appeared episodically in a manner that was task dependent. Very recently, it has been found that during the Sternberg task (Figure 9.7B) the onset and offset of theta is tightly linked to the beginning and end of each of trial (Lisman et al., submitted). These results strongly support the idea that theta oscillations play an important role in organizing STM.

Transfer of Information From an Oscillatory STM Buffer to a Hippocampal LTM Store by NMDA-Mediated LTP

■ **At Which Hippocampal Synapses Are Contextual Association, Autoassociation, and Heteroassociation Stored?** Identification of the synapses in the brain where particular information is stored is a major goal of neuroscience. It is generally agreed that episodic memory is stored in the hippocampus, at least during initial phases of LTM. So much is known about the architecture and function of the hippocampus that it is possible to make an educated guess about the function of different subregions and the type of information stored at different synaptic connections. As shown in Figure 9.10, the hippocampal region is composed of three networks, the dentate, CA1, and CA3 region (the subiculum is not considered here). A model

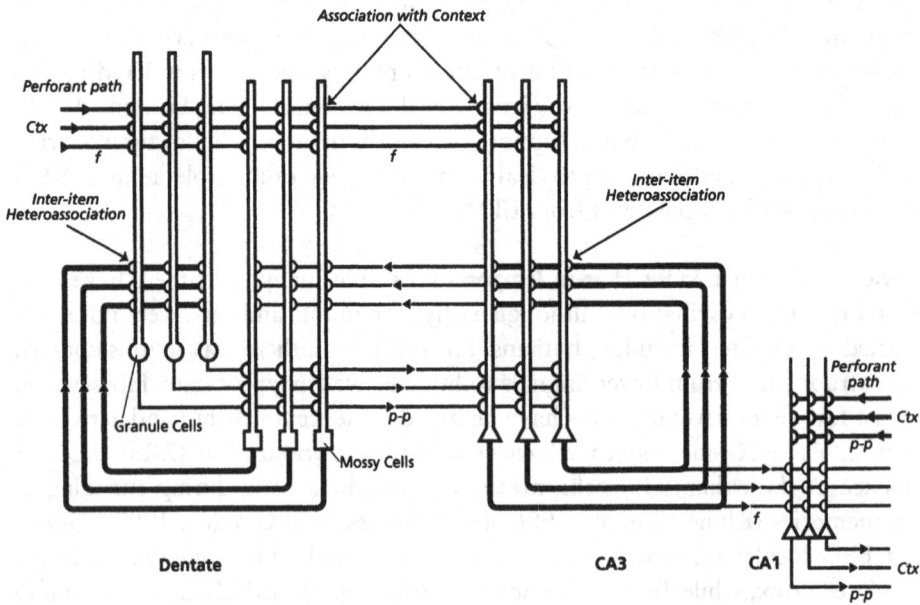

Figure 9.10. The hippocampal network and possible storage sites of different kinds of LTM associations during list learning.

developed by one of us (Lisman, 1999) proposes how the dentate and CA3 regions work together to store and recall episodic memory sequences in context. List learning is an excellent example of sequence learning.

The starting point of the model is an explanation of the function of the two bidirectionally connected recurrent networks, the dentate and CA3. The model builds on previous work on abstract neural networks (Kleinfeld, 1986; Sompolinsky and Kanter, 1986), showing how optimal recall of memory sequences requires the interaction of heteroassociative and autoassociative information. In the absence of autoassociative information, sequence recall by a heteroassociative network becomes problematic (Figure 9.2B) because of the concatenation of errors [the cells representing memory A stimulate the cells representing memory B but with errors resulting in memory B′ (the number of primes is used to designate the degree of error)]. If memory B′ is used to excite the cell that encode memory C, the resulting prediction is even worse, C′. However, a well established capability of autoassociative networks is to correct a degraded memory; thus B′ can be corrected to B. Thus, a sequence can be accurately recalled through the reciprocal interaction of an autoassociative and heteroassociative network, as illustrated in Figure 9.2E. In the model of Figure 9.10, the autoassociative information is stored in the recurrent connections of the dentate while the heteroassociative interitem links are in the recurrent collaterals of CA3. It is proposed that the lists can be accurately recalled through the reciprocal interaction of the CA3 and dentate.

The model also proposes to explain how contextual information is handled. Context refers to aspects of the environment that are more stable than the sudden burst of information that constitutes a memory item. A key observation regarding the encoding of context in the rat hippocampus is that there are no cells that continuously fire when the animal is a certain context (in this case, the particular experimental chamber in which the animal is tested). Rather, context exerts its influence by enabling a particular subset of place cells to be fired by more specific information (i.e., when the rat enters a place field). According to the model, contextual input arrives at CA3 (and probably also at hilar mossy cells) through the perforant path from the entorhinal cortex. This input is on the most distal dendrites and is therefore inefficient at firing the neuron. However, it may bring the membrane potential near enough to threshold so that the cell can be fired by a single giant synaptic input from a dentate granule cell. Without this depolarizing bias, the dentate input generates a large excitatory postsynaptic potential (EPSP), which is nevertheless too small to fire the cell. The specific CA3 cells that fire are thus determined not only by item information, carried by granule cells, but also by contextual information that arrives through the perforant path. In this way, item information is encoded in context. Redundant context information need not be continuously recorded in detail and may be filtered out by depressing synapses at the perforant path synapses onto granule cells. Based on these considerations, one can tentatively argue that the presentation of items strengthens item autoassociations in the dentate recurrent network, that interitem heteroassociations are formed in the CA3 recurrent synapses, and that contextual–item autoassociations are formed in the perforant path connections to CA3 and hilar mossy cells (Figure 9.10).

Simulations of this bidirectional interaction would clearly be desirable, but have not yet been undertaken. In the next section we describe simulations of the much simpler case where a heteroassociative network is unidirectionally driven by an autoassociative buffer network during learning. This is sufficient to reveal some interesting properties of the network and how they depend on the properties of LTP.

■ **The Theta/Gamma Buffer Allows NMDA-Mediated LTP to Form Interitem Linkage Between Events with Large Temporal Separation.** We now turn to the question of how the information actively maintained by a theta/gamma buffer could encode information in an LTM network by NMDA-mediated LTP. What we demonstrate in Figure 9.9 is that the buffer allows interitem association to be formed, even if items are presented many seconds apart. To explain this point, it is first necessary to define the time window of LTP. Although it is commonly stated that for LTP to occur there must be simultaneous firing of the postsynaptic and presynaptic cells (as postulated by Hebb), this is not exactly true. It has been shown that after the presynaptic cell fires, there is a time window of about 100 msec during which LTP will be induced if the postsynaptic cell fires (Markram et al., 1997). For this reason, if cell A is driven by sensory input from one item and cell B is driven by sensory input from a second item presented 100 msec later, the synaptic connection from cell A to cell B will be strengthened. This is an asymmetric change since the connection from B to A will not be strengthened. In the absence of a buffer, this mechanism could not form interitem links between events separated by more than 100 msec. If a theta/gamma buffer is operative, however, events that occurred seconds apart are represented by cells that fire in successive gamma cycles, that is, with a temporal separation of 25 msec (Figures 9.7A and 9.9). This is within the time window of LTP. Thus interitem linkages will form even if items were presented seconds apart. A simulation of this process is shown in Figure 9.9. The demonstration that the network has successively encoded the sequence is demonstrated by presenting the first two items in the list, which then triggers recall of the remainder of the list.

Several further aspects of this simulation are noteworthy. First the strengthening is asymmetric (see the synaptic weight matrix in Figure 9.9, bottom left): the nth item will be linked to the n+1 item, with relatively little linkage in the reverse direction. This may be related to the asymmetric aspect of the CPR curve (Figure 9.3). Second, the strengthening is not just between consecutive items (between the n and n+1 item); a smaller but significant strengthening occurs between the nth item and n+2 item (and even the n+3 item). This occurs because the window of LTP is considerably longer than a single gamma cycle. These more complex linkages mean that when a memory becomes active, it will not just be because of input from the n−1 item (a simple pairwise process) but also because of input from the n−2 and n−3 items. This is called *multiple cueing*. The reader can demonstrate this property of his or her memory by recalling the letter in the alphabet that comes after the single cue, *N*. For most people it is much easier to name the next letter if multiple cues are given, for example, What is the letter that comes after *LMN?* The existence of multiple cueing has been verified by formal psychophysical analysis (Kahana and Caplan, submitted).

If LTP causes heteroassociative synaptic modifications, how then can autoassociative changes occur? In a theta/gamma buffer, this requires that the window of LTP by quite short, specifically less than the duration of a gamma cycle. In a previous article it was argued that the window was determined by the deactivation time of NMDA channels and that autoassociative networks might have NMDA channels with very fast deactivation times (Jensen and Lisman, 1996a). However, recent experimental studies suggest that factors in addition to the deactivation time can also influence the time window (Bi and Poo, 1998).

■ **Enhancement of LTM Formation by Intent; Enhancement of LTP by Cholinergic Modulation.** How long does it take to get information into LTM and how long does it take to induce LTP? If these numbers were similar, it would lend support for the idea that LTP underlies LTM formation. Unfortunately, neither the behavioral literature nor the physiologic literature has anything definitive to say about this. Both fields have had to struggle with the same issue, that of behavioral state.

The psychological literature shows quite clearly that intention to learn can have dramatic effects on memory storage. For example, without intention to learn, the duration of repetition has no effect on the strengthening of interitem associations. Item-specific information, however, is strengthened even under conditions of unintentional encoding. This can be seen in both recognition memory tests and priming tests. Interestingly, these forms of learning are largely spared in subjects with temporal lobe amnesia.

The physiologic literature shows that the amount of LTP induced and the duration of stimulation required to induce it depend strongly on the neuromodulatory state. It now seems clear that the standard slice preparation does not give us correct insight into quantitative questions about how LTP occurs *in vivo* because the neuromodulatory inputs from the basal forebrain and brain stem structures have been cut off. Indeed, the slice preparation most resembles that of slow wave sleep, when all neuromodulatory systems are inactive. These neuromodulatory inputs can affect synaptic plasticity. The most dramatic example of this is the ability of cholinergic modulation to enhance theta oscillations, and the consequent changes in the rules and sensitivity of synaptic plasticity. Winson and Pavlides (Pavlides et al., 1988) were the first to show that the phase of arrival of synaptic inputs during theta determined whether LTP could be induced. This work was extended by Huerta and Lisman (1993), who showed that if stimulation is given at the peak of theta, strengthening occurs; if the same stimulus falls at the trough, then previously potentiated synapses are weakened (Figure 9.11). This work was done *in vitro,* but subsequent work showed similar results *in vivo* (see Chapter 7). The rules that determine the sign of synaptic modification in the presence of neuromodulators may thus be quite different

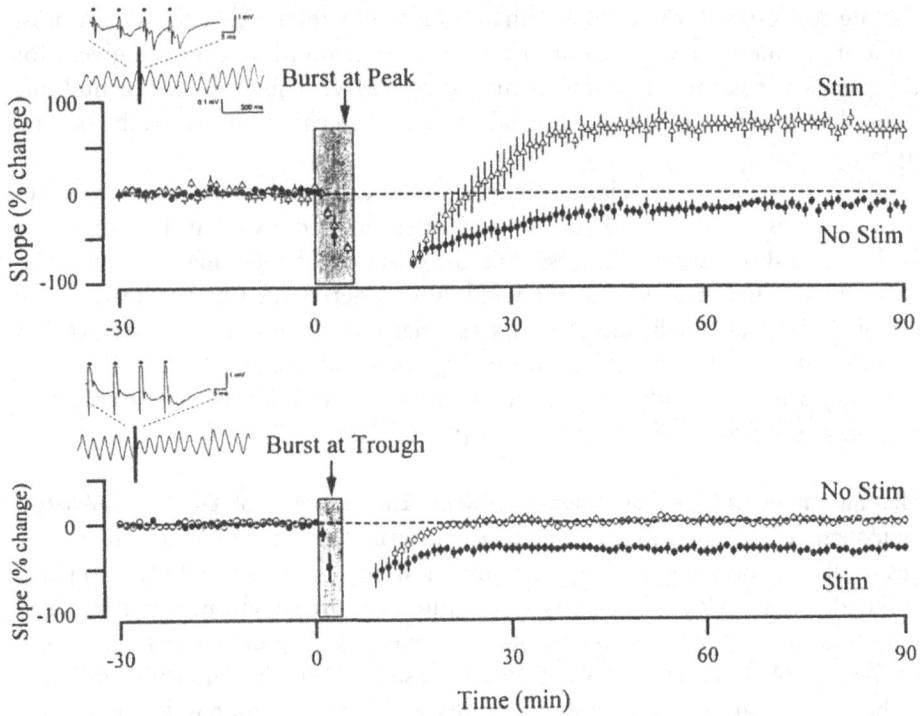

Figure 9.11. Cholinergic modulation induces theta oscillations, enhances synaptic plasticity, and makes the sign of synaptic modification dependent on theta phase. A single brief burst of four action potentials (see inset) evoked LTP if the burst is given at the peak of theta (**top**) or produces depotentiation if the burst is given at the trough (**bottom**). Such bursts produce no plasticity if given without carbachol. Experiments were done on a hippocampal slice with two pathways, one of which was stimulated with a burst (Stim), and one of which was not (No Stim). The gray region is the period during which 50 micromolar carbachol was applied. Application of carbachol induced theta and depressed the field EPSP, the size of which is quantified by the slope of the rise edge.

from those in the absence, where it is the frequency of stimulation that determines the sign of synaptic modification.

In addition to affecting the rules of synaptic modulations, the cholinergic induction of theta oscillations greatly enhances the sensitivity of plasticity. In the presence of carbachol-induced theta, a single burst of only three stimuli at 100 Hz is sufficient to induce LTP. Such bursts induce on LTP at all in the absence of carbachol (typically 100 stimuli at 100 Hz are used to induce LTP). Bursts of this kind can be considered natural stimuli since they are commonly observed *in vivo*. These results provided the strongest evidence to date that cholinergic modulation during *in vivo* theta may provide such a strong enhancement of plasticity that it may be considered a requirement for LTP induction by natural stimuli. This could then explain the strong amnestic effects of cholinergic antagonists and, in particular, the reduction of the pre-recency region of the serial position curve attributable to LTM (Figure 9.5B).

Future Prospects

With recent advances for studying the physiologic basis of learning in humans, the already established behavioral results on human memory take on added importance. These results provide a good starting place for elucidating physiologic mechanisms. We hope we have made clear that there are already interesting proposals that relate mechanisms to behavior and that further efforts in this direction are warranted.

What are the most important questions that need to be answered? Perhaps foremost is to rigorously settle the issue of whether there is a multi-item STM buffer. The proposal for such a buffer emerged from psychological findings and yet remains controversial. We have reviewed the physiologic evidence that favors such a buffer, but the evidence remains indirect. Definitive evidence would be the demonstration of the validity of Figure 9.7A, which shows that cells encoding different items fire persistently, but with different theta phase. It may be possible to obtain such evidence using single unit recording on epileptic patients.

With the clear demonstration of human theta, it will now be possible to learn much more about these oscillations and to test the linkage between theta oscillations and STM. The use of intracranial and MEG methods should elucidate the spatial distribution of theta, its timing during memory tasks, and whether theta amplitude or frequency depends on memory load.

It has not been generally noted that the pharmacological work on humans supports the idea that LTM is modified within seconds, as postulated by the Atkinson-Shiffrin model. Moreover, the available data appear consistent with the properties of LTP. This is an exciting idea that needs to be more rigorously examined. If true, it would mean that simple free-recall experiments provide a behavioral assay of *in vivo* LTP. The prospect for understanding the pharmacologic modulation of this process could then be pursued using a data set that has not been exploited: drug companies give standard memory tests to a very large number of subjects in the course of the drug approval process. Of particular importance would be further tests of the effect of NMDA antagonists.

More generally, we urge a closer link between the physiologic and psychological study of memory. These fields have been too isolated. The time has come to bring them together.

REFERENCES

Atkinson, R.C., and Shiffrin, R.M. (1968). Human memory: A proposed system and its control processes. In K.W. Spence and J.T. Spence (Eds.), *The psychology of learning and motivation* (Vol. 2, pp. 89–105). New York: Academic Press.

Baddeley, A.D. (1996). The concept of working memory. In S.E. Gathercole (Ed.), *Models of short term memory* (pp. 1–22). East Sussex, United Kingdom: Psychology Press.

Baddeley, A.D., and Warrington, E.K. (1970). Amnesia and the distinction between long- and short-term memory. *J. Verbal Learning Verbal Behav.* 9: 176–189.

Barch, D.M., Braver, T.S., Nyström, L.E., Forman, S.D. et al. (1997). Dissociating working memory from task difficulty in human prefrontal cortex. *Neuropsychologia* 35: 1373–1380.

Berger, T.W., Rinaldi, P.C., Weisz, D.J., and Thompson, R.F. (1983). Single-unit analysis of different hippocampal cell types during classical conditioning of rabbit nictitating membrane response. *J. Neurophysiol.* 50: 1197–1219.

Bi, G.Q., and Poo, M.M. (1998). Synaptic modifications in cultured hippocampal neurons: Dependence on spike timing, synaptic strength, and postsynaptic cell type. *J. Neurosci.* 18: 10464–10472.

Bjork, R.A., and Whitten, W.B. (1974). Recency-sensitive retrieval processes in long-term free recall. *Cogn. Psychol.* 6: 173–189.

Bragin, A., Jando, G., Nadasdy, Z., Hetke, J. et al. (1995). Gamma (40-100 Hz) oscillation in the hippocampus of the behaving rat. *J. Neurosci.* 15: 47–60.

Braver, T.S., Cohen, J.D., Nyström, L.E., Jonides, J. et al. (1997). A parametric study of prefrontal cortex involvement in human working memory. *Neuroimage* 5: 49–62.

Burgess, A.P., and Gruzelier, J.H. (1997). Short duration synchronization of human theta rhythm during recognition memory. *Neuroreport* 8: 1039–1042.

Burkart, M., Heun, R., and Benkert, O. (1998). Serial position effects in dementia of the Alzheimer type. *Dement. Geriatr. Cogn. Disord.* 9: 130–136.

Burrows, D., and Okada, R. (1973). Parallel scanning of semantic and formal information. *J. Exp. Psychol.* 97: 254–257.

Cave, C.B., and Squire, L.R. (1992). Intact verbal and nonverbal short-term memory following damage to the human hippocampus. *Hippocampus* 2: 151–163.

Chappell, M., and Humphreys, M. (1994). An auto-associative network for sparse representations: Analysis and application to models of recognition and cued-recall. *Psychol. Rev.* 101: 103–128.

Clifton, C., and Birenbaum, S. (1970). Effects of serial position and delay of probe in memory scan task. *J. Exp. Psychol.* 86: 69–70.

Cohen, J.D., Nyström, L.E., Sabb, F.W., Braver, T.S. et al. (1997a). Tracking the dynamics of fMRI activation in humans under manipulations of duration and intensity of working memory processes. *Soc. Neurosci.* 23: 1678.

Cohen, J.D., Perlstein, W.M., Braver, T.S., Nyström, L.E. et al. (1997b). Temporal dynamics of brain activation during a working memory task. *Nature* 386: 604–608.

Colombo, M., and Gross, C.G. (1994). Responses of inferior temporal cortex and hippocampal neurons during delayed matching to sample in monkeys (Macaca fascicularis). *Behav. Neurosci.* 8: 443–455.

Craik, F.I.M. (1970). The fate of primary memory items in free recall. *J. Verbal Learning Verbal Behav.* 9: 143–148.

Craik, F.I., Gardiner, J.M., and Watkins, M.J. (1970). Further evidence for negative recency effect in free recall. *J. Verbal Learning Verbal Behav.* 9: 554–560.

Crannell, C.W., and Parrish, J.M. (1957). A comparison of immediate memory span for digits, letters, and words. *J. Psychol.* 44: 319–327.

Drachman, D.A. (1978). Central cholinergic system and memory. In M.A. Lipton, A. DiMascio, and K.P. Killam (Eds.), *Psychopharmacology: A generation of progress.* (pp. 651–662). New York: Raven Press.

Drachman, D.A., and Arbit, J. (1966). Memory and the hippocampal complex. II. Is memory a multiple process? *Arch. Neurol.* 15: 52–61.

Forrin, B., and Cunningham, K. (1973). Recognition time and serial position of probed item in short-term memory. *J. Exp. Psychol.* 99: 272–279.

Frith, C.D., Richardson, J.T.E., Samuel, M., Crow, T.J. et al. (1984). The effects of intravenous diazepam and hyoscine upon human memory. *Q. J. Exp. Psychol.* 36A: 133–144.

Gevins, A., Smith, M.E., McEvoy, L., and Yu, D. (1997). High-resolution EEG mapping of cortical activation related to working memory: Effects of task difficulty, type of processing, and practice. *Cereb. Cortex* 7: 374–385.

Ghoneim, M.M., Hinrichs, J.V., Mewaldt, S.P., and Petersen, R.C. (1985). Ketamine: Behavioral effects of subanesthetic doses. *J. Clin. Pharmacol.* 5: 70–77.

Gillund, G., and Shiffrin, R.M. (1984). A retrieval model for both recognition and recall. *Psychol. Rev.* 91: 1–67.

Givens, B. (1996). Stimulus-evoked resetting of the dentate theta rhythm: Relation to working memory. *Neuroreport* 8: 159–163.

Glenberg, A.M., Bradley, M.M., Stevenson, J.A., Kraus, T.A. et al. (1980). A two-process account of long-term serial position effects. *J. Exp. Psychol. Hum. Learn. Mem.* 6: 355–369.

Greene, R.L. (1986). A common basis for recency effects in immediate and delayed recall. *J. Exp. Psychol. Learn. Mem. Cogn.* 12: 413–418.

Greene, R.L., and Crowder, M. (1984). Effects of semantic similarity on long-term recency. *Am. J. Psychol.* 97: 441–449.

Hampson, R.E., Squires, N.K., and Deadwyler, S.A. (1993). Hippocampal cell firing correlates of delayed-match-to-sample performance in rat. *Behav. Neurosci.* 107: 715–739.

Howard, M., and Kahana, M.J. (1999). Contextual variability and serial position effects in free recall. *J. Exp. Psychol. Learn. Mem. Cogn.* 25: 923–941.

Huerta, P.A., and Lisman, J.E. (1993). Heightened synaptic plasticity of hippocampal CA1 neurons during a cholinergically induced rhythmic state. *Nature* 364: 723–725.

Jensen, O., Idiart, M.A.P., and Lisman, J.E. (1996). Physiologically realistic formation of autoassociative memory in networks with theta/gamma oscillations: Role of fast NMDA channels. *Learn. Mem.* 3: 243–256.

Jensen, O., and Lisman, J.E. (1996a). Novel lists of 7±2 known items can be reliably stored in an oscillatory short-term memory network: Interaction with long-term memory. *Learn. Mem.* 3: 257–263.

Jensen, O., and Lisman, J.E. (1996b). Theta/gamma networks with slow NMDA channels learn sequences and encode episodic memory: Role of NMDA channels in recall. *Learn. Mem.* 3: 264–278.

Jensen, O., and Lisman, J.E. (1998). An oscillatory short-term memory buffer model can account for data on the Sternberg task. *J. Neurosci.* 18: 10688–10699.

Kahana, M. (1996). Associative retrieval processes in free recall. *Mem. Cogn.* 24: 103–109.

Kahana, M.J., Sekuler, R., Caplan, J.B., Kirschen, M. et al. (1999). Human theta oscillations exhibit task dependence during virtual maze navigation. *Nature* 399: 781–784.

Kleinfeld, D. (1986). Sequential state generation by model neural networks. *Proc. Natl. Acad. Sci. USA* 83: 9469–9473.

Klimesch, W., Dopplemayr, M., Russegger, H., and Pachinger, T. (1996). Theta band power in the human scalp EEG and the encoding of new information. *Neuroreport* 7: 1235–1240.

Klimesch, W., Doppelmayr, M., Schimke, H., and Ripper, B. (1997). Theta synchronization and alpha desynchronization in a memory task. *Psychophysiology* 34: 169–176.

Koppenaal, L., and Glanzer, M. (1990). An examination of the continuous distractor task and the long-term recency effect. *Mem. Cogn.* 18: 183–195.

Krystal, J.H., Karper, L.P., Seibyl, J.P., Freeman, G.K. et al. (1994). Subanesthetic effects of the noncompetitive NMDA antagonist, ketamine, in humans. Psychotomimetic, perceptual, cognitive, and neuroendocrine responses. *Arch. Gen. Psychiatry* 51: 199–214.

Levy, W.B., Wu, X., and Baxter, R.A. (1995). Unification of hippocampal function via computational/encoding considerations. In D.J. Amit, P. del Guidice, B. Denby, E.T. Rolls et al. (Eds.), *Proceedings of the third workshop on neural networks: From biology to high energy physics. Int. J. Neural Syst.* (Suppl.) 6: 71–80. Singapore: Scientific Publishing.

Linn, R.T., Wolf, P.A., Bachman, D.L., Knoefel, J.E. et al. (1995). The 'preclinical phase' of probable Alzheimer's disease. A 13-year prospective study of the Framingham cohort. *Arch. Neurol.* 52: 485–490.

Lisman, J.E. (1999). Relating hippocampal circuitry to function: Recall of memory sequences by reciprocal dentate-CA3 interactions. *Neuron* 22: 233–242.

Lisman, J.E., and Idiart, M.A.P. (1995). Storage of 7±2 short term memories in oscillatory subcycles. *Science* 267: 1512–1515.

Malhotra, A.K., Pinais, D.A., Weingartner, H., Sirocco, K. et al. (1996). NMDA receptor function and human cognition: The effects of ketamine in healthy volunteers. *Neuropsychopharmacology* 14: 301–307.

Mandler, G., Rabinowitz, J.C., and Simon, R.A. (1981). Coordinate organization: The holistic representation of word pairs. *Am. J. Psychol.* 92: 209–222.

Manoach, D.S., Schlaug, G., Siewart, B., Darby, D.G. et al. (1997). Prefrontal cortex fMRI signal changes are correlated with working memory load. *Neuroreport* 8: 545–549.

Markram, H., Lubke, J., Frotscher, M., and Sakmann, B. (1997). Regulation of synaptic efficacy by coincidence of postsynaptic Aps and EPSPs. *Science* 275: 213–215.

Marshall, P.H., and Werder, P.R. (1972). The effects of the elimination of rehearsal on primacy and recency. *J. Verbal Learning Verbal Behav.* 11: 649–653.

McElree, B., Dolan, P.O., and Jacoby, L.L. (1999). Isolating the contributions of familiarity and source information to item recognition: A time course analysis. *J. Exp. Psychol. Learn. Mem. Cogn.* 25: 563–582.

Mecklinger, A., Kramer, A.F., and Strayer, D.L. (1992). Event-related potentials and EEG components in a semantic memory search task. *Psychophysiology* 29: 104–119.

Mecklinger, A., and Pfeifer, E. (1996). Event-related potentials reveal topographical and temporal distinct neuronal activation patterns for spatial and object working memory. *Cogn. Brain Res.* 4: 211–224.

Metcalfe, J. (1991). Recognition failure and the composite memory trace in CHARM. *Psychol. Rev.* 98: 529–553.

Murdock, B.B. (1962). The serial position effect of free recall. *J. Exp. Psychol.* 64: 482–488.

Murdock, B.B. (1982). A theory for the storage and retrieval of item and associative information. *Psychol. Rev.* 89: 609–626.

Murdock, B.B. (1997). Context and mediators in a theory of distributed associative memory (TODAM2). *Psychol. Rev.* 1997: 839–862.

Murdock, B.B., and Walker, K.D. (1969). Modality effects in free recall. *J. Verbal Learning Verbal Behav.* 8: 665–676.

Newcomer, J.W., Farber, N.B., Jevtovic-Todorovic, V., Selke, G. et al. (1999). Ketamine-induced NMDA receptor hypofunction as a model of memory impairment and psychosis. *Neuropsychopharmacology* 20: 106–118.

O'Keefe, J., and Recce, M.L. (1993). Phase relationship between hippocampal place units and the EEG theta rhythm. *Hippocampus* 3: 317–330.

Ostfeld, A.M., and Aruguete, A. (1962). *J. Pharmacol. Exp. Ther.* 137: 133–139.

Paulesu, E., Frith, C.D., and Frackowiak, R.S.J. (1993). The neural correlates of the verbal component of working memory. *Nature* 362: 342–343.

Pavlides, C., Greenstein, Y.J., Grudman, M., and Winson, J. (1988). Long-term potentiation in the dentate gyrus is induced preferentially on the positive phase of theta-rhythm. *Brain Res.* 439: 383–387.

Postman, L., and Phillips, L. (1965). Short-term temporal changes in free recall. *Q. J. Exp. Psychol.* 17: 132–138.

Raaijmakers, J.G.W., and Shiffrin, R.M. (1981). Search of associative memory. *Psychol. Rev.* 88: 93–134.

Rockstroh, S., Emre, M., Tarral, A., and Pokorny, R. (1996). Effects of the novel NMDA-receptor antagonist SDZ EAA 494 on memory and attention in human. *Psychopharmacology* 124: 261–266.

Rypma, B., and D'Esposito, M. (1999). The roles of prefrontal brain regions in components of working memory: Effects of memory load and individual differences. *Proc. Natl. Acad. Sci. USA* 96: 6558–6563.

Rypma, B., Prabhakaran, V., Desmond, J.E. Glover, G.H. et al. (1999). Load-dependent roles of frontal brain regions in the maintenance of working memory. *Neuroimage* 9: 216–226.

Shallice, T., and Warrington, E.K. (1970). Independent functioning of verbal memory stores: A neuropsychological study. *Q. J. Exp. Psychol.* 22: 261–273.

Smith, E.E., and Jonides, J. (1998). Neuroimaging analyses of human working memory. *Proc. Natl. Acad. Sci. USA* 95: 12061–12068.

Sompolinsky, H., and Kanter, I. (1986). Temporal association in asymmetric neural networks. *Phys. Rev. Lett.* 57: 2861–2864.

Sternberg, S. (1966). High-speed scanning in human memory. *Science* 153: 652–654.

Tesche, C.D., and Karhu, J. (1999). Characterization of theta oscillations in normal human hippocampus during a working memory task. *Neuroimage* 9: S973.

Thapar, A., and Greene, R. (1993). Evidence against a short-term-store account of long-term recency effects. *Mem. Cogn.* 21: 329–337.

Vallar, G., and Shallice, T. (Eds). (1990). Neuropsychological impairments of short-term memory. Cambridge: Cambridge University Press.

Vinogradova, O.S. (1984). Functional organization of the limbic system in the process of registration of information: Facts and hypothesis. In R.L. Isaakson and K.H. Pribram (Eds.), The hippocampus. (pp. 1–69). New York: Plenum Press

Watkins, M.J., Watkins, O.C., and Crowder, R.G. (1974). The modality effect in free and serial recall as a function of phonological similarity. *J. Verbal Learning Verbal Behavior* 13: 430–447.

Watkins, M.J., Neath, I., and Sechler, E.S. (1989). Recency effect in recall of a word list when an immediate memory task is performed after each word presentation. *Am. J. Psychol.* 102: 265–270.

Yonelinas, A.P. (1999). Recognition memory ROCs and the dual-process signal-detection model: Comment on Glanzer, Kim, Hilford, and Adams. *J. Exp. Psychol. Learn. Mem. Cogn.* 25: 514–521.

CHAPTER TEN

Neuronal Networks, Synaptic Plasticity, and Memory Systems in Primates

Edmund T. Rolls

SUMMARY

Synapse-specific increases and decreases in synaptic strength that depend on the activity of the presynaptic and postsynaptic neuron are central to modern theories of how networks in the brain operate in setting up sensory representations of the world, in memory, and in producing appropriate motor responses. The goals of this chapter are to show how different features of these synaptic modifications are crucial to the operation of different types of network, and to the operation of several different brain systems. The types of network considered will be three that are fundamental to brain function, namely pattern associators, autoassociators, and competitive networks. Each performs a different type of operation for the brain. Then the ways in which these types of synaptic modification are implicated in the operation of the hippocampus and related cortical areas in memory (see the section The Primate Hippocampus), and the cerebral neocortex in visual object recognition (see the section Synaptic Modification Rules) and short-term memory (see the section Short-Term Memory) will be described. The points made apply to any synapse-specific modification process in the brain, regardless of whether that process happens to be long-term potentiation/depression (LTP/LTD). More formal descriptions of the operation of some of the networks introduced here are provided by Rolls and Treves (1998), and by Hertz et al. (1991). Ways in which these architectures may be specified genetically are suggested by Rolls and Stringer (2000b).

The author has worked with A. Treves, G. Wallis, and P. Foldiak on some of the investigations referred to here, and their contribution is sincerely acknowledged. Different parts of the research described were supported by the Medical Research Council, PG9826105; by a Human Frontier Science Program grant; by an EC Human Capital and Mobility grant; by the MRC Oxford Interdisciplinary Research Centre in Cognitive Neuroscience; and by the Oxford McDonnell-Pew Centre in Cognitive Neuroscience.

Pattern Associators

A fundamental operation of most nervous systems is to learn to associate a first stimulus with a second that occurs at about the same time, and to retrieve the second stimulus when the first is presented. The first stimulus might be the sight of food, and the second stimulus the taste of food. After the association has been learned, the sight of food would enable its taste to be retrieved. In classical conditioning, the taste of food might elicit an unconditioned response of salivation, and if the sight of the food is paired with its taste, then the sight of that food would by learning come to produce salivation. More abstractly, if one idea is associated by learning with a second, then when the first idea occurs again, the second idea will tend to be associatively retrieved. Areas of the brain in which such pattern associators may be present include the amygdala and orbitofrontal cortex (for learning associations between, e.g., the sight of food and its taste, or more generally in stimulus-reinforcement association learning and emotion; see Rolls, 1990c, 1999a, 2000a, 2000b; Davis, 1992; Rolls and Treves, 1998) and in corticocortical backprojections.

Architecture and Operation

The prototypical network for pattern association is shown in Figure 10.1. What we have called the second or unconditioned stimulus pattern (**u**) is applied through unmodifiable synapses to produce vector force firing of the output neurons (**r**). (In this notation, **u** refers to the vector of firing of the unconditioned input stimulus, that is the firing rates u_i of the N input neurons i, which are indexed by $i = 1, N$. Details of the use of simple linear algebra in defining the operation of such networks are provided by Rolls and Treves, 1998.) The first or conditioned stimulus pattern **r'** present on the horizontally running axons in Figure 10.1 is applied through modifiable synapses *(w)* to the dendrites of the output neurons. The synapses are modifiable in such a way that if there is presynaptic firing on an input axon r'_j paired during learning with postsynaptic activity on neuron r_i, then the strength or weight w_{ij} between that axon and the dendrite increases. This simple learning rule is often called the Hebb rule, after Donald Hebb, who in 1949 formulated the hypothesis that if the firing of one neuron was regularly associated with another, then the strength of the synapse or synapses between the neurons should increase in strength. After learning, presenting the pattern **r'** on the input axons will activate the dendrite through the strengthened synapses. If the cue or conditioned stimulus pattern is similar to that learned, then there will be some activation of the postsynaptic neuron produced by each of the firing axons afferent to a synapse strengthened by the previous learning. The total activation h_i of each postsynaptic neuron i is then the sum of such individual activations. (This is a process intended to model simple summation of inputs by graded depolarization in the postsynaptic neuron.) In this way, just the correct output neurons are strongly activated, and the second or unconditioned stimulus is effectively recalled. The recall is best when only strong activation of the

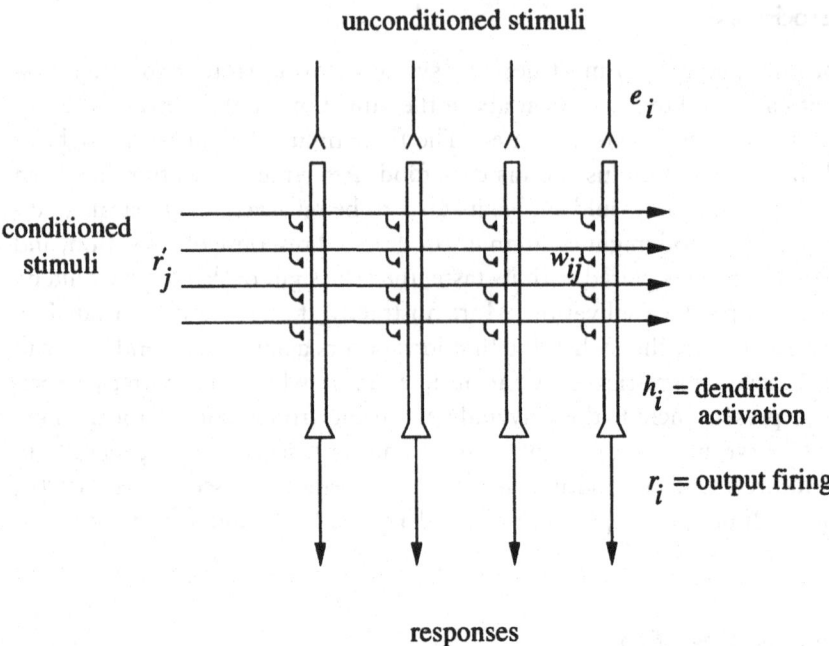

Figure 10.1. The architecture of a network for pattern association (see text).

postsynaptic neuron produces firing, that is if there is a threshold for firing, just like real neurons. The reasons for this arise when many associations are stored in the memory, as will soon be shown.

A more precise description of pattern association memory will now be introduced, in order to help us to understand more exactly how pattern associators operate. We have denoted above a conditioned stimulus input pattern as $\mathbf{r}'$. Each of the axons has a firing rate, and if we count or index through the axons using the subscript j, the firing rate of the first axon is r'_1, of the second r'_2, of the jth r'_j, etc. The whole set of axons forms a vector, which is just an ordered (1, 2, 3 etc.) set of elements. The firing rate of each axon r'_j is one element of the firing rate vector $\mathbf{r}'$. Similarly, using i as the index, we can denote the firing rate of any output neuron as r_i, and the firing rate output vector as $\mathbf{r}$. With this terminology, we can then identify any synapse onto neuron i from neuron j as w_{ij} (see Figure 10.1). In this chapter, the first index, i, always refers to the receiving neuron (and thus signifies a dendrite), while the second index, j, refers to the sending neuron (and thus signifies an axon in Figure 10.1). We can now specify the learning and retrieval operations as follows.

■ **Learning.** The firing rate of every output neuron is forced through strong unmodifiable synapses to a value determined by the forcing or unconditioned stimulus input. That is, for any one neuron $i, r_i = u_i$ (see Figure 10.1).

The Hebb rule can then be written as follows:

$$\delta w_{ij} = k \cdot r_i \cdot r'_j \tag{1}$$

where w_{ij} is the change of the synaptic weight w_{ij}, which results from the simultaneous (or conjunctive) presence of presynaptic firing r'_j and postsynaptic firing r_i (or strong depolarization), and k is a learning rate constant that specifies how much the synapses alter on any one pairing. The presynaptic and postsynaptic activity must be present approximately simultaneously (to within perhaps 100 msec), or even with the presynaptic activity just before the postsynaptic activation, which may often be the situation behaviorally when associations are learned.

The Hebb rule is expressed in this multiplicative form to reflect the idea that *both* presynaptic and postsynaptic activity must be present for the synapses to increase in strength. The multiplicative form also reflects the idea that strong pre- and postsynaptic firing will produce a larger change of synaptic weight than smaller firing rates. The Hebb rule thus captures what is typically found in studies of associative long-term potentiation (LTP). It is also assumed for now that before any learning takes place, the synaptic strengths are small in relation to the changes that can be produced during Hebbian learning. We will see that this assumption can be relaxed later when a modified Hebb rule is introduced that can lead to a reduction in synaptic strength (long-term depression, LTD) under some conditions.

■ **Recall.** When the conditioned stimulus is present on the input axons, the total activation h_i of a neuron i is the sum of all the activations produced through each strengthened synapse w_{ij} by each active neuron r'_j. We can express this as

$$h_i = \Sigma_j \, r'_j \cdot w_{ij} \tag{2}$$

where Σ_j indicates that the sum is over the N input axons indexed by j. The multiplicative form here indicates that activation should be produced by an axon only if it is firing, and only if it is connected to the dendrite by a strengthened synapse. It also indicates that the strength of the activation reflects how fast the axon r'_j is firing, and the strength of the synapse w_{ij}. The sum of all such activations expresses the idea that summation (of synaptic currents in real neurons) occurs along the length of the dendrite to produce activation at the cell body, where the activation h_i is converted into firing r_i. This conversion can be expressed as

$$r_i = f(h_i) \tag{3}$$

which indicates that the firing rate is a function of the postsynaptic activation. The function is called the activation function in this case. The function at its simplest could be linear, so that the firing rate would be proportional to the activation (see Figure 10.2a). Real neurons have thresholds, with firing occurring only if the activation is above the threshold. A threshold linear activation function is shown in Figure 10.2b. This has been useful in formal analysis of the properties of neural networks. Neurons also have firing rates that become saturated at a maximum

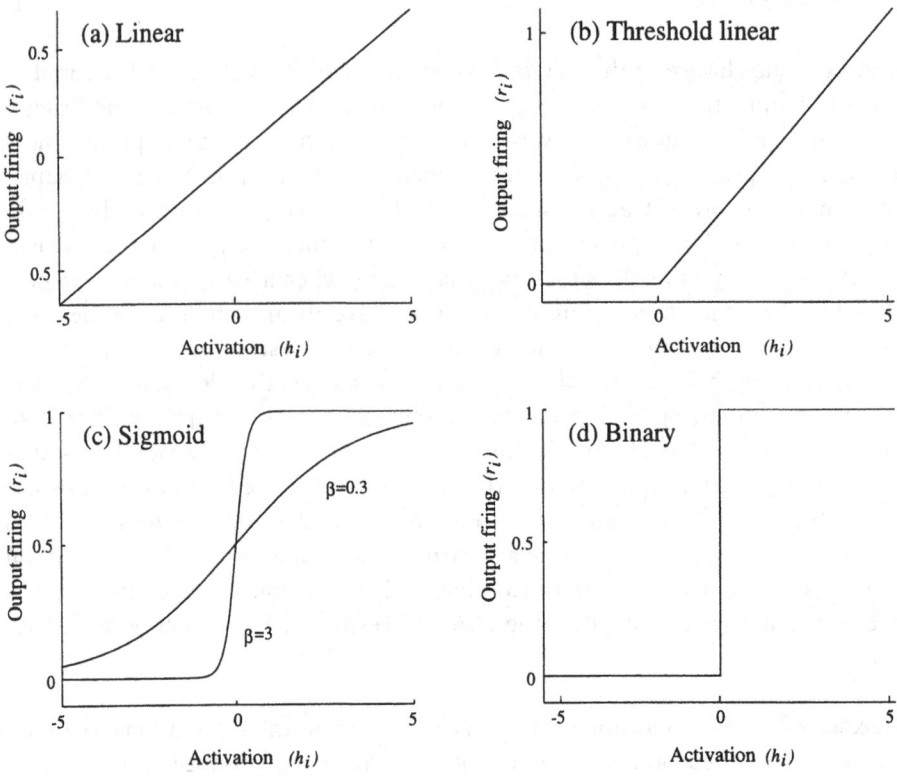

Figure 10.2. A set of different activation functions of neurons (see text). Each activation function shows a relationship between the activation of the neuron by its inputs (abscissa), and the output firing of the neuron (ordinate).

rate, and we could express this as the sigmoid activation function shown in Figure 10.2c. Another simple activation function, used in some models of neural networks, is the binary threshold function (Figure 10.2d), which indicates that if the activation is below threshold, there is no firing, and that if the activation is above threshold, the neuron fires maximally. Some nonlinearity in the activation function is an advantage, for it enables small activations produced by interfering memories to be minimized, and it can enable neurons to perform logical operations, such as fire only if two or more sets of inputs are present simultaneously.

With networks of this type, many associations between different conditioned and unconditioned stimuli can be learned, as described shortly. These networks also have many very biologically attractive features, including generalization across similar conditioned input stimuli, and graceful degradation of performance if some of the input axons or the synapses in the network are damaged, or are not available during development. These properties arise only if the input patterns are represented across an ensemble of axons (distributed encoding), because then similarity can be represented by correlations of one pattern of input with another, as described fully by Rolls and Treves (1998).

Relevance of Different Aspects of the Synaptic Modification Used

■ **Local Learning Rule.** The learning used in pattern association neural networks [Eq. (1)] is a local learning rule in that the information required to specify the change in synaptic weight is available locally at the synapse, as it is dependent only on the presynaptic firing rate r'_j available at the synaptic terminal, and the postsynaptic activation or firing r_i available on the dendrite of the neuron receiving the synapse. This is a property of LTP and LTD. This makes the learning rule biologically plausible, in that the information about how to change the synaptic weight does not have to be carried from a distant source where it is computed to every synapse. (Such a nonlocal learning rule would not be biologically plausible, in that there are no appropriate connections known in most parts of the brain to bring in the synaptic training signal to every synapse; see Rolls and Treves, 1998, and compare McLeod et al., 1998.)

Another useful property of real neurons in relation to Eq. (1) is that the postsynaptic term, r_i, is available on much of the dendrite of a cell, if (as is the case for many large cells in the brain, e.g., pyramidal cells) the electrotonic length of the dendrite is short (see Koch, 1999). Thus if a neuron is strongly activated with a high value for r_i, then any active synapse onto the cell will be capable of being modified. This enables the cell to learn an association between the pattern of activity on all its axons and its postsynaptic activation. If in contrast a group of coactive axons made synapses close together on a small dendrite, then the local depolarization might be intense, and these synapses only would modify onto the dendrite. (A single distant active synapse would not modify in this type of neuron, because of the long electronic length of the dendrite.) The computation in this case is described as Sigma-Pi, to indicate that there is a local product computed, and then the output of the neuron can reflect the sum of such local multiplications (see further Rolls and Treves, 1998).

■ **Capacity** (see Rolls and Treves, 1990). The number of different associations that can be stored in a pattern associator is proportional to the number C of independently modifiable synapses on the dendrite of each output neuron. It is for this reason that a synapse-specific modification rule is desirable. If one synapse adjacent to another with the appropriate pre- and postsynaptic activity for synapse modification also showed synapse modification, then the number of different pattern associations that could be stored would be halved. The details of the number of different memories that can be stored in pattern association networks with different types of activation function are described elsewhere (Rolls and Treves, 1998) and summarized next, but the important conclusion is that just stated.

Linear Associative Neuronal Networks. These networks have a linear activation function, and are trained by a Hebb (or similar) associative learning rule. The capacity of these networks is C different input vectors ($\mathbf{r'}$, where $r'_j = 1$, C) mapped to an output $\mathbf{r}$. For no interference, the conditioned stimulus input vectors $\mathbf{r'}$ must be orthogonal (i.e., they must be uncorrelated). If the CS input pattern vectors are not orthogonal, then the dot product of them is not 0, and an output neuron activated by one of the vectors will be activated by the other. The capacity in this case will be less than C.

The Use of LTD to Remove the Correlation between Different Input Patterns with the Firing Rate of Each Axon Greater Than or Equal to Zero. If the input firing rates on the axons are in the range $(0,+x)$ (where x is the maximum firing rate in, e.g., spikes/s, as they will be for real neurons, then the different input vectors will be correlated. Because each neuron effectively calculates the correlation (or more strictly the inner or dot product) of the different input vectors r' with the weight vectors on each dendrite w_i, two different input vectors with positive only firing rates will always produce correlated outputs (i.e., the correlation between any two such vectors will be positive). This will produce interference between the different memories stored in the network (see Rolls and Treves, 1998). A solution to this issue that arises with input vectors r' that can only assume positive values (e.g., firing rates) is to use a modified learning rule of the following form:

$$\delta w_{ij} = k \cdot r_i \cdot (r'_j - c) \tag{4}$$

where c is a constant. This learning rule includes (in proportion to r_i) increasing the synaptic weight if $(r'_j - c)$ is greater than 0 (long-term potentiation), and decreasing the synaptic weight if $(r'_j - c)$ is less than 0 (heterosynaptic long-term depression). If c is the average activity of an input axon r'_j across patterns, then n input vectors can still be learned by the network [provided for linear networks that the resulting vectors $(r'_j - c$, with $j = 1, C)$ are mutually orthogonal]. (In large networks, c can be the average activity of the input vector r', which would be more plausible in the brain; see Rolls and Treves, 1990.)

This modified (Hebbian) learning rule will be described in more detail, in terms of a contingency table showing the synaptic strength modifications produced by different types of learning rule, where LTP indicates an increase in synaptic strength (long-term potentiation), and LTD indicates a decrease in synaptic strength (long-term depression). In Table 10.1, 0 for the postsynaptic activation or the presynaptic firing should be read as low, and 1 as high.

Heterosynaptic long-term depression is so-called because it is the decrease in synaptic strength that occurs to a synapse that is *other than* that through which the postsynaptic cell is being activated. This heterosynaptic depression is the type of change of synaptic strength that is required (in addition to LTP) for effective subtraction of the average presynaptic firing rate, in order to make the CS vectors appear more orthogonal to the pattern associator. The rule is sometimes called the Singer-Stent rule, after work by Singer (1987) and Stent (1973). Evidence that this type of LTD is found in the hippocampus was described by Levy (Levy, 1985; Levy and Desmond, 1985; see Brown et al., 1990). Homosynaptic long-term depression is so-called because it is the decrease in synaptic strength that occurs to a synapse that is (the *same as* that which is) active. For it to occur, the postsynaptic neuron must simultaneously have only low activity, which might be below its mean activity, as formalized in Eq. (8). (This rule is sometimes called the BCM rule after the paper of Bienenstock, Cooper, and Munro, 1982.)

Table 10.1. Effects of pre- and postsynaptic activity on synaptic modification

		Post-synaptic Activation	
		0	High
Presynaptic firing	0	No Change	Heterosynaptic LTD
	High	homosynaptic LTD	LTP

The value of heterosynaptic LTD in associative neuronal networks is thus that it enables the correlation between CS input patterns induced by the positive-only firing rates to be removed. This enables interference between different CSs induced by this factor to be removed. It enables the theoretical limit for the number of patterns to be associated in such networks to be achieved. This limit is in the case of linear associative networks c patterns if the patterns are orthogonal, and somewhat less than c patterns if they are not orthogonal (see Rolls and Treves, 1990, 1998).

Associative Neuronal Networks with Nonlinear Neurons. With nonlinear neurons, for example, with a threshold in the output activation function so that the output firing r_i is 0 when the activation h_i is below the threshold, or with a sigmoid activation function, then the capacity can be measured in terms of the number of (conditioned stimulus) input patterns r′ that can produce different outputs in the network. As with the linear counterpart, in order to remove the correlation that would otherwise occur between the patterns because the elements can take only positive values, it is useful to use a modified Hebb rule

$$\delta w_{ij} = k \cdot r_i \cdot (r'_j - c) \qquad \text{(Eq. 4 above)}$$

With fully distributed orthogonal (after subtracting the mean using the term c above) input patterns r′, it is possible to store, as with linear associative networks, C different patterns where there are C inputs per dendrite.

If sparse (distributed) input patterns r are used (for the output neurons, see Rolls and Treves, 1998), then many more than C patterns can be stored, even when the patterns are random (e.g., each element is set on or off at random). [A local representation is a representation in which the information that a particular stimulus or event occurred is provided by the activity of one of the elements in the vector, e.g., by one of the nodes or neurons in the network. A (fully) distributed representation is one in which the activity of all the elements in the vector is needed to specify which stimulus or event occurred. A sparse (distributed) representation is one in which only a proportion *(a)* of the C input axons r'_j are active (>0) at any one time. The sparseness is then *a* (for binary neurons). The activity of this subset of nodes is sufficient to identify which stimulus or event was present in such a sparse distributed representation.] Indeed, the number of different patterns or prototypes P that can be stored is

$$P \approx C/[a_o \log(1/a_o)] \tag{5}$$

where a_o is the sparseness of the *output* firing pattern r produced by the unconditioned stimulus. P can in this situation be much larger than C (see Rolls and Treves, 1990, 1998). This is an important result for encoding in pattern associators, because it means that provided that the activation functions are nonlinear (which is the case with real neurons), there is a very great advantage to using sparse encoding, for then many more than C pattern associations can be stored. Sparse representations may well be present in brain regions involved in associative memory for this reason (see Rolls and Treves, 1998).

■ **Overwriting Old Memories; Forgetting.** As additional memories are added to a network, it can be helpful to overwrite old memories. One of the advantages of this is that associative neuronal networks have a limited capacity, noted above, and if this capacity is exceeded, recall of any of the memories from the network can be impaired. Heterosynaptic LTD effectively allows gradual overwriting of old memories, in that synapses strengthened by old memories might be required according to Eq. (4) to be decreased onto an active dendrite from inactive synapses. If the pattern association must be reversed (e.g., pattern 1 is no longer associated with a taste or reward), then the ability to show heterosynaptic LTD enables the output neurons to stop responding to pattern 1.

■ **Synaptic Strength Resolution.** In the associative networks described, the information that can be utilized per synapse is in the order of 0.2 to 0.4 bits. (One bit might correspond to the synapse being either strong or weak/absent. Two bits might correspond to four levels of synaptic strength.) This implies that the number of different levels of synaptic strength that would need to be implemented by a synaptic modification process such as LTP/LTD when applied to associative networks might be only two to four levels. Much can be achieved if there are only two levels of synaptic strength (absent/weak and strong), as shown in the original analyses of Willshaw and Longuet-Higgins (1969). The implication is that for this type of memory, little precision of synaptic modification is needed (see Rolls and Treves, 1998).

■ **Nonlinear Operations in the Postsynaptic Neuron — NMDA Receptors.** The nonlinear property of the NMDA receptors means that synaptic modification would only occur onto the most strongly activated postsynaptic neurons in an associative network. This has led to the notion of cooperativity, in that only postsynaptic neurons with several moderately active presynaptic inputs will have sufficient depolarization for any synaptic modification. This means that effectively the postsynaptic neuron would store the correlation between several conjunctively active inputs (and later respond to any one of the inputs alone). This effect is equivalent to nonlinearity on the output activation function of neurons. It tends (by making the representations stored effectively sparser than the representations received) to increase the number of memories that can be stored in the network [see Eq. (5) above], at the expense of some (nonlinear) distortion of the inputs stored (see Rolls, 1989c; Rolls and Treves, 1990; Treves and Rolls, 1991; Rolls and Treves, 1998).

Autoassociation Memory

Autoassociative memories, or attractor neural networks, store memories, each one of which is represented by a pattern of neural activity. They can then recall the appropriate memory from the network when provided with a fragment of one of the memories. This is called *completion*. Many different memories can be stored in the network and retrieved correctly. The network can learn each memory in one trial. Because of its "one-shot" rapid learning, and ability to complete, this type of network is well suited for episodic memory storage, in which each past episode must be stored and recalled later from a fragment, and kept separate from other episodic memories. An autoassociation memory can also be used as a short-term memory, in which iterative processing around the recurrent collateral connection loop keeps a representation active until another input cue is received.

Architecture and Operation

The prototypical architecture of an autoassociation memory is shown in Figure 10.3. The external input e_i is applied to each neuron i by unmodifiable synapses. This produces firing r_i of each neuron, or a vector of firing on the output neurons **r**. Each output neuron i is connected by a recurrent collateral connection to the other neurons in the network, via modifiable connection weights w_{ij}. This architecture effectively enables the output firing vector **r** to be associated during learning with itself. Later on, during recall, presentation of part of the external input will force some of the output neurons to fire, but through the recurrent collateral axons and the modified synapses, other neurons in r can be brought into activity. This process can be repeated a number of times, and recall of a complete pattern may be perfect. Effectively, a pattern can be recalled or recognized because of associations formed between its parts. This requires distributed representations.

Next I introduce a more precise and detailed description of the above, and describe the properties of these networks. A formal description of the operation of these networks is provided in Appendix 3 of Rolls and Treves (1998), and by Hertz et al. (1991).

■ **Learning.** The firing of every output neuron i is forced to a value r_i, determined by the external input e_i. It is sometimes overlooked that there must be a mechanism for ensuring that during learning r_i does approximate e_i, and must not be influenced much by the recurrent collateral connections; otherwise the new external pattern **e** will not be stored in the network, but instead something that is influ-

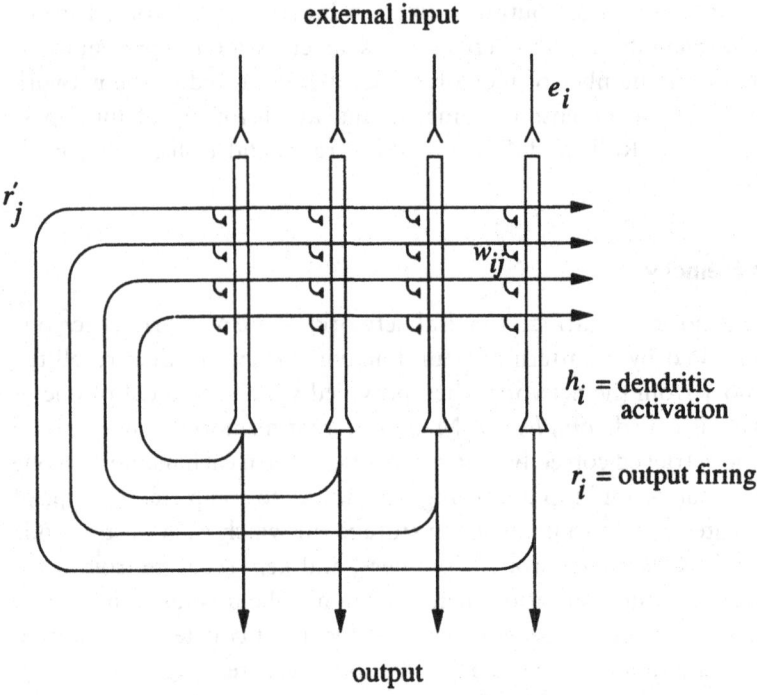

Figure 10.3. The architecture of a network for autoassociation (see text).

enced by the previously stored memories. It is thought that in some parts of the brain, such as the hippocampus, there are processes such as the effect of the mossy fiber inputs to the CA3 pyramidal neurons that help the external connections to dominate the firing during learning (see below and Rolls, 1989b, 1989c; Treves and Rolls, 1992; Rolls and Treves, 1998). In addition, synaptic transmission in the recurrent collaterals may be reduced during learning (Hasselmo et al., 1995).

$$\delta w_{ij} = k \cdot r_i \cdot r'_j \qquad \text{(Hebb rule)} \qquad \text{(Eq. 1 above)}$$

■ **Recall.** During recall the external input e_i is applied and produces output firing, operating through the nonlinear activation function described below. The firing is fed back by the recurrent collateral axons shown in Figure 10.2, to produce activation of each output neuron through the modified synapses on each output neuron. The internal activation h_i produced by the recurrent collateral effect on the ith neuron is the sum of the activations produced in proportion to the firing rate of each axon r'_j operating through each modified synapse w_{ij}, that is,

$$h_i = \Sigma_j r'_j \cdot w_{ij} \qquad \text{(Eq. 2 above)}$$

where Σ_j indicates that the sum is over the C input axons indexed by j.

The output firing r_i is a function of the activation produced by the recurrent collateral effect (internal recall) and by the external input (e_i):

$$r_i = f(h_i + e_i) \tag{6}$$

The output activation function f must be nonlinear, and may be, for example, binary threshold, linear threshold, sigmoid, etc. (see Figure 10.2). A nonlinear activation function is used to minimize interference between the pattern being recalled and other patterns stored in the network, and to ensure that what is a positive feedback system remains stable. The network can be allowed to repeat this recurrent collateral loop a number of times. Each time the loop operates, the output firing becomes more like the originally stored pattern; this progressive recall is usually complete within five to fifteen iterations.

Properties

The internal recall in autoassociation networks involves multiplication of the firing vector of neuronal activity by the vector of synaptic weights on each neuron. This inner product vector multiplication allows the similarity of the firing vector to previously stored firing vectors to be provided by the output (as effectively a correlation), if the patterns learned are distributed. As a result of this type of correlation computation performed if the patterns are distributed, many important properties of these networks arise, including pattern completion (because part of a pattern is correlated with the whole pattern), and graceful degradation (because a damaged synaptic weight vector is still correlated with the original synaptic weight vector). These properties are described in more detail by Rolls and Treves (1998).

Relevance of Different Aspects of the Synaptic Modification Used

■ **Local Learning Rule.** The learning used in autoassociation neural networks, a version of the Hebb rule, is as follows:

$$\delta w_{ij} = k \cdot r_i \cdot r'_j \qquad \text{(Eq. 1 above)}$$

The same points apply as described above for pattern associators.

■ **Positive-Only Firing Rates.** As with pattern associators, if positive-only firing rates are used, then the correlation this induces between different pattern vectors can be removed by subtracting the mean of the presynaptic activity from each presynaptic term, using a type of LTD. This can be specified as

$$\delta w_{ij} = k \cdot r_i \cdot (r'_j - c) \qquad \text{(Eq. 4 above)}$$

where c is a constant. This learning rule includes (in proportion to r_i) increasing the synaptic weight if $(r'_j - c)$ is greater then 0 (long-term potentiation), and decreasing the synaptic weight if $(r'_j - c)$ is less than 0 (heterosynaptic long-term depression). This procedure works optimally if c is the average activity of an input axon r'_j across patterns. One implication of this is that if the postsynaptic activity is high, and the presynaptic activity is below average, then LTD might be predicted if the networks are involved in autoassociation (or pattern association).

■ **Capacity (see Treves and Rolls, 1991).** The number of different memories that can be stored in autoassociators is (as with pattern associators) proportional to the number C of independently modifiable synapses on the dendrite of each neuron. It is for this reason that a synapse-specific modification rule is desirable. Some further details are provided next, but what has just been stated is the most important point in relation to synapse specificity.

With the nonlinear neurons used in the network, the capacity can be measured in terms of the number of input patterns r that can be stored in the network and recalled later with a stable basin of attraction. With fully distributed orthogonal (after subtracting the mean) input patterns **r** (see pattern associators), it is possible to store C different patterns, where there are C inputs to each neuron in the network, each neuron having C synaptic weights. With fully distributed random binary patterns in a fully connected autoassociation network, the number of patterns that can be learned is $0.14C$ (Hopfield, 1982). Treves and Rolls (1991) have been able to extend this analysis to autoassociation networks that are much more biologically relevant by having diluted connectivity (missing synapses), and neurons with graded (continuously variable) firing rates. The number of different patterns P that can be stored is then

$$P \simeq \frac{C}{a\ln(1/a)} k \tag{7}$$

where C is the number of synapses on each dendrite devoted to the recurrent collaterals from other neurons in the network, and k is a factor that depends weakly on the detailed structure of the rate distribution, on the connectivity pattern, and so forth, but is roughly in the order of 0.2 to 0.3. a is the sparseness of the representation, which for binary neurons can be measured by the proportion of neurons that are firing. (For neurons with real firing rates, the corresponding measure is

$$a = (\Sigma_{i=1,N} r_i/N)^2 / \Sigma_{i=1,N} (r_i^2/N)$$

where r_i is the firing rate of the i'th neuron in the set of N neurons.

■ **Overwriting Old Memories.** As additional memories are added to an autoassociative network, it can be helpful to overwrite old memories. One of the advantages of this is that autoassociative neuronal networks have a limited capacity, noted above, and if this capacity is exceeded, recall of any of the memories from the network is impaired. Heterosynaptic LTD effectively allows gradual overwriting of old memories, in that synapses strengthened by old memories might be required according to Eq. (4) to be decreased onto an active dendrite from inactive synapses. Homosynaptic LTD may also contribute to this useful forgetting.

■ **Synaptic Strength Resolution.** In the autoassociative networks described, the information that can be utilized per synapse is in the order of 0.2 to 0.4 bits (Treves and Rolls, 1991; Rolls and Treves, 1998). This implies that the number of different levels of synaptic strength that would need to be implemented by a synaptic modification process such as LTP/LTD when applied to associative networks might be only two to four levels.

■ **Nonlinear Operations in the Postsynaptic Neuron—NMDA Receptors.** The nonlinear property of the NMDA receptors means that synaptic modification would only occur onto the most strongly activated postsynaptic neurons in an autoassociative network. This effect is equivalent to nonlinearity in the output activation function of neurons. It tends (by making the representations stored effectively sparser that the representations received) to increase the number of memories that can be stored in the network [see Eq. (7)], at the expense of some (nonlinear) distortion of the memories stored (see Rolls, 1989c; Treves and Rolls, 1991; Rolls and Treves, 1998).

■ **Covariance Learning Rule versus LTD.** In a covariance learning rule, the means of both the pre- and the postsynaptic factor are subtracted, as indicated in Eq. (8).

$$\delta w_{ij} = k \cdot (r_i - \mu_i) \cdot (r'_j - \mu_j) \tag{8}$$

where μ_i is the mean of the postsynaptic activity of the output neuron, and μ_j is the mean of the presynaptic terminal j. This rule was effectively used in the original Hopfield (1982) autoassociation network. An implication of this rule is that with both the presynaptic and the postsynaptic activity low, the synapse will be strengthened, which seems neurobiologically unnatural. In heterosynaptic LTD, only the mean of the presynaptic activity μ_j is subtracted. Autoassociation networks operate well if only heterosynaptic LTD is present. The term $(r_i - \mu_i)$ in Eq. (8) would allow homosynaptic LTD if the presynaptic rate is high and the postsynaptic activity r_i is low.

Competitive Networks

Function

Competitive neural nets learn to categorize input pattern vectors. Each category of inputs activates a different output neuron (or set of output neurons; see below). The categories formed are based on similarities between the input vectors. Similar – that is correlated – input vectors activate the same output neuron. In that the learning is based on similarities in the input space and there is no external teacher that forces classification, this is an unsupervised network. The term *categorization* is used to refer to the process of placing vectors into categories based on their similarity.

The categorization produced by competitive nets is of great potential importance in perceptual systems. Each category formed reflects a set or cluster of active inputs r'_j, which occur together. This cluster of coactive inputs can be thought of as a feature, and the competitive network can be described as building feature analyzers, where a feature can now be defined as a correlated set of inputs. During learning, a competitive network gradually discovers these features in the input space, and the process of finding these features without a teacher is referred to as *self-organization*. Another important use of competitive networks is to remove redundancy from the input space, by allocating output neurons to reflect a set of inputs that co-occur. Another important aspect of competitive networks is that they separate patterns that are somewhat correlated in the input space, to produce outputs for the different patterns that are less correlated with each other, and may indeed easily be made orthogonal to each other. This has been referred to as orthogonalization. Another important function of competitive networks is that partly by removing redundancy from the input information space, they can produce sparse output vectors, without losing information. We may refer to this as sparsification.

These latter operations are useful as preprocessing operations before signals are applied to associative networks, which benefit from sparse, noncorrelated input patterns if they are to store large numbers of memories (see above and Rolls and Treves, 1998).

Architecture and Algorithm

■ **Architecture.** The basic architecture of a competitive network is shown in Figure 10.4. It is a one-layer network with a set of inputs $\mathbf{r}'$ that make modifiable excitatory synapses w_{ij} with the output neurons. The output cells compete with each other (for example, by mutual inhibition) in such a way that the most strongly activated neuron or neurons win the competition and are left firing strongly. The synaptic weights, w_{ij}, are initialized to random values. The absence of some of the synapses (for example, producing randomly diluted connectivity), is not a problem for such networks, and can even help them (see below).

In the brain, the inputs arrive through axons, which make synapses with the dendrites of the output or principal cells of the network. The principal cells are typically pyramidal cells in the cerebral cortex. In the brain the principal cells are typically excitatory, and mutual inhibition between them is implemented by inhibitory interneurons, which receive excitatory inputs from the principal cells. The inhibitory interneurons then send their axons to make synapses with the pyramidal cells, typically using GABA (gamma-amino butyric acid) as the inhibitory transmitter. An algorithm that can be thought to represent this follows.

1. Apply an input vector $\mathbf{r}'$ and calculate the output activation h_i of each neuron

$$h_i = \Sigma_j \, r'_j \cdot w_{ij} \qquad\qquad\qquad\qquad \text{(Eq. 2 above)}$$

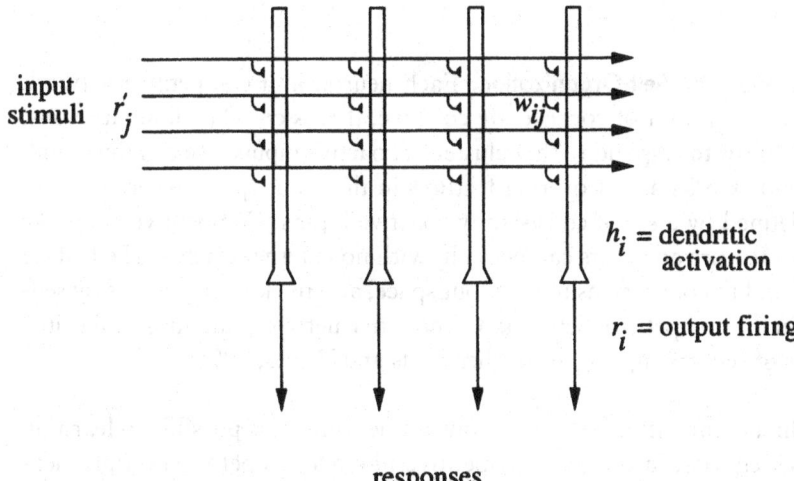

input
stimuli r'_j

w_{ij}

h_i = dendritic
      activation

r_i = output firing

responses

Figure 10.4. The architecture of a competitive network (see text).

where the sum is over the C input axons, r'_j.
(It is useful to normalize the length of each input vector $\mathbf{r}'$.)
The output firing $r1_i$ is a function of the output activation

$$r1_i = f(h_i) \tag{9}$$

This function can be linear, sigmoid, monotonically increasing, and so forth.

2. Allow competitive interaction between the output neurons by a mechanism such as lateral or mutual inhibition, to produce a contrast-enhanced version of r1

$$\mathbf{r} = f_{comp}(\mathbf{r}1) \tag{10}$$

This is typically a nonlinear operation, and in its most extreme form may be a winner-take-all function, in which after the competition one neuron may be "on" and the others "off."

3. Apply the Hebb learning rule

$$\delta w_{ij} = k \cdot r_i \cdot r'_j \tag{Eq. 1 above}$$

4. Normalize the length of the synaptic weight vector on each dendrite to prevent the same few neurons always winning the competition.

$$\Sigma_j (w_{ij})^2 = 1 \tag{11}$$

5. Repeat steps 1 to 4 for each different input stimulus $\mathbf{r}'$ in random sequence a number of times.

Properties

■ **Feature Discovery by Self-Organization.** Each neuron in a competitive network becomes activated by a set of consistently coactive, that is correlated, input axons, and gradually learns to respond to that cluster of coactive inputs. We can thus think of competitive networks as discovering features in the input space, where features can now be defined by a set of consistently coactive inputs. Competitive networks thus show how feature analyzers can be built, with no external teacher. The feature analyzers respond to correlations in the input space, and the learning occurs by self-organization in the competitive network. Competitive networks are thus well suited to the analysis of sensory inputs (see further Rolls and Treves, 1998).

■ **Capacity.** In a competitive net with N output neurons, it is possible to learn up to N output categories, in that the competitive interactions between output neurons are first order. (That is, the competition between the output neurons is uniform in that they are not connected in such a way that pairs, triples, etc. can act together to force themselves apart from other pairs, triples, etc. of output neurons.) It is thus the number of output neurons, rather than the number of input connections per neuron, that determines the number of categories that can be formed. The output neurons need not operate in a winner-take-all manner (to produce local or grandmother cell representations), but instead can operate with soft competition to leave a number of neurons still active after the mutual (lateral) inhibition.

■ **Normalization of the Length of the Synaptic Weight Vector on Each Dendrite—A Role for Heterosynaptic LTD.** Normalization is necessary to ensure that one or a few neurons do not always win the competition. (If the weights on one neuron were increased by simple Hebbian learning, and there was no normalization of the weights on the neuron, then it would tend to respond strongly in the future to patterns with some overlap with patterns to which that neuron has previously learned, and gradually that neuron would capture a large number of patterns.) A biologically plausible way to achieve this weight adjustment is to use a modified Hebb rule:

$$\delta w_{ij} = k \cdot r_i \left(r'_j - w_{ij} \right) \tag{12}$$

where k is a constant, and r'_j and w_{ij} are in appropriate units. This implements a Hebb rule that increases synaptic strength according to conjunctive pre- and post-synaptic activity, and also allows the strength of each synapse to decay in proportion to the firing rate of the postsynaptic neuron (as well as in proportion to the existing synaptic strength). This is an important computational use of heterosynaptic LTD. This rule can maintain the sums of the synaptic weights on each neuron to be very similar without any need for explicit normalization of the synaptic strengths, and is useful in competitive nets. [The rule given in Eq. (12) strictly maintains the sum of the weights on a neuron to be constant if the neurons are linear.] This rule was used by Willshaw and von der Malsburg (1976).

If explicit weight normalization is needed (i.e., keeping the vector length, that is, the square root of the sum of the squares of the synaptic strengths, constant), the appropriate form of the modified Hebb rule (again for linear neurons) is

$$\delta w_{ij} = k \cdot r_i \, (r'_j - r_i w_{ij}) \tag{13}$$

This rule, formulated by Oja (1982), makes weight decay proportional to r_i^2, normalizes the synaptic weight vector (see Hertz, et al., 1991), is still a local learning rule, and is known as the Oja rule.

In both these rules, the important point is that the degree of LTD and LTP depend on the existing synaptic strength. If the synaptic strength is low (e.g., before any LTP has been induced), then LTP should be (other things being equal) large. If LTP has already been induced, further LTP might be expected to be smaller. Conversely, LTD should be especially evident when LTP has previously been induced. These effects, which are frequently found in experiments on LTP and LTD, therefore should not necessarily be regarded as spurious effects, but may be related to this fundamental design feature needed in competitive neuronal networks.

■ **Nonlinearity in the Learning Rule.** Nonlinearity in the learning rule can assist competition (Rolls, 1989c). In the brain, LTP typically occurs only when strong activation of a neuron has produced sufficient depolarization for the voltage-dependent NMDA receptors to become unblocked, allowing Ca^{2+} to enter the cell. This means that synaptic modification occurs only on neurons that are strongly activated, effectively assisting competition to select few winners. The learning rule can be written

$$\delta w_{ij} = k \cdot m_i \, (r'_j - w_{ij}) \tag{14}$$

where m_i is a nonlinear function of r_i, which mimics the operation of the NMDA receptors in learning.

Brain Systems in Which Competitive Networks May Be Used for Orthogonalization and Sparsification

One system is the hippocampus, in which the dentate granule cells may operate as a competitive network in order to prepare signals for presentation to the CA3 autoassociative network. In this case, the operation is enhanced by expansion recoding, in that (in the rat) there are approximately three times as many dentate granule cells as there are cells in the preceding stage, the entorhinal cortex (see section The Primate Hippocampus). This expansion recoding will itself tend to reduce correlations between patterns (cf. Marr, 1969).

Also in the hippocampus, the CA1 neurons are thought to act as a competitive network that recodes the separate representations of each of the parts of an episode that must be separately represented in CA3, into a form more suitable for the recall by pattern association performed by the backprojections from the hippocampus to the cerebral cortex (see section Backprojections to the Neocortex).

The granule cells of the cerebellum may perform a similar function, but in this case the principle may be that each of the very large number of granule cells receives a very small random subset of inputs, so that the outputs of the granule cells are decorrelated with respect to the inputs (Marr, 1969; see Rolls and Treves, 1998).

Competitive Networks Using LTP and Homosynaptic LTD

A different learning rule that has been proposed to account for plasticity changes during development of the visual system has, in addition to Hebbian increments (synaptic strength increases when there is high pre- and postsynaptic activity), decrements in synaptic strength if the postsynaptic firing is below a certain threshold T_c and there is presynaptic activity. These decrements would correspond to homosynaptic LTD. In Bienenstock et al.'s investigation (1982) of this rule, the threshold (T_c) referred to above was a function of the average activation of the neuron, and varied in such a way that the average activation of different neurons was kept approximately equal. This BCM rule prevents domination by any one dendrite, by adjusting its sensitivity (using T_c) according to its mean response to the input stimulus set. A very active neuron will develop a very high threshold, causing reduction of weights and thus reduced response to future stimuli. It is correspondingly impossible for a neuron not to react to at least one of the stimuli, and so all output neurons become allocated to one category or another. A further analysis of networks taught with this rule is provided by Rolls and Treves (1998).

The Primate Hippocampus

Evidence from the effects of damage to the hippocampus, and from recording the activity of neurons in it, indicates that it is involved in the formation of memories about particular events, especially when they involve a spatial component (see Rolls, 1999b). These are formed rapidly, and frequently involve associating together a number of spatial inputs (where the event happened) with visual (e.g., the sight of a person) inputs and perhaps auditory, taste, and olfactory inputs. It is suggested that the memory for such episodes is formed in the hippocampus, which allows convergence of all these signals into one network, that of the CA3 pyramidal cells. This network has extensive recurrent connections between the different CA3 pyramidal cells, which are associatively modifiable (Urban et al., 1996). It has therefore been suggested that the CA3 cells operate as an autoassociative network, which can store such episodic memories, and then recall each memory from a part of it (see Rolls, 1987, 1989b, 1989c, 1990b). This analysis of the role of the primate hippocampus in memory is described next.

Effects of Damage to the Hippocampus and Connected Structures on Memory

In monkeys, damage to the hippocampus or to some of its connections such as the fornix produces deficits in learning about where objects are and where responses must be made (see Rolls, 1996b). For example, macaques and humans with damage to the hippocampus or fornix are impaired in object–place memory tasks in which not only the objects seen, but where they were seen, must be remembered (Gaffan and Saunders, 1985; Parkinson et al., 1988; Smith and Milner, 1981). Such object–place tasks require a whole-scene or snapshot-like memory (Gaffan, 1994). Also, fornix lesions impair conditional left–right discrimination learning, in which the visual appearance of an object specifies whether a response is to be made to the left or the right (Rupniak and Gaffan, 1987). A comparable deficit is found in humans (Petrides, 1985). Fornix-sectioned monkeys are also impaired in learning on the basis of a spatial cue a to which object to choose (e.g., if two objects are on the left, choose object A, but if the two objects are on the right, choose object B) (Gaffan and Harrison, 1989a). Further, monkeys with fornix damage are also impaired in using information about their place in an environment. For example, Gaffan and Harrison (1989b) found learning impairments when the position of the monkey in the room determined which of two or more objects the monkey had to choose. Rats with hippocampal lesions are impaired in using environmental spatial cues to remember particular places (see Jarrard, 1993, 1995), and it has been argued that the necessity to utilize allocentric spatial cues (Cassaday and Rawlins, 1997), to utilize spatial cues or bridge delays (Jackson et al., 1998), or to perform relational operations on remembered material (Eichenbaum, 1997), may be characteristic of the deficits. In recent experiments in which hippocampal cells have been damaged with ibotenic acid leaving intact fibers of passage, deficits can still be found on spatial tasks, with a particular impairment found, for example, in a "whole scene" task in which the monkey must touch a particular location in a "spatial scene" shown on a video monitor (E.Murray, personal communication).

One way of relating the impairment of spatial processing to other aspects of hippocampal function (including the memory of recent events or episodes in humans) is to note that this spatial processing involves a snapshot type of memory, in which one whole scene with its often unique set of parts or elements must be remembered. This memory may then be a special case of episodic memory, which involves an arbitrary association of a set of spatial and/or nonspatial events that describe a past episode. For example, the deficit in paired associate learning in humans (see Squire, 1992) may be especially evident when this involves arbitrary associations between words, for example window–lake.

It appears that the deficits in "recognition" memory (tested, for example, for visual stimuli seen recently in a delayed match to sample task) produced by damage to this brain region are related to damage to the perirhinal cortex, which receives from high order association cortex and has connections to the hippocampus (see Figure 10.4) (Zola-Morgan et al., 1989, 1994; Suzuki and Amaral, 1994a, 1994b). Given that some topographic segregation is maintained in the afferents to the hippocampus through the perirhinal and parahippocampal cortices (Amaral and Witter, 1989; Suzuki and Amaral, 1994a, 1994b), it may be that these areas are able to subserve memory within one of these topographically separated areas. The final convergence afforded by the hippocampus into a single network in CA3, which may operate by autoassociation (see Figure 10.4 and below), allows arbitrary associations between any of the inputs to the hippocampus, for example, spatial, visual object, auditory, and idiothetic cues such as whole body motion and eye position, which may all be involved in typical episodic memories (see below and Rolls, 1996b; Rolls and Treves, 1998). The perirhinal cortex may also play a role in learning invariant representations of objects by implementing continuing neuronal activity to provide a short-term memory trace (see below).

Neurophysiology of the Primate Hippocampus and Connected Areas

In the rat, many hippocampal pyramidal cells fire when the rat is in a particular place, as defined, for example, by the visual spatial cues in an environment such as a room (O'Keefe, 1990; 1991; Kubie and Muller, 1991). There is information from the responses of many such cells about the place where the rat is in the environment. When a rat enters a new environment B connected to a known environment A, there is a period in the order of 10 minutes in which as the new environment is learned, some of the cells that formerly had place fields in A develop instead place fields in B. It is as if the hippocampus sets up a new spatial representation that can map both A and B, keeping the proportion of cells active at any one time approximately constant (Wilson and McNaughton, 1993). Some rat hippocampal neurons are found to be more task-related, responding, for example, to olfactory stimuli to which particular behavioral responses must be made (Eichenbaum, 1997), and some of these neurons may in different experiments show place-related responses.

It was recently discovered that in the primate hippocampus, many spatial cells have responses not related to the place where the monkey is, but instead related to the place where the monkey is looking (Rolls et al., 1997a; Rolls, 1999b). These are called *spatial view cells*. These cells encode information in allocentric (world-related, as contrasted with egocentric) coordinates (Rolls et al., 1998; Georges-François et al., 1999). They can in some cases respond to remembered spatial views in that they respond when the view details are obscured, and use idiothetic cues including eye position and head direction to trigger this memory recall operation (Robertson et al., 1998). Another idiothetic input that drives some primate hippocampal neurons is linear and axial whole body motion (O'Mara et al., 1994), and in addition, the primate presubiculum has been shown to contain head direction cells (Robertson et al., 1999).

Part of the interest of spatial view cells is that they could provide the spatial representation required to enable primates to perform object-place memory (e.g., remembering where they saw a person or object, which is an example of an episodic memory) and indeed similar neurons in the hippocampus respond in object-place memory tasks (Rolls et al., 1989b). Associating together such a spatial representation with a representation of a person or object could be implemented by an autoassociation network implemented by the recurrent collateral connections of the CA3 hippocampal pyramidal cells (Rolls, 1989b, 1989c, 1996b; Rolls and Treves, 1998). Some other primate hippocampal neurons respond in the object-place memory task to a combination of spatial information and information about the object seen (Rolls et al., 1989b). Further evidence for this convergence of spatial and object information in the hippocampus is that in another memory task for which the hippocampus is needed, learning where to make spatial responses when a picture is shown, some primate hippocampal neurons respond to a combination of which picture is shown, and where the response must be made (Miyashita et al., 1989; Cahusac et al., 1993).

These primate spatial view cells are thus unlike place cells found in the rat (O'Keefe, 1979; Muller et al., 1991). Primates, with their highly developed visual and eye movement control systems, can explore and remember information about what is present at places in the environment without having to visit those places. Such spatial view cells in primates would thus be useful as part of a memory system, in that they would provide a representation of a part of space that would not depend on exactly where the monkey or human was, and that could be associated with items that might be present in those spatial locations. An example of the utility of such a representation in humans would be remembering where a particular person had been seen. The primate spatial representations would also be useful in remembering trajectories through environments, of use, for example, in short-range spatial navigation (O'Mara et al., 1994; Rolls, 1999b).

The representation of space in the rat hippocampus, which is of the place where the rat is, may be related to the fact that with a much less developed visual system than the primate, the rat's representation of space may be defined more by the olfactory and tactile as well as distant visual cues present, and may thus tend to reflect the place where the rat is. An interesting hypothesis on how this difference could arise from essentially the same computational process in rats and monkeys is as follows (see Rolls, 1999b). The starting assumption is that in both the rat and the primate, the dentate granule cells and the CA3 and CA1 pyramidal cells respond to combinations of the inputs received. In the case of the primate, a combination of visual features in the environment will over a typical viewing angle of perhaps 10 to 20 degrees result in the formation of a spatial view cell, the effective trigger for which will thus be a combination of visual features within a relatively small part of space. In contrast, in the rat, given the very extensive visual field that may extend over 180 to 270 degrees, a combination of visual features formed over such a wide visual angle would effectively define a position in space, that is, a place. The actual processes by which the hippocampal formation cells would come to respond to feature combinations could be similar in rats and monkeys, involving, for example, competitive learning in the dentate granule cells, autoassociation learning in CA3 pyramidal cells, and competitive learning in CA1 pyramidal cells (see Rolls, 1989b, 1989c, 1996b; Treves and Rolls, 1994; Rolls and Treves, 1998). Thus spatial view cells in primates and place cells in rats might arise by the same computational process but be different by virtue of the fact that primates are foveate and view a small part of the visual field at any one time, whereas the rat has a very wide visual field. Although the representation of space in rats therefore may be in some ways analogous to the representation of space in the primate hippocampus, the difference does have implications for theories, and modeling, of hippocampal function. In rats, the presence of place cells has led to theories that the rat hippocampus is a spatial cognitive map, and can perform spatial computations to implement navigation through spatial environments (O'Keefe and Nadel, 1978; O'Keefe, 1991; Burgess et al., 1994). The details of such navigational theories could not apply in any direct way to what is found in the primate hippocampus. Instead, what is applicable to both the primate and rat hippocampal recordings is that hippocampal neurons contain a representation of space (for the rat, primarily where the rat is; and for the primate, primarily of positions "out there" in space) that is a suitable representation for an episodic memory system. In primates, this would enable one to remember, for example, where an object was seen. In rats, it might enable memories to be formed of where particular objects (for example, those defined by olfactory, tactile, and taste inputs) were found. Thus, at least in primates, and possibly also in rats, the neuronal representation of space in the hippocampus may be appropriate for forming memories of events (which usually in these animals have a spatial component). Such memories would be useful for spatial navigation, for which according to the present hypothesis the hippocampus would implement the memory component but not the spatial computation component. Evidence that what neuronal recordings have shown is represented in the nonhuman primate hippocampal system may also be present in humans is that regions of the hippocampal formation can be activated when humans look at spatial views (Epstein and Kanwisher, 1998; O'Keefe et al., 1998).

Given these hypotheses, we have developed a computational theory of the operation of the hippocampus (see Rolls, 1987, 1989b, 1989c, 1990a, 1990b, 1996b; Rolls and Treves, 1998; Treves and Rolls, 1991, 1992, 1994). The ways in which LTP and LTD are thought to contribute to the operation of different parts of the hippocampal circuitry are now described, to show how the three types of networks described above may be used in this brain system.

Hippocampal Circuitry (see Fig. 10.5)

Projections from the entorhinal cortex reach the granule cells (of which there are 10^6 in the rat) in the dentate gyrus (DG) via the perforant path (pp). The granule cells project to CA3 cells via the mossy fibers (MF), which provide a *sparse* but possibly powerful connection to the 3×10^5 CA3 pyramidal cells in the rat. Each CA3 cell receives approximately 50 MF inputs, so that the sparseness of this connectivity is thus 0.005 percent. By contrast, there are many more—possibly weaker—direct pp inputs onto each CA3 cell, in the rat of the order of 4×10^3. The largest number of synapses (about 1.2×10^4 in the rat) on the dendrites of CA3 pyramidal cells is, however, provided by the (recurrent) axon collaterals of CA3 cells themselves (rc). It is remarkable that the recurrent collaterals are distributed to other CA3 cells throughout the hippocampus (Ishizuka et al., 1990; Amaral

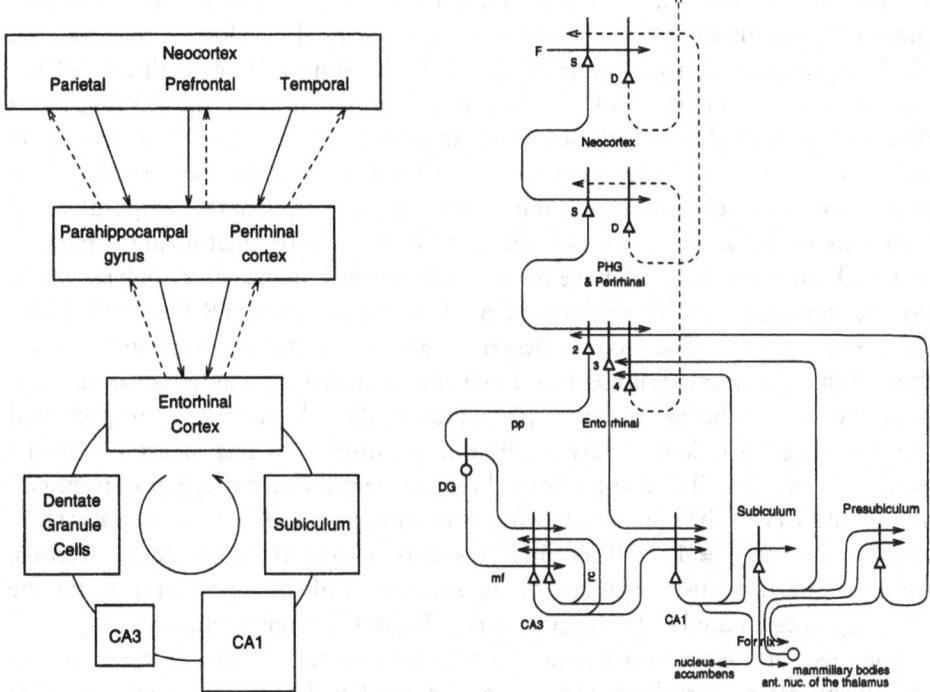

Figure 10.5. Forward connections (**solid lines**) from areas of cerebral association neocortex via the parahippocampal gyrus and perirhinal cortex, and entorhinal cortex, to the hippocampus; and backprojections (**dashed lines**) via the hippocampal CA1 pyramidal cells, subiculum, and parahippocampal gyrus to the neocortex. There is great convergence in the forward connections down to the single network implemented in the CA3 pyramidal cells, and great divergence again in the backprojections. **Left:** block diagram. **Right:** more detailed representation of some of the principal excitatory neurons in the pathways. D, Deep pyramidal cells; DG, dentate granule cells; F, forward inputs to areas of the association cortex from preceding cortical areas in the hierarchy; mf, mossy fibers; PHG, parahippocampal gyrus and perirhinal cortex; pp, perforant path; rc, recurrent collateral of the CA3 hippocampal pyramidal cells; S, superficial pyramidal cells. 2, pyramidal cells in layer 2 of the entorhinal cortex; 3, pyramidal cells in layer 3 of the entorhinal cortex. The thick lines above the cell bodies represent the dendrites.

and Witter, 1989; Amaral et al., 1990), so that effectively the CA3 system provides a single network, with a connectivity of approximately 2 percent between the different CA3 neurons given that the connections are bilateral.

CA3 As an Autoassociation Memory

Many of the synapses in the hippocampus show associative modification as shown by LTP, and this synaptic modification appears to be involved in learning (Morris, 1989). On the basis of the evidence summarized above, Rolls (1987, 1989a, 1989b, 1989c, 1990a, 1990b, 1991a, 1991b) has suggested that the CA3 stage acts as an autoassociation memory that enables episodic memories to be formed and stored for an intermediate term in the CA3 network, and that subsequently the extensive recurrent collateral connectivity allows for the retrieval of a whole representation to be initiated by the activation of some small part of the same representation (the cue). The hypothesis is that because the CA3 operates effectively as a single network, it can allow arbitrary associations between inputs originating from very different parts of the cerebral cortex to be formed. These might involve associations between information originating in the temporal visual cortex about the presence of an object, and information originating in the parietal cortex about where it is. We have therefore performed quantitative analyses of the storage and retrieval processes in the CA3 network (Treves and Rolls, 1991, 1992; Rolls et al., 1997b). The analysis described above (see Autoassociation Memory) showed that the number of memories that can be stored in an autoassociation network such as that believed to be implemented by the CA3 neurons is proportional to the number of independently modifiable synapses onto each neuron from the other CA3 neurons. The computational requirement is thus for synapse specificity of LTP and LTD if the number of different memories stored in the network is to be maximized. For $C = 12,000$ modifiable synapses from the recurrent collaterals, and $a = 0.02$ (a realistic estimate of the sparseness of the representation for the rat), p_{max} is calculated to be approximately 36,000 different memories.

For this autoassociation to operate without interference due to the positive-only firing rates of real neurons, it is also predicted that heterosynaptic LTD should be demonstrable in the CA3 to CA3 associatively modifiable synapses (Debanne et al., 1998).

In an argument developed elsewhere, we hypothesize that the mossy fiber inputs force efficient information storage by virtue of their strong and sparse influence on the CA3 cell firing rates (Treves and Rolls, 1992; Rolls, 1989a, 1989b). On the basis of this, we predict that the mossy fibers may be necessary for new learning in the hippocampus, but may not be necessary for recall of existing memories from the hippocampus. The nonassociative LTP of the mossy fiber to CA3 cell synapses is suggested to enhance the signal-to-noise ratio of the mossy fiber input: consistently firing mossy fibers will tend to produce large effects on the postsynaptic neuron (see Treves and Rolls, 1994). Experimental evidence consistent with this prediction about the role of the mossy fibers in learning has been described in mice without mossy fiber LTP associated with a lack of the mGluR1 receptor (Conquet et al., 1994; see also Lassalle et al., 2000). The issue here is that during learning it is useful to minimize (relative to the external inputs) the activation of the output neurons produced by the recurrent collaterals (because the recurrent collateral effect reflects previous memories, but not the new representations to be learned), and at the same time to increase the learning rate of the recurrent collateral synapses. Hasselmo et al. (1995), in a model that is in other respects very similar to the model just described, suggests that the cholinergic inputs to the hippocampus may have these beneficial effects.

We have also presented reasons why the direct perforant path system to CA3 (see Figure 10.5), which itself needs to be associatively modifiable, is the one involved in relaying the cues that initiate retrieval (Treves and Rolls, 1992). This set of synapses does show LTP. This perforant path to CA3 projection is hypothesized to operate effectively as a pattern associator, associating whatever firing the mossy fibers produce in the CA3 neurons with the concurrent activity on the direct perforant path inputs. Later, a fragment of the original perforant path input can act as a good retrieval cue to initiate retrieval in the CA3 autoassociation network (Treves and Rolls, 1992; Rolls, 1995).

The theory is developed elsewhere that the dentate granule cell stage of hippocampal processing acts to produce during learning the sparse yet efficient (i.e., nonredundant) representation in CA3 neurons that is required for the autoassociation to perform well (Rolls, 1989a, 1989b, 1989c; see also Treves and Rolls, 1992). One way in which it may do this is by acting as a competitive network to remove redundancy from the inputs producing a more orthogonal, sparse, and categorized set of outputs (Rolls, 1987, 1989a, 1989b, 1989c, 1990a, 1990b). This is the hypothesized function of LTP onto dentate granule cells from the perforant path input. Heterosynaptic LTD is also predicted to be here, because of its importance in competitive networks (see above).

It is suggested that the CA1 cells, given the separate parts of each episodic memory that must be separately represented in CA3 ensembles, can allocate neurons, by competitive learning, to represent at least larger parts of each episodic memory (Rolls, 1987, 1989a, 1989b, 1989c, 1990a, 1990b). This implies a more efficient representation, in the sense that when eventually after many further stages, neocortical neuronal activity is recalled (as discussed below); each neocortical cell need not be accessed by all the axons carrying each component of the episodic memory as represented in CA3, but instead by fewer axons carrying larger fragments (see Treves and Rolls, 1994).

Some of the cells with spatial responses in the primate hippocampus and presubiculum (see Rolls, 1999b) could be involved in functions other than purely episodic memory. For example, head direction and whole body motion neurons could be useful as part of a system for remembering the compass bearing (head direction) and distance traveled, to enable one, for example, to find one's way back to the origin, even with a number of sectors of travel, and over a number of minutes. This is referred to as *path integration*, and uses idiothetic cues. Spatial memory and navigation can also benefit from visual information about places being looked at, which can be used as landmarks, and spatial view cells added to the head direction cells and whole body motion cells would provide the basis for a good memory system useful in navigation. Another possibility is that primate head direction cells are part of a system for computing during navigation which direction to head toward next. For this, not only would a memory system be needed of the type elaborated elsewhere (Rolls, 1989a, 1989b, 1996a; Treves and Rolls, 1994; Rolls and Treves, 1998) that can store spatial information of the type found in the hippocampus, but also an ability to use this information in spatial computation of the appropriate next bearing would be needed. Such a system might be implemented using a hippocampal memory system that associated together spatial views, whole body motion, and head direction information. The findings described by Rolls (1999b) and Robertson et al. (1999) certainly implicate the hippocampus in the update of spatial view cells' firing produced in the dark by idiothetic cues including eye position and head direction signals. The system would be different from that in the rat (Burgess et al., 1994; McNaughton et al., 1996; Samsonovich and McNaughton, 1997), in that spatial view is represented in the primate hippocampus. In primates, the CA3 system might as part of its autoassociation function maintain firing in a continuous attractor of spatial view neurons when the spatial view is obscured (see Robertson et al., 1999), and this spatial view representation might be updated by idiothetic cues arising during eye movements and whole body motion, and anchored by visual cues when available (see Rolls, 1999b).

Although hippocampal theta-wave activity is prominent in the rat hippocampus and can influence LTP, theta is not a clear feature of hippocampal activity in macaques, even during active locomotion, as shown by field potential recordings and by autocorrelation analyses of neuronal activity (Rolls et al., 2000).

Backprojections to the Neocortex

Once information is stored in the hippocampus, it will be necessary to retrieve it at some time (as otherwise the stored information would not be useful). The retrieval may involve reinstating activity back in the cerebral neocortex corresponding to that during the storage. For example, the hippocampus may be able to recall the whole of a previously stored episode for a period of days, weeks, or months after the episode, when even a fragment of the episode is available to start the recall. This recall from a fragment of the original episode would take place particularly as a result of completion produced by the autoassociation implemented in the CA3 network. It would then be the role of the hippocampus to reinstate in the cerebral neocortex the whole of the episodic memory. The cerebral cortex would then, with the whole of the information in the episode now producing firing in the correct sets of neocortical neurons, be in a position to use the information to initiate action, or to use the recalled episodic information to contribute to the formation of new structured semantic memories.

It is suggested that during recall, the connections from CA3 via CA1 (and the subiculum) would allow activation of at least the pyramidal cells in the deep layers of the entorhinal cortex (see Figure 10.5). These neurons would then, by virtue of their backprojections to the parts of cerebral cortex that originally provided the inputs to the hippocampus, terminate in the superficial layers of those neocortical areas, where synapses would be made onto the distal parts of the dendrites of the cortical pyramidal cells (see Rolls, 1989a, 1989b, 1989c; Rolls and Treves, 1998).

The architecture with which this would be achieved is shown in Figure 10.5. The feedforward connections from association areas of the cerebral neocortex (solid lines in Figure 10.5) show major convergence as information is passed to CA3, with the CA3 autoassociation network having the smallest number of neurons at any stage of the processing. The backprojections allow for divergence back to neocortical areas. The way in which it is suggested that the backprojection synapses are set up to have the appropriate strengths for recall is as follows (see Rolls, 1989a, 1989b; Treves and Rolls, 1994). During the setting up of a new episodic memory, there would be strong feedforward activity progressing toward the hippocampus. During the episode, the CA3 synapses would be modified, and via the CA1 neurons (and the subiculum), a pattern of activity would be produced on the backprojecting synapses to the entorhinal cortex. Here the backprojecting synapses from active backprojection axons onto pyramidal cells being activated by the forward inputs to entorhinal cortex would be associatively modified. A similar process would be implemented at some at least of the preceding stages of neocortex, that is, in the parahippocampal gyrus/perirhinal cortex stage, and in association cortical areas.

How many backprojecting fibers does one need to synapse on any given neocortical pyramidal cell, in order to implement the mechanism outlined above? Treves and Rolls (1994) have shown that the maximum number of independently generated memory patterns that can be retrieved is given, essentially, by the same formula as that which applies to autoassociation networks [Eq. (7)] above

$$p \approx \frac{C}{a\ln(1/a)} k' \tag{7'}$$

where, however, a is now the sparseness of the representation at any given stage, and C is the average number of (back-) projections each cell of that stage receives from cells of the previous one (Treves and Rolls, 1991, 1994) (k' is a similar slowly varying factor to that introduced above). This shows that there should be very many backprojection fibers; in fact, there are as many as the forward projecting fibers. It is suggested that the reason for this is so that as many representations can be recalled by backprojections as can be produced by the forward inputs (Rolls, 1989a, 1989b, 1989c; Treves and Rolls, 1994). The recall process could also only operate if the backprojections are associatively modifiable, and this is therefore a prediction. It is also predicted that heterosynaptic LTD will be demonstrable in the backprojection pathways, because of its importance in what is a pattern association architecture. In addition, it also follows that the backprojection pathway should be multistage, for otherwise each CA3 (or CA1) cell would have to contact an enormous number of neocortical neurons.

It is suggested that the hippocampus is able to recall the whole of a previously stored episode for a period of days, weeks, or months after the episode, when even a fragment of the episode is available to start the recall. This recall from a fragment of the original episode would take place particularly as a result of completion produced by the autoassociation implemented in the CA3 network. It would then be the role of the hippocampus to reinstate in the cerebral neocortex the whole of the episodic memory. The cerebral cortex would then, with the whole of the information in the episode now producing firing in the correct sets of neocortical neurons, be in a position to use the information to initiate action or to use the recalled episodic information to contribute to the formation of new structured semantic memories, as described in more detail by Rolls (1996b) and Rolls and Treves (1998).

In systems of the type shown in Figure 10.5 with backprojecting synapses, not only can recall occur, but there can also be interaction between the different stages of the system. Renart et al. (1999a, 1999b) have analyzed the storage properties of such systems, and have shown that the top-down projections can usefully support the retrieval of memories in earlier stages of the system if the ratio of the strengths of the backprojection synapses to the within-layer (recurrent collateral) synapses is kept within defined bounds. This implies that LTP and LTD will need to operate with approximately similar strengths of synapses, and of synaptic modification, for the recurrent collateral and backprojection synapses.

Synaptic Modification Rules Useful in Learning Invariant Representations in the Cerebral Cortex

Neurophysiologic findings indicate that neurons in the temporal visual cortical areas can respond to objects such as faces relatively independently of where on the retina the face is shown, of its size, and even in some cases relatively independently of the view of the face (see Rolls, 1992, 1994, 1997; Wallis and Rolls, 1997; Booth and Rolls, 1998). It is suggested that these invariant representations are formed using a multilayer competitive network architecture in which each layer corresponds to one of the visual cortical areas (see Figure 10.6). In order to learn about the invariances that are characteristic of objects in the real world, it is suggested that a modified Hebb rule is used in the competitive networks. The modification involves a short-term averaging process, operating over a period in the order of 0.5 seconds. This would enable the network to associate together inputs produced by the same object seen in rapid succession on different places on the retina, in different sizes, in different views, and so forth. Because this trace of previous activation would last for only approximately 0.5 seconds, the representations of different objects would not be associated together, due to the statistics of viewing of the world. (One object is typically inspected for a short period, then the eyes move to another, etc.) The prediction described below is that in the temporal cortical areas concerned with forming invariant representations, a modified Hebbian learning rule would be present, which would include a trace of previous activation because of its utility in learning invariant representations.

To test and clarify the hypotheses just described about how the visual system may operate to learn invariant object recognition, we have performed a simulation that implements hypotheses about how the visual cortex could operate. The network simulated can perform object, including face, recognition in a biologically plausible way, and after training shows, for example, translation and view invariance (Wallis et al., 1993; Wallis and Rolls, 1997).

The synaptic learning rule used can be summarized as follows:

$$\delta w_{ij} = k \cdot m_i \cdot r'_j \tag{15}$$

and

$$m_i^t = (1 - \eta) \, r_i^{(t)} + \eta m_i^{(t-1)} \tag{16}$$

a

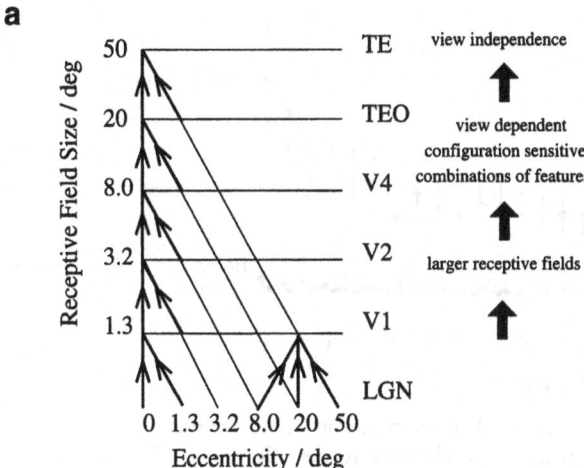

b

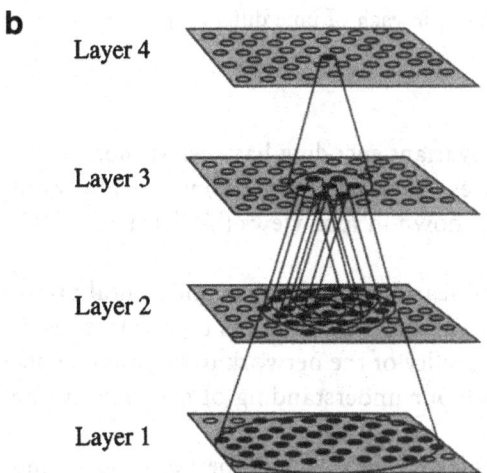

Figure 10.6. (a) Schematic diagram showing convergence achieved by the forward projections in the visual system, and the types of representation that may be built by competitive networks operating at each stage of the system from the primary visual cortex (V1) to the inferior temporal visual cortex (area TE) (see text). LGN, lateral geniculate nucleus. Area TEO forms the posterior inferior temporal cortex. The receptive fields in the inferior temporal visual cortex (for example, in the TE areas) cross the vertical midline (not shown). (b) Hierarchical network structure of VisNet.

where r'_j is the jth input to the neuron, r_i is the output of the ith neuron, w_{ij} is the jth weight on the ith neuron, η governs the relative influence of the trace and the new input (typically 0.4 to 0.6), and $m_i^{(t)}$ represents the value of the ith cell's memory trace at time t. In our simulations the neuronal learning was bounded by normalization of each cell's dendritic weight vector, as in standard competitive learning. The results of the simulations show that networks trained with the trace learning rule do have neurons with high values of the discrimination factor that measures how well a neuron discriminates between stimuli independently of loca-

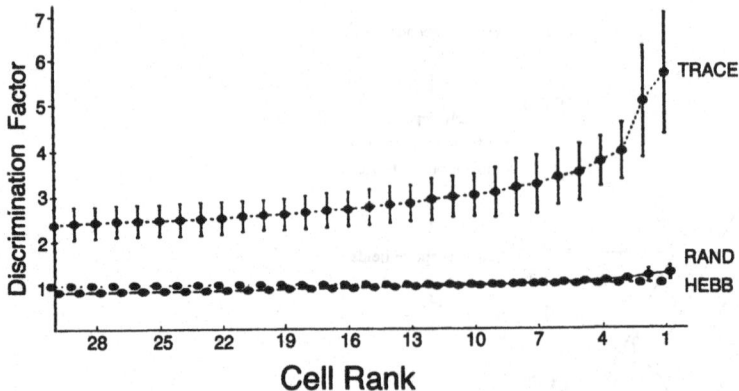

Figure 10.7. Comparison of VisNet network discrimination when trained with the trace learning rule, with a Hebb rule (No trace), and when not trained (Random). The discrimination factor, showing how well each neuron discriminated between the stimuli independently of location (see Wallis and Rolls, 1997), for the 32 most invariant neurons is shown. The network was trained with three letters (L, T, and +) in each of nine different positions on the retina.

tion (see Figure 10.7). Similar position invariant encoding has been demonstrated for a stimulus set consisting of eight faces. View invariant coding has also been demonstrated for a set of five faces each shown in four views (Wallis et al., 1993; Wallis and Rolls, 1997; Rolls, 1997).

These results show that the proposed learning mechanism and neural architecture can produce cells with responses selective for stimulus type with considerable position or view invariance. The ability of the network to be trained with natural scenes may also help to advance our understanding of encoding in the visual system.

The hypothesis is that because objects have continuous properties in space and time in the world, an object at one place on the retina might activate feature analyzers at the next stage of cortical processing, and when the object was translated to a nearby position, because this would occur in a short period (e.g., 0.5 seconds), the membrane of the postsynaptic neuron would still be in its "Hebb-modifiable" state (caused, for example, by calcium entry as a result of the voltage-dependent activation of NMDA receptors), and the presynaptic afferents activated with the object in its new position would thus become strengthened on the still-activated postsynaptic neuron. It is suggested that the short temporal window (e.g., 0.5 seconds) of Hebb-modifiability helps neurons to learn the statistics of objects moving in the physical world, and at the same time to form different representations of different feature combinations or objects, as these are physically discontinuous and present less regular correlations to the visual system. One idea here is that the temporal properties of the biologically implemented learning mechanism are such that it is well suited to detecting the relevant continuities in the world of real objects. Another suggestion is that a memory trace for what has been seen in the last 300 msec appears to be implemented by a mechanism as simple as continued firing of inferior temporal neurons after the stimulus has disappeared, as was found in the masking experiments described by Rolls and Tovee (1994) and Rolls et al. (1994; see Rolls and Treves, 1998). I also suggest that other invariances, for example, size, spatial frequency, and rotation invariance, could be learned by a comparable process. (Early processing in V1 that enables different neurons to represent inputs at different spatial scales would allow combinations of the outputs of such neurons to be formed at later stages. Scale invariance would then result from detecting at a later stage which neurons are almost conjunctively active as the size of an object alters.) It is suggested that this process takes place at each stage of the multiple-layer cortical processing hierarchy, so that invariances are learned first over small regions of space, and then over successively larger regions. This limits the size of the connection space within which correlations must be sought.

The trace process operating in conjunction with LTP/LTD described here would be useful in cortical areas involved in learning invariant representations. In the primate brain, this is the ventral visual system projecting via V1, V2, and V4 to the temporal cortical visual areas. It would not be useful in cortical mechanisms involved in motion detection, in which temporal smearing of this type might interfere with the need for precise dynamics in the system. Motion analysis operates especially in the dorsal visual system projecting from V1 via MT to MST and so forth. It is therefore predicted that a temporal trace in the synaptic modification rules may be less evident in the dorsal than the ventral visual system. The requirement for a different type of synaptic modification rule might indeed be one of the fundamental computational reasons for separation of visual processing into these two partially separate processing streams.

There have been a number of recent investigations to explore this type of learning further. In one investigation, Parga and Rolls (1998) and Elliffe et al. (2000) incorporated the associations between exemplars of the same object in the recurrent synapses of an autoassociative ("attractor") network, so that the techniques of statistical physics could be used to analyze the storage capacity of a system implementing invariant representations in this way. They showed that such networks did have an "object" phase in which the presentation of any exemplar (e.g., view) of an object would result in the same firing state as other exemplars of the same object, and that the number of different objects that could be stored is proportional to the number of synapses per neuron divided by the number of "views" of each object. Rolls and Milward (2000) explored the operation of the trace learning rule used in the VisNet architecture further, and showed that the rule operated especially well if the trace incorporated activity from previous presentations of the same object, but no contribution from the current neuronal activity being produced by the current exemplar of the object. The explanation for this is that this temporally asymmetric rule (the presynaptic term from the current exemplar, and the trace from the preceding exemplars) encourages neurons to respond to the current exemplar in the same way as they did to previous exemplars. It is of interest to consider whether intracellular processes related to LTP might implement an approximation of this rule, given that it is somewhat more powerful than the standard trace learning rule described above. Rolls and Stringer (2000a) went on to show that part of the power of this type of trace rule can be related to gradient descent and temporal difference (see Sutton and Barto, 1998) learning.

Consistent with this hypothesis, there is evidence that rapid learning is implemented in the inferior temporal visual cortex. For example, Rolls et al. (1989a) showed that neurons rapidly adjusted their responses (in 1 to 2 seconds for each stimulus) into a profile of firing to a new set of faces that enabled the neurons to discriminate between the faces, and Tovee et al. (1996) showed that neurons came to respond to ambiguous black and white images that contained faces with just a few seconds of viewing the same pictures in gray scale images in which the faces could be clearly seen. In studies designed to investigate the neural basis of semantic memory, Miyashita and colleagues (see Higuchi and Miyashita, 1996; Miyashita, 1999) have shown that inferior temporal cortex neurons can have similar responses to pairs of visual stimuli that regularly occur separated from each other by 1 to 3 seconds, and that the learning of these associations may depend on the perirhinal cortex, which has backprojections to the inferior temporal visual cortex, and which could help to produce maintained firing in response to a stimulus in the inferior temporal visual cortex (see Figure 10.4). The delays involved in these experiments are longer than those needed for learning invariant representations of objects (in which the time taken to transform from one view to another might be 100 to 500 msec), but nevertheless the fact that at least entorhinal cortex neurons can help to bridge delay periods by maintaining firing for a short period after a stimulus has disappeared (Suzuki et al., 1997) may be useful in the learning of view-invariant representations. Indeed, Buckley et al. (1998) have shown that perirhinal lesions may impair the learning of new view-invariant representations of objects. A useful hypothesis here is that the perirhinal cortex may implement a short-term attractor memory that may be useful in setting up the trace required for invariant learning, and that view invariances are either learned in the perirhinal cortex or utilize backprojections from it to enable its memory trace to support a memory trace in the inferior temporal visual cortex to implement invariance learning there.

Short-Term Memory

A common method that the brain uses to implement a short-term memory is to maintain the firing of neurons during a short memory period after the end of a stimulus. In the inferior temporal cortex this firing may be maintained for a few hundred milliseconds even when the monkey is not performing a memory task (Rolls and Tovee, 1994; Rolls et al., 1994, 1999; cf. Desimone, 1996). In more ventral temporal cortical areas such as the entorhinal cortex the firing may be maintained for longer periods in delayed match to sample tasks (Suzuki et al., 1997), and in the prefrontal cortex for even tens of seconds (see Fuster, 1997). In the dorsolateral and inferior convexity prefrontal cortex the firing of the neurons may be related to the memory of spatial responses or objects (Wilson et al., 1993;

Goldman-Rakic, 1996) or both (Rao et al., 1997), and in the principal sulcus/frontal eye field/arcuate sulcus region to the memory of places for eye movements (Funahashi et al., 1989). The firing may be maintained by the operation of associatively modified recurrent collateral connections between nearby pyramidal cells producing attractor states in autoassociative networks (Amit, 1995; Rolls and Treves, 1998; see Figure 10.3c). For the short-term memory to be maintained during periods in which new stimuli are to be perceived, there must be separate networks for the perceptual and short-term memory functions, and indeed two coupled networks, one in the inferior temporal visual cortex for perceptual functions, and another in the prefrontal cortex for maintaining the short-term memory during intervening stimuli, provides a precise model of the interaction of perceptual and short-term memory systems (Renart et al., 2000). To set up a new short-term memory attractor, synaptic modification is needed to form the new stable attractor. Once the attractor is set up, it may be used repeatedly when triggered by an appropriate cue to hold the short-term memory state active by continued neuronal firing even without any further synaptic modification (see Kesner and Rolls, 2000). Thus agents that impair LTP may impair the formation of new short-term memory states, but not the use of previously learned short-term memory states (see Kesner and Rolls, 2000).

Conclusion

The importance of some of the different properties of LTP and LTD for understanding *how* different parts of the brain compute has been described. A number of predictions about the properties of LTP and LTD in biological systems have been made. If LTP and LTD are not involved in learning, then another type of very similar synapse-specific modification of synaptic strength would be needed in the brain to implement memory and perceptual learning in the ways described here. In different brain regions the duration of LTP may be different, in order to implement, for example, long-term semantic memory in the cerebral cortex, episodic memory in the hippocampus, which may be overwritten by processes involving LTD, and short-term memory.

REFERENCES

Amaral, D.G., and Witter, M.P. (1989). The three-dimensional organization of the hippocampal formation: A review of anatomical data. *Neuroscience* 31: 571–591.

Amaral, D.G., Ishizuka, N., and Claiborne B. (1990). Neurons, numbers and the hippocampal network. *Prog. Brain Res.* 83: 1–11.

Amit, D.J. (1995). The Hebbian paradigm reintegrated: Local reverberations as internal representations. *Behav. Brain Sci.* 18: 617–657.

Bennett, A. (1990). Large competitive networks. *Network* 1: 449–462.

Bienenstock, E.L., Cooper, L.N., and Munro, P.W. (1982). Theory for the development of neuron selectivity: Orientation specificity and binocular interaction in visual cortex. *J. Neurosci.* 2: 32–48.

Booth, M.C.A., and Rolls, E.T. (1998). View-invariant representations of familiar objects by neurons in the inferior temporal visual cortex. *Cereb. Cortex* 8: 510–523.

Brown, T.H., Kairiss, E.W., and Keenan, C.L. (1990). Hebbian synapses: Biophysical mechanisms and algorithms. *Ann. Rev. Neurosci.* 13: 475–511.

Buckley, M.J., Booth, M.C.A., Rolls, E.T., and Gaffan, D. (1998). Selective visual perception deficits following perirhinal cortex ablation in the macaque. *Soc. Neurosci. Abstr.* 24: 18.

Burgess, N., Recce, M., and O'Keefe, J. (1994). A model of hippocampal function. *Neural Networks* 7: 1065–1081.

Cahusac, P.M.B., Rolls, E.T., Miyashita, Y., and Niki, H. (1993). Modification of the responses of hippocampal neurons in the monkey during the learning of a conditional spatial response task. *Hippocampus* 3: 29–42.

Cassaday, H.J., and Rawlins, J.N. (1997). The hippocampus, objects, and their contexts. *Behav. Neurosci.* 111: 1228–1244.

Conquet, F., Bashir, Z.I., Davies, C.H., Daniel, H. et al. (1994). Motor deficit and impairment of synaptic plasticity in mice lacking mGluR1. *Nature* 372: 237–243.

Davis, M. (1992). The role of the amygdala in conditioned fear. In J.P. Aggleton (Ed.), *The amygdala* (Ch. 9, pp. 255–305). New York: Wiley-Liss.

Debanne, D., Gahwiler, B.H., and Thompson, S.M. (1998). Long-term plasticity between pairs of individual CA3 pyramidal cells in rat hippocampal slice cultures. *J. Physiol.* 507.1: 237–247.

Desimone, R. (1996). Neural mechanisms for visual memory and their role in attention. *Proc. Natl. Acad. Sci. USA* 93: 13494–13499.

Eichenbaum, H. (1997). Declarative memory: Insights from cognitive neurobiology. *Ann. Rev. Psychol.* 48: 547–572.

Elliffe, M.C.M., Rolls, E.T., Parga, N., and Renart, A. (2000). A recurrent model of transformation invariance by association. *Neural Networks.* 13: 225–237.

Epstein, R., and Kanwisher, N. (1998). A cortical representation of the local visual environment. *Nature* 392: 598–601.

Funahashi, S., Bruce, C.J., and Goldman-Rakic, P.S. (1989). Mnemonic coding of visual space in monkey dorsolateral prefrontal cortex. *J. Neurophysiol.* 61: 331–349.

Fuster, J.M. (1997). *The Prefrontal Cortex* (3rd ed., p. 333). New York: Raven Press.

Gaffan, D. (1994). Scene-specific memory for objects: A model of episodic memory impairment in monkeys with fornix transection. *J. Cogn. Neurosci.* 6: 305–320.

Gaffan, D., and Saunders, R.C. (1985). Running recognition of configural stimuli by fornix transected monkeys. *Q. J. Exp. Psychol.* 37B: 61–71.

Gaffan, D., and Harrison, S. (1989a). A comparison of the effects of fornix section and sulcus principalis ablation upon spatial learning by monkeys. *Behav. Brain Res.* 31: 207–220.

Gaffan, D., and Harrison, S. (1989b). Place memory and scene memory: Effects of fornix transection in the monkey. *Exp. Brain Res.* 74: 202–212.

Georges-François, P., Rolls, E.T., and Robertson, R.G. (1999). Spatial view cells in the primate hippocampus: Allocentric view not head direction or eye position or place. *Cereb. Cortex* 9: 197–212.

Goldman-Rakic, P.S. (1996). The prefrontal landscape: Implications of functional architecture for understanding human mentation and the central executive. *Phil. Trans. R. Soc. London B* 351: 1445–1453.

Hasselmo, M.E., Schnell, E., and Barkai, E. (1995). Dynamics of learning and recall at excitatory recurrent synapses and cholinergic modulation in rat hippocampal region CA3. *J. Neurosci.* 15: 5249–5282.

Hertz, J., Krogh, A., and Palmer, R.G. (1991). *Introduction to the Theory of Neural Computation.* Wokingham, UK: Addison-Wesley.

Higuchi, S., and Miyashita, Y. (1996). Formation of mnemonic neuronal responses to visual paired associates in inferotemporal cortex is impaired by perirhinal and entorhinal lesions. *Proc. Natl. Acad. Sci. USA* 95: 739–743.

Hopfield, J.J. (1982). Neural networks and physical systems with emergent collective computational abilities. *Proc. Natl. Acad. Sci. USA* 79: 2554–2558.

Ishizuka, N., Weber, J., and Amaral, D.G. (1990). Organization of intrahippocampal projections originating from CA3 pyramidal cells in the rat. *J. Comp. Neurol.* 295: 580–623.

Jackson, P.A., Kesner, R.P., and Amann, K. (1998). Memory for duration: Role of hippocampus and medial prefrontal cortex. *Neurobiol. Learn Mem.* 70: 328–348.

Jarrard, E.L. (1993). On the role of the hippocampus in learning and memory in the rat. *Behav. Neural Biol.* 60: 9–26.

Jarrard, L.E. (1995). What does the hippocampus really do? *Behav. Brain Res.* 71: 1–10.

Kesner R.P., and Rolls, E.T. (2000). Role of long term synaptic modification in short term memory. *Hippocampus.*

Koch C. (1999). *Biophysics of Computation.* Oxford: Oxford University Press.

Kohonen, T. (1984). *Self-Organization and Associative Memory.* Berlin: Springer-Verlag.

Kubie, J.L., and Muller, R.U. (1991). Multiple representations in the hippocampus. *Hippocampus* 1: 240–242.

Lassalle, J.M., Bataille, T., and Halley, H. (2000). Reversible inactivation of the hippocampal mossy fiber synapses in mice impairs spatial learning, but neither consolidation nor memory retrieval, in the Morris navigation task. *Neurobiology of Learning and Memory.* 73: 243–257.

Levy, W.B. (1985). Associative changes in the synapse: LTP in the hippocampus. In W.B. Levy, J.A. Anderson, and S. Lehmkuble (Eds.), *Synaptic modification, neuron selectivity, and nervous system organization* (Ch. 1, pp. 5–33). Hillsdale, NJ: Erlbaum.

Levy, W.B., and Desmond, N.L. (1985). The rules of elemental synaptic plasticity. In W.B. Levy, J.A. Anderson, and S. Lehmkuhle (Eds.), *Synaptic modification, neuron selectivity, and nervous system organization* Ch. 6, pp. 105–121. Hillsdale, NJ: Erlbaum.

Marr, D. (1969). A theory of cerebellar cortex. *J. Physiol.* 202: 437–470.

McLeod, P., Plunkett, K., and Rolls, E.T. (1998). *Introduction to Connectionist Modelling of Cognitive Processes.* Oxford: Oxford University Press.

McNaughton, B.L., Barnes, C.A., Gerrard, J.L., Gothard, K. et al. (1996). Deciphering the hippocampal polyglot: The hippocampus as a path integration system. *J. Exp. Biol.* 199: 173–185.

Miyashita, Y. (1999). Visual associative long-term memory: Encoding and retrieval in inferotemporal cortex of the primate. In M. Gazzaniga (Ed.), *The cognitive neurosciences* (Ch. 27, pp. 379–392). Cambridge, MA: MIT Press.

Miyashita, Y., Rolls, E.T., Cahusac, P.M.B., Niki, H. et al. (1989). Activity of hippocampal neurons in the monkey related to a conditional spatial response task. *Behav. Brain Res.* 33: 229–240.

Morris, R.G.M. (1989). Does synaptic plasticity play a role in information storage in the vertebrate brain? In R.G.M. Morris (Ed.), *Parallel distributed processing: Implications for psychology and neurobiology* (Ch. 11, pp. 248–285). Oxford: Oxford University Press.

Muller, R.U., Kubie, J.L., Bostock, E.M., Taube, J.S. et al. (1991). Spatial firing correlates of neurons in the hippocampal formation of freely moving rats. In J. Paillard (Ed.), *Brain and space.* pp. 296–333. Oxford: Oxford University Press.

Oja, E. (1982). A simplified neuron model as a principal component analyzer. *J. Math. Biol.* 15: 267–273.

O'Keefe, J. (1979). A review of the hippocampal place cells. *Prog. Neurobiol.* 13: 419–439.

O'Keefe, J. (1990). A computational theory of the cognitive map. *Prog. Brain Res.* 83: 301–312.

O'Keefe, J. (1991). The hippocampal cognitive map and navigational strategies. In J. Paillard (Ed.), *Brain and space* (pp. 273–295). Oxford: Oxford University Press.

O'Keefe, J., and Nadel, L. (1978). *The Hippocampus as a Cognitive Map.* p. 570. Oxford: Clarendon Press.

O'Keefe, J., Burgess, N., Donnett, J.G., Jeffery, K.J. et al. (1998). Place cells, navigational accuracy, and the human hippocampus. *Phil. Trans. R. Soc. London* B 353: 1333–1340.

O'Mara, S.M., Rolls, E.T., Berthoz, A., and Kesner, R.P. (1994). Neurons responding to whole-body motion in the primate hippocampus. *J. Neurosci.* 14: 6511–6523.

Parga, N., and Rolls, E.T. (1998). Transform invariant recognition by association in a recurrent network. *Neural Comp.* 10: 1507–1525.

Parkinson, J.K., Murray, E.A., and Mishkin, M. (1988). A selective mnemonic role for the hippocampus in monkeys: Memory for the location of objects. *J. Neurosci.* 8: 4059–4167.

Petrides, M. (1985). Deficits on conditional associative-learning tasks after frontal- and temporal-lobe lesions in man. *Neuropsychologia* 23: 601–614.

Renart, A., Parga, N., and Rolls, T. (1999a). Backprojections in the cerebral cortex: Implications for memory storage. *Neural Comp.* 11: 1349–1388.

Renart, A., Parga, N., and Rolls, E.T. (1999b). Associative memory properties of multiple cortical modules. *Network* 10: 237–255.

Renart, A., Parga, N., and Rolls, E.T. (2000). A recurrent model of the interaction between the prefrontal cortex and inferior temporal cortex in delay memory tasks. *Advances in Neural Information Processing Systems* 12. (In Press).

Robertson, R.G., Rolls, E.T., and Georges-François, P. (1998). Spatial view cells in the primate hippocampus: Effects of removal of view details. *J. Neurophysiol.* 79: 1145–1156.

Robertson, R.G., Rolls, E.T., Georges-François, P., and Panzeri S. (1999). Head direction cells in the primate pre-subiculum. *Hippocampus* 9: 206–219.

Rolls, E.T. (1987). Information representation, processing and storage in the brain: Analysis at the single neuron level. In J.-P. Changeux and M. Konishi (Eds.), *The neural and molecular bases of learning* (pp. 503–540). Chichester: Wiley.

Rolls, E.T. (1989a). Information processing in the taste system of primates. *J. Exp. Biol.* 146: 141–164.

Rolls, E.T. (1989b). Functions of neuronal networks in the hippocampus and neocortex in memory. In J.H. Byrne and W.O. Berry (Eds.), *Neural models of plasticity: Experimental and theoretical approaches* (pp. 240–265). San Diego: Academic Press.

Rolls, E.T. (1989c). Parallel distributed processing in the brain: Implications of the functional architecture of neuronal networks in the hippocampus. In R.G.M. Morris (Ed.), *Parallel distributed processing: Implications for psychology and neurobiology* (Ch. 12, pp. 286–308). Oxford: Oxford University Press.

Rolls, E.T. (1990a). Principles underlying the representation and storage of information in neuronal neuronal networks in the primate hippocampus and cerebral cortex. In S.F. Zornetzer, J.L. Davis, and C. Lau (Eds.), *An introduction to neural and electronic networks* (Ch. 4, pp. 73–90). San Diego: Academic Press.

Rolls, E.T. (1990b). Theoretical and neurophysiological analysis of the functions of the primate hippocampus in memory. *Cold Spring Harbor Symp. Quant. Biol.* 55: 995–1006.

Rolls, E.T. (1990c). A theory of emotion, and its application to understanding the neural basis of emotion. *Cogn. Emot.* 4: 161–190.

Rolls, E.T. (1991a). Functions of the primate hippocampus in spatial and non-spatial memory. *Hippocampus* 1: 258–261.

Rolls, E.T. (1991b). Functions of the primate hippocampus in spatial processing and memory. In J. Paillard (Ed.), *Brain and space* (pp. 353–376). Oxford: Oxford University Press.

Rolls, E.T. (1992). Neurophysiological mechanisms underlying face processing within and beyond the temporal cortical visual areas. *Phil. Trans. R. Soc.* 335: 11–21.

Rolls, E.T. (1994). Brain mechanisms for invariant visual recognition and learning. *Behav. Proc.* 33: 113–138.

Rolls, E.T. (1995). A model of the operation of the hippocampus and entorhinal cortex in memory. *Int. J. Neural Syst.* 6 (Suppl):51–70.

Rolls, E.T. (1996a). The orbitofrontal cortex. *Phil. Trans. R. Soc. London B* 351: 1433–1444.

Rolls, E.T. (1996b). A theory of hippocampal function in memory. *Hippocampus* 6: 601–620.

Rolls, E.T. (1997). A neurophysiological and computational approach to the functions of the temporal lobe cortical visual areas in invariant object recognition. In M. Jenkin and L. Harris (Eds.), *Computational and psychophysical mechanisms of visual coding* (pp. 184–220). Cambridge: Cambridge University Press.

Rolls, E.T. (1999a). *The Brain and Emotion.* Oxford: Oxford University Press.

Rolls, E.T. (1999b). Spatial view cells and the representation of place in the primate hippocampus. *Hippocampus* 9: 467–480.

Rolls, E.T. (2000a). Memory systems in the brain. *Ann. Rev. Psychol.* 51: 599–630.

Rolls, E.T. (2000b). The orbitofrontal cortex and reward. *Cerebral Cortex.* 10: 284–294.

Rolls, E.T., and Milward, T. (2000). A model of invariant object recognition in the visual system: Learning rules, activation functions, lateral inhibition, and information-based performance measures. *Neural Comp.* 12(10): (In press).

Rolls, E.T., and Stringer, S.M. (2000a). Invariant object recognition in the visual system with error correction and temporal difference learning.

Rolls E.T., and Stringer S.M. (2000b). On the design of neural networks in the brain by genetic evolution. *Progress in Neurobiology* 61:557–579.

Rolls, E.T., and Tovee, M.J. (1994). Processing speed in the cerebral cortex and the neurophysiology of visual masking. *Proc. R. Soc. B* 257: 9–15.

Rolls, E.T., and Treves, A. (1990). The relative advantages of sparse versus distributed encoding for associative neuronal networks in the brain. *Network* 1: 407–421.

Rolls, E.T., and Treves, A. (1998). *Neural Networks and Brain Function.* Oxford: Oxford University press.

Rolls, E.T., Baylis, G.C., Hasselmo, M.E., and Nalwa, V. (1989a). The effect of learning on the face-selective responses of neurons in the cortex in the superior temporal sulcus of the monkey. *Exp. Brain Res.* 76: 153–164.

Rolls, E.T., Miyashita, Y., Cahusac, P.M.B., Kesner, R.P. et al. (1989b). Hippocampal neurons in the monkey with activity related to the place in which a stimulus is shown. *J. Neurosci.* 9: 1835–1845.

Rolls, E.T., Tovee, M.J., Purcell, D.G., Stewart, A.L. et al. (1994). The responses of neurons in the temporal cortex of primates, and face identification and detection. *Exp. Brain Res.* 101: 474–484.

Rolls, E.T., Robertson, R.G., and Georges-François, P. (1997a). Spatial view cells in the primate hippocampus. *Eur. J. Neurosci.* 9: 1789–1794.

Rolls, E.T., Treves, A., Foster, D., and Perez-Vicente, C. (1997b). Simulation studies of the CA3 hippocampal subfield modelled as an attractor neural network. *Neural Networks* 10: 1559–1569.

Rolls, E.T., Treves, A., Robertson, R.G., Georges-François, P. et al. (1998). Information about spatial view in an ensemble of primate hippocampal cells. *J. Neurophysiol.* 79: 1797–1813.

Rolls, E.T., Tovee, M.J., and Panzeri, S. (1999). The neurophysiology of backward visual masking: Information analysis. *J. Cogn. Neurosci.* 11: 335–346.

Rolls, E.T., Georges-François, P., and Robertson, R.G. (2000). The activity of interneurons in the primate hippocampus.

Rupniak, N.M.J., and Gaffan, D. (1987). Monkey hippocampus and learning about spatially directed movements. *J. Neurosci.* 7: 2331–2337.

Samsonovich, A., and McNaughton, B. (1997). Path integration and cognitive mapping in a continuous attractor neural network model. *J. Neurosci.* 17: 5900–5920.

Singer, W. (1987). Activity-dependent self-organization of synaptic connections as a substrate for learning. In J.-P. Changeux and M. Konishi (Eds.), *The neural and molecular bases of learning,* (pp. 301–335). Chichester: Wiley.

Smith, M.L., and Milner, B. (1981). The role of the right hippocampus in the recall of spatial location. *Neuropsychologia* 19: 781–793.

Squire, L.R. (1992). Memory and the hippocampus: A synthesis from findings with rats, monkeys and humans. *Psychol. Rev.* 99: 195–231.

Stent, G.S. (1973). A psychological mechanism for Hebb's postulate of learning. *Proc. Natl. Acad. Sci.* 70: 997–1001.

Sutton, R.S., and Barto, A.G. (1998). *Reinforcement Learning.* p. 322. Cambridge, MA: MIT Press.

Suzuki, W.A., and Amaral, D.G. (1994a). Perirhinal and parahippocampal cortices of the macaque monkey — cortical afferents. *J. Comp. Neurol.* 350: 497–533.

Suzuki, W.A., and Amaral, D.G. (1994b). Topographic organization of the reciprocal connections between the monkey entorhinal cortex and the perirhinal and parahippocampal cortices. *J. Neurosci.* 14: 1856–1877.

Suzuki, W.A., Miller, E.K., and Desimone, R. (1997). Object and place memory in the macaque entorhinal cortex. *J. Neurophysiol.* 78: 1062–81.

Tovee, M.J., Rolls, E.T., and Ramachandran, V.S. (1996). Rapid visual learning in neurones of the primate temporal visual cortex. *Neuroreport* 7: 2757–2760.

Treves, A., and Rolls, E.T. (1991). What determines the capacity of autoassociative memories in the brain? *Network* 2: 371–397.

Treves, A., and Rolls, E.T. (1992). Computational constraints suggest the need for two distinct input systems to the hippocampal CA3 network. *Hippocampus* 2: 189–199.

Treves, A., and Rolls, E.T. (1994). A computational analysis of the role of the hippocampus in memory. *Hippocampus* 4: 374–391.

Treves, A., Rolls, E.T., and Simmen, M. (1997). Time for retrieval in recurrent associative memories. *Physica D* 107: 392–400.

Urban, N.N., Henze, D.A., Lewis, D.A., and Barrionuevo, G. (1996). Properties of LTP induction in the CA3 region of the primate hippocampus. *Learn. Mem.* 3: 86–95.

Wallenstein, G.V., Eichenbaum, H., and Hasselmo, M.E. (1998). The hippocampus as an associator of discontiguous events. *Trends Neurosci.* 21: 317–323.

Wallis, G., Rolls, E.T., and Foldiak, P. (1993). Learning invariant responses to the natural transformations of objects. *Int. Joint Conference Neural Networks* 2: 1087–1090.

Wallis, G., and Rolls, E.T. (1997). Invariant face and object recognition in the visual system. *Prog. Neurobiol.* 51: 167–194.

Willshaw, D.J., and Longuet-Higgins, H.C. (1969). The holophone—recent developments. In D. Michie (Ed.), *Machine intelligence 4* Edinburgh: Edinburgh University Press.

Willshaw, D.J., and von der Malsburg, C. (1976). How patterned neural connections can be set up by self-organization. *Proc. R. Soc. London B* 194: 431–445.

Wilson, M.A., and McNaughton, B.L. (1993). Dynamics of the hippocampal ensemble code for space. *Science* 261: 1055–1058.

Wilson, F.A.W., O'Sclaidhe, S.P., and Goldman-Rakic, P.S. (1993). Dissociation of object and spatial processing domains in primate prefrontal cortex. *Science* 260: 1955–1958.

Zola-Morgan, S., Squire, L.R., Amaral, D.G., and Suzuki, W.A. (1989). Lesions of perirhinal and parahippocampal cortex that spare the amygdala and hippocampal formation produce severe memory impairment. *J. Neurosci.* 9: 4355–4370.

Zola-Morgan, S., Squire, L.R., and Ramus, S.J. (1994). Severity of memory impairment in monkeys as a function of locus and extent of damage within the medial temporal lobe memory system. *Hippocampus* 4: 483–494.

CHAPTER ELEVEN

Revisiting the LTP Orthodoxy

Plasticity versus Pathology

Jill C. McEachern and Christopher A. Shaw

SUMMARY

Long-term potentiation (LTP) continues to be the most intensely studied model of neuroplasticity, and is viewed by many as a substrate of learning. Other potential roles of LTP, however, have not received widespread discussion in the field. In this chapter, we will evaluate the LTP phenomena, discuss the putative connection to learning, and expand the discussion to include the participation of LTP and kindling in some forms of neuronal pathology. The available evidence appears to support a role for LTP in a continuum of events reflecting different levels of neural activity ranging from long-term depression (LTD) through LTP and kindling and culminating in cellular degeneration. In place of LTP as the substrate of learning at a neuronal level, we outline a model in which multiple levels of neural organization exert mutual control such that activity and modifiability at any level are controlled by those levels above and below.

Research is essentially a dialogue with Nature. The important thing is not to wonder about Nature's answer—for she is always honest—but to closely examine your question to her.

A. Szent-Gyorgi

Introduction

It is now over a quarter of a century since long-term potentiation (LTP) was first described (Bliss and Lomo, 1973). Initially it was viewed, rightly with great excitement, as an interesting phenomenon possibly linked to learning. Now it is

This work was supported by grants from the British Columbia Health Research Foundation and the MITACS Centre of Excellence. We thank Dr. C. Hölscher for helpful comments on an earlier version of this manuscript.

frequently declared in unqualified terms to be the "cellular basis of learning and/or memory" (e.g., "LTP is a learning mechanism," Fanselow, 1997) and its study virtually dominates the field of neuronal plasticity. Those new to the neurosciences would be forgiven for assuming that this transition occurred because the relationship between LTP and learning or memory had been experimentally demonstrated. This is not the case. The reality is a bit stranger, and may tell us more about the nature of twentieth-century science than about the mechanisms underlying learning and memory. The fact is, once the formula "LTP = memory" was written, for most neuroscientists there was no turning back and almost no attempt to question first principles (e.g., what is LTP really and, if not the basis for learning and memory, what is it?). A generation of students has passed into academia accepting the linkage of LTP to learning and memory as dogma. A few dissenting voices have been raised, but in context to literally thousands of articles on the subject, they are largely ignored. The strongest focus in today's LTP research is to understand molecular mechanisms involved in induction and maintenance processes rather than to question the physiologic relevance of a phenomenon that is typically induced artificially. Despite the technical wizardry of many of the current studies, many of the initial questions raised by the pioneers of LTP research are still being debated. Could the reason for this lie not in the failure or inadequacy of experimental technique, but rather in the questions being asked?

A reevaluation of LTP is long overdue. In 1996, we published two reviews on the LTP phenomena (McEachern and Shaw, 1996a, 1996b) and laid open to scrutiny the fundamental assumptions in the field. Since then, others have repeated these queries and proposed alternatives (Barnes, 1995; Shors and Matzel, 1997); for a comprehensive review, see also Cain, 1997; McEachern and Shaw, 1999). And, while many investigators have responded in a positive way to the challenges to orthodoxy, others have taken refuge in the repetition of familiar litanies or in overt statements of faith.

A fundamental goal of our previous articles was to address selected sources of controversy in the LTP literature in order, first, to assess the progress that had been made in understanding the molecular mechanisms of LTP, and second, to sift compelling correlations between LTP and learning or memory from vagaries of experimental technique. What we discovered, however, was that a synthesis of the LTP research was nearly impossible due to the fact that very different experimental techniques and preparations were used by different groups, and worse, variables absolutely crucial to experimental outcome were often disregarded. For example, studies frequently failed to account for the nonspecific effects of drugs, gene deletion, temperature, and motor activity; many ignored the effects of age-dependent variability; and the great majority lacked controls for the effects of test stimulus intensity. These factors, combined with the contradictory results in virtually all areas of the field, left little room to draw firm conclusions about either the function or the underlying mechanisms of LTP. In our view, the situation has not changed since that time, and to date the extent of homology between observed types of LTP, the site and nature of the alteration, the temporal progression and duration of the potentiation, and the relationship of LTP to learning and memory all remain issues of contention.

Still, it is hard to circumvent the fact that changes in synaptic strength and/or number seem to be a prerequisite for a memory model based on a population of neurons that does not show a net increase over time, even though it has proven difficult to establish this point with any certainty. Further, the previous dogma that neurons are not generated in the adult brain seems itself to be undergoing massive revision (Gould et al., 1998). This last notwithstanding, it is certainly true that various attributes of LTP make it an attractive candidate memory mechanism. It can be relatively durable, has associative properties (but see Gallistel, 1995), can be induced by stimuli approximating endogenous activity patterns, and similar increases in synaptic response may occur as a result of learning. However, a model of learning or memory with LTP as a substrate will need to account for a variety of other properties of the phenomenon.

In the following sections we will briefly attempt to deal with the issues raised above. For a more comprehensive overview of the vast LTP literature, the reader is referred to the various reviews cited in the text and the chapters in this volume (Chapters 7 and 13). We will, in addition, provide a detailed discussion of evidence supporting our contention that LTP is part of a continuum of neural events ranging from long-term depression (LTD) to neuronal degeneration. In place of the conventional view of LTP as the basis of learning, we offer a brief description of a model for neural plasticity and stability.

LTP Characteristics Pertinent to a Model of Learning or Memory: A Critique

In a recent commentary, Abraham (1997) (see also Fanselow, 1997) has reiterated some of the articles of faith that purportedly link LTP to learning and memory. In brief, they are the three key characteristics of input/synapse specificity, associativity, and persistence. Leaving aside the question of whether these characteristics are even required for learning (see Gallistel, 1995), what do their presence or absence imply for LTP either as the substrate of learning, or in other roles, for example, pathology? We will discuss these in order.

■ **Input/Synapse Specificity.** This would seem desirable in a memory mechanism, and, as cited by Abraham, often, but not always occurs for LTP. Accepting that cases where LTP is not input specific can be attributed to spread or diffusion of the effect to nonstimulated synapses or circuits, LTP would appear to satisfy this criterion. We note, however, that this does not preclude other roles for LTP. The examples of nonspecific LTP are consistent with our contention that there is a continuum of effects from more to less specific and from possibly beneficial to pathologic.

■ **Associativity.** Learning is often described as requiring the association of stimulus and response; hence if LTP underlies learning it might also show this property. Again, based on Gallistel (1995), it may or may not matter much that this is not always the case. Further, does the presence of associativity, when it does occur for LTP, mean that LTP subserves learning rather than another function? In answer, we observe that associative mechanisms are *not* unique to learning and memory, rather they are involved in various other events, including pathologic ones. For example, the ability of certain compounds to act as excitotoxins requires the simultaneous cooperative effects of different molecules in a form of chemical synergy (see Olney et al., 1990); likewise, associative processes are important in behavioral and physiologic sensitization to the effects of drugs (Wolf, 2000).

■ **Persistence.** The literature is replete with examples of different forms of potentiation, ranging from short-term to long-term. Although with some induction methods LTP is fairly long lasting, it is not permanent (Jeffery et al., 1990; Abraham et al., 1994, 1995). These observations would seem to argue against LTP *in itself* acting as a lasting physical change underlying long-term memory. Impermanence is not necessarily a fatal strike against LTP as a memory mechanism, however. The problem can be circumvented in a variety of ways, for example: (1) it can be postulated that a relatively transient form of LTP could, before decaying, trigger lasting alterations in downstream circuit behavior (e.g., through a morphologic change) that then act as the substrate for memory; (2) the argument can be made that the function of the hippocampus in memory may be most significant early on, and subsequently its role may diminish while that of other structures, possibly the cortex, becomes more important. Hippocampal LTP may be sufficiently stable to reflect the time course of this type of relationship; however, studies of cortical LTP indicate that it is not permanent either (Doyere et al., 1993), although recent studies by Trepel and Racine (1998) suggest otherwise. A problem with the latter, however, is that the field potentials recorded before and after LTP-inducing stimuli do not have the same shape. In consequence, measurements at set time intervals after the test stimuli may not measure the same responses, making comparisons in the different conditions difficult to interpret. The authors choose to interpret their data as suggesting that various late components of the field potentials are potentiated for very long periods. We think that the method of measurement used in this study makes this conclusion at best uncertain; (3) we might admit that human memories are neither permanent nor invariant across the life span (Bartlett, 1932), and mechanisms for reinvigorating molecules involved in synaptic modifications could provide the basis for the longevity of certain memories (Kavanau, 1994). If LTP were to be periodically refreshed, or alternatively, served as a transient triggering mechanism for downstream changes, then it would be more compatible with the durability of memory.

In regard to the issue of persistence, one must also address the long-term physiologic consequences of a persistent increase in response amplitude which in other circumstances appears to be pathologic, for example, as occurs in kindling and with excitotoxic stimulation (for primary references see citations in McEachern and Shaw, 1999). Overall, the characteristic of persistence for LTP in relation to memory remains uncertain at best in most circumstances and likely to prove pathologic in others.

Taken together, these criteria linking LTP with learning seem ambiguous: nice to have when present, loose enough to steer around when not present. Moreover, these criteria are not inconsistent with other very different roles of LTP, including developmental and/or pathologic actions.

In addition to these three often mentioned key criteria, other characteristics and issues must be adequately explained in any theory of LTP-based learning or memory. These are briefly discussed below.

■ **Depotentiation/Reversal of LTP.** The fact that LTP can be depotentiated (reversed) is pertinent to the issue of the permanence and hence suitability of LTP as a memory mechanism. LTP induced *in vitro* and *in vivo* in the hippocampus (Larson et al., 1993; Holscher et al., 1997a,b; Martin, 1998) and *in vivo* in the afferent system to the prefrontal cortex (Burette et al., 1997) can be reversed by various patterns of low-frequency stimulation, and within time windows varying from only minutes to the longest experimental time point measured (hours). In some of these experiments (Larson et al., 1993; Holscher et al., 1997a,b), LTP reversal was possible with theta-frequency stimulation. The ability of the theta rhythm, a pattern of neural activity that accompanies certain forms of activity in the behaving animal, to both induce and reverse LTP suggests that if LTP is to serve a role in memory, then either safeguards must protect against LTP reversal except in special conditions, or, as we suggest, LTP is meant to persist only transiently before being reversed by ongoing neural activity and regulatory processes. Others suggest that the return of a subset of potentiated synapses to baseline activity levels might function to enhance detail in newly encoded representations (Larson et al., 1993) or to prevent "saturation" of synaptic plasticity (Doyere et al., 1993). Whatever the postulated function of LTP reversal, a theory of LTP-based long-term memory must be capable of accounting for the seeming instability of a process previously considered essentially irreversible during the maintenance phase.

■ **Distribution and Nature of LTP.** The prototypical form of LTP is the NMDA receptor-dependent version first discovered in the hippocampus. Joining this "classical" form we now have various NMDA- and non–NMDA-dependent forms in the hippocampus and many other structures, including, in mammals, spinal cord (Randic et al., 1993), superior cervical ganglion (Burgos et al., 1994), and medial geniculate nucleus (Gerren and Weinberger, 1983). Furthermore, LTP-like increases in neural response are observed in anoxia (Hammond et al., 1994), kindling (Racine and Cain, 1991), and drug addiction (Wolf, 2000). The discovery that LTP can be induced in structures and circumstances not conventionally associated with higher vertebrate learning and memory function means either that the definitions of these processes must be broad enough to encompass such atypical forms, or that if LTP occurs physiologically, it serves functions other than, or in addition to, learning and memory.

■ **Saturation of Plasticity.** One problem in linking LTP, a potentiated response, to learning is that of saturation (i.e., what happens when the system is fully potentiated?). It is difficult from reading most articles on LTP to avoid the impression that the mechanisms of LTP magnitude are viewed as analogous to information storage in a computer hard drive: once full, the system can receive no more information and memory must be deleted (or stored elsewhere; see below). For LTP does this mean that no further modifications are possible for both the synapse and cell, and what does that imply for the saturation of learning? In answer to this, we note that experiments on learning that employed massive synaptic stimulation to saturate LTP have given inconclusive results (for primary citations, see Chapter 7 in this volume; see also Cain, 2000). As in other cases cited in the previous sections, one can make various ad hoc hypotheses to avoid what is an obvious problem for learning based on a mechanism that employs magnitude of response size/activity, particularly if the latter has a potentially pathologic consequence at the high end. One could, for example, cite evidence for morphologic alterations that follow as downstream consequences of short-term alterations in activity, and claim that the latter, not the former is the substrate of learning. Indeed, this could well be correct, but does little to address the problem of LTP saturation. In fact, such an explanation would further serve to de-link LTP as the substrate of learning. The same critique holds for attempts to argue that LTP is initially expressed at one site, but that the information (learning) is distributed to another site (e.g., hippocampus versus cortex). In summary, a direct link between LTP and learning would require saturation of both LTP and learning. In turn, depotentiation should reset both to lower levels. Even if experimental data existed to support these points, the overall problem of saturation for learning would not be solved. In contrast, alterations in morphology or distribution would allow an "out" for the latter, but would lend support to our contention that LTP and learning are not strictly linked.

Exploring the "Nuts and Bolts" of Potential Synaptic Modifications in LTP: Implications

Leaving aside for the moment the relevance of LTP at the behavioral level, it may be valuable to consider the types of modification that may be possible at the synaptic level, and the potential consequences of each. When thinking about signal transduction at a chemical synapse (comprising the majority of synapses between neurons in the brain), the choices for modification fall into a limited number of categories. Basically, alterations can be presynaptic, postsynaptic, both, or "extra-synaptic" (e.g., sprouting or activating new or silent synapses or new cell birth). Of the presynaptic changes, the choices are alterations in neurotransmitter released, by increases in quantal size or rate, or both. Postsynaptically, the choice is between alterations in neurotransmitter receptor characteristics (number, affinity, location, active versus nonactive, etc.) or in structural modifications of the postsynaptic membrane acting to make transmission more effective. The debate over site of modification has raged for as long as LTP has been known, with no resolution to date. Some parties have favored presynaptic modifications, some postsynaptic changes, both receptor-based and structural, and some have tried to incorporate both pre- and postsynaptic elements. The issue is not resolved and contradictory data have accumulated for each position (see references in McEachern and Shaw, 1996a). In spite of this, or maybe because of it, few investigators have explored the implications of such possible modifications for long-term cellular function. In the following, we address this issue.

■ **Presynaptic Modifications.** Presynaptic modifications in quantal size or frequency could account for alterations in response amplitude such as those observed with LTP. However, presynaptic alterations would not occur *in vacuo* and thus would have "downstream" consequences for synaptic function as a whole. Specifically, we would expect that alterations in neurotransmitter release would, over time, induce regulation of target postsynaptic receptor populations. As a general rule, such regulation appears to be homeostatic (see Pasqualotto and Shaw, 1996, for discussion and citations; see also McEachern and Shaw, 1999), decreasing receptor number when neurotransmitter release is high, and increasing receptor number when it is low. In brief, greater neurotransmitter stimulation, as would occur when quantal size and/or frequency increases should lead to a decrease in receptor number in adult neurons. Hence the consequence of such enhanced release might initially be a larger amplitude response on the postsynaptic side, but only until receptor regulation gets switched on. Since receptor regulation, at least when mediated by phosphorylation reactions, occurs within a time frame of seconds to minutes, the induced potentiation should decrease over the same time frame. Indeed, for some forms of LTP (see above), this appears to be the case. Two other forms of receptor regulation might also be expected to result from increased transmitter release, notably channel desensitization and altered mRNA expression for receptor protein (see Pasqualotto and Shaw, 1996, for citations), both of which appear to operate with much the same feedback logic. In brief, it is difficult to see how the system could avoid such regulatory modulation if the initial event were a change in neurotransmitter release. One possibility that must be considered, however, is a small change in quantal release that might affect excitatory postsynaptic potential (EPSP) "failure rate" rather than general synaptic amplitude (Stevens and Wang, 1994). Thus one of three major possibilities must arise: (1) Whatever LTP is or induces, it escapes or violates normal feedback mechanisms observed to control receptor characteristics that occur at higher levels of quantal release; (2) a subset of this first possibility may be that age-related differences in the direction of regulation allow such modifications to be induced in young animals; or (3) the mechanism of LTP is not primarily one of presynaptic alterations in neurotransmitter release. In regard to (1) and (2), we have previously reported such age-dependent alterations in regulation that could, in principle, account for an upregulation of receptors in the presence of increased neurotransmitter in "young" neurons (Shaw et al., 1994), and we note that many LTP experimenters indeed use young animals (see McEachern and Shaw, 1996a; see also below). Of course, this explanation would not account for LTP in adults. The overall consequence of a failure to homeostatically regulate receptor number is the potentially harmful consequence of increased current flux into affected neurons: AMPA receptors flux primarily sodium ions (with some calcium ions), which in hydrated form will lead to cell swelling; NMDA receptors will carry calcium into the cell, activating various protein kinases and proteolytic enzymes, and so forth (Obrenovich and Urenjak, 1997). Any cell with maintained, excessive, current flow would be at risk for death (McEachern and Shaw, 1999).

The last of the above possibilities is that presynaptic alterations are not involved in LTP generation, leading to the following.

■ **Postsynaptic Modifications.** As above, two possibilities arise: receptor function is enhanced by increasing receptor number or affinity, or postsynaptic structural modifications are induced; either or both could augment synaptic current flow (i.e., increased synaptic EPSP response amplitude more rapidly reaching spike threshold and likely culminating in an increase in neuronal response rate). As above, increased postsynaptic receptor function could lead to excitotoxicity and cell death, depending on how close the range of activation brings the neuron to the pathologic levels of current influx. Structural changes affecting the shape of synaptic elements and configurations could also lead to larger amplitude EPSP/rate of response, but data in support of this possibility remain controversial (Geinisman et al., 1995; Sorra and Harris, 1998).

■ **"Extra-synaptic" Modification.** Whether or not LTP is associated with the creation of "new infrastructure," e.g., activation of silent synapses, sprouting, or new cell birth, is another contentious subject (e.g., Geinisman et al., 1991, vs. Sorra and Harris, 1998). But as long as such changes do not produce a net current exceeding excitotoxic tolerance, they might provide a viable method of enhancing neural activity. This idea is discussed in greater detail below (p. 278).

■ **Kindling, LTP, and Receptor Regulation.** It may be instructive to consider the phenomenon of kindling, which could be thought of as an extreme form of plastic alteration along a continuum of LTP-like effects. First described by Goddard (1967), kindling is observed in animals given repeated electrical stimuli in any of various brain nuclei. The electrical stimuli are delivered at an intensity below that which can initially induce seizures, yet as the number of stimuli accumulates over the course of days, seizure activity begins to be manifest as epileptic-like neural discharges and motor symptoms of increasing severity. Behaviorally, the animals appear to mimic many of the stages of temporal lobe epilepsy. Once animals have received upward of 150 electrical stimuli, seizures may become "spontaneous," that is, they occur even in the absence of an externally initiated stimulus. Once induced, the kindling-related effects are long-lasting, and motor seizures can be reevoked even following an extended period in the absence of further electrical stimuli. Kindling thus appears to represent a long-term synaptic/circuit modification of neural response following repeated stimulation. Some of the modifications that occur in kindling may involve cell death (Cavazos et al., 1994).

In many respects, kindling resembles LTP, a point made by other investigators (for citations, see McEachern and Shaw, 1996a; Teskey and Valentine, 1998). In regard to this, we have attempted to place LTP and kindling into a continuum of events ranging from transient neural potentiations all the way through to excitotoxic cell death. Correct or not, the similarities between LTP and kindling are strong enough to be worth examining in more detail, particularly at the "nuts and bolts" level. Much of our recent work has attempted to extend the correlations between LTP and kindling to changes in ionotropic receptor characteristics. Just as questions have been raised about the potential for receptor modifications to underlie LTP, the more massive effects of kindling suggest that receptor modifications, if they occur, should be even more pronounced than might be expected for LTP (see McEachern and Shaw, 1999). For kindling, the literature is also divided on this point, but most studies to date have used kindling paradigms of less than 100 stimuli. We have reexamined the issue for the various ionotropic receptors that govern both fast excitatory (AMPA and NMDA) and inhibitory (GABA$_A$) synaptic transmission in rats with varying numbers of stimuli to the amygdala and we observed the following: For AMPA receptors, the first five stimuli give the largest change in receptor number, with a total decrease of approximately 30 percent. Animals given more stimuli show a general trend to smaller levels of regulation (McEachern and Shaw, 1999). While various interpretations are possible for these data, what they resemble is a "normal" homeostatic form of receptor regulation that we have previously observed for AMPA receptors in a slice preparation (Pasqualotto et al., 1996). In other words, the excitatory stimulations initially lead to a decrease in receptor number. As the downregulation of the receptors wanes with continuing stimulation, the seizures become more pronounced. This result suggests that increasing numbers of stimuli override the normal mechanisms of homeostatic receptor regulation such that the progressive failure allows the development of an increasingly pathologic form of plasticity in which seizures and perhaps cell death result.

Overall, the above discussion should have raised concerns about the consequences of particular ways of altering synaptic machinery, in particular the potential to generate excitotoxic events. But if not one of these, how can synapses be altered to reflect alterations in synaptic input? In the last section of this chapter we will touch on what we believe to be the answer to this question, namely by a transient, rather than permanent, modification in synaptic properties that is manifest as an alteration in the response of the cell and circuit in which it resides.

Relevance of LTP to Learning/Memory

The property of LTP that has perhaps received relatively less overall experimental attention than it warrants, especially given its importance, is its potential relevance to behavior, this last generally taken to refer to learning and/or memory. We previously raised the following points on this subject (McEachern and Shaw, 1996a), which to our knowledge remain unanswered by those who continue to make definitive statements about the connection between LTP and learning or memory: Much of the experimental evidence cited as the strongest support for a link between LTP and learning or memory is rendered inconclusive due to failure to account for critical experimental variables such as animal age, and nonspecific effects of pharmacologic, genetic, or behavioral manipulations. We will leave most of this discussion to the other authors of this volume (e.g., see Chapter 7), but will consider a few points we consider most crucial.

■ **Correlations Based on Pharmacologic Manipulations.** Pharmacologic interventions with NMDA receptor antagonists that block both LTP and learning or memory in certain tasks seemed to provide a promising correlation between molecular and behavioral neuroplasticity (e.g., Morris et al., 1986; Robinson et al., 1989; Staubli et al., 1989). However, upon close inspection, the drugs used in these studies were found to cause insurmountable nonspecific effects on neural activity (Keith and Rudy, 1990; Hargreaves and Cain, 1992). More recently, two sets of findings have further weakened the correlation between LTP and learning/memory based on the ability of drugs to block both simultaneously. First, it has been found that pretraining the sensory and motor elements of a spatial learning task allowed rats to overcome what was previously assumed to be a deficit in both LTP and (as a result) spatial learning (Bannerman et al., 1995; Saucier and Cain, 1995). Second, pharmacologic *dissociation* of LTP and learning has been observed, where LTP is blocked and learning is unaffected, or vice versa (Riedel et al., 1995; Hölscher et al., 1996). Overall, no rightful claim can be made either that learning/memory and the underlying molecular substrates were specifically blocked, or that an unambiguous link between LTP and learning/memory has been demonstrated in these experiments.

■ **Correlations Based on Genetic Manipulations.** Similarly, various genetic deletion models have been created in which animals develop without the gene encoding a protein considered important in neuroplastic processes, for instance, a receptor subtype or a protein kinase (Grant et al., 1992; Silva et al., 1992a, 1992b; Aiba et al., 1994). Again, an LTP-learning/memory link was proclaimed based on the corresponding failure of measures of both LTP and learning or memory in the mutants. Once again, the nonspecific effects prevent such a conclusion: Thorough testing of the mutants in various experiments demonstrated severe changes in morphologic, electrophysiologic, and behavioral attributes as a result of gene deletion during development (Grant et al., 1992; Butler et al., 1993; Aiba et al., 1994; McNamara, 1994; Stevens et al., 1994). This should not be all that surprising given that genes and their products directly and indirectly mediate multiple functions and regulatory processes, both during development and in the mature brain, and that gene deletion disrupts all of these. An additional confound of developmental gene deletion is that it will not be possible to untangle effects of deletion on normal development from effects on adult nervous system function and plasticity. However, these experiments continue to be cited as proof that LTP is the substrate of learning and/or memory despite the ambiguity of their interpretation. A recent improvement in this technique is the genetic "knock-down," which eliminates the developmental effects of gene deletion, putting the experimental results on par with those from pharmacologic blockade correlation experiments (see arguments presented above).

■ **Spurious Correlations.** LTP is now so closely associated with NMDA receptor action and response increase that it is sometimes forgotten that they are not necessarily synonymous. The necessity for NMDA receptor function during a learning or memory task is often equated with the necessity for LTP, in some cases even when neural activity is not measured. Similarly, the label "LTP" is often put on any observed increase in response, regardless of whether there is any measurement of its longevity (e.g., Izquierdo, 1994; Fanselow, 1997).

Age Dependence and LTP

Much of the neuroplasticity literature suffers from a fundamental and, we believe, fatal flaw; namely, the failure to treat age as a critical variable in studies of LTP phenomenology and possible behavioral relevance. This flaw produces two sets of problems. The first arises as a result of the fact that experimental age has an enormous impact upon several characteristics of LTP, including ease of induction, amount, duration, and induction of LTD versus LTP by a given stimulation. Furthermore, the molecular mechanisms underlying LTP expression differ at different ages (for primary citations, see McEachern and Shaw, 1996a, 1999). Because experimental age is not standard among researchers, any attempt to synthesize the vast literature into an overall view of the nature and mechanisms of LTP is precluded.

The second set of problems is due to the likelihood that neuroplastic modifications serve a developmental function in young animals in addition to or even *separate* from their actions in the adult central nervous system (CNS). The problem, then, is dissociating developmental plasticity subserving genetically programmed and activity-dependent "wiring-up" processes from the concomitant neuroplastic changes subserving learning and memory in young animals. That is, it will be difficult to correlate any LTP effect observed in a young animal specifically to learning and/or memory, as is often claimed in the literature. The following discussion will develop these points in greater detail.

In much of the LTP literature, the assumption that LTP is the substrate of various types of behavioral neuroplasticity is taken for granted. While we do not accept this view, we will for the moment allow it to stand. Just how important is the variable of age to neuroplasticity? We note, first, that age-dependent forms of neuroplasticity have been widely documented in a great number of mammalian neural circuits and systems (for a review see Shaw et al., 1994). Early postnatal life often contains various "critical periods," and it is in just such periods that the dynamics of neuronal modification appear to be most pronounced. It is quite widely acknowledged that age-dependent modifications of neuronal activity and function occur in large part because of the very dramatic alterations in neuronal structure and biochemistry that occur during development and aging. Included in a partial list of differences between young and adult CNS are fluctuations in synaptic number and distribution (Aghajanian and Bloom, 1967; Blue and Parnavelas, 1983), growth and/or retraction of dendritic branches (see Movshon and Van Sluyters, 1981), modifications of the postsynaptic density (Rao et al., 1998), and a vast array of changes in pre- and postsynaptic receptor characteristics (see Shaw, 1996). To expand upon just the latter, age-dependent receptor modifications can involve a range of rather fundamental features, each of which would be expected to have a major impact on neuronal functions involved in activity-dependent modifications. Of these, receptor modifications leading to changes in cell sensitivity (e.g., number and affinity) are obvious. Additionally, however, many receptor populations undergo rather profound alterations in overall regional and cellular distribution. In concert with alterations in number, changing distributions affect the ratios of the various populations, leading inevitably to alterations in cellular response properties. Further, channel kinetics and ionic dependence may be developmentally affected, often by changes in subunit composition (Burnashev et al., 1992). Not least, second messenger type and coupling to receptors appear to be in flux during development as do the activities of the various protein kinases and phosphatases that act to modulate receptor function. This last has as an immediate consequence a major effect on amount and *direction* of receptor regulation. As we have described elsewhere (Shaw et al., 1994), similar stimuli produce *opposite* effects on a number of receptor populations as a function of age. To illustrate, sustained cellular depolarization reduces excitatory AMPA receptors and increases inhibitory $GABA_A$ receptors in adult rat cortex, yet in young cortex the same stimulus increases AMPA and reduces $GABA_A$ receptor numbers. In other words, the effects of such stimulation will be to reduce excitability in the adult cortex while increasing it in the young. It is rather difficult to imagine that such age-dependent dynamics could fail to have a significant impact on the short- and long-term neuronal response to LTP-inducing stimulation. The rather routine need to suppress $GABA_A$ receptor function before inducing LTP in many adult neural circuits would seem to support this point (see, for example, Artola and Singer, 1987). While the above example has provided details only for age-dependent differences in the regulation of receptors, equally profound modifications of features of neuronal structure, biochemistry, and function can also be found in abundance.

Without question, such differences must be addressed by those attempting to find the underlying mechanism and physiologic role of LTP, and must call into question any simple assumption that LTP in its various forms and underlying mechanisms can be studied independently of age. Given this, it is remarkable that many in the LTP field choose to proceed as if this were not the case. As cited in our previous reviews (McEachern and Shaw, 1996a, 1999), some workers in the field routinely ignore the issue altogether, mixing experimental ages or even failing to cite them. Young animals are preferred for neuroplasticity research because of the greater ease of manipulation and preparation of tissue from these animals, and because of the apparently greater viability of the tissue in acute experiments. In addition, young brain tissues usually give more robust, clearer LTP. The reasons for this are not clear, but it may be due to less anoxic damage during preparation, a legitimately greater level of LTP, or both. What makes this situation even more remarkable is that workers in the field can hardly be ignorant of the widespread descriptions of age-dependent LTP (Harris and Teyler, 1984; Kamal et al., 1998; Ito et al., 1999), which appears to display properties in young that differ in important ways from adults. The net result of all of this is that there is no way to determine from the current literature if LTP in adult neurons is closely related to that in younger animals in either induction parameters, durability, amount, mechanism, or function. Rather, the few studies that do exist in which young and adult LTP are compared suggest significant differences (McEachern and Shaw, 1996a, 1999). Regarding induction, some workers would clearly hope that age differences could be resolved simply (e.g., by the notion that optimum parameters of stimulation may vary as a function of age while leaving the basic mechanisms and function the same). This may, in fact, be true, but experiments have not to our knowledge been done to demonstrate it. The absence of such experiments leaves open the real prospect that LTP mechanisms and function studied in developing animals may bear little or no relation to that in adults. As such, the nature and mechanisms of LTP in young animals should not be presented as a general template of neuroplasticity, as is the case when age is not reported. A concerted effort should also be made to more systematically compare LTP induced at different developmental stages. A few recent studies have made an effort to address this issue (Norris et al., 1996; Kamal et al., 1998; Ito et al., 1999).

The attempt to formulate strong correlations between LTP and learning or memory based on studies in young animals is problematic is because aspects of development add many nonspecific variables to the equation, only one of which is activity-dependent neuroplasticity. It is clear that developmental alterations in neuronal function are not solely activity-dependent. Rather, neuroplastic modifications in development play out against a background of evolving genetic instruction in dynamic interplay with experience. Developmental alterations of the nervous system involve large-scale remodeling of synapses and neural cells, during which both synapses and neurons are added and removed as an animal develops. In contrast, large-scale neural death and remodeling in adulthood is considered to be a consequence of pathology and, although it now seems that neurons are born continuously in some regions of the nervous system throughout life (Gould et al., 1998), it will be obvious that replacing some neurons in a circuit is not the same as the large-scale process of circuit formation in the young brain.

LTP and Learning/Memory: Conclusions

The results from many of the correlational experiments attempting to link LTP and learning/memory are highly ambiguous due to the nonspecific effects of animal age, and genetic and pharmacologic manipulations. But what is the alternative? In our view, it is to take advantage of protocols that study plasticity mechanisms used by intact animals performing a behaviorally relevant task. Some carefully performed experiments are making strides toward understanding naturally occurring plasticity mechanisms, either by investigating lasting behavioral learning-induced changes later *in vitro* (McKernan and Shinnick-Gallagher, 1997), or by using multisite recording *in vivo* in behaving animals (Freeman, 1994; Chrobak and Buzsaki, 1998). Such protocols are a rich potential source of data on contextually relevant changes in neuroplasticity at multiple levels of organization from behavior, natural brain wave activity, and sensory map alterations down to synaptic mechanisms.

Relationship of LTP and LTD to Plasticity and Pathology: A Continuum Model

The following section presents a brief review of the plasticity-pathology continuum model. A more detailed version can be found in McEachern and Shaw (1999).

■ **Overview.** A close look at the literature led us to believe that the terms LTP and LTD are used as a catch-all to encompass a spectrum of activity-potentiating and -depressing phenomena of varying function, duration, and underlying biochemical substrates. While artificially induced forms of LTP and LTD may serve many functions, or none, in the behaving animal, researchers may have tapped into a range of naturally occurring processes that serve to adjust synaptic strength in a multitude of ways, and which contribute to a variety of processes, both beneficial and pathologic. LTP- and LTD-like alterations in synaptic efficacy may be employed throughout the CNS in whatever context is required (Teyler, 2000), including neuronal migration, synaptic connection, and setting response levels during early development; laying down sensory and motor schemata; repairing damage; as well as recording experience.

■ **Plasticity-Pathology Relationship.** Interestingly, many of the characteristics and molecular mechanisms involved in LTP and LTD, considered by many to be substrates of beneficial behavioral outcomes such as learning and memory, are strikingly similar to the underlying pathologic changes that may lead to epileptogenesis. The concept of a link between physiologic and pathologic plasticity is not new. Parallels have previously been recognized between LTP and neuronal degeneration (Lynch and Seubert, 1989); among LTP, cell migration, trophic interactions, seizures, and ischemia (Hammond et al., 1994; Ben Ari, 1995); and between mechanisms that mediate neuronal sprouting during normal development and those described in Alzheimer's disease (Cotman et al., 1990; Neill, 2000). Parallels between LTD, LTP, and kindling exist at many levels. For example, similar patterns of high-frequency stimulation trains lead in each case to persistent alterations in synaptic activity levels. Further, the mechanisms involved in induction and maintenance of all three phenomena include elements of the glutamatergic excitatory transmission system and associated intracellular signaling cascades. Recruitment of the NMDA receptor (but note that NMDA receptor-independent forms of each exist) and an elevation of internal calcium ion concentration are often important in the induction phase, and AMPA receptor activity contributes to the expression of each (Bliss and Collingridge, 1993). The activity of mGlu receptors (Linden, 1994); protein kinases (Stevens et al., 1994); phosphatases (Mulkey et al., 1994); neurotrophic factors (Sazgar et al., 1995); gene transcription (Qian et al., 1993); and synthesis of new protein (Abraham and Otani, 1991; Bliss and Collingridge, 1993) have been implicated in all three forms of neuroplasticity. In addition, the various forms of neuroplasticity and the cellular response to trauma all appear to stimulate activation of some of the same immediate early genes and gene products (Hughes et al., 1999). Additional lines of support indicate an overlap of biochemical mechanisms subserving LTD and LTP. First, there is a parallel time course of onset and maintenance, and, more convincingly, saturation of LTP can be fully reversed by subsequent induction of LTD, and vice versa, without affecting the maximal level of either. Were the initial induction mechanisms distinct, at most a partial reversal would be achieved and the attainable ceiling for each would be altered by serial inductions (Dudek and Bear, 1993).

The relationship between LTP and kindling is a subject of ongoing investigation. The discovery that electrical (Sutula and Steward, 1986) and chemical kindling are accompanied by a lasting potentiation of measures of synaptic efficacy in a manner thought by some to resemble "classical" LTP (Ben Ari and Gho, 1988) led to the proposal that LTP might serve as the cellular mechanism of kindling (Collingridge and Bliss, 1987). In addition, the morphologic synaptic modifications accompanying some forms of LTP and kindling are similar (Geinisman et al., 1991). However, a variety of sources report discrepancies between the two phenomena; the most important in our view is the fact that repeated induction of LTP without an after-discharge does not induce kindling (Sutula and Steward, 1987).

These and other observations indicate that LTP is alone insufficient to explain the mechanisms of kindling. Kindling is, however, a multifaceted phenomenon measured in part by behavioral criteria including motor seizures. Nevertheless, it is evident that LTP can contribute to kindling. When LTP is first induced in the perforant path, the number of stimulations subsequently required to induce kindling is diminished (Sutula and Steward, 1986). It has also been discovered that kindling can both be prevented from developing and reversed by low-frequency stimulation similar to that used to induce LTD or depotentiation of LTP (Weiss et al., 1995). Like LTP, there are multiple forms of kindling with distinct characteristics (Lothman and Williamson, 1994), possibly reflecting different protocols and sites of delivery of kindling stimulation and subserved by cascades with unique molecular components or interactions.

In view of the mutual facilitation between LTP and kindling, we speculate that the induction of certain forms of LTP can contribute directly to kindling of abnormal activity, or can trigger processes that increase susceptibility to kindling under the influence of additional factors. Interpolating back to the overlap between mechanisms of LTP and LTD, we are presented with the conundrum that activation of an initially similar subset of the cellular "machinery" (i.e., the glutamatergic system) can produce widely divergent effects on synaptic activity. These range from depressed activity (LTD) and an intermediate degree of enhancement (LTP), to the pathologic case of excessive, synchronous firing (kindling). The physiologic basis for the divergence in outcome is unknown, and cannot be simply related to the magnitude of the rise in internal calcium (McEachern and Shaw, 1996a, 1999).

■ **Plasticity-Induced Neuronal Degeneration: Kindling and LTP.** As indicated above, the kindling process can result in neuronal death. The damage can be mediated by the kindling stimulation itself when the protocol employs intense stimulations and short interstimulus intervals (rapid kindling), or can be caused or exacerbated by seizure activity (Wasterlain and Shirasaka, 1994). A persistent enhancement of synaptic activity level as a result of induction of some forms of LTP may also trigger changes that, especially in combination with other stressors (see below), contribute to neuronal degeneration. At this point it becomes necessary to be more precise in our treatment of the "umbrella term" LTP. This is because the specific *underlying mechanism* of response enhancement in LTP is very relevant from the standpoint of possible pathologic outcome. Neuronal damage is well known to occur as a result of excitotoxic overactivation of receptors mediating excitatory neurotransmission (Cavazos et al., 1994; Lipton and Rosenberg, 1994; Wasterlain and Shirasaka, 1994) and the concomitant increase in intracellular ion levels. Excessive influx of sodium ions (Na^+) can pull in water molecules and result in lysis of neuronal membranes (Obrenovitch and Urenjak, 1997) and high intracellular calcium (Ca^{2+}) levels activate potentially fatal degradative processes (Lipton and Rosenberg, 1994). Neuronal degeneration may also proceed through extended activation of "death genes" reputed to figure in apoptosis (Represa et al., 1995), including local dendritic apoptosis (Sugimori et al., 1995). We would therefore predict that a neural change that results in greater excitatory receptor activation and higher internal Ca^{2+} and Na^+ levels would leave the neuron vulnerable to degenerative processes. Such is the case when response magnitude at a synapse is persistently increased and maintained via increased glutamatergic system function; as a result there is the potential to unleash the cascade of excitotoxic/apoptotic processes just described. In addition, synaptic activity appears to increase the generation of free radicals in neuronal mitochondria (Bindokas et al., 1998). Maintenance of this form of potentiation, *particularly long-term*, could result in neural dysfunction or death. Experimental support exists for the idea that LTP based on an increased magnitude of glutamatergic activation may be pathologic. Yamada (1998) studied the effects of benzoylpiperidine 1 (1-BCP) on hippocampal neurons in culture. 1-BCP increases field EPSP peak and duration in hippocampal slices, and is also known to facilitate LTP and to improve learning and memory performance in rats and humans. Yamada found that AMPA receptor function potentiated by 1-BCP resulted in AMPA receptor-mediated excitotoxic death of a significant proportion of the hippocampal neurons. Free-radical–mediated oxidative stress may also be a causal mechanism of neural degeneration in various of the age-related neurologic disorders (for references, see Bains and Shaw, 1997).

Regulatory processes designed to cause the decay of this type of LTP may be important safeguards against a pathologic outcome. In contrast to the possibly detrimental result of an increase in synaptic response magnitude, we predict that response potentiation achieved by activating "new infrastructure" (e.g., creation of new synapses or activation of previously quiescent ones; Isaac et al., 1995) is the only way to improve neuronal response properties without pushing cells closer to the line between physiologic and pathologic levels of excitation. Other means of synaptic potentiation, including an increased magnitude or duration of postsynaptic response, a greater "probability of hits" (decreased failure rate at a synapse), or a decreased threshold (successfully responding to a weaker stimulus) would all seem to run the danger of building up excessive ionic fluxes and free radical production. This is particularly true because LTP has a positive feed-forward nature, in that strong synaptic activation resets the response to a higher level. As such, there is an inherent danger that the process could cycle beyond limits of neuronal tolerance. This would have the greatest likelihood of inducing pathology when the following conditions apply: (1) The alteration is maintained long-term; (2) it is induced in neurons with selective vulnerability, due, for example, to a low complement of calcium-binding proteins or antioxidant molecules; or (3), when combined with any other stressor that compromises energy metabolism or antioxidant defense (e.g., trauma, hypoxia, etc.).

Does this mean that the brain avoids the use of the above-mentioned "potentially dangerous" modes of strengthening synapses? Presumably, this would depend on the margin of safety separating the *physiologic* range of excitation from the *pathologic*. For example, what is the difference in the magnitude of glutamate activation leading to Ca^{2+} and Na^+ fluxes that causes excitotoxic damage compared to that measured in baseline physiologic activity or following LTP induction? A large difference in magnitude would suggest that neuronal protective mechanisms such as neurotransmitter uptake, ion pumps, and Ca^{2+} buffering would be sufficient to prevent damage except in the face of other stressors. Conversely, a small margin of safety would make it unlikely that such high-risk methods of synaptic enhancement would be feasible as permanent substrates for learning or memory. A transient potentiation that initiates "downstream" changes and then decays, on the other hand, would be less likely to have pathologic consequences, although these might occur if induction coincided with severe neural trauma. It is this type of transient potentiation that we believe might be useful for beneficial changes, for example, in the early stages of a synaptic mechanism that acts as a building block for learning or memory.

Implications of Shared Molecular Mechanisms in Neuroplasticity and Neuropathology

There are a number of very significant implications to a plasticity-pathology relationship. As we have seen, elements of the glutamatergic system and the related internal ionic buildup are involved in both plastic alterations such as LTD and LTP and pathologic alterations such as kindling and excitotoxic/apoptotic neural degeneration. Therefore, the neural "plasticity machinery" is not distinct from the "pathology machinery," and neural dysfunction and death need not necessarily result from changes that are alien to the normal brain (e.g., plaques and tangles). More important, the fact that the same molecular machinery is involved in both neuroplastic and neuropathologic alternations means that the ability of neurons to undergo molecular and functional modification (plasticity) has a price: It leaves them vulnerable to pathology. Susceptibility to pathologic changes would be exacerbated by induction of a form of LTP that produces a persistent increase in postsynaptic response magnitude via increased ionic fluxes, and would be mitigated or avoided by the decay of this type of synaptic potentiation and maintenance of improved response instead of by a morphologic alteration. We must emphasize, though, that morphologic changes can have the same negative impact as other forms of neuroplasticity when inappropriately induced. To illustrate, we refer to two articles that detail a specific change in synaptic morphology, the so-called perforated synapse. The first review notes that perforated synapse formation follows LTP induction (Geinisman et al., 1991). The second (Wolff et al., 1995) discusses the dynamics of synaptic stabilization, during which the development of the perforated synapse is a transient event that sometimes results in the loss of the affected synapse. If indeed perforated synapse creation underlies both LTP and synaptic pruning, the possibility that LTP reflects a pathologic process must again be considered.

A greater chance of causing detrimental effects no doubt exists when plasticity is induced by artificial stimulation paradigms, since they can most likely overcome many of the normal safeguards that would be present *in vivo*. Protective responses may be bypassed in any number of ways, for example by using the $GABA_A$ antagonist bicuculline to depress inhibition, by employing nonphysiologic stimulation and/or pathways in the absence of normal connections and context, and so forth. In addition there is the possibility that what is being studied in such experiments is the brain's response to injury, caused by electrode implantation or tissue sectioning. In contrast, natural learning- or memory-induced plasticity in the intact animal will reflect a very tightly controlled balance between the dynamics of appropriately changing neural response versus the regulatory processes that prevent those changes from going beyond the range of cellular tolerance.

■ **Pathologic Extremes of the Plasticity-Pathology Continuum.** The above section has presented the case for recognizing the negative side of neural modifications such as kindling and some forms of LTP. We therefore extend the continuum of plasticity-pathology relationships to include neuronal degeneration as an extreme outcome that may occur at both ends of the spectrum when plastic alterations go awry. While some forms of LTP might increase the likelihood that a neuron will succumb to disorders of overexcitation, persistent depression of neural activity could possibly have equally detrimental effects. At the extreme low end of activity, we hypothesize that there is a "disuse degeneration" phenomenon resulting from severely diminished or inappropriate activity in a neuron that has been deprived of normal afferent or target activation as a consequence of functional and/or morphologic disconnection. This type of perturbation could conceivably result in loss of the benefits of neurotrophic factors, molecules that play a key role in neuronal survival and repair (Oppenheim, 1989), and whose trophic action may be derived from appropriate neural activity.

Although speculative, this process has a precedent of sorts in the developmental elimination of neurons that make insufficient or inappropriate synaptic contacts (Clarke, 1985; Oppenheim, 1989). In ocular dominance plasticity, for example, geniculostriate afferents from an occluded eye become disconnected from their target neurons in cortical layer IV during a critical period in early development

(Movshon and Van Sluyters, 1981; Collingridge and Singer, 1991). More importantly from the perspective of our model, apoptosis also appears to occur in adult neurons as a result of abnormal afferent input caused by a noninvasive manipulation. Adult mice housed on a slowly revolving (0.8 rev./min) turntable had significant numbers of dying neurons in the vestibular nuclei after only 48 hours, compared to nonrotated controls (Mitchell et al., 1995). Observations from another source may also bear upon the idea of disuse-related degeneration. The apoptosis of specific neurons in the dentate gyrus occurring as a result of adrenalectomy can be prevented by low-intensity electroconvulsive stimulation, which increases the expression of mRNAs for certain trophic factors (Masco et al., 1995). The rescue of deprived neurons by compensatory overactivity is a feature that would be predicted by our model. We speculate that disuse degeneration may occur as LTD devolves to a more severe curtailment of appropriate or relevant activity. As was true for a postulated LTP-pathology link, the move from LTD to pathology would depend on its underlying mechanism, persistence, the coincidence of additional stressors, and the margin of safety between physiologic and detrimental decreases in neural activity.

We note also that hyperexcitation and disuse processes may occur simultaneously for interactive neural populations in disease states, with both processes leading to neural degeneration, albeit with different underlying molecular mechanisms and time courses. This is because degeneration of neurons either by excitotoxic/apoptotic processes or through disuse could lead to further disuse degeneration in synaptically associated cells that become disconnected. This process is perhaps reflected in the progressive nature of many neurodegenerative diseases. Sprouting of new connections to deprived neurons may retard the loss of cells due to underactivity. Alternatively, they may cause further pathology (Wasterlain and Shirasaka, 1994), possibly by contributing to abnormal activation patterns. Certain circuits (e.g., cortex) appear to possess strong safeguards designed to prevent inappropriate plastic modifications from occurring. This could serve the dual function of limiting superfluous information storage and susceptibility to pathologic disruptions.

What Determines Whether the Outcome of Neural Modification Is Beneficial or Pathologic?

We postulate that the effect along the continuum that results from a given modification event depends on a variety of factors, including the nature of the inducing stimulus, the selective vulnerability of the neurons, and the ability of the circuit to re-regulate to maintain safe limits of activity. We briefly discuss these in the following.

■ **Stimulation Effects.** The nature of the stimulus may include characteristics of intensity, frequency, duration, number of repetitions, level of postsynaptic depolarization, magnitude of rise in internal Ca^{2+} and Na^+, spatiotemporal pattern of stimulation, not to mention as yet unknown factors. Stimulus-dependent induction of synaptic response changes ranging from LTD to LTP has been observed by various groups. Dudek and Bear (1992) found that stimulation at a frequency of 1 to 3 Hz produced a lasting synaptic depression in hippocampal CA1 neurons, at 10 Hz there was no net change in response, but stimulation at 50 Hz produced a persistent potentiation. Similarly, the same tetanic stimulus that induces LTP can induce LTD under conditions of (1) low postsynaptic depolarization (Artola et al., 1990); (2) decreased extracellular Ca^{2+} (Mulkey and Malenka, 1992); or (3) synaptic activation delayed relative to postsynaptic depolarization. As an added complication, the nature of the plastic outcome also depends on the previous history of the activity in the synapse (e.g., Freeman, 1981, 1983), a previous observation recently named *metaplasticity* (Abraham and Tate, 1997).

The next stages in the continuum are achieved with stronger stimulation. Kindling is induced by stimulation trains in a comparable frequency range to that used to induce LTD and LTP but at a greater intensity (typically defined by the capability to elicit an after-discharge), and with a greater number of repetitions. Neuronal degeneration results from rapid kindling and frequent perforant path stimulation using long trains and a short interstimulus interval, also in the same frequency range (Sloviter, 1987). Therefore, the plastic outcome in a circuit is uniquely dependent on variations in induction stimulus that are for the most part poorly understood.

■ **Selective Vulnerability of Neurons: Neuron and Circuit Characteristics, Trauma, Age and Ability to Regulate.** The predisposition of neurons or neuronal circuits to exhibit plastic or pathologic alterations may also be dictated by neuronal phenotype and circuit characteristics. Several phenotypical attributes of neurons may make them selectively vulnerable to pathologic outcomes of modification. This includes factors such as the specific complement of neurotransmitter receptors, ion channels, Ca^{2+}-binding proteins, and free-radical scavenging mechanisms. For example, a paucity of two calcium-binding proteins, calbindin and parvalbumin, has been observed both in hippocampal neurons particularly sensitive to seizure-activity–induced degeneration (Sloviter, 1989) and in motor neurons that degenerate in the early stages of amyotrophic lateral sclerosis (ALS) (Alexianu et al., 1994). Circuit characteristics that determine selective vulnerability may include developmental changes in the number and type of connections, and sprouting of new connections as a reaction to injury.

Any perturbation that affects normal neural function, especially by compromising energy state and maintenance of membrane potentials (e.g., ischemia, anoxia), will have great influence on the outcome of a plastic alteration. Under these conditions, even normal levels of neural activity can cause neural degeneration by excitotoxicity (Meldrum, 1993) or activation of a cell death program; the effects of prolonged synaptic potentiation would be expected to be worse (Gozlan et al., 1995).

Many of the traits of neurons and circuits, their ability to undergo plastic modification, and their vulnerability and response to injury are age dependent. As discussed in detail above, widespread differences in "hardware" and function result in significant age-related differences in plasticity. Age-dependent changes in magnitude and/or ease of induction are documented for LTD (Mulkey and Malenka, 1992; Dudek and Bear, 1993), LTP (Harris and Teyler, 1984; Bronzino et al., 1994), and kindling (Trommer et al., 1994; Geinisman et al., 1995), with greater plasticity reported in young versus adult or aged animals. It is also a well-established observation that the type and severity of neuronal injury that results from various forms of CNS trauma is age-dependent (Moshe, 1998; Villablanca et al., 1998). To illustrate, a number of features make the immature hippocampus hyperexcitable, and hence highly susceptible to kindling and epileptogenesis (Wasterlain and Shirasaka, 1994), including an NMDA receptor isoform with decreased voltage dependence (Ben Ari et al., 1988), an excess of recurrent excitatory connections (Swann et al., 1991), and the early excitatory action of GABA (Cherubini et al., 1990). Unique age-dependent attributes of the young brain can also confer resistance to insult. For example, the neuronal damage resulting from seizures is less severe relative to that produced in the adult, as a result of a greatly diminished metabolic rate and the immaturity of certain aspects of the excitatory neurotransmission system (Wasterlain and Shirasaka, 1994; Moshe, 1998). The fact that such age dependence exists in recovery from injury may also reflect the ability of the young nervous system to rebuild and compensate for damage in a manner unavailable in the adult. These observations make it all the more remarkable that age is often not treated as a critical variable in LTP experiments, as discussed above in the section on age dependence.

An additional factor that may determine whether a particular modification leads to pathology is the ability of the affected neurons to rebalance activity to a safe level. A common response of dynamic systems to perturbation is homeostatic regulation, and the wide range of homeostatic processes observed throughout biology may act as protective mechanisms in this regard. Determining how the brain maintains homeostasis while undergoing change, and understanding how it fails, are fundamental challenges of neuroplasticity research.

■ **Summary and Implications of the Plasticity-Pathology Continuum.** In conclusion, neurons are in no way homogeneous in their plastic response to stimuli nor in their degree of susceptibility to damage. Some of the factors that determine whether the response to a given perturbation will be a beneficial plastic alteration (such as might underlie learning or memory) or a pathologic alteration (such as might underlie various neural diseases) include the nature of the stimulation and the selective neuronal vulnerability due to phenotype, traumatic influences, age, and ability to regulate.

Various possibilities seem to exist regarding the behavioral relevance of LTP in relation to this continuum: One is that long-term potentiation of the magnitude of glutamatergic function at a synapse is exceedingly risky, and the brain either does not make use of this mechanism for beneficial plastic alterations or quickly reverses it. A second is that the margin of safety between tolerable and pathologic levels of synaptic activity is sufficiently large that this form of synapse strengthening is only pathologic in combination with other stressors. A third is that certain neuronal subsets are uniquely suited for the demands of potentiated activity through highly efficient "clean-up" mechanisms and/or the ability to replace degenerated neurons by new cell birth, an effect recently noted to occur in adult hippocampus (Gould et al., 1998). Regions of the hippocampus could, for example, be designed to act as "hair-trigger" zones for plastic change. Greater mortality of neurons in such structures would be balanced by a relatively high level of cell birth. Replacing neurons in a circuit that transiently triggered the lasting changes that were maintained elsewhere would seemingly be less complex than replacing cells in a circuit related to "long-term information storage" (e.g., cortical?). A new "trigger circuit" neuron would only be required to take on relatively general properties of circuit function, whereas complex connections and interrelationships would most likely need to be regained by a new "information storage circuit" neuron. This distinction is speculative, and is not meant to be interpreted to the literal extreme that there is a strict separation between some kinds of neurons that are modifiable "disposable" neurons and others that are "storage bins." However, a certain amount of specialization of function would be a beneficial way to manage the potentially neuropathologic consequences of exhibiting a high degree of plasticity. An additional implication is that the search for the most durable changes should not be in the initial "trigger" site, but at downstream locations.

Neural Plasticity and Stability Across Levels of Organization: Outline of a Model

For LTP to be able to serve as a substrate for learning or memory a number of criteria would have to be fulfilled. Key among these, as discussed in the previous sections, is the crucial requirement that LTP should have a clear behavioral outcome: LTP induction should go hand in hand with a learned response, such that inducing the former should provide the latter. The opposite should also be true, that is, molecular or other events that block learning should also prevent LTP. As supported by the citations in the above sections and in other chapters in this volume (Chapters 7 and 13), data supporting the former relationship have been difficult to obtain and, in our view, in most cases the available evidence is not convincing. Manipulations that block both LTP and learning are abundant, but nonspecific. Recent data suggesting that NR2B gene expression enhances learning may contribute to the debate (Tang et al., 1999), particularly if it can be demonstrated that LTP increases and decreases accompany higher or lower levels of behavioral learning *as well as* neurotransmitter receptor expression. These criteria, in particular, must be satisfied in adult animals. Note that the difficulty of obtaining clear evidence for LTP in learning/memory in most cases does not mean that it does not function in this role in any circumstance. Rather, we believe the above sections make clear that the various forms of LTP may have a number of roles, some potentially related to beneficial (plastic) neural modifications, others to forms of artificial pathologic response.

As we have stated above, it is difficult to avoid the notion that some form of change in response characteristics or magnitude, at either a synaptic or cellular level, must participate in learning. Simultaneously, as we have shown, prolonged events, such as some forms of LTP, can be pathologic. This leads to a need for a transient form of synaptic modification that does not last long enough to elicit pathologic processes, yet that provides the basis for a more durable modification in neural response leading to effects on behavior. Superficially, transience would appear to be at odds with a mechanism in which stability is required. However, we believe that there is a way around this constraint and in the following we will briefly outline some thoughts on what such a mechanism might look like, and how it might be maintained or altered.

The basic idea of the model is that activity and the modification or stability of that activity does not occur only at one level of organization, but rather at numerous levels. For example, while LTP is usually induced and measured at a synaptic or cellular level, these levels are only some of those that clearly exist in a continuum from genetic instruction to behavior. Between these extremes are synaptic, cellular, neural circuit, neural system, and coordination between systems, to mention but a few of the major delineations. Activity at each level is dependent on the ones above *and* below. Taking again the example of the synaptic level, synaptic strengths and activities are controlled, in part, by the expression of various proteins (e.g., structural elements, receptors, kinases, and phosphatases). Much of the latter is under genetic control, which determines what molecules are expressed, how they are transported, where they are used, and so forth. In turn, synaptic activity can affect genomic expression of such molecules via negative and positive feedback processes. Although much is still unknown about the mutual interactions between genetic expression and the activity of the synapse, it is quite clear that such interactions exist and regulate overall synaptic activity (e.g., receptor regulation). Above the synaptic level is the level of the individual neuron whose net activity is determined by the individual activity of hundreds or thousands of individual synapses. The activity at a cellular level impacts on the activity at the synapse, thus establishing yet another feedback mechanism between levels (see Desai et al., 2000). Such mutually reinforcing activity can be viewed as a specific trajectory of change that leads across all levels of organization. Viewed in this way, external stimuli and behavior, if they are sufficiently strong, make their way down across levels to ultimately impact genomic function and expression.

Similarly, genetic information is expressed progressively across levels, culminating in systems level activity and, finally, behavior. Each level contains powerful negative feedback mechanisms that normally serve to control alterations in overall activity. For example, at the synapse, receptors are regulated by the opposing action of protein kinases and phosphatases: Overstimulation is normally followed by receptor downregulation (Pasqualotto and Shaw, 1996). Negative feedback *between* levels serves the same function: Overstimulation at a synapse causes downregulation of genomic receptor expression (Kim et al., 1996) and initiates homeostatic controls at the cellular level (Desai et al., 2000). The net consequence of such feedback is twofold: First, only the "strongest" stimuli have a trajectory across all levels. Second, by traversing all levels, the stimulus is distributed to make the new activity mutually reinforcing across levels. Another consequence of the above is that stimuli that exceed the built-in constraints can induce pathology. In our view, LTP as typically induced out of context in *in vitro* preparations provides such an example: By exceeding constraints of longevity and/or strength, it induces pathologic processes. Transient potentiation, in contrast, serves to reset the other levels of organization, ultimately leading to altered behavior. The altered behavior, in turn, reinforces the lower levels. The latter may serve to explain why the durability of a behavioral modification (e.g., spatial learning) may not have an obvious electrophysiologic modification linked to a particular anatomic locus (e.g., LTP in dentate gyrus). For example, once distributed to a larger system (cortex), alterations in neural activity in hippocampal circuits can shortly return to near prestimulation levels and thus avoid a potential excitotoxic outcome. It is interesting to speculate that normal *in vivo* activity may occasionally exceed the tolerance of the system and induce cell death. We noted above in regard to the latter that dentate shows neuronal birth in adulthood (Gould et al., 1998), suggesting the possibility that new neurons are added to this "hair-trigger" circuit to replace those killed in normal activity.

Other speculative aspects of the model include the following in relation to the changing nature of plasticity during aging, with different levels of neural organization making differing contributions: (1) Early in life, genetic information contributes more significantly than environmental input in order to structure the developing neural levels. The genetic contribution may include instructions for the various molecules present at the synapse, for neuronal sprouting, and for synaptogenesis, etc. (2) During the critical periods for various neurons, environmental influences combine with genetic instructions to provide major modifications in long-term neural activity. Included in this stage is the peak of synaptogenesis and receptor proliferation, both regulated by external stimuli (see above section on age dependence for references). (3) Beyond the critical periods (for most well-studied neural circuits, occurring after puberty), environmental influences become the greatest factor for changing neural activity, albeit to a lesser extent than during the critical period. At this stage homeostatic regulation of receptors and synapses becomes paramount and the alterations that do occur reflect "fine tuning" of neuronal function that nevertheless can amount to significant alterations in behavior when amplified across neuronal levels of organization. In contrast to young neurons, in the adult, large-scale changes in neuron number or connectivity reflect a pathologic process that may arise in response to injury or gene dysfunction.

Neuronal plasticity thus reflects restructuring of activity across levels; neuronal stability reflects the homeostatic controls at each level. Large-scale changes in connectivity may be more likely to occur in the young nervous system, which may lack certain feedback controls (e.g., inhibitory processes; see Cherubini et al., 1990); stability against large-scale alterations may be more a feature of adult nervous systems where only fine tuning is required and that occurs only under precisely defined and controlled conditions.

The above is intended as a brief introduction to a way of viewing neuronal plasticity and stability as a consequence of mutually reinforcing processes that occur between levels of organization of the nervous system. A full treatment of this model and its implications for LTP and neuroplasticity as a whole are presented in Shaw and McEachern (2000).

Conclusions

1. Now, as when our original review was written, we take exception to the dogmatic adherence by many in the field to the view that a relationship between LTP and learning/memory has been established unequivocally.
2. In our opinion, this stance has largely prevented other possible roles for LTP-like plasticity from being examined. For example, correlations between LTP and certain *pathologic* forms of neuroplasticity may be as striking as any between LTP and learning or memory; this is an area of inquiry that may have had more attention if not for preconceptions in the field.
3. We propose a quite different model in which we emphasize that interactions across multiple levels of neural organization may be required for understanding the dynamic interplay between plasticity/pathology and stability in the nervous system, in contrast to the current focus on an isolated level of organization (e.g., synaptic LTP) as the basis of learning.

REFERENCES

Abraham, W.C. (1997). Keeping faith with the properties of LTP. *Behav. Brain Sci.* 20: 614.

Abraham, W.C., and Otani, S. (1991). Macromolecules and the maintenance of long-term potentiation. In F. Morrell (Ed.), *Kindling and synaptic plasticity: The legacy of Graham Goddard* (pp. 92–109). Boston: Birkhauser.

Abraham, W.C., and Tate, W.P. (1997). Metaplasticity: A new vista across the field of synaptic plasticity. *Prog. Neurobiol.* 52: 303–323.

Abraham, W.C., Christie, B.R., Logan, B., Lawlor, P. et al. (1994). Immediate early gene expression associated with the persistence of heterosynaptic long-term depression in the hippocampus. *Proc. Natl. Acad. Sci. USA* 91: 10049–10053.

Abraham, W.C., Masonparker, S.E., Williams, J., and Dragunow, M. (1995). Analysis of the decremental nature of LTP in the dentate gyrus. *Mol. Brain Res.* 30: 367–372.

Aghajanian, G.K., and Bloom, F.E. (1967). The formation of synaptic junctions in developing rat brain: A quantitative electron microscopic study. *Brain Res.* 6: 716–727.

Aiba, A., Chen, C., Herrup, K., Rosenmund, C. et al. (1994). Reduced hippocampal long-term potentiation and context-specific deficit in associative learning in mGluR1 mutant mice. *Cell* 79: 365–375.

Alexianu, M.E., Ho, B.K., Mohamed, A.H., Labella, V. et al. (1994). The role of calcium-binding proteins in selective motoneuron vulnerability in amyotrophic lateral sclerosis. *Ann. Neurol.* 36: 846–858.

Artola, A., and Singer, W. (1987). Long-term potentiation and NMDA receptors in rat visual cortex. *Nature* 330: 649–652.

Artola, A., Brocher, S., and Singer, W. (1990). Different voltage-dependent thresholds for inducing long-term depression and long-term potentiation in slices of rat visual cortex. *Nature* 347: 69–72.

Bains, J.S., and Shaw, C.A. (1997). Neurodegenerative disorders in humans: The role of glutathione in oxidative stress-mediated neuronal death. *Brain Res. Rev.* 25: 335–358.

Bannerman, D.M., Good, M.A., Butcher, S.P., Ramsay, M. et al. (1995). Distinct components of spatial learning revealed by prior training and NMDA receptor blockade. *Nature* 378: 182–186.

Barnes, C.A. (1995). Involvement of LTP in memory: Are we "searching under the street light"? *Neuron* 15: 751–754.

Bartlett, F.C., (1932). *Remembering: A study in Experimental and Social Psychology.* London: Cambridge University Press.

Ben-Ari, Y. (1995). Activity-dependent forms of plasticity. *J. Neurobiol.* 26: 295–298.

Ben-Ari, Y., and Gho, M. (1988). Long-lasting modification of the synaptic properties of rat CA3 hippocampal neurons induced by kainic acid. *J. Physiol.* (London) 404: 365–384.

Ben-Ari, Y., Cherubini, E., and Krnjevic, K. (1988). Changes in voltage dependence of NMDA currents during development. *Neurosci. Lett.* 94: 88–92.

Bindokas, V.P., Lee, C.C., Colmers, W.F., and Miller, R.J. (1998). Changes in mitochondrial function resulting from synaptic activity in rat hippocampal slice. *J. Neurosci.* 18: 4570–4587.

Bliss, T.V.P, and Collingridge, G.L. (1993). A synaptic model of memory: Long-term potentiation in the hippocampus. *Nature* 361: 31–39.

Bliss, T.V.P., and Lomo, T. (1973). Long-lasting potentiation of synaptic transmission in the dentate area of the anaesthetized rabbit following stimulation of the perforant path. *J. Physiol.* (London) 232: 331–356.

Blue, M.E., and Parnavelas, J.G. (1983). The formation and maturation of synapses in the visual cortex of the rat. II. Quantitative analysis. *J. Neurocytol.* 12: 697–712.

Bronzino, J.D., Abuhasaballa, K., Austinlafrance, R.J., and Morgane, P.J. (1994). Maturation of long-term potentiation in the hippocampal dentate gyrus of the freely moving rat. *Hippocampus* 4: 439–446.

Burette, F., Jay T.M., and Laroche, S. 1997. Reversal of LTP in the hippocampal afferent fiber system to the prefrontal cortex in vivo with low-frequency patterns of stimulation that do not produce LTP. *J. Neurophysiol.* 78: 1155–1160.

Burgos, G.R.G., Biali, F.I., Siri, L.C.N., and Cardinali, D.P. (1994). Effect of gamma-aminobutyric acid on synaptic transmission and long-term potentiation in rat superior cervical ganglion. *Brain Res.* 658: 1–7.

Burnashev, N., Monyer, H., Seeburg, P.H., and Sakmann, B. (1992). Divalent ion permeability of AMPA receptor channels is dominated by the edited form of a single subunit. *Neuron* 8: 189.

Butler, L., Silva, A., Tonegawa, S., and McNamara, J.O. (1993). Enhanced seizure susceptibility yet impairment of kindling development in alpha-calcium calmodulin kinase II mutant mice. *Soc. Neurosci. Abstr.* 19: 1030.

Cain, D.P. (1997). LTP, NMDA, genes and learning. *Curr. Opin. Neurobiol.* 7: 235–242.

Cain, D.P. (2000). Synaptic models of neuroplasticity: What is LTP? In C.A. Shaw and J.C. McEachern (Eds.), *Toward a theory of neuroplasticity.* Philadelphia: Taylor & Francis. (in press)

Cavazos, J.E., Das, I., and Sutula, T.P. (1994). Neuronal loss induced in limbic pathways by kindling: Evidence for induction of hippocampal sclerosis by repeated brief seizures. *J. Neurosci.* 14: 3106–3121.

Cherubini, E., Rovira, C., Gaiarsa, J.L., Corradetti, R. et al. (1990). GABA mediated excitation in immature rat CA3 hippocampal neurons. *Int. J. Devl. Neurosci.* 8: 481–490.

Chrobak, J.J., and Buzsáki, G. (1998). Gamma oscillations in the entorhinal cortex of the freely behaving rat. *J. Neurosci.* 18: 388–398.

Clarke, G.R.G. 1985. Neuronal death in the development of the vertebrate nervous system. *Trends Neurosci.* 8: 345–349.

Collingridge, G.L., and Bliss, T.V.P. (1987). NMDA receptors—their role in long-term potentiation. *Trends Neurosci.* 10: 288–293.

Collingridge, G.L., and Singer, W. 1990. Excitatory amino acid receptors and synaptic plasticity. *Trends Pharmacol. Sci.* 11: 290–296.

Cotman, C.W., Geddes, J.W., Ulas, J., and Klein, M. (1990). Plasticity of excitatory amino acid receptors: Implications for aging and Alzheimer's disease. *Prog. Brain Res.* 86: 55–61.

Desai, N.S., Nelson, S.B., and Turrigiano, G.G. (2000). Homeostatic regulation of cortical networks. In C.A. Shaw and J.C. McEachern (Eds.), *Toward a theory of neuroplasticity.* Philadelphia: Taylor & Francis. in press.

Doyere, V., Burette, F., Redini-Del Negro, C., and Laroche, S. (1993). Long-term potentiation of hippocampal afferents and efferents to prefrontal cortex: Implications for associative learning. *Neuropsychologia* 3: 1031–1053.

Dudek, S.M., and Bear, M.F. (1992). Homosynaptic long-term depression in area CA1 of hippocampus and effects of N-methyl-D-aspartate receptor blockade. *Proc. Natl. Acad. Sci. USA* 89: 4363–4367.

Dudek, S.M., and Bear, M.F. (1993). Bidirectional long-term modification of synaptic effectiveness in the adult and immature hippocampus. *J. Neurosci.* 13: 2910–2918.

Faneslow, M.S. (1997). Without LTP the learning circuit is broken. *Behav. Brain Sci.* 20: 616.

Freeman, W.J. (1981). A physiological hypothesis of perception. *Perspect. Biol. Med.* 24: 561–592.

Freeman, W.J. (1983). The physiological basis of mental images. *Biol. Psychiatr.* 18: 1107–1125.

Freeman, W.J. (1994). Neural networks and chaos. *J. Theor. Biol.* 171: 13–18.

Gallistel, R.C. (1995). Is LTP a plausible basis for memory? In J.L. McGaugh, N.M. Weinberger, and G. Lynch (Eds.), *Brain and memory: modulation and mediation of neuroplasticity* (pp. 328–337). New York: Oxford University Press.

Geinisman, Y., De Toledo-Morrell, L., and Morrell, F. (1991). Structural synaptic substrates of kindling and long-term potentiation. In F. Morrell (Ed.), *Kindling and synaptic plasticity* (pp. 124–159). Boston: Birkhauser.

Geinisman, Y., De Toledo-Morrell, L., Morrell, F., and Heller, R.E. (1995). Hippocampal markers of age-related memory dysfunction: Behavioral, electrophysiological and morphological perspectives. *Prog. Neurobiol.* 45: 223–252.

Gerren, R.A., and Weinberger, N.M. (1983). Long-term potentiation in the magnocellular medial geniculate nucleus of the anaesthetized cat. *Brain Res.* 265: 138–142.

Goddard, G.V. (1967). Development of epileptic seizures through brain stimulation at low intensity. *Nature* 214: 1020–1021.

Gould, E., Tanapat, P., McEwen, B.S., Flugge, G. et al. (1998). Proliferation of granule cell precursors in the dentate gyrus of adult monkeys is diminished by stress. *Proc. Natl. Acad. Sci. USA* 95: 3168–3171.

Gozlan, H., Khazipov, R., and Ben-Ari, Y. (1995). Multiple forms of long-term potentiation and multiple regulatory sites of N-methyl-D-aspartate receptors: Role of the redox site. *J. Neurobiol.* 26: 360–369.

Grant, S.G.N., O'Dell, T.J., Karl, K.A., Stein, P.L. et al. (1992). Impaired long-term potentiation, spatial learning, and hippocampal development in fyn mutant mice. *Science* 258: 1903–1910.

Hammond, C., Crepel, V., Gozlan, H., and Ben-Ari, Y. (1994). Anoxic LTP sheds light on the multiple facets of NMDA receptors. *Trends Neurosci.* 17: 497–503.

Hargreaves, E.L., and Cain, D.P. (1992). Hyperactivity, hyper-reactivity, and sensorimotor deficits induced by low doses of the N-methyl-D-aspartate non-competitive channel blocker MK801. *Behav. Brain Res.* 47: 23–33.

Harris, K.M., and Teyler, T.J. (1984). Developmental onset of long-term potentiation in area CA1 of the rat hippocampus. *J. Physiol.* (London) 346: 27–48.

Hölscher, C., Annyl, R., and Rowan, M. (1997a). Stimulation on the positive phase of hippocampal theta rhythm induces long-term potentiation which can be depotentiated by stimulation on the negative phase in area CA1 in vivo. *J. Neurosci.* 17: 6470–6477.

Hölscher, C., McGlinchey, L., Anwyl, R., and Rowan, M.J. (1997b). HFS-induced long-term potentiation and LFS-induced depotentiation in area CA1 of the hippocampus are not good models for learning. *Psychopharmacology* 130: 174–182.

Hölscher, C., McGlinchey, L., Anqyl, R., and Rowan, M.J. (1996). 7-Nitro indazole, a selective neuronal nitric oxide synthase inhibitor in vivo, impairs spatial learning in the rat. *Learn Mem.* 2(6): 267–78.

Hughes, P.E., Alexi, T., Walton, M., Williams, C.E. (1999). Activity and injury-dependent expression of inducible transcription factors, growth factors and apoptosis-related genes within the central nervous system. *Prog. Neurobiol.* 57: 421–450.

Isaac, J.T.R., Nicoll, R.A., and Malenka, R.C. (1995). Evidence for silent synapses—implications for the expression of LTP. *Neuron* 15: 427–434.

Izquierdo, I. (1994). Pharmacological evidence for a role of long-term potentiation in memory. *FASEB J.* 8(14): 1139–45.

Ito, K-I., Skinkle, K.L., and Hicks, T.P. (1999). Age-dependent, steroid-specific effects of oestrogen on long-term potentiation in rat hippocampal slices. *J. Physiol.* 515(Pt. 1): 209–220.

Jeffery, K.J., Abraham, W.C., Dragunow, M., and Mason, S.E. (1990). Induction of Fos-like immunoreactivity and the maintenance of long-term potentiation in the dentate gyrus of unanesthetized rats. *Mol. Brain Res.* 8: 267–274.

Kamal, A., Biessels, G.J., Gispen, W.H., and Urban, I.J.A. (1998). Increasing age reduces expression of long-term depression and dynamic range of transmission plasticity in CA1 field of the rat hippocamus. *Neuroscience* 83: 707–715.

Kavanau, J.L. (1994). Sleep and dynamic stabilization of neural circuitry: A review and synthesis. *Behav. Brain Res.* 63: 111–126.

Keith, J.R., and Rudy, J.W. (1990). Why NMDA-receptor-dependent long-term potentiation may not be a mechanism of learning and memory: Reappraisal of the NMDA-receptor blockade strategy. *Psychobiology* 18: 251–257.

Larson, J., Xiao, P., and Lynch, G. (1993). Reversal of LTP by theta frequency stimulation. *Brain Res.* 600: 97–102.

Linden, D.J. (1994). Long-term synaptic depression in the mammalian brain. *Neuron* 12: 457–472.

Lipton, S.A., and Rosenberg, P.A. (1994). Excitatory amino acids as a final common pathway for neurologic disorders. *N. Engl. J. Med.* 330: 613–622.

Lothman, E.W., and Williamson, J.M. (1994). Closely spaced recurrent hippocampal seizures elicit two types of heightened epileptogenesis: A rapidly developing, transient kindling and a slowly developing, enduring kindling. *Brain Res.* 649: 71–84.

Lynch, G., and Seubert, P. (1989). Links between long-term potentiation and neuropathology. An hypothesis involving calcium-activated proteases. *Ann. NY Acad. Sci.* 568: 171–180.

Martin, S.J. (1998). Time-dependent reversal of dentate LTP by 5Hz stimulation. *NeuroReport* 9: 3775–3781.

Masco, D., Sahibzada, N., and Gale, K. (1995). Electroconvulsive shock prevents apoptotic and excitotoxic cell death. *Soc. Neurosci. Abstr.* 21: 811.

McEachern, J.C., and Shaw, C.A. (1996a). An alternative to the LTP orthodoxy: A plasticity-pathology continuum model. *Brain Res. Rev.* 22: 51–92.

McEachern, J.C., and Shaw, C.A. (1996b). Does LTP correlate with memory or neuropathology? Or what happens when homeostatic receptor regulation fails? In C.A. Shaw (Eds.), *Receptor dynamics in neural development* (pp. 253–301). Boca Raton, FL: CRC Press.

McEachern, J.C., and Shaw, C.A. (1999). The plasticity-pathology continuum: Defining a role for the LTP phenomenon. *J. Neurosci. Res.* 58: 42–61.

McKernan, M.G., and Shinnick-Gallagher, P. (1997). Fear conditioning induces a lasting potentiation of synaptic currents in vitro. *Nature* 390: 607–611.

McNamara, J.O. (1994). Cellular and molecular basis of epilepsy. *J. Neurosci.* 14: 3413–3425.

Meldrum, B. (1993). Amino acids as dietary excitotoxins: A contribution to understanding neurodegenerative disorders. *Brain Res. Rev.* 18: 293–314.

Mitchell, I.J., Cooper, A.J., Brown, G.D.A., and Waters, C.M. (1995). Apoptosis of neurons in the vestibular nuclei of adult mice results from prolonged change in the external environment. *Neurosci. Lett.* 198: 153–156.

Morris, R.G.M., Anderson, E., Lynch G.S., and Baudry, M. (1986). Selective impairment of learning and blockade of long-term potentiation by N-methyl-D-aspartate receptor antagonist, AP5. *Nature* 319: 774–776.

Moshe, S.L. (1998). Brain injury with prolonged seizures in children and adults. *J. Child Neurol.* 13 (Suppl. 1): S3–6.

Movshon, J.A., and Van Sluyters, R.C. (1981). Visual neural development. *Annu. Rev. Psychol.* 32: 477–522.

Mulkey, R.M., and Malenka, R.C. (1992). Mechanisms underlying induction of homosynaptic long-term depression in area CA1 of the hippocampus. *Neuron* 9: 967–975.

Mulkey, R.M., Endo, S., Shenolikar, S., and Malenka, R.C. (1994). Involvement of a calcineurin/inhibitor-1 phosphatase cascade in hippocampal long-term depression. *Nature* 369: 486–488.

Neill, D. (2000). Maladaptive and dysfunctional synaptoplasticity in relation to Alzheimer's disease and schizophrenia. In C.A. Shaw and J.C. McEachern (Eds.), *Toward a theory of neuroplasticity*. Philadelphia: Taylor & Francis. in Press.

Norris, C.M., Korol, D.L., and Foster, T.C. (1996). Increased susceptibility to induction of long-term depression and long-term potentiation reversal during aging. *J. Neurosci.* 16: 5382–5392.

Obrenovitch, T.P., and Urenjak, J. (1997). Altered glutamatergic transmission in neurological disorders: From high extracellular glutamate to excessive synaptic efficacy. *Prog. Neurobiol.* 51: 39–87.

Olney, J.W., Zorumski, C., Price, M.T., and Labruyere, J. (1990). L-cysteine, a bicarbonate-sensitive endogenous excitotoxin. *Science* 248: 569–599.

Oppenheim, R.W. (1989). The neurotrophic theory and naturally occurring motoneuron death. *Trends Neurosci.* 12: 252–255.

Pasqualotto, B.A., and Shaw, C.A. (1996). Regulation of ionotropic receptors by protein phosphorylation. *Biochem. Pharmacol.* 51: 1417–1425.

Qian, Z., Gilbert, M.E., Colicos, M.A., Kandel, E.R. et al. (1993). Tissue-plasminogen activator is induced as an immediate early gene during seizure, kindling and long-term potentiation. *Nature* 361: 453–457.

Racine, R.J., and Cain, D.P. (1991). Kindling-induced potentiation. In F. Morrell (Ed.), *Kindling and synaptic plasticity* (pp. 39–53). Boston: Birkhauser.

Randic, M., Jiang, M.C., and Cerne, R. (1993). Long-term potentiation and long-term depression of primary afferent neurotransmission in the rat spinal cord. *J. Neurosci.* 13: 5228–5241.

Rao, A., Kim, E., Sheng, M., and Craig, A.M. (1998). Heterogeneity in the molecular composition of excitatory postsynaptic sites during development of hippocampal neurons in culture. *J. Neurosci.* 18: 1217–1229.

Riedel, G., Wetzel, W., Kozikowski, A.P., and Reymann, K.G. (1995). Block of spatial learning by mGluR agonist tADA in rats. *Neuropharmacology* 34: 559–561.

Represa, A., Niquet, J., Pollard, H., and Ben-Ari, Y. (1995). Cell death, gliosis, and synaptic remodeling in the hippocampus of epileptic rats. *J. Neurobiol.* 26: 413–425.

Robinson, G.S., Jr., Crooks, G.B., Jr., Shinkman, P.G., and Gallagher, M. (1989). Behavioral effects of MK-801 mimic deficits associated with hippocampal damage. *Psychobiology* 17: 156–164.

Sazgar, M., Chick, B.A., Rashid, K., Van der Zee, C.E.E.M. et al. (1995). Role of nerve growth factor in kindling and kindling-induced mossy fiber sprouting. *Soc. Neurosci. Abstr.* 21: 1973.

Saucier, D., and Cain, D.P. (1995). Spatial learning without NMDA receptor-dependent long-term potentiation. *Nature* 378: 186–189.

Shaw, C.A. (1996). Age-dependent expression of receptor properties and function in CNS development. In C.A. Shaw (Ed.), *Receptor dynamics in neural development* (pp. 3–17). Boca Raton, FL: CRC Press.

Shaw, C.A., Lanius, R.A., and van den Doel, K. (1994). The origin of synaptic neuroplasticity: Crucial molecules or a dynamical cascade? *Brain Res. Rev.* 19: 241–263.

Shaw, C.A., and McEachern, J.C. (2000). Traversing levels of organization: Neural plasticity and stability. In C.A. Shaw and J.C. McEachern (Eds.), *Toward a theory of neuroplasticity*. Philadelphia: Taylor & Francis. in Press.

Shors, T.J., and Matzel, L.B. (1997). Long-term potentiation: What's learning got to do with it? *Behav. Brain Sci.* 20: 597–655.

Silva, A.J., Paylor, R., Wehner, J.M., and Tonegawa, S. (1992a). Impaired spatial learning in (alpha-calcium calmodulin kinase II mutant mice. *Science* 257: 206–211.

Silva, A.J., Stevens, C.F., Tonegawa, S., and Wang, Y. (1992b). Deficient hippocampal long-term potentiation in alpha-calcium-calmodulin kinase II mutant mice. *Science* 257: 201–206.

Sloviter, R.S. (1987). Decreased hippocampal inhibition and a selective loss of interneurons in experimental epilepsy. *Science* 235: 73–76.

Sloviter, R.S. (1989). Calcium-binding protein (Calbindin-D28K) and parvalbumin immunocytochemistry: Localization in the rat hippocampus with specific reference to the selective vulnerability of hippocampal neurons to seizure activity. *J. Comp. Neurol.* 280: 183–196.

Sorra, K.E., and Harris, K.M. (1998). Stability in synapse number and size at 2 hr after long-term potentiation in hippocampal area CA1. *J. Neurosci.* 18: 658–671.

Staubli, U., Thibault, O., DiLorenzo, M., and Lynch, G. (1989). Antagonism of NMDA receptors impairs acquisition but not retention of olfactory memory. *Behav. Neurosci.* 103: 54–60.

Stevens, C.F., and Wang, Y. (1994). Changes in reliability of synaptic function as a mechanism for plasticity. *Nature* 371: 704–707.

Stevens, C.F., Tonegawa, S., and Wang, Y. (1994). The role of calcium-calmodulin kinase II in three forms of synaptic plasticity. *Curr. Biol.* 4: 687–693.

Sugimori, M., Cherksey, B.D., and Llinas, R. (1995). Dendritic apoptosis: A new mechanism for restricted neuroal death. *Soc. Neurosci. Abstr.* 21: 2019.

Sutula, T., and Steward, O. (1986). Quantitative analysis of synaptic ptoentiation during kindling of the perforant path. *J. Neurophysiol.* 56: 732–746.

Sutula, T., and Steward, O. (1987). Facilitation of kindling by prior induction of long-term potentiation in the perforant path. *Brain Res.* 420: 109–117.

Swann, J.W., Smith, K.L., and Brady, R.J. (1991). Age-dependent alterations in the operations of hippocampal neural networks. *Ann. NY Acad. Sci.* 627: 264–276.

Szent-Gyorgi, A. (1996). Cited in L.E. Limbird, *Cell surface receptors: A short course in theory and methods* (2nd ed). Boston: Kluwer Academic Publishers.

Tang, Y.-P., Shimizu, E., Dube, G.R., Rampon, C. et al. (1999). Genetic enhancement of learning and memory in mice. *Nature* 401: 63–69.

Teskey, G.C., and Valentine, P.A. (1998). Post-activation potentiation in the neocortex of awake freely-moving rats. *Neurosci. Behav. Rev.* 22: 195–207.

Teyler, T.J. (2000). LTP and the superfamily of synaptic plasticities. In C.A. Shaw and J.C. McEachern (Eds.), *Toward a theory of neuroplasticity*. Philadelphia: Taylor & Francis. in press.

Trepel, C., and Racine, R.J. (1998). Long-term potentiation in the neocortex of the adult, freely moving rat. *Cereb. Cortex* 8: 719–729.

Trommer, B.L., Pasternak, J.F., Nelson, P.J., Colley, P.A. et al. (1994). Perforant path kindling alters dentate gyrus field potentials and paired pulse depression in an age-dependent manner. *Dev. Brain Res.* 79: 115–121.

Villablanca, J.R., Carlson-Kuhta, P., Schmanke, T.D., and Houda, D.A. (1998). A critical maturational period of reduced brain vulnerability to developmental injury. I. Behavioral studies in cats. *Dev. Brain Res.* 105: 309–324.

Wasterlain, C.G., and Shirasaka, Y. (1994). Seizures, brain damage and brain development. *Brain Dev.* 16: 279–295.

Weiss, S.R.B., Li, X.L., Rosen, J.B., Li, H. et al. (1995). Quenching: Inhibition of development and expression of amygdala kindled seizures with low frequency stimulation. *Neuroreport* 6: 2171–2176.

Wolf, M.E. (2000). The neuroplasticity of addiction. In C.A. Shaw and J.C. McEachern (Eds.), *Toward a theory of neuroplasticity.* Philadelphia: Taylor & Francis, in press.

Wolff, J.R., Laskawi, R., Spatz, W.B., and Missler, M. (1995). Structural dynamics of synapses and synaptic components. *Behav. Brain Res.* 66: 13–20.

Yamada, K. (1998). AMPA receptor activation potentiated by the AMPA modulator 1-BCP is toxic to cultured rat hippocampal neurons. *Neurosci. Lett.* 249: 119–122.

CHAPTER TWELVE

Long-Term Potentiation and Associative Learning

Can the Mechanism Subserve the Process?

Louis D. Matzel and Tracey J. Shors

SUMMARY

In several forms in the mammalian brain, long-term potentiation (LTP) displays certain neurophysiologic characteristics that are commonly regarded as evidence that this mechanism for neuronal plasticity subserves the induction and/or storage of associative memories. In particular, the associative nature of LTP (induction by conjoint pre- and postsynaptic activity) and its dependence on relatively short interstimulus intervals between pre- and postsynaptic activity suggest certain qualitative similarities between LTP induction and the processes that define associative learning. Despite the popular acceptance of this cursory evidence, the processes that govern the formation and expression of associative memories are far more malleable and heterogeneous than those suggested by such mechanistic analogies. Here we describe in some detail the fundamental characteristics of the associative learning process, with an emphasis on those characteristics that are relevant to the assertion that LTP is an appropriate device for the storage of associative memories. With this as our point of reference, we are left to conclude that the mechanistic properties of LTP are in some instances irrelevant, and in some cases contraindicate, a role for LTP in the induction or storage of associative memories.

Introduction

Associative learning, an example of which is classical conditioning, is often described as a "simple" form of learning, limited in application to the modifica-

This work was supported by the National Institute of Mental Health (NIMH; MH48387) of the U.S. Public Health Service, the Charles and Johanna Busch Memorial Fund, and the James McKeen Cattell Fund (to LDM), and NIMH (MH59970), the National Science Foundation (IBN-9511027), and the National Alliance on Schizophrenia and Depression (to TJS). Thanks are extended to Chet Ghandi for comments on an earlier version of the manuscript and to Ralph Miller for helpful discussions.

tion of reflexive behaviors. This colloquial description is an unfortunate charac-terization of the phenomenon that misrepresents the fundamental nature and range of influence of associative learning. The insights that could be derived from a complete appreciation of the associative learning process were obvious to Ivan Pavlov, the Nobel Prize winner in 1904 for his studies on the physiology of diges-tion. Pavlov used a rudimentary behavioral response as salivary secretion to index the acquisition of learned associations, and chose it not only because it was con-venient (as a gastric physiologist he was well prepared to measure salivation), but also in order to understand the annoying habit of his dogs to salivate before they were actually fed (i.e., at the very sight of the lab technician who delivered their food). This "psychic reflex" intrigued Pavlov, and he viewed this "conditional reflex" not as an opportunity to further study salivary excretion, but rather as a means to study the brain. The conditioned response provided an opportunity to make inferences about the function of an organ that was otherwise impenetrable in his era.

But what of saliva? Is classical conditioning relevant only to the modification of this and other visceral responses? Not in Pavlov's view. Some of his earliest exper-iments indicated that classical conditioning was not simply a mechanism for the modification of reflexive behaviors. For instance, Pavlov observed that if a hungry dog were conditioned to salivate in response to a click that preceded the delivery of food, it would cease responding to the click if the test occurred after the dog was allowed to free feed. If tested again after a subsequent period of food depri-vation, the dog would again salivate when presented with the click. Thus the con-ditioned reflex was not reflexive at all. Rather, it was an expression of the interaction between what the dog had learned about a stimulus with the condi-tions under which the animal was tested. Over the past century of research on classical conditioning, this characteristic of associative learning has been recog-nized as a fundamental feature of the process, so much so that contemporary investigators and theoreticians might describe classical conditioning as "the learn-ing of relations among events so as to allow the organism to represent its environ-ment" (Rescorla, 1988b). Note that this contemporary description of the associative learning process makes no reference whatsoever to a behavioral response, much less the modification of a simple reflex.

Despite the observations of Pavlov and the subsequent researchers, there is still a tendency by those outside of the immediate discipline to describe classical con-ditioning as the modification of a reflexive response, or at the level of the nervous system, of a reflex arc (i.e., motor pathway). Moreover, it is common to misrepre-sent or oversimplify the circumstances that produce associative memories, the content of those memories, or the translation of those memories into the observed conditioned response. Were these misrepresentations without consequence, they would merely be the fodder for an intellectual curiosity. However, these misrepre-sentations can have grave consequences if one were to attempt to describe the learning process at a mechanistic level. For instance, long-term potentiation (LTP), a long-lasting increase in synaptic efficacy in the mammalian brain, possesses cer-tain neurophysiologic characteristics that have led many to assert that it is a mechanism for the storage of associative memories. This common assertion is based on several central observations. First, the induction of LTP is facilitated by conjoint pre- and postsynaptic activity; thus it is said to have an "associative" quality resembling the stimulus pairings (e.g., the click and the food) that define classical conditioning. That is, the synaptic connections between cells are strengthened to create an association between input and output events. In addition, the induction of associative LTP requires that a relatively short interval intervene between the onset of activity in the pre- and postsynaptic neurons. Again, it is recognized that relatively short interstimulus intervals (ISIs) between a conditioned stimulus (CS, e.g., Pavlov's click) and an unconditioned stimulus (US, e.g., Pavlov's food) are often efficacious in producing associative memories. But is classical conditioning really so simple that it can be adequately captured by the simple assertions that it is "associative" and dependent on a short ISI? As we will describe, neither statement begins to capture the essence of associative learning and memory. Thus any mechanism that provides a nominal description of these features of associative learning may be wholly inadequate as the basis for a more comprehensive description of the actual process.

In this chapter we have several goals. First, we will review some of the fundamental properties of associative learning. This review is not intended to be exhaustive, as more exhaustive reviews and theoretical treatments have appeared in recent years (e.g., Rescorla, 1988a; Wasserman and Miller, 1997). Instead, we will focus on those characteristics of associative learning that are most relevant to the question of whether LTP can subserve the induction or storage of associative memories. Second, we will describe some of the neurophysiologic characteristics of LTP and compare those characteristics to those of associative learning. Minimally, we anticipate that such a comparison will raise questions about the assertion that LTP is a substrate for associative learning, but more significantly, that a more complete appreciation of the learning process will serve as the heuristic foundation for further empirical advances.

Associative Learning: A Multidimensional Process

As a form of associative learning, classical conditioning is most simply described as the learning that occurs when an animal is exposed to two or more stimuli, which as a function of their orderly arrangement are perceived by the animal to be related. As noted above, Rescorla (1988b) describes this as a process by which an animal develops an appreciation of stable relationships in its environment, and as a consequence, is able to adopt strategies for the successful negotiation of its world. In this regard, the common supposition that classical conditioning or associative learning is a "lower" form of learning and unrelated to higher "cognitive" function appears somewhat languid, that is, does not capture the fact that association formation is of pervasive relevance to simple and complex behaviors and memories. This circumscribed view of associative learning is in part a reflection of the procedures used in classical conditioning and the way these procedures are often described in popular literature and introductory textbooks. In a typical experiment of Pavlov's, a dog might be exposed to a tone (the conditioned stimulus; CS) after which a portion of meat powder (the unconditioned stimulus; US) is delivered to its oral cavity. Prior to this experience, the animal is unresponsive to the tone (it is said to be behaviorally "neutral"), but displays excitement, including salivation, in response to the meat. After several "pairings" of the CS and US, the animal begins to salivate in response to the sound of the tone, that is, before the meat is delivered. On the surface, it is hard for the casual observer to imagine the importance of studying a gastric reflex such as salivation (at least its relevance might appear rather limited). But spit is but a tool, and the conditioned response (CR) is but an indication of what the animal has learned about a relationship between two stimuli. It is obviously critical that we have objective ways to measure what the animal has learned, but equally critical that we appreciate that the behavioral response does not necessarily represent what has been learned and is not necessarily the sole consequence of that learning. It is important to remember what may be intuitively obvious outside of the laboratory; learning need not have an overt behavioral consequence and the expression of learning may depend on the conditions under which an animal is tested.

Since Pavlov's early descriptions of associative learning, literally dozens of behavioral responses have served as indices of learning in animals ranging from invertebrates to humans. Popularly employed conditioning preparations include the conditioned eyeblink response (e.g., in response to a tone that has been previously paired with an air puff or shock to the eye), conditioned heart rate changes (e.g., in response to a light paired with foot shock), conditioned "emotional" responses such as behavioral immobility or "freezing" (an indication of fear following paired presentation of a CS with shock or other stressor), conditioned analgesic responses (to a place or "context" associated with pain), and conditioned taste aversions (to some flavor that preceded the onset of an illness). Although data derived from these various approaches have provided much insight into the nature of learning, they have also indicated that associative learning and conditioned responses are not easily described by a static set of rules. To illustrate this point, we will first review some of characteristics of associative learning that most exemplify its flexibility, complexity, and functional utility.

The Learning "Curve" and Strengthening through Repetition

Classical conditioning was historically conceived of as learning that occurred as a consequence of exposure to repeated pairings (or trials) of stimuli (Hilgard, 1948; Klatsky, 1980). The expression of learning during associative training often conforms to the classic negatively accelerating learning curve, and the generation of this curve is integral to eminent formal models of classical conditioning (e.g., Rescorla and Wajner, 1972; Pearce and Hall, 1980). However, associative learning and its lasting expression does not require multiple trials. Depending on the conditions, learning may be asymptotic (or nearly so) following a single trial (Annau and Kamin, 1961; Smith and Roll 1967). Although mathematical descriptions of association formation predict incremental learning under some circumstances, they also allow for asymptotic one-trial learning under a broad range of conditions, for example, during the paired presentation of intense (high salience) CSs and USs. Likewise, the rate of acquisition of a CR is influenced by the interval between the onset of the CS and the onset of the US (Gibbon and Balsam, 1981). Moreover, the environmental niche that an animal fills influences the rate at which it acquires a given CS-US association. For example, rats rapidly (often with a single trial) learn to associate a flavor with illness, but are slow to learn the association between the same flavor and a foot shock (Garcia and Koelling, 1966). Thus, a number of circumstances can interact to influence the rate at which an animal learns. Moreover, the conditioning arrangements that characteristically require extensive training for asymptotic performance may not reflect an underlying slow rate of learning per se, but instead some difficulty in expressing the learned response. For instance, rabbits are notoriously slow to acquire the conditioned eyeblink response, often requiring hundreds of trials to reach asymptotic levels of performance (Schneiderman and Gormezano, 1964). However, if the experimenter simultaneously records the acquisition of conditioned heart rate and eyeblink responses to the same CS, the learned modifications of heart rate are asymptotic within ten trials (Black and Black, 1967). Thus, for the same CS and US combination, the apparent rate of "learning" does not represent the actual rate of acquisition, but instead, can reflect a constraint imposed by the response system that is monitored. In theoretical approaches to this issue, it has been suggested that the eyeblink response is slowly acquired because of the precise timing necessary to emit a blink just prior to the onset of the US. Thus while the animal might recognize the CS-US relationship early in training, the generation of an appropriate conditioned response requires a level of temporal precision that is slowly acquired (Cantor, 1981). As a further consideration, different rates of acquisition of even a single response might differ across species or between sexes within a species. For example, rats acquire the conditioned eyeblink response much more rapidly than rabbits (Servatius and Shors, 1996) and females more rapidly than males (Wood and Shors, 1998; Shors et al., 2000).

Based on the above, it is clear that the rate at which an associative memory is acquired is not determined by a single, invariant underlying mechanism, but is instead a product of an interaction between the training procedure, stimulus properties, and the response requirements of the task.

The Interstimulus Interval and the Efficacy of Learning

Pavlov recognized that the classically conditioned response was acquired more rapidly when the interval between the onset of the CS and the onset of the US (the interstimulus interval or ISI) was relatively short. Using his standard training procedure, dogs learned well with ISIs of several seconds, but exhibited relatively slower learning when the ISI was extended to several minutes. This observation (among others) led Pavlov to advocate that temporal contiguity was the principal determinant of association formation. Qualitative support came from later experiments. In the earliest eye blink conditioning experiments (conducted on humans), it was observed that very short ISIs (<1 second) supported good learning, while longer ISIs supported progressively weaker learning. Based on these and similar observations (Schneiderman and Gormezano, 1964), it is often asserted that "short" ISIs are most effective in inducing the formation of associations, and moreover, that there exists a generic "optimal" ISI for the formation of learned associations. However, these assumptions regarding the ISI are not well founded. Even Pavlov recognized that "shorter" was not necessarily better, noting that extremely short ISIs impaired learning in the same manner as did extremely long ISIs. This observation was disconcerting to Pavlov, since it indicated that temporal contiguity alone was not sufficient for associative learning; if it were, shorter ISIs would necessarily produce more efficacious learning. Since these early studies, it has become apparent that the efficacy of an ISI is determined by the conditioning procedure, by the response requirements of the task, and as a function of the inter-action between the ISI and the length of the session in which the training trials are presented. The optimal ISI ranges from several hundred milliseconds in the rabbit eyeblink preparation, to several seconds in rabbit conditioned bradycardia (Black and Black, 1967), to tens of seconds for many conditioned emotional responses (Annau and Kamin, 1961), to hours for conditioned taste aversions. In fact, in the case of conditioned taste aversions, ISIs of less than an hour significantly impair learning, and good learning can be obtained with intervals as long as 2 days (Smith and Roll, 1967). Thus not only is there no universally effective ISI for all learning tasks, even within a single task the range of effective ISIs can vary over several orders of magnitude.

Perhaps more striking is the observation that effectiveness of the ISI varies as a function of the time spent in the conditioning context. In a series of experiments, Kaplan (1984) exposed pigeons to paired presentations of a key light and food, with a fixed interval intervening between the offset of the key light and the presentation of food (i.e., a "trace" interval). When the ISI (i.e., the trace interval) between a key light (CS) and food (US) was short relative to the length of the conditioning session, Kaplan's birds rapidly acquired an "excitatory" conditioned response, that is, they approached and pecked the key when it was illuminated. However, if the conditioning session was shortened and the ISI was unchanged, no conditioned response to the key light emerged. If the conditioning session was shortened still more, such that it was only marginally longer than the still constant ISI, the birds withdrew from the lit key, indicative of the key having acquired "inhibitory" or aversive qualities. A common interpretation of these findings is that during the long conditioning session, the lit key served as a good predictor of food, isolating it in time. In the short conditioning session, the key light was perceived by the bird to signal a period when food was not available, thus acquiring an aversive quality. These results indicate that the effectiveness of a given ISI is not fixed, but rather is a function of the time that the CS tells the animal that it must wait for US delivery relative to the time that the animal would wait for the US if the CS were simply omitted (Gibbon and Balsam, 1981).

Temporal-Order Effects

As noted, Pavlov believed that temporal contiguity was the principal determinant of association formation and thus the order in which a nominal CS and US were presented should have no bearing on the acquisition of a conditioned response. Moreover, he anticipated that the simultaneous presentations of a CS and US would produce better learning than either the forward (CS prior to US) or backward (US prior to CS) presentations of the same stimuli. Pavlov was surprised to find simultaneous and backward conditioning arrangements supported vastly inferior learning than did the forward arrangement, a result that has led to the common belief that classical conditioning requires the forward arrangement of a CS and US. However, it is now clear that weak excitatory conditioning can be obtained following backward training, particularly following the first training trial (Shurtleff and Ayres, 1981; for review, see Spetch et al., 1981). More important, it is now appreciated that with sufficient training, the backward CS acquires inhibitory properties, suggesting that it is perceived by the animal to predict the *absence* of the US (Siegal and Domjan, 1971; Maier et al., 1976). In this later case, the animal's behavior is said to reflect an inhibitory association between the CS and US. Following this inhibitory learning, any subsequent attempt to make the backward CS excitatory (e.g., through forward conditioning) will progress at a "retarded" rate, and the inhibitory CS will oppose excitatory responses if it is presented in compound with another CS that has known excitatory value. In conclusion, backward conditioning does not fail to produce learning, but rather produces a form of learning that cannot be detected in typical tests of excitation.

The failure of simultaneous conditioning to produce clear evidence of learning and the distinct type of learning induced by backward conditioning have led some to conclude that classical conditioning is not merely the culmination of some automatic process that follows mechanically from the contiguous occurrence of two stimuli. Rather, the conditioned response is said to emerge from an animal's appreciation of stimulus relationships, and as such, is said to reflect the information provided to the animal by a particular stimulus (Rescorla, 1988a, 1988b).

It should be noted that this "informational" account of associative learning is a matter of some current debate. In a protracted series of experiments, Miller and his colleagues (e.g., Matzel et al., 1988; Miller and Barnett, 1993) have come to a different conclusion regarding the sufficiency of contiguity to support learning. In a typical experiment, rats are trained to associate two stimuli that are nominally described as CSs (e.g., a tone and a light; CS1 and CS2). Following forward pairings of CS1 and CS2, CS2 is then paired simultaneously with a shock US. On subsequent tests, CS2 evokes no conditioned fear, indicative of the simultaneous conditioning "deficit." However, when CS1 is tested, it evokes a strong fear response. To Miller, these results suggest that simultaneous pairings of CS2 and shock produced good learning, but that CS2 evokes no response given that it has no predictive value (or might in fact elicit from the animal a state analogous to "relief" when it is tested in the absence of the shock). In contrast, CS1 is said to evoke fear by virtue of its predictive relationship with CS2 (which the animal has learned, co-occurs with shock). According to Miller, simultaneous conditioning (e.g., between CS2 and shock) is sufficient to support the formation of an association, but as is the case with backward conditioning, does not evoke a response that is evident as excitation. Regardless of the interpretation, it is clear that contiguity alone is of little value in describing the acquisition of classically conditioned responses. Rather, the temporal order of CS and US presentations has a direct influence on either the form of learning and/or the nature of the conditioned response to that CS.

Contextual Learning and Temporal Invariance

A major advance in our appreciation of learning processes followed from the observation that a place, or conditioning "context" can acquire associative strength in much the same manner as punctate CSs, that is, the context in which a US (e.g., shock or food) was presented could come to evoke conditioned responses appropriate for that US (McAllister and McAllister, 1962; Rescorla, 1968; for reviews, see Balsam and Tomie, 1985). As an example, a rat might be placed in a distinct enclosure in which USs (e.g., shocks) are presented on a random basis with no discrete signal to predict them (i.e., they are not preceded by a punctate CS). Following such an experience, the rats will exhibit fear when they are subsequently returned to that context. This fear might be evident by the animal's "freezing" upon being placed in the enclosure (Fanselow and Tighe, 1988), or by the reluctance of the animals to consume water in that context (Matzel et al., 1987). This appreciation of contextual learning was a principal impetus for the influential model of associative learning described by Rescorla and Wagner in 1972. In their model, it was posited that the conditioning context is functionally equivalent to punctate CSs, and as such, acquires associative strength and can compete with discrete CSs for associative strength if they are trained in that context. This formulation has been enormously successful in describing and predicting a range of conditioning phenomena (described below).

It may not be surprising that a context can serve to predict a US, but we were slow to recognize the role of context conditioning, as by its nature, it is not easily accounted for by the contiguity-based views of classical conditioning that once dominated the field. To illustrate the problem, consider the following experiment (Matzel et al., 1987). Rats were exposed to six unsignaled shocks (500 msec duration) that were randomly distributed throughout a 60-minute session in a context referred to as "A." Up to 30 days after this experience (the last test session), water-deprived animals exhibited abnormally long latencies (approximately 1,000 sec) to initiate drinking in that context. This contextual learning was demonstrated to be associative in nature, since rats exposed to shock in a different context (Context "B") were quick to drink in Context A (approximately 6 seconds) and rats shocked in Context A and subsequently exposed to that context without shock presentations (i.e., the context was "extinguished") also drank without hesitation (7 seconds). Associative in nature, this form of conditioning is not operationally homologous to more typical Pavlovian procedures. First, the average interval between shocks in this example was approximately 10 minutes (i.e., six unsignaled shocks occurred in a 60-minute session). If one considers the context similar in nature to a discrete CS, this is analogous to an exceedingly long ISI of 10 minutes. Moreover, the context is present for approximately 10 minutes in the complete absence of shock (i.e., during the intershock interval). By strict contiguity theory, it should undergo substantial extinction during the 10-minute interval in which shock does not occur. Lastly, the shocks were randomly distributed throughout the session, and thus unlike a discrete CS, the context was not particularly useful in isolating the occurrence of any particular shock. It is clear that contiguity-based descriptions of associative learning would have great difficulty in accommodating this temporally invariant form of learning (Talk et al., 1999). Nevertheless, context conditioning is readily obtained under a wide range of experimental conditions. So ubiquitous is its influence, contemporary studies of associative learning are replete with strategies to control its affects.

Associative Memories Can Persist Indefinitely

It is commonly assumed that memories fade in a regular manner, becoming monotonically and progressively weaker with the passage of time. However, this is not universally true and there is some debate regarding the nature of this "forgetting" process. In everyday life, one encounters numerous examples in which an elderly relative or acquaintance can vividly recall seemingly inconsequential events from their early childhood. It should not be surprising then that in the laboratory, one can easily demonstrate the potential for relatively stable memories (for extensive reviews and discussion, see Spear, 1978; Spear et al., 1990). It was noted above that a rat's memory for contextual associations can persist intact for at least 30 days (Matzel et al., 1987). Although 30 days represents only a fraction of the rat's life span, others have demonstrated intact retention over considerably longer intervals. In one early study on the time course of "forgetting," Wendt (1937) was clearly dismayed by his observation that after a 2.5-year retention interval, his dogs displayed only marginal forgetting. Even after 2.5 years, they still responded to 80 percent of the CS presentations. Likewise, Hoffman et al. (1963) found virtually no loss of conditioned fear among a group a pigeons tested more than 2 years after initial training. Despite the stability of memory under many conditions, it is also obvious that all memories are not expressed with equal efficacy across an animal's life span. Again, anecdotal evidence clearly indicates that retention is often quite fragile, and concurring evidence can be found in the laboratory. For instance, infant rats can exhibit complete forgetting after only 3 hours (Miller et al., 1989). Moreover, different aspects of what was learned during original training can be forgotten at significantly different rates (McAllister and McAllister, 1971). However, even in cases where behavioral responses indicate that complete forgetting has occurred, it is commonly observed that forgetting can be alleviated by exposure to some component of the original training events, even while explicitly preventing new learning. For example, although infant rats quickly forget the relationship between a CS paired with shock, simply exposing the animals to the shock (a "reminder") long after forgetting appears complete is often sufficient to reinstate the memory for the CS (Campbell and Jaynes, 1966). This reinstatement of apparently lost memories is observed in many instances, and when attempted, the reinstatement of forgotten memories is far more typical than not (for reviews, see Miller et al., 1986; Spear et al., 1990). These results indicate to some that forgetting represents the failure to retrieve stored memories, not the actual decay of the memory itself. Thus while the expression of associative memories can weaken over time, they may in many instances persist intact across exceedingly long retention intervals, even for a lifetime.

Failed and Extinguished Associative Memories Are Easily Relearned

Forgotten memories and previously extinguished associations are universally observed to be relearned at a facilitated rate relative to original acquisition. Extinction differs from forgetting in that the memory is deliberately modified after initial learning. For example, after exposing a dog to pairings of a tone CS with a food US, the tone might be repeatedly presented alone such that the original conditioned response (e.g., salivation) dissipates, culminating in a dog that no longer salivates in response to the tone. Pavlov conceived of extinction as a form of "unlearning." However, even Pavlov recognized the inadequacy of this description, given that following extinction, his dogs relearned the conditioned response at a facilitated rate relative to during initial acquisition, an effect that has been replicated under diverse conditions as well as after apparent "forgetting" (e.g., Konorski and Szwejkowska, 1950; Matzel et al., 1992; Napier et al., 1992). Modern theories assume that this process of response diminution (via forgetting or extinction) and the potential for rapid relearning would be invaluable to organisms living in environments subject to regular, cyclic variations (Spear, 1978).

The Nature of Learning During Classical Conditioning

One of the most aggressive debates this century among learning theorists was whether animals learned responses per se, or whether they learned stimulus relationships, which in turn determined the nature of the response. The principals in this debate were the eminent theorists Clark Hull and Edward Tolman. According to Hull, during paired presentations of a CS and US an animal's response to the CS was modified through a process analogous to reflex substitution. Following training, the animal did not consider the "meaning" of a CS, but rather responded reflexively to it, in much the same manner that it responded to the US. Hull's view was characterized as a description of a stimulus-response (S-R) process whereby the CS directly evoked a conditioned response. This view of learning was notably devoid of any reliance on animal "cognition." In contrast, Tolman asserted that during CS-US presentations, animals learned about the relationship between the two events. This characterization of learning was referred to as a stimulus-stimulus (S-S) model, specifying that one stimulus evoked a representation of the other. In contrast to Hull, Tolman's view required that an animal appreciate stimulus relationships, which would in turn allow it to develop flexible response strategies. The debate between Hull and Tolman (and their proponents) dominated psychology for nearly two decades. Although the debate was never entirely resolved, Tolman's view prevails today.

Because it is most directly relevant to our later discussion of LTP and learning, we will briefly review some of the data that support Tolman's S-S model. As discussed above, Pavlov observed that the CR to a CS was not an inevitable (reflexive) consequence of CS-US (click-food) pairings, but rather was dependent on the dog's state of deprivation at the time of testing. It is not clear how Pavlov interpreted this result, as he advocated the view that conditioned responses were reflexive and represented the "transfer" of response-evoking properties of the US (e.g., food) to the initially neutral CS. Likewise, this result is not so easily accounted for by an S-R model, wherein it would be stipulated that the CS evokes a reflexive response as a consequence of having been paired with the US. In contrast, Tolman would be quite comfortable with such an observation, arguing that the CS evoked in the animal a "representation" or "expectation" of food, and that the response to this expectation was influenced by the animal's state of hunger.

Results like Pavlov's have been observed under diverse conditions. For instance, Rescorla (1973) observed that a rat's fear of a tone that had been paired with a horn US (a naturally aversive stimulus) would diminish if after conditioning, the animal's fear response to the horn was habituated. In conceptually related experiments, Bouton and his colleagues (Bouton and Peck, 1989; Bouton, 1991) have repeatedly found that the response to an extinguished CS can be modulated by the context in which it is ultimately tested. For instance, if a CS was trained in a context referred to as "A" and extinguished in that context, the CS will elicit no response (by definition, the end result of extinction). However, if the CS were trained in Context A and extinguished in a distinct context referred to as "B," the CS will elicit an intact conditioned response if it is subsequently tested in Context A, or in another, novel location. Thus the same CS may elicit different responses depending only on where it is tested. In direct contradiction of Hull's S-R model, these findings indicate that the learned response to a CS is not reflexive, but instead may take expressly different forms depending on the conditions under which the animal tested and the current affective value of the US that it predicts.

To explicitly test Tolman's S-S view of learning, Brogden (1939) employed a procedure that he referred to as "sensory preconditioning." In these experiments, Brogden's dogs were exposed to repeated pairings of a light (S1) and a buzzer (S2), each of which were behaviorally neutral (i.e., did not evoke any overt behavioral response). As one would expect, following pairings of the light and buzzer, presentations of the light (S1) alone elicited no behavioral response. Subsequently, the dogs received conditioning trials in which the buzzer (S2) was paired with foot shock (S3), culminating in the development of a leg-flexion CR to the buzzer. Of particular interest was the response to the light (S1) when it was tested after the buzzer (S2) had been paired with shock (S3). The light now elicited leg flexion in a manner similar to that of the buzzer. Brogden argued that during the initial phase of training, the light had been associated with the buzzer (S1-S2), followed by an association of the buzzer with shock (S2-S3). When the light is finally tested, it evokes a memory of the buzzer, which in turns evokes a memory of shock, eliciting a conditioned response appropriate for an impending shock (i.e., S1-S2-S3). Brogden's results have since been replicated with other conditioning tasks and procedures. It has been determined that the response to S1 is dependent on an intact association between it and S2 at the time of test, and that S2 must elicit some memory of S3 at the time of test, that is, both associations must be intact if S1 is to elicit an overt response at the time of testing (Rizley and Rescorla, 1972; Rescorla, 1980; Matzel et al., 1988). Since S1 is paired only with S2, S1 should according to Hull elicit the "reflex" learned during that training, that is, S1 should elicit no response regardless of later manipulations of S2. However, Tolman would argue that the representation of S2 elicited by S1 and the representation of a biologically salient US by S2 should engender (through S-S learning) S1 with the capacity to elicit a response appropriate for that US at the time of testing. These experiments provide clear support for Tolman's view of associative learning.

Based on Pavlov's view of associative learning, it is often stated that classical conditioning requires the pairing of a biologically neutral CS with a biologically significant US, after which the CS comes to evoke a response similar to that native (unconditioned) response to the US. Sensory preconditioning experiments and others like them have led some contemporary theorists to suggest that the use of terms such as "unconditioned stimulus" and "biologically significant" are misleading with regard to the conditions that underlie the development of associations (Dickinson, 1980). As the preceding experiments clearly indicate, associations can be formed between any stimuli and sequences of stimuli, regardless of their affective qualities. Accordingly, associative learning is a process by which animals record the relationships between stimuli and events in their world so that they might use that information in a flexible manner appropriate for the prevailing environmental conditions.

Associations Are Not the Automatic Consequence of Temporal Contiguity

Despite its obvious inadequacy, contiguity theory persisted as the principal explanatory tool in the description of associative learning. During the decade of the 1960s, an array of conceptually related experiments was reported that led to a complete reassessment of the nature of associative learning. One experiment in particular foreshadowed the decade's more prominent work. Egger and Miller (1962) trained rats with paired presentations of a short-duration (1.5 seconds) CS (referred to as S2) and food. However, for some of their animals, the onset of a second, longer (2 second) CS (S1) preceded the onset of S2 by 0.5 seconds. On subsequent tests, S2 evoked a CR only in those animals for which it was trained in the absence of S1. Egger and Miller argued that although S2 was reliably paired with food for each group of animals, S2 was rendered redundant and ignored when it was preceded by S1. Since S2 provided no uniquely useful information, it was said that the contiguous relationship between S2 and food did not support learning.

Experiments in the following years were at least as important in illustrating the inadequacy of simple contiguity to support associative learning. In Kamin's (1969) "blocking" experiments, a CS such as a tone was paired with a shock US. Normally, Kamin's rats quickly learned that the tone predicted shock, and came to exhibit conditioned fear (suppression of bar pressing for food) during presentations of the tone. However, if rats were trained with a stimulus compound composed of the tone and a light that had been previously paired with shock, the animals failed to learn about the tone (i.e., later tests of the tone in isolation revealed only weak conditioned fear). Kamin suggested that during compound training of the light and tone, the light adequately predicted shock such that the animals were not "surprised" by it. Consequently, the animals did not attend to the conditioning stimuli and thus did not learn about the relationship of the tone with shock.

In conceptually similar experiments, Rescorla (1968, 1969) and Wagner (1969) reported that the degree of correlation between a CS and US, not merely the contiguous occurrence of the two events, determined the degree to which an association would form between them. In fact, Rescorla reported that despite occasional contiguous occurrences of a tone and shock, the tone would acquire inhibitory properties if the context in which it was trained was a more reliable predictor of shock (i.e., if the tone predicted a decrease in shock likelihood relative to that predicted by the training context).

The seminal experiments of the 1960s clearly indicated that the contiguous relationship between a CS and US was not sufficient to establish an association between them, but rather that animals assessed the predictive value of a stimulus relative to other stimuli present during a training session. In so doing, animals were presumed to take a more active role in the learning process. This shift in emphasis away from the role of temporal contiguity has engendered a number of influential theories regarding the nature of associative learning. Foremost among them was the formal model of Rescorla and Wagner (1972), in which it is stipulated that stimuli compete for the associative strength that a given US can support. As it becomes well predicted, a US can support no additional learning. Consequently, redundant, less informative, or less salient stimuli do not easily enter into associations. Similarly, others have posited that associative learning is an attention-based process whereby the attention devoted to a CS progressively diminishes as a given US becomes increasingly well predicted, diverting attention away from stimuli that provide less valid or more ambiguous information about a US (Pearce and Hall, 1980). It should be noted that not all contemporary models reject contiguity as the basis for associative learning. Rather, a class of "performance-based" models assume that contiguity is sufficient for the establishment of an association between stimuli (e.g., a CS and US), but that factors related to the relative capacities of stimuli to elicit a response determine the nature and strength of that response (Gibbon and Balsam, 1981; Miller and Matzel, 1988). The virtues of these various approaches are reviewed in detail elsewhere (Delamater and LoLordo, 1989). Although all of these various formulations of the associative learning process have proven to be inadequate in some respects, they share the common assumption that this "simple" form of learning cannot be characterized as "reflexive," and that conditioned responses do not follow as a mechanical consequence of an animal's passive exposure to environmental events.

The Form of the Conditioned Response

Based on his observations, Pavlov thought that through associative pairings with the US, the CS would acquire the response-evoking properties of the US. That is, the affective quality of the US was "transferred" to the CS. This seemed a reasonable assessment since conditioned salivation was observed in response to a CS paired with food and conditioned limb withdrawal in response to a CS paired with shock to that limb. However, Pavlov's view of the conditioned response cannot account for many (or most) associatively trained responses, and was based on his serendipitous choice of conditioning procedures. For instance, in the earliest studies of fear conditioning (Estes and Skinner, 1941), it was observed that the unconditioned response of rats to a foot shock US induced behavior marked by a state of agitation or anxiety and characterized by jumping in place, indiscriminate running, and intense vocalization. In contrast, the conditioned response to a CS that had been paired with the foot shock was observed to suppress overt behavior (i.e., "freezing"). Similarly, in response to a shock US, a rat's heart rate increases dramatically, while the CR to a CS that predicts shock is a heart rate decrease (Schneiderman, 1972). In these instances, the unconditioned and conditioned responses could be characterized as being "opposite" one another.

Conditioned responses may in some instances mimic the unconditioned response to the US. For instance, an aversive shock induces the rapid onset of an opioid-dependent form of analgesia in rats. In a similar manner, a context that was previously associated with shock can evoke a conditioned analgesic response that is attenuated by prior administration of opioid antagonists (Matzel et al., 1987; Maier and Warren, 1988; Matzel et al., 1989; Fanselow et al., 1991). A rabbit's unconditioned response to periorbital shock is a closure of its nictitating membrane and eyelid. Likewise, a CS that has been paired with the periorbital shock induces a conditioned nictitating membrane closure and an eyeblink. Even in these cases of apparent reflex transfer, the CS does not actually elicit the same response as the US. For instance, the periorbital shock elicits a membrane closure that peaks rapidly after the onset of the shock and is maintained for the shock's duration. In contrast, the conditioned membrane closure does not develop until late in the CS interval, ultimately occurring at a time just prior to the onset of the US (Schneiderman et al., 1964). Adding further to the complexity of the CR, Holland (1977) has reported that the conditioned response evoked by a CS can reflect a combination of responses appropriate for both the CS and US. After CS-US pairings, the response elicited by the initial onset of the CS may reflect innate response-evoking qualities of that stimulus (e.g., a rapid head-turn toward a tone CS), while later during the CS, responses emerge that may be more appropriate for the specific US that the CS predicts, for example, freezing if the CS predicts shock or approaching a food cup if the CS predicts food delivery.

To account for the diverse nature of conditioned responses, Perkins (1968) developed the "preparatory response hypothesis," which states that the form of the CR is determined by the nature of the US, and is a manifestation of a coping (preparatory) response elicited by the CS. Thus, the CS prepares the animal for the impending US. For example, the compensatory response (e.g., hypertension) elicited by a context in which morphine had been administered is thought to protect the animal against acute deleterious effects of the drug, raising the threshold for potential overdose (Siegal, 1989).

One of the great successes of the preparatory response hypothesis came from the common observation that rats preferred signaled to unsignaled shock, a result that was commonly interpreted to reflect the capacity of the signal (CS) to elicit responses that might reduce the perceived intensity of shock. To directly test this hypothesis, Miller et al. (1999) developed a procedure in which rats were required to rate the relative intensities of shocks that were either preceded by a signal or which were unsignaled. Despite exhibiting a clear preference for the signaled shock, the rats rated the unsignaled shock as less intense. In contradiction to the predictions of the preparatory response hypothesis, these data indicate that rats perceive a signaled shock as more intense than an identical shock that is unsignaled. Nevertheless, Miller et al. were disposed to accept the general validity of the preparatory response hypothesis and noted that as a consequence of the evolutionary influences exerted by its environment, an animal comes to prefer signaled over unsignaled danger. Unlike in the laboratory, an animal in its natural habitat might employ successful responses to deter the danger.

It is clear from the above discussion that it is often difficult to make a priori predictions about the form of the conditioned response. It can take many forms, and is determined by an interaction of the CS and US, the nature of the test, and the animal's innate predispositions. It is clearly inadequate to describe the conditioned response as the consequence of a transfer of the reflex-eliciting qualities of the US to the CS.

Can LTP Subserve the Process of Associative Memory?

Although "LTP" can take many forms and is often used as an acronym for any observation of synaptic facilitation, we will limit the present discussion to particular forms of LTP that have been described in the mammalian hippocampus. In particular, we will focus on the NMDA receptor-dependent forms of LTP that are expressed in dentate gyrus granule neurons in response to stimulation of the perforant pathway, and in area CA1 pyramidal cells in response to stimulation of the Schaffer collaterals (the branches of the axons of CA3 pyramidal neurons). This approach is warranted because of the relative wealth of information about these two subtypes of LTP, and also because these forms are widely asserted to possess characteristics suitable for the storage of associative memories (Collingridge and Bliss, 1995; Martinez and Derrick, 1996; Miller and Mayford, 1999). We will not provide a comprehensive description of the mechanisms underlying LTP or the experiments that purport to demonstrate a role for LTP in memory, as we have already written extensively on these topics (Shors and Matzel, 1997) and detailed reviews appear in this volume and elsewhere (Malenka and Nicoll, 1999). Instead, we will assess the degree to which the properties of LTP parallel characteristics of the learning process.

In our previous critique of the LTP-learning hypothesis (Shors and Matzel, 1997), we were criticized in several accompanying commentaries for assuming that neurophysiologic properties of single cells or synapses (as represented by LTP) should correspond with the properties of a "systems-level" process such as memory. In doing so, we were said to have built a "straw house," the weak foundation of which could only lead to the inevitable conclusion that LTP was not suitable for this purpose. While a reasonable charge, it is at the same time an indictment of more widely accepted presumptions. We must stress that the purported mechanistic similarities between LTP and associative learning provide the principal basis for common and typically unquestioned assertions that LTP *is* an appropriate device for the storage of associative memories. If the properties of LTP serve as the basis for these assertions, then it is imperative to ask whether empirical evidence supports the conclusion. In the absence of such scrutiny, the superficial similarities between LTP and memory will persist as the basis for a conclusion that is not warranted.

The pervasive emphasis on the role of hippocampal LTP in associative memory is curious in some respects. First, the hippocampus is not generally thought to play a necessary role in the induction or generation of many classically conditioned responses. The hippocampus is, however, required for a certain class of conditioned responses where the task is more demanding, such as during trace conditioning where the CS and US are temporally disparate (Solomon et al., 1986; McEchron et al., 1998; Beylin et al., 1999; Gould et al., 1999a, 1999b). As will become evident below, the temporal constraints on LTP are poorly suited to subserve trace conditioning. Of greater conceptual concern is its role in spatial memory, a form of memory that is dependent on the hippocampus for learning and expression (Riedel et al., 1999). Spatial learning is impaired by manipulations that disrupt the induction of hippocampal LTP (Morris et al., 1991; Davis et al., 1992) and can be accompanied by a facilitation of synaptic responses that are qualitatively similar to that induced by LTP (Jeffery and Morris, 1993). Although this line of research is perhaps the best evidence for a role of LTP in learning, it is commonly asserted that spatial learning does not represent an associative process (Morris, 1981). If we accept this assertion, then the associative nature of LTP is of little use in describing the mechanism by which spatial memories are stored (cf. Wallenstein et al., 1998). Thus, the conceptual basis for assertions that LTP contributes to these various forms of memory is somewhat tenuous.

Associative LTP and Associative Learning

Given that the conceptual fit between LTP and associative learning is tenuous, one might ask why a presumed connection between the two is so commonly asserted. In part, this assertion reflects a theoretical derivative; LTP is in certain respects consistent with the Hebbian principle of synaptic facilitation. In *The Organization of Behavior,* his classic treatment of behavioral neuroscience, Hebb (1949) speculated that "When an axon of cell A ... excite(s) cell B and repeatedly or persistently takes part in firing it, some growth process or metabolic change takes place in one or both cells so that A's efficiency as one of the cells firing B is increased." This speculation of Hebb's, commonly referred to as "Hebb's Rule," resembles the operations and consequences of LTP induction and is frequently submitted as the fundamental basis for the conclusion that associative (or "Hebbian") LTP subserves associative learning. Although Hebb's comments were offered purely as an example of the type of hypothesis that might direct empirical investigations, his "rule" has been widely adopted by the neuroscience community as the foundation from which the mechanism of memory storage should emerge. Although viable as a hypothesis, we must stress that a role for Hebbian synaptic facilitation in learning or memory has never been established, and in fact, has been contradicted by certain data (e.g., Carew et al., 1984).

LTP is typically defined as a persistent increase in synaptic efficacy in response to brief tetanic (high-frequency) stimulation of an afferent pathway (Bliss and Gardner-Medwin., 1973; Bliss and Lømo, 1973). Following LTP induction, a fixed amount of presynaptic stimulation induces a "potentiated" postsynaptic response, for example, an increase in spread and amplitude of the excitatory postsynaptic potential (EPSP). A defining feature of LTP is its dependence on high levels of postsynaptic calcium. Induction of LTP is prevented by a postsynaptic injection of calcium chelators (Lynch et al., 1983), and LTP can be mimicked by artificially loading postsynaptic cells with calcium (Malenka et al., 1988). Evidence indicates that during LTP induction, the primary (or at least sufficient) source of intracellular calcium arises from current flow through a calcium-selective ion channel that is coupled to the NMDA subtype of glutamate receptor (e.g., Collingridge et al., 1983; Harris et al. 1984; Jahr and Stevens, 1987). This receptor is unique in that both glutamate binding and a moderate level of depolarization are required for its activation. At normal resting potentials ($\gg$ −70 mV), the channel is blocked by magnesium, and glutamate binding alone is insufficient to dispel the block. However, at depolarized membrane potentials (> −40 mV), magnesium is expelled from the channel such that glutamate binding is then sufficient to induce a flow of calcium ions through the channel. Thus, the NMDA receptor channel is said to be dually regulated by both the transmitter ligand and membrane voltage.

The cofactors required to open the NMDA channel (i.e., calcium and voltage) can be recruited through several means. First, a relatively long and intense burst of presynaptic activity (such as a high-frequency train of depolarizing stimulation) can induce LTP by releasing glutamate onto the postsynaptic receptor while simultaneously depolarizing the postsynaptic cell through stimulation of non-NMDA classes of glutamate receptors. Second, shorter and more physiologically relevant levels of presynaptic activity can induce hippocampal LTP if the postsynaptic cell is independently depolarized during the binding of glutamate, such as might occur in response to input from a second afferent pathway. This dual regulation is one of the features of LTP that has encouraged the idea that LTP is associative in nature; that is, two events (presynaptic activity and postsynaptic depolarization) must occur in close temporal proximity in order for potentiation to occur. These two biophysical events are often cited as analogous to the CS and US that characterize associative learning. LTP is said to be "associative" in nature, in that roughly contiguous, low-intensity stimulation of two pathways, or higher intensity stimulation of weak inputs that converge on the same postsynaptic target are effective in inducing LTP when stimulation of neither pathway alone is sufficient (Levy and Steward, 1979; Barrionuevo and Brown, 1983). For the successful induction of associative LTP, the two converging inputs onto the postsynaptic target must be stimulated in close temporal contiguity (i.e., within approximately 100 msec or less). Thus LTP may not result from normal activity in a single pathway, but rather might be reserved for purposes of "coincidence detection," for instance, between a CS and US.

As described above, the operation underlying the induction of associative LTP suggests a mechanism that is nominally similar to that described by Hebb's Rule. At this point, it is important to note that the associative nature of LTP reflects the dependence of LTP on sufficient levels of postsynaptic activity (McNaughton et al., 1978) and is presumed to reflect the additive effects of multiple postsynaptic calcium signals. This suggests that the "associative" feature of LTP is simply the successful expression of what might occur nonassociatively, that is, with sufficient stimulation of a single afferent fiber (and is thus conceptually analogous to sensitization). This raises questions regarding the application of this associative feature of LTP to associative learning, which is not generally considered to reflect the amplification of some nonassociative process (Pearce and Dickinson, 1975). Thus in itself, the potential for LTP induction by "associative" stimulation protocols provides little support for its presumed role in the induction of associative memories.

Acquisition Kinetics of LTP and Associative Memory

The synaptic potentiation expressed during LTP induction is characteristically incremental in nature, that is, it accumulates across successive bouts of stimulation. Once asymptotic, additional bouts of stimulation will produce no further synaptic potentiation, indicative of a physiologic upper limit on LTP (Shors and Dryver, 1994). Of particular interest, the expression of synaptic potentiation following the stimulation protocol is slow to develop, typically requiring tens of seconds if not minutes to reach its stable asymptotic level. How do these features of LTP induction compare to the acquisition of associative memories? Although the conditioned response that emerges during associative learning can increase incrementally with successive training trials, conditioned responses are often robust and can be asymptotic and enduring after a single training event. Thus, while LTP is characterized as exhibiting "strength through repetition," this characteristic is not a defining feature of associative learning. Moreover, CRs can be observed "immediately" (at the earliest possible retention test) following a training event, consistent with the common-sense expectation that the memory of an event begins upon termination of the inducing event (if not before). In contrast, stable LTP emerges gradually after stimulation. Thus the mechanism of LTP is not well suited to subserve either one-trial learning or immediate retention.

Trial-Spacing Influences on the Induction of LTP and Associative Memory

The acquisition of associative memories follows characteristic rules of trial spacing. That is, acquisition is facilitated when trials are widely distributed relative to when they are closely spaced. In the most extreme examples, exposure to one trial a day over repeated days results in much faster learning than the same number of trials presented in a single session. Within a single training session, relatively longer intertribal intervals support faster acquisition than shorter intervals. In contrast, synaptic facilitation accruing from LTP stimulation protocols is severely impaired if successive stimulations are presented at long interstimulation intervals (de Jonge and Racine, 1985). While narrowly spaced periods of stimulation can produce an acquisition curve for LTP that is superficially similar to the acquisition curve that can be observed during associative learning, more widely distributed periods of stimulation often result in no accumulation of LTP. This in part reflects the rapid decay of LTP during the interstimulation interval. Thus, the effects of trial spacing on the induction of LTP and associative memories are diametrically opposite one another.

Effective Interstimulus Intervals for the Induction of LTP and Associative Memory

More than any other feature, the short forward delay between pre- and postsynaptic activity that is required for the induction of associative LTP is offered as evidence that this form of synaptic plasticity is well suited for the storage of associative memories. At a qualitative level, this is a reasonable assertion, given that classical conditioning is often believed to require a short, forward interval between the CS and US for successful learning. While this characterization dominates colloquial views of associative learning, it is an erroneous description of the actual phenomenon. As described previously, associations are formed between stimuli that are nominally referred to as a "CS" and "US" when those stimuli are trained with a backward or simultaneous arrangement. Thus the potential for backward conditioning appears incongruent with the mechanism of associative LTP. One could argue that this incongruence is artificial and reflects a misplaced (and literal) reliance on arbitrary labeling systems that assign specific significance to stimuli designated as a CS or US. As we discussed earlier, many contemporary accounts of learning are based on the supposition that animals make stimulus-stimulus associations, and assign no special significance to descriptors such as "CS" or "US" (Dickinson, 1980). In this respect, the analogy between the pre- and postsynaptic events that underlie LTP induction to the CS and US used during classical conditioning could be said to be no more than a semantic convenience, and as such, the mechanism of LTP might easily account for potential for backward conditioning. However, if one were to adopt this position, then the "forward" ISI that is required for the induction of associative LTP should not be interpreted either as support or repudiation of LTP's role in associative learning.

Although the seeming inability of associative LTP to allow for backward associations can be easily disregarded, a more veritable disparity between LTP and associative learning emerges when we compare the "short" ISI that supports associative LTP to the range of ISIs that underlie associative learning. As was described above, the ISI between pre- and postsynaptic stimulation that gives rise to associative LTP ranges from 0 to 100 msec and ISIs of more than 100 msec are ineffective (Gustafsson et al., 1987). In contrast, the optimal ISI between the CS and US during classical conditioning varies from several hundred milliseconds in the rabbit eyeblink preparation, to several seconds in rabbit conditioned bradycardia, to tens of seconds for many conditioned emotional responses, to many hours for conditioned taste aversions. More significantly, ISIs far in excess of the "optimal" are quite effective in supporting associations. For instance, in typical conditioned fear or appetitive autoshaping procedures, ISIs of 10 seconds between the CS and aversive US are quite effective in supporting learning, but ISIs as long as 3 minutes are commonly reported to support good learning. Although the CR is slower to develop with these longer ISIs, the ultimate level of conditioned response can be quite similar in the two extreme cases (e.g., Durlach, 1983).

A still greater incongruity between the ISIs that support LTP and associative learning is reflected in the observation that a single ISI can result in either inhibitory or excitatory learning depending on the overall duration of the conditioning session. These dichotomous effects of a single ISI presumably reflect the temporal isolation of the US by the CS relative to that of the contextual stimuli in which CS-US training occurs (Gibbon and Balsam, 1981).

A final disparity that is encountered when we compare the ISI functions of LTP and associative learning is that robust conditioned responding can be observed in response to a context in which USs were delivered in the absence of a discrete CS. This conditioned response to the context develops even in those instances where there is no regular temporal relationship between the contextual cues (i.e., the conditioning context) and the US delivered in that context, and where the interval between successive USs is quite long (e.g., >10 minutes).

In all, the short forward ISI (0 to 100 msec) that is effective in inducing LTP fails to account for the range and affects of ISIs on associative learning and conditioned responding. We might then ask whether the short ISI that supports associative LTP can account for *any* known instance of associative learning. Not to our knowledge. In fact, this interval is far shorter than is optimal for any behavioral conditioning procedure that has ever been described. Despite these apparent failures of LTP, it should be noted that near simultaneity of stimuli has been suggested to support efficient learning in Pavlovian paradigms, while the behavioral expression of that learning is determined by an interaction of the specific ISI with the response system that is being observed (Matzel et al. 1988; Rescorla, 1980). Were this the case, LTP might still be an appropriate induction mechanism for learning. Despite this caveat, any analogy between associative LTP and associative learning that is based on allusions to "similar" ISI functions is based on a mischaracterization of the learning process.

From our discussion thus far, it is apparent that numerous incongruities arise when attempting to relate the properties of LTP to the process of associative learning. While many of these incongruities have been previously described (Keith and Rudy, 1990; Vanderwolf and Cain, 1994; Shors and Matzel, 1997; Wallenstein et al., 1998), little empirical effort has been directed toward their resolution. There have, however, been attempts to address the discrepancies related to the ISI functions that subserve LTP and associative learning. For instance, Brown and colleagues (Canli and Brown, 1996; Lam et al., 1996; Faulkner and Brown, 1999) have identified cells in the amygdala and perirhinal cortex that exhibit long latencies to fire a spike during periods of prolonged depolarization. In some cases, the latency to fire can be as long as several seconds. Thus, it has been proposed that the availability of a distribution of cells with a range of firing latencies could account for the range of ISIs that support different types of associative learning. Although provocative, it is still unclear how the appropriate cell would "know" its involvement in any particular association, unless the cell that represents the CS (and that exhibits an appropriate firing latency) projected onto a vast number of postsynaptic targets, one of which was experiencing a US-induced depolarization. Accordingly, a pair of such cells (or populations of cells) would need to exist for every possible pair of CSs and USs and every possible "optimal" ISI. Although unlikely, this possibility cannot be entirely dismissed. Even so, this kind of formulation cannot account for the observation that the optimal ISI for any CS-US pair is not fixed, but rather varies as a function of the duration of the training session. Moreover, the firing latencies of several seconds that have been described by Brown are inadequate to account for many effective ISI functions (that can range from minutes to hours) that support associative learning. In all, we are left to conclude that the temporal kinetics of LTP induction are in only the most perfunctory sense analogous to those that underlie associative learning (see also Diamond and Rose, 1994).

We must consider one final complication, one for which no empirical resolution is forthcoming. Animals are capable of associating stimuli that are temporally discontinuous as evidenced by their capacity for trace conditioning. Even in the most temporally constrained forms of conditioning such as exemplified by the rabbit eyeblink preparation, the rabbits acquire conditioned responses when the CS offset precedes the US onset by hundreds of milliseconds. (Note also that conditioning is observed in other preparations with trace intervals as long as many hours.) This is a particularly important observation with regard to the role of LTP, as trace conditioning is regarded to involve the hippocampus (Solomon et al., 1986; McEchron et al., 1998; Beylin et al., 1999; Gould et al., 1999a,b). This dependence of trace conditioning on the hippocampus and ubiquitous expression of associative LTP in the hippocampus has led to the common conclusion that LTP is well suited to subserve this form of learning. However, as noted, associative LTP requires nearly contiguous pre- and postsynaptic activity, and intervals longer than 100 msec are ineffective. Thus, like delay conditioning, the temporal constraint on associative LTP does not account for learning when a trace intervenes between the CS and US. Moreover, since the CS offset occurs long before the US onset, a scheme such as that proposed by Brown (described above) does not describe this type of learning, as even long-latency spikes in the afferent (CS) fiber would occur well before postsynaptic depolarization. In this one case where hippocampal LTP is most clearly applicable to the acquisition of a classically conditioned response, the mechanism fails to account for the temporal parameters of learning.

The Persistence of LTP and Associative Memories

One of the most commonly asserted reasons for LTP's promotion as a memory device is its persistence (i.e., it is "long lasting"). It is intriguing in that prior to its description, synaptic facilitation lasting more than seconds had not been observed in the mammalian nervous system. However, "persistence", as used to describe synaptic plasticity, refers to a time frame that is vastly different from that used to describe memory. In the most comprehensive analysis, it was reported that LTP could persist for over a week following repetitive *in vivo* inductions in area CA1 (a median of 10.5 days in CA1; Staubli and Lynch, 1987). In the mouse, LTP in the dentate gyrus has been observed 24 hours, but not 10 days, after induction (Davis et al., 1997). In commonly studied *in vitro* preparations of the hippocampal slice, maintenance of LTP beyond 8 hours is not typically observed (Reymann et al., 1985), although this more rapid decay may reflect the inherent instability of this preparation. There have been no reports of nondecremental LTP, that is, when LTP is assessed over time, it always decays, and usually does so quite rapidly. To enhance its persistence, some have used multiple stimulating tetani, sometimes exceeding 100 high-frequency trains distributed over days or weeks (e.g., Castro et al., 1989). Even with such extensive (excessive?) "training," a characteristic decay of the synaptic response to baseline levels is observed within days to a week. To account for the relatively rapid decay of LTP, it has been proposed that competing phenomena such as long-term depression (LTD) can supplant previous induction of potentiation (Pavlides et al., 1988; Sejenowski, 1990). Thus, in addition to its inherent decay, LTP may be reversed because of the natural occurrence of LTD in subsets of potentiated synapses. This disparity between the persistence of LTP and of stable associative memories should not be overlooked. Many of the failures of LTP to account for memory induction or storage might be disregarded as being the product of an unreasonable expectation that the properties of single synapses should account for memories, the expression of which is a systems-level process. Regardless of the complexity of the system, however, any underlying storage device must be able to maintain those memories over an appreciable portion (if not the entirety) of an animal's life span. LTP clearly fails to meet this most fundamental requirement.

"Forgetting" and Facilitated Reacquisition of LTP and Associative Memories

As described, the strength of an associatively conditioned response can in some instances decay spontaneously over time (i.e., they are "forgotten"). Likewise, the conditioned response can be extinguished by posttraining presentations of the CS alone. Both "forgotten" and extinguished conditioned responses exhibit facilitated reacquisition, that is, they are relearned more efficiently than was the case during initial acquisition. As discussed, the magnitude of LTP is dependent on the number of stimuli that are delivered. With more stimulation, greater magnitudes of LTP are observed, until some asymptotic level is attained (Shors and Dryver, 1994). One could view this observation as analogous to strengthening through repetition during memory induction, in which case a memory can be enhanced by repeated training events. However, in order for LTP to increase in magnitude with repeated exposure to the tetani, the tetani must be delivered before the prior potentiation decays back to baseline, that is, the acquisition curve associated with LTP induction develops only under conditions of short interstimulation (trial) intervals. Following a decay to baseline, LTP is neither more easily induced nor more persistent than it was after previous inductions (de Jonge and Racine, 1985). Thus the savings effect that is so characteristic of forgotten conditioned responses cannot be accounted for by underlying LTP.

With regard to extinction, it is not entirely clear what an extinction protocol might resemble following induction of associative LTP. Following pairings of pre- and postsynaptic stimulation, one might imagine a procedure where afferent stimulation (analogous to a CS) was presented in the absence of postsynaptic stimulation (analogous to the absence of a US). In fact, it is possible to induce "depotentiation" by stimulating afferent fibers at a much slower rate than that used for the initial induction of LTP. However, given that LTP can be induced in a nonassociative form (i.e., in response to afferent stimulation alone) it seems unlikely that a rate of afferent stimulation like that used during the induction of LTP could ever result in a loss of LTP. The important point here is that synaptic depression or "LTD" (Ito, 1989) can *only* be induced with rates of afferent stimulation orders of magnitude slower than that which induces LTP. Of course, the extinction of a behaviorally conditioned CR does not require that the CS-alone presentations occur at a slower rate than was used during initial CS-US training. Thus not only does LTP not exhibit facilitated acquisition or an acquisition function that is similar to that which accompanies associative learning, it has characteristics that are fundamentally incompatible with the basic property of extinction.

Network Properties of LTP and Associative Memory

As it is commonly conceived, synaptic facilitation that characterizes LTP alters the flow of current through a neural network, biasing the network toward some "response" that would not otherwise occur. To imagine how such an alteration of current flow might account for associative learning, we must recall the nature of the network that subserves the induction and expression of associative LTP. During the stimulation protocol that induces associative LTP, an afferent pathway is activated just prior to postsynaptic depolarization. In this network, the afferent cell(s) are conceived of as coding for the CS while the postsynaptic target codes the US (Kelso and Brown, 1986; Gustafsson and Wigstrom, 1988; Brown et al., 1990). After a CS-US pairing (and the induction of associative LTP), the cells responding to the CS will more efficiently depolarize those cells that code the US. As a consequence, those cells that code the US will stimulate some efferent set of motor pathways that subserve the native response to that US. Thus, via the induction of LTP, the CS will have acquired the ability to evoke that response that was previously evoked only by the US. Accordingly, the conditioned response should necessarily take the form of the unconditioned response. This conceptualization is not intended as a literal description of associative learning, as its advocates do not actually intend to imply that complex events such as a CS are processed in single cells or homogeneously across a population of cells. Nevertheless, this kind of formulation, expanded to a systems level, is the foundation by which it has been assumed that LTP is used in the formation of learned responses. Despite its appeal and simplicity, this description of a hypothetical neural network for the generation of conditioned responses fails at several levels. Most important, the conditioned response to a CS does not necessarily resemble the response to the US, and in fact may take a form that is "opposite" to that evoked by the US. As a further complication, the response to a CS may often reflect a compendium of behaviors that represent the interaction of that particular CS with the specific US that it predicts. Likewise, the conditioned response will vary as a function of the constraints imposed on the animal by the testing situation and is not fixed by the conditions that prevailed at the time of training.

The complexity of the conditioned response is to some extent a likely reflection of the process that underlies associative learning. As will be recalled, under a wide range of circumstances, classically conditioned responses were said to be the product of an animal having formed S-S associations. That is, the animal learns about stimulus relationships, and the nature of the relationships and the conditions under which the animal is tested determine the form of the conditioned response. Necessarily, descriptions of classical conditioning that are based on the assumption that associative LTP serves as the storage mechanism are a description of a process that is S-R in nature. In short, the neural network that underlies a conditioned response based on the induction of associative LTP is in essence the description of the modification of reflex arcs (i.e., motor pathways). From the prior discussion of classical conditioning it should be clear that this form of learning cannot be adequately or accurately described simply as the modification of reflexive behavior.

One simple and clear example of the errors engendered by the assertion that the associative LTP can subserve associative learning is warranted. In a hypothetical experiment, an animal might be trained with a tactile CS (vibration of the animal's skin) paired with a shock US in a context that we will refer to as "A." In a second context referred to as "B," the animal is exposed to the same CS, but in this context, the CS is not reinforced. (One might wonder if a CS can actually be the "same" when perceived in two distinct locations. While this is difficult to determine with complete certainty, a tactile CS such as used in this hypothetical experiment would not be obviously affected by the environment and so would likely to be perceived as the same stimulus, impinging on the same receptors and sensory systems.) After several sessions in which the CS is reinforced in Context A and not reinforced in Context B, the animal will exhibit strong conditioned responding in the former but not the later context. Thus, the animal has made a simple discrimination that in turn guides the conditioned response, a process that is ubiquitous and fundamentally important in the generation of appropriate responses to stimuli. Although of a rudimentary nature, the hypothetical experiment described above cannot be accommodated by models of conditioned response that are based on the modification of reflex pathways by associative LTP. The response to a common CS varies dramatically depending on whether it is tested in Context A (where it has been paired with shock) or Context B (where it was presented without reinforcement). The real problem arises when one considers that in both cases the CS stimulates the same receptors that must impinge on those cells that activate the response to the US, that is, the pre- and postsynaptic units that undergo LTP are the same regardless of the animals' immediate location. Thus, a simple network model of conditioned response that is based on associative LTP predicts no differential responding in the two conditions. Instead, an intermediate level of response (the average of the reinforced and nonreinforced trials) should be expressed in response to the CS in both contexts (cf., Rogers and Steinmetz, 1998).

We do not view this particular example as illustrating a fatal flaw in the hypothesis that LTP serves as the storage mechanism for associative memories. Rather, it reflects the prevalent tendency to oversimplify the associative learning process. Neurophysiological descriptions of conditioned response generation are often based on the presumption that modifications of a response pathway are the result of the facilitation of the synaptic interaction between the cell (or group of cells) that code the CS and the cell (or group of cells) that codes the US. It is simple enough to presume that the response to a CS can be modulated by other stimuli present during training or testing such that the response may differ under different testing conditions. This can be accomplished regardless of whether LTP or some other device (cf. Matzel et al., 1998) serves as the substrate mechanism for the storage of the associative memory. The critical point is that current models of associative conditioning that purport to account for conditioned responses by the LTP-induced modification of a reflex pathway are based on erroneous assumptions about associative learning and can only account for the most elementary conditioned response under severely limited conditions.

Conclusions, Resolutions, and Future Directions

At numerous levels, associative LTP fails to fulfill the minimum criterion required of a neural mechanism to support associative learning. Properties of its induction cannot account for the conditions that induce associative learning, its characteristics are unsuited for the maintenance of that memory, and neural networks that depend on LTP as a storage device do not adequately describe the form of learned conditioned responses. Many of these failures of this purported memory mechanism reflect an oversimplification of the phenomenon, and as such could be resolved by more comprehensive models that place the mechanism of LTP within a larger neural system in which stimulus relationships are encoded and from which complex, adaptive, and flexible behaviors might emerge. Other failures of the mechanism to account for learning processes are not so easily attributable to oversimplifications of the process, but instead reflect immutable characteristics of the mechanism. These failures, such as the inherently decremental nature of LTP and the facilitation of LTP induction by massed training (massed stimulation), would seem to exclude LTP from serious consideration as an associative memory mechanism.

Based on our analysis, we must conclude that the common presumption that LTP is the underlying storage device for associative memories is untenable. Two principal problems follow from our continued focus on LTP as a memory storage mechanism. One is that we have limited our ability to recognize other functional roles that LTP may play within the nervous system. Given that synapses throughout the mammalian brain undergo potentiation using protocols similar to those that induce LTP, it is quite reasonable to assume that synaptic facilitation does play *some* role in the induction or expression of memories, for instance, as a gain control device that influences the rate of learning (Shors and Matzel, 1997). The second and perhaps more dangerous consequence of the continued focus on LTP as a memory device is that it deters efforts to elucidate other mechanisms that might be better suited to subserve the complex process of associative memory.

REFERENCES

Annau, Z., and Kamin, L.J. (1961). The conditioned emotional response as a function of intensity of the US. *J. Comp. Physiol. Psychol.* 54: 428–432.

Barrionuevo, G., and Brown, T.H. (1983). Associative long-term potentiation in hippocampal slices. *Proc. Natl. Acad. Sci. USA* 80: 7347–7351.

Beylin, A.V., Talk, A.C., Gandhi, C.C., Wood, G.F. et al. (1999). Acquisition but not performance of trace eyeblink conditioning is dependent on the hippocampus. *Soc. Neurosci. Abst.* 25: 89.

Black, R.W., and Black, P.E. (1967). Heart rate conditioning as a function of interstimulus interval in rats. *Psychonom. Sci.* 8: 219–220.

Bliss, T.V., and Gardner-Medwin, A.R. (1973). Long-lasting potentiation of synaptic transmission in the dentate area of the unanesthetized rabbit following stimulation of the perforant path. *J. Physiol. (London)* 232: 357–374.

Bliss, T.V., and Lømo, T. (1973). Long-lasting potentiation of synaptic transmission in the dentate area of the anaesthetized rabbit following stimulation of the perforant path. *J. Physiol. (London)*, 232: 331–356.

Bouton, M.E. (1991). Context and retrieval in extinction and in other examples of interference in simple associative learning. In L. Dachowski and C. F. Flaherty (Eds.), *Current topics in animal learning* (pp. 25–53). Hillsdale, NJ: Erlbaum.

Bouton, M.E., and Peck, C.A. (1989). Context effects on conditioning, extinction, and reinstatement in an appetitive conditioning preparation. *Animal Learning Behav.* 17: 188–198.

Brogden, W.J. (1939). Sensory pre-conditioning. *J. Exp. Psychol.* 25: 323–332.

Brown, T.H., Kairiss, E.W., and Keenan, C.L. (1990). Hebbian synapses: Biophysical mechanisms and algorithms. *Annu. Rev. Neurosci.* 13: 475–511.

Campbell, B.A., and Jaynes, J. (1966). Reinstatement. *Psychol. Rev.* 73: 478–480.

Canli, T., and Brown, T.H. (1996). Amygdala stimulation enhances the rat eyeblink reflex through a short- latency mechanism. *Behav. Neurosci.* 110: 51–59.

Cantor, M.B. (1981). Information theory: A solution to two big problems in the analysis of behavior. In P. Harzem and M.D. Zeiler (Eds.), *Predictability, correlation, and contiguity* (pp. 287–320). New York: John Wiley and Sons.

Carew, T.J., Hawkins, R.D., Abrams, T.W., and Kandel, E.R. (1984). A test of Hebb's postulate at identified synapses which mediate classical conditioning in *Aplysia. J. Neurosci.* 4: 1217–1224.

Castro, C.A., Silbert, L.H., McNaughton, B.L., and Barnes, C.A. (1989). Recovery of spatial learning deficits following decay of electrically-induced synaptic enhancement in the hippocampus. *Nature* 342: 545–548.

Collingridge, C.L., and Bliss, T.V.P. (1995). Memories of NMDA receptors and LTP. *Trends Neurosci.* 18: 54–56.

Collingridge, G.L., Kehl, S.J., and McLennan, H. (1983). Excitatory amino acids in synaptic transmission in the Schaeffer-commissural pathway of the rat hippocampus. *J. Physiol. (London)* 443: 33–46.

Davis, S., Butcher, S.P., and Morris, R.G.M. (1992). The NMDA receptor antagonist D-2-amino-5-phosphonopentanoate (D-AP5) impairs spatial learning and LTP in vivo at intracerebral concentrations comparable to those that block LTP in vitro. *J. Neurosci.* 12: 21–34.

Davis, S., Bliss, T.V.P., Dutrieux, D., Laroche, S. et al. (1997). Induction and duration of long-term potentiation in the hippocampus of the freely moving mouse. *J. Neurosci. Res.* 75: 75–80.

de Jonge, M., and Racine, R.J. (1985). The effects of repeated induction of long-term potentiation in the dentate gyrus. *Brain Res.* 328: 181–185.

Delamater, A.R., and LoLordo, V.M. (1991). Event revaluation procedures and associative structures in Pavlovian conditioning. In L. Dachowski and C.F. Flaherty (Eds.), *Current topics in animal learning.* Hillsdale: Erlbaum.

Diamond, D.M., and Rose, G.M. (1994). Does associative LTP underlie classical conditioning? *Psychobiology* 22: 263–269.

Dickinson, A. (1980). *Contemporary Animal Learning Theory.* Cambridge, England: Cambridge University Press.

Durlach, P.J. (1983). Effect of signaling intertrial unconditioned stimuli in autoshaping. *J. Exp. Psychol. Anim. Behav. Proc.* 9: 374–389.

Egger, M.D., and Miller, N.E. (1962). Secondary reinforcement in rats as a function of information value and reliability of the stimulus. *J. Exp. Psychol.* 64: 97–104.

Esters, W.K., and Skinner, B.F. (1941). Some quantitative properties of anxiety. *J. Exp. Psychol.* 29: 390–400.

Fanselow, M.S., and Tighe, T.J. (1988). Contextual conditioning with massed versus distributed unconditional stimuli in the absence of explicit conditional stimuli. *J. Exp. Psychol. Anim. Behav. Proc.* 14: 187–199.

Fanselow, M.S., Kim, J.J., Young, S.L., Calcagnetti, D.J. et al. (1991). Differential effects of selective opioid peptide antagonists on the acquisition of Pavlovian fear conditioning. *Peptides* 12: 1033–1037.

Faulkner, B., and Brown, T.H. (1999). Morphology and physiology of neurons in the rat perirhinal-lateral amygdala area. *J. Comp. Neurol.* 411: 613–642.

Garcia, J., and Koelling, R.A. (1966). Relation of cue to consequence in avoidance learning. *Psychonom. Sci.* 4: 123–124.

Gibbon, J., and Balsam, P. (1981). Spreading association in time. In L.C. Locurto, H.S. Terrace, and J. Gibbon (Eds.), *Autoshaping and conditioning theory* (pp. 219–253). New York: Academic Press.

Gould, E., Beylin, A.V., Tanapat, P., Reeves, A. et al. (1999a). Learning enhances adult neurogenesis in the adult hippocampal formation. *Nat. Neurosci.* 2: 260–265.

Gould, E., Tanapat, P., Hastings, N., and Shors, T.J. (1999b). Neurogenesis in adulthood: A possible role in learning. *Trends Cognitive Sci.* 3: 186–192.

Gustafsson, B., and Wigstrom, H. (1988). Physiological mechanisms underlying long-term potentiation. *Trends Neurosci.* 11: 156–162.

Gustafsson, B., Wigstrom, H., Abraham, W.C., and Huang, Y.Y. (1987). Long-term potentiation in the hippocampus using depolarizing current pulses as the conditioning stimulus to single volley synaptic potentials. *J. Neurosci.* 7: 774–780.

Harris, E.W., Ganong, A.H., and Cotman, C.W. (1984). Long-term potentiation in the hippocampus involves activation of N-methyl-D-aspartate receptors. *Brain Res.* 323: 132–137.

Hebb, D.O. (1949). *The Organization of Behavior.* New York: Wiley-Interscience.

Hilgard, E.R. (1948). *Theories of Learning.* New York: Appleton-Century-Crofts.

Hoffman, H.S., Flesher, M., and Jensen, P. (1963). Stimulus aspects of aversive controls: The retention of conditioned suppression. *J Exp. Anal. Behav.* 6: 575–583.

Holland, P.C. (1977). Conditioned stimulus as a determinant of the form of the Pavlovian conditioned response. *J. Exp. Psychol. Anim. Behav. Proc.* 3: 77–104.

Ito, M. (1989). Long-term depression. *Ann. Rev. Neurosci.* 12: 85–102.

Jahr, C.E., and Stevens, C.F. (1987). Glutamate activates multiple single channel conductances in hippocampal neurons. *Nature* 325: 522–525.

Jeffery, K.J., and Morris, R.G.M. (1993). Cumulative long-term potentiation in the rat dentate gyrus correlates with, but does not modify, performance in the water maze. *Hippocampus* 3: 133–140.

Kaplan, P.S. (1984). Temporal parameters in trace autoshaping: From excitation to inhibition. *J. Exp. Psychol. Anim. Behav. Proc.* 10: 113–126.

Kamin, L.J. (1969). Predictability, surprise, attention, and conditioning. In R.M. Church and B. A. Campbell (Eds.), *Punishment and aversive behavior* (pp 52–91). New York: Appleton-Century-Crofts.

Keith, J.R., and Rudy, J.W. (1990). Why NMDA-receptor-dependent long-term potentiation may not be a mechanism of learning and memory: Reappraisal of the NMDA-receptor blockade strategy. *Psychobiology* 18: 251–257.

Kelso, S.R., and Brown, T.H. (1986). Differential conditioning of associative synaptic enhancement in hippocampal brain slices. *Science* 232: 85–87.

Klatsky, R. (1980). *Human Memory* (2nd ed.). San Francisco: Freeman.

Konorski, J., and Szwejkowska, G. (1950). Chronic extinction and restoration of conditioned reflexes: I. Extinction against the excitatory background. *Acta Biol. Exp.* 15: 155–170.

Lam, Y.W., Wong, A., Canli, T., and Brown, T.H. (1996). Conditioned enhancement of the early component of the rat eyeblink reflex. *Neurobiol. Learn. Mem.* 66: 212–220.

Levy, W.B., and Steward, O. (1979). Synapses as associative memory elements in the hippocampus. *Brain Research,* 175: 233–245.

Lynch, G., Larson, J., Kelso, S., Barrionuevo, G. et al. (1983). Intracellular injections of EGTA block induction of hippocampal long-term potentiation. *Nature* 305: 719–721.

Maier, S.F., Rapaport, P., and Wheatley, K.L. (1976). Conditioned inhibition and the UCS-CS interval. *Anim. Learn. Behav.* 4: 217–220.

Maier, S.F., and Warren, D.A. (1988). Controllability and safety signals exert dissimilar proactive effects on nociception and escape performance. *J. Exp. Psychol. Anim. Behav. Proc.* 14: 18–25.

Malenka, R.C., and Nicoll, R.A. (1999). Long-term potentiation—a decade of progress? *Science* 17: 1870–1874.

Malenka, R.C., Kauer, J.A., Zucker, R.S., and Nicoll, R.A. (1988). Postsynaptic calcium is sufficient for potentiation of hippocampal synaptic transmission. *Science* 242: 81–84.

Martinez, J.L., and Derrick, B.E. (1996). Long-term potentiation and learning. *Ann. Rev. Psychol.* 47: 173–203.

Matzel, L.D., and Miller, R.R. (1987). Recruitment time of conditioned opioid analgesia. *Physiol. Behav.* 39: 135–140.

Matzel, L.D., and Miller, R.R. (1989). Development of shock-induced analgesia: A search for hyperalgesia. *Behav. Neurosci.* 103: 850–856.

Matzel, L.D., Brown, A.M., and Miller, R.R. (1987). Associative effects of US preexposure: Modulation of conditioned responding by an excitatory training context. *J. Exp. Psychol. Anim. Behav. Proc.* 13: 65–72.

Matzel, L.D., Held, F.P., and Miller, R.R. (1988). Information and expression of simultaneous and backward associations: Implications for contiguity theory. *Learn. Motiv.* 19: 317–344.

Matzel, L.D., Collin, C., and Alkon, D.L. (1992). Biophysical and behavioral correlates of memory storage, degradation, and reactivation. *Behav. Neurosci.* 106: 954–963.

Matzel, L.D., Talk, A.C., Muzzio, I., and Rogers, R.F. (1998). Ubiquitous molecular substrates for associative learning and activity-dependent neuronal facilitation. *Rev. Neurosci.* 9: 129–168.

McAllister, W.R., and McAllister, D.E. (1962). Role of the CS and of apparatus cues in the measurement of acquired fear. *Psychol. Rep.* 11: 749–756.

McAllister, W.R., and McAllister, D.E. (1971). Behavioral measurement of conditioned fear. In F.R. Brush (Ed.), *Aversive conditioning and learning* (pp. 105–179). New York: Academic Press.

McEchron, M.D., Bouwmeester, H., Tseng, W., Weiss, C. et al. (1998). Hippocampectomy disrupts auditory trace fear conditioning and contextual fear conditioning in the rat. *Hippocampus* 8: 638–646.

McNaughton, B.L., Douglas, R.M., and Goddard, G.V. (1978). Synaptic enhancement in fascia dentata: Cooperativity among coactive afferents. *Brain Res.* 157: 277–293.

Miller, R.R., and Barnet, R.C. (1993). The role of time in elementary associations. *Curr. Dir. Psychol. Sci.* 2: 106–111.

Miller, R.R., and Matzel, L.D. (1988). Generation of acquired responses. In G.H. Bower (Ed.), *Psychology of learning and motivation* (Vol. 22., pp. 51–92). Orlando: Academic Press.

Miller, S., and Mayford, M. (1999). Cellular and molecular mechanisms of memory: The LTP connection. *Curr. Opin. Genet. Dev.* 9: 333–337.

Miller, R.R., Kasprow, W.J., and Schachtman, T.R. (1986). Retrieval variability: Sources and consequences. *Am. J. Psychol.* 99: 145–218.

Miller, J.S., Jagielo, J.A., and Spear, N.E. (1989). Age-related differences in short-term retention of separable elements of an odor aversion. *J. Exp. Psychol. Anim. Behav. Proc.* 15: 194–201.

Miller, R.R., Greco, C., Vigorito, M., and Marlin, N.A. (1999). Similar tailshock is perceived as similar to a stronger unsignalled tailshock: Implications for a functional analysis of classical conditioning. *J. Exp. Psychol. Anim. Behav. Proc.* 9: 105–131.

Morris, R.G.M. (1981). Spatial localization does not require the presence of local cues. *Learn. Motiv.* 12: 239–260.

Morris, R.G.M., Davis, S., and Butcher, S.P. (1991). Hippocampal synaptic plasticity and NMDA receptors: A role in information storage. In J.R. Krebs and G. Horn (Eds.), *Behavioral and neural aspects of learning and memory* (pp. 89–106) Oxford: Clarendon Press.

Napier, R.M., Macrae, M., and Kehoe, E.J. (1992). Rapid reacquisition in conditioning of the rabbit's nictitating membrane response. *J. Exp. Psychol. Anim. Behav. Proc.* 18: 182–192.

Pavlides, C., Greenstein, Y.J., Grudman, M., and Winson, J. (1988). Long-term potentiation in the dentate gyrus is induced preferentially on the positive phase of theta-rhythm. *Brain Res.* 439: 383–387.

Pearce, J.M., and Dickinson, A. (1975). Pavlovian counterconditioning: Changing the suppressive properties of shock by association with food. *J. Exp. Psychol. Anim. Behav. Proc.* 1: 170–177.

Pearce, J.M., and Hall, G. (1980). A model for Pavlovian learning: Variations in the effectiveness of conditioned but not of unconditioned stimuli. *Psychol. Rev.* 87: 532–552.

Perkins, C.C. (1968). An analysis of the concept of reinforcement. *Psychol. Rev.* 75: 155–172.

Rescorla, R.A. (1968). Probability of shock in the presence and absence of CS in fear conditioning. *J. Comp. Physiol. Psychol.* 66: 1–5.

Rescorla, R.A. (1969). Conditioned inhibition of fear resulting from negative CS-US contingencies. *J. Comp. Physiol. Psychol.* 67: 504–509.

Rescorla, R.A. (1973). Effect of US habituation following conditioning. *J. Comp. Physiol. Psychol.* 82: 137–143.

Rescorla, R.A. (1980). Simultaneous and successive associations in sensory preconditioning. *J. Exp. Psychol. Anim. Behav. Proc.* 6: 207–216.

Rescorla, R.A. (1988a). Behavioral studies of Pavlovian conditioning. *Ann. Rev. Neurosci.* 11: 329–352.

Rescorla, R.A. (1988b). Pavlovian conditioning. It's not what you think it is. *Am. Psychol.* 43: 151–160.

Rescorla, R.A., and Wagner, A.R. (1972). A theory of Pavlovian conditioning: Variations in the effectiveness of reinforcement. In A.H. Black and W.F. Prokasy (Eds.), *Classical conditioning II: Current research and theory* (pp. 64–99). New York: Appleton-Century-Crofts.

Reymann, K.G., Malisch, R., Schulzeck, K., Brodemann, R. et al. (1985). The duration of long-term potentiation in the CA1 region of the hippocampal slice preparation. *Brain Res. Bull.* 15: 249–255.

Riedel, G., Micheau, J., Lam, A.G.M., Roloff, E.V.L. et al. (1999). Reversible neural inactivation reveals hippocampal participation in several memory processes. *Nat. Neurosci.* 2: 898–905.

Rizley, R.C., and Rescorla, R.A. (1972). Associations in second-order conditioning and sensory preconditioning. *Journal of Comparative and Physiological Psychology,* 81: 1–11.

Rogers, R.F., and Steinmetz, J.E. (1998). Contextually based conditional discrimination of the rabbit eyeblink response. *Neurobiol. Learn. Mem.* 69: 307–319.

Schneiderman, N. (1972). Response system divergencies in aversive classical conditioning. In A.H. Black and W.F. Prokasy (Eds.), *Classical conditioning II: Current research and theory* (pp. 341–376). New York: Appleton-Century-Crofts.

Schneiderman, N., and Gormezano, I. (1964). Conditioning of the nictitating membrane of the rabbit as a function of CS-US interval. *J. Comp. Physiol. Psychol.* 57: 188–195.

Sejenowski, T.J. (1990). Homosynaptic long-term depression in hippocampus and neocortex. *Sem. Neurosci.* 2: 355–363.

Servatius, R.J., and Shors, T.J. (1996). Early acquisition but not retention of the classically conditioned eyeblink response is N-methyl-d-aspartate (NMDA) receptor dependent. *Behav. Neurosci.* 110: 1040–1048.

Shors, T.J., and Dryver, E. (1994). Effect of stress and long-term potentiation on subsequent LTP and the theta burst response in the dentate gyrus. *Brain Res.* 666: 232–238.

Shors, T.J., and Matzel, L.D. (1997). Long-term potentiation: What's learning got to do with it? *Behav. Brain Sci.* 20: 597–655.

Shors, T.J., Beylin, A.V., and Gould, E. (2000). The modulation of Pavlovian memory. *Behav. Brain Res.,* in press.

Shurtleff, D., and Ayres, J.J.B. (1981). One trial backward excitatory fear conditioning in rats: Acquisition, retention, extinction, and spontaneous recovery. *Anim. Learn. Behav.* 9: 65–74.

Siegal, S. (1989). Pharmacological conditioning and drug effects. In A.J. Goudie and E. Oglesby (Eds.), *Psychoactive drugs: Tolerance and sensitization* (pp. 115–180). Clifton, NJ: Humana Press.

Siegal, S., and Domjan, M. (1971). Backward conditioning as an inhibitory procedure. *Learn. Motiv.* 2: 1–11.

Smith, J.C., and Roll, D.L. (1967). Trace conditioning with X-rays as an aversive stimulus. *Psychonom. Sci.* 9: 12.

Solomon, P.R., van der Schaaf, E.R., Weisz, D., and Thompson, R.F. (1986). Hippocampus and trace conditioning of the rabbit's classically conditioned nictitating membrane response. *Neuroscience* 100: 729–744.

Spear, N.E. (1978). *The Processing of Memories: Forgetting and Retention.* Hillsdale, NJ: Erlbaum.

Spear, N.E., Miller, J.S., and Jagielo, J.A. (1990). Animal memory and learning. *Ann. Rev. Psychol.* 41: 169–211.

Spetch, M.L., Wilkie, D.M., and Pinel, J. (1981). Backward conditioning: A reevaluation of the empirical evidence. *Psychol. Bull.* 89: 163–175.

Staubli, U., and Lynch, G. (1987). Stable hippocampal long-term potentiation elicited by 'theta' pattern stimulation. *Brain Res.* 435: 227–234.

Talk, A.C., Muzzio, I.A., and Matzel, L.D. (1999). Neurophysiological substrates of context conditioning suggest a temporally invariant form of activity-dependent neuronal facilitation. *Neurobiol. Learn. Mem.* 72: 95–117.

Vanderwolf, C.H., and Cain, D.P. (1994). The behavioral neurobiology of learning and memory: A conceptual reorientation. *Brain Res. Rev.* 19: 264–297.

Wagner, A.R. (1969). Stimulus validity and stimulus selection. In W.K. Honig, and N.J. Mackintosh (Eds.), *Fundamental issues in associative learning.* Halifax: Dalhousie University Press.

Wallenstein, G.V., Eichenbaum, H., and Hasselmo, M.E. (1998). The hippocampus as an associator of discontiguous events. *Trends Neurosci.* 21: 317–323.

Wasserman, E.A., and Miller, R.R. (1997). What's elementary about associative learning? *Ann. Rev. Psychol.* 48: 573–607.

Wendt, G.R. (1937). Two and one-half year retention of a conditioned response. *J. Gen. Psychol.* 17: 178–180.

Wood, G.E., and Shors, T.J. (1998). Stress facilitates classical conditioning in males, but impairs classical conditioning in females through activational effects of ovarian hormones. *Proc. Natl. Acad. Sci.* 95: 4066–4071.

Setting the Stage for Memory Formation

Stress, Arousal, and Attention

CHAPTER THIRTEEN

Strategies for Studying the Role of LTP in Spatial Learning

What Do We Know? Where Should We Go?

Donald P. Cain

SUMMARY

Recent data from research on spatial learning mechanisms with the water maze are discussed, with emphasis on the role of NMDA receptor-dependent long-term potentiation (LTP). Detailed analysis of behavior in the water maze has indicated a need to distinguish among different components of this seemingly simple task. Nonspatial pretraining allows for the separation of behavioral strategy learning and learning the spatial location of the hidden platform. Nonspatially pretrained rats can learn the location of a hidden platform as quickly as controls despite being treated with any of a variety of pharmacologic agents. When a water maze task of conventional difficulty is used, nonspatially pretrained rats given an NMDA receptor antagonist to block hippocampal LTP can learn the location of the hidden platform as quickly as controls. When an especially difficult water maze task is used, involving repeated one-trial learning with repeated reversal learning, blockade of hippocampal LTP produces a spatial memory impairment for long but not short retention intervals in nonspatially pretrained rats. These and other experiments point to an important issue of task difficulty in the research. It should prove useful to systematically vary experimental treatments and task difficulty as a means of identifying specific brain circuits that are important for specific components of the water maze or other tasks. This information can then be used to further evaluate the role of LTP in the learning.

This work was supported by a grant from the Natural Science and Engineering Research Council of Canada. I thank Ron Racine for helpful discussions.

Christian Hölscher, editor, *Neuronal Mechanisms of Memory Formation.* © 2001 Cambridge University Press. Printed in the United States of America. All rights reserved.

Introduction

Long-term potentiation (LTP) has properties of central nervous system change that are inherently interesting and that could be relevant to a variety of behavioral phenomena. Chief among these is its relevance to systematic and enduring behavioral change, or learning and memory. In the decades since Bliss and Lomo's (1973) pioneering work, LTP has received an enormous amount of attention as a laboratory model of learning. From the beginning there was enthusiasm for LTP as more than simply a formal learning model, to be studied in the brain slice, for example. This enthusiasm is quite understandable in view of the remarkably close fit between the properties of LTP and Hebb's (1949) hypothetical synapse. If LTP is not a neural learning mechanism, it should be.

Is LTP a learning mechanism? Does it play a required, causal role in establishing enduring memory for any form of learning? Early research through the late 1980s supported a role for LTP in learning and memory, and some recent research still does. However, in the last decade a number of studies have failed to support much of the original optimism about LTP as a general memory mechanism. I shall discuss some of those studies here, but space constraints dictate that I focus mainly on selected studies that deal with NMDA receptor-dependent LTP in spatial learning. Spatial learning was selected because perhaps more work with LTP has been done on this topic than any other, and because the ability to navigate effectively is essential for survival in mammals, making spatial learning ethologically relevant.

A great deal is known about the neural mechanisms of various forms of LTP; most of this has come from work with the brain slice. The question of which form of LTP one is studying in any particular experiment is an important one (McEachern and Shaw, 1996). Long-term depression (LTD; Heynen et al., 1996) has also been described and may be highly relevant to learning, but little research on learning has been done with these phenomena. The slice technique has limitations for answering the questions related to behavioral learning posed in this chapter, so the discussion will focus mostly on research with awake, behaving animals.

Recent studies show that understanding the exact relations between LTP and learning or memory is not a simple and straightforward undertaking. The difficulties and ambiguities of the research, some of which are discussed below, attest to this. It has become clear that in this effort close attention must be paid to behavioral aspects of the research if we are to be confident of the conclusions. The reasons for this will become clearer below, but for now we take it as a given that as much effort needs to be made in the behavioral aspects of the research as in the strictly neural ones.

A goal of this chapter is to analyze selected research results and to provide comments on research strategies that may prove useful for answering the question of a causal role of LTP in spatial learning and memory. There have been a number of strategies used in studies of LTP and learning, each of which has both advantages and limitations. No single strategy can provide definitive answers. We begin with the strategy that was used first.

The Correlation Strategy

The correlation strategy involves documenting the occurrence of LTP in intact animals or in brain slices taken from animals that have learned a task, or relating the strength of inducible electrophysiologic LTP to the speed or permanence of learning in the same animal. As two prominent researchers put it, "no amount of research studying whether LTP is necessary for learning will ever be persuasive in the absence of studies definitively establishing that LTP occurs naturally during learning. Uncomfortable as it is, we have to face up to the complications of demonstrating that this synaptic mechanism is actually engaged during learning" (Morris and Davis, 1994).

This strategy was used by a number of laboratories with rats that learned standard laboratory tasks, some of which were spatial in nature. The first such study found a positive correlation between the accuracy of navigation to a hole on a large circular board that led to a dark goal box underneath, and the amount of hippocampal LTP that could be induced separately in the same rat (Barnes, 1979). Other studies reported the occurrence of hippocampal LTP as a result of behavioral training in a variety of nonspatial tasks (Ruthrich et al., 1982; Weisz et al., 1982; Skelton et al., 1987), or from exploring a novel complex environment (Sharp et al., 1985), which would be expected to have a spatial learning component. However, since hippocampal damage does not seem to interfere with learning or performance of the tasks it is not clear that hippocampal LTP would necessarily be expected to occur.

An important caveat in LTP research with intact behaving animals is the fact that physiologic processes other than learning and memory can affect the amplitude and other properties of the evoked field potentials that are used to document LTP. Field potential changes due to factors unrelated to learning or memory are so much like those that occur in laboratory LTP that they are easily mistaken for genuine LTP. One cause of such changes is the brain activation that occurs during locomotion and postural shifts, and that alters the properties of field potentials in the hippocampus and neocortex whether the animal is learning something or not. Thus, evoked field potentials are larger when the animal is immobile than when it is moving (Winson and Abzug, 1978; Vanderwolf et al., 1987). The problem for LTP-learning research is that behavioral learning necessarily involves, and is documented by, systematic changes in behavior. Often an element of the systematic behavioral change is a reduction in exploratory and other movements as the animal learns to perform the specifically rewarded behaviors in an efficient manner. Since the relation between the occurrence of behavioral movement and field potential amplitude is inverse, this kind of systematic behavioral change would have the effect of increasing field potential amplitude, whether or not LTP plays a causal role in the learning. This kind of change could easily be mistaken for learning-induced LTP when the possibility exists that a different neural mechanism underlies the learning.

Another cause of changes in field potentials is the slight increase in body and brain temperature that results from behavioral movement, due to the metabolic events taking place in muscular contraction (Moser et al., 1993; Cain et al., 1994).

Even heating or cooling from external sources can affect field potentials (Moser et al., 1993; Cain et al., 1994). Again, the changes can be misinterpreted as learning-induced LTP when they have nothing to do with learning mechanisms, and they are fully reversible as the brain regains its original temperature (Moser et al., 1993).

None of the learning studies mentioned above used controls for these two confounds. The confounds can be eliminated by holding behavior constant while the potentials are being recorded, for example, by delivering test pulses only when the animal is immobile, or by subtracting the effects of brain temperature change from any changes in evoked potential magnitude that might have resulted from learning a task. When these control measures were used in studies involving radial arm maze, avoidance, and water maze tasks, hippocampal and neocortical potentials did not change after the training (Cain et al., 1993; Moser et al., 1993; Hargreaves et al., 1990; Beiko and Cain, 1998). However, in one study involving controls for brain temperature changes, exploration of novel objects in an open field led to increases in hippocampal field potentials (Moser et al., 1994). Although the above studies recorded LTP in brain structures in which the most prominent form of electrically induced LTP requires NMDA receptor activity, none of them actually confirmed that the field potentials were NMDA receptor-dependent and that the neural mechanisms of the field potential changes were the same as those that occur in laboratory LTP.

Recent work with a nonspatial task, fear conditioning, which depends on auditory circuits projecting to the amygdala, has shown that increases in the response to auditory conditioned stimuli, and LTP resulting from electrical stimulation of the auditory thalamus, are identical in their field potential properties (McKernan and Shinnick- Gallagher, 1997; Rogan et al., 1997). Control procedures ruled out confounds due to ongoing behavior. Unfortunately, attempts to determine whether these effects were dependent on activation of NMDA receptors, and thus might relate to NMDA receptor-dependent LTP, were unsuccessful because antagonism of NMDA receptors greatly reduced the baseline field potential in the amygdala (Rogan, personal communication). This is an example of the multiple functions of NMDA receptors in sensory processing and normal synaptic conduction, in addition to any role they have in LTP (Daw et al., 1993; see Cain, 1997a). The fact that NMDA receptors are involved in so many aspects of brain function makes it extremely difficult to determine the specific functional contribution of NMDA receptor-dependent LTP to learning (Cain, 1997a). Indeed, there is evidence that NMDA receptor mechanisms are involved in the generation of complex natural behaviors such as grooming (Robertson et al., 1999). Moreover, as with all correlations, concluding that an association between potentiation and behavioral events proves causality is not possible. Other strategies, to be discussed below, must be used to arrive at conclusions about causality.

Improving the Correlation Strategy

The discovery of LTD and depotentiation of LTP (Staubli and Lynch, 1990) suggests that a modified approach might be useful in the search for electrophysiologic correlates of learning and memory. Much current thought and data support the idea that information in the form of altered synaptic weights might be stored in a distributed manner (McNaughton and Morris, 1987), in the hippocampus and neocortex among other regions. If this is true, the use of field potentials evoked by single test pulses as an assay for potentiation due to natural learning may not yield unambiguous information. This is because we have no a priori reason to think that information is stored only, or even preferentially, as an increase in synaptic weight. It is just as likely stored as a decrease in synaptic weight, either as LTD or as depotentiation of existing LTP. Given that baseline (prelearning) synaptic weights in the target structure can be expected to differ at different synapses at any given moment, if changes in synaptic weight in either direction can store information, changes in either direction are likely to occur at different synapses in the circuit during learning. It is possible that LTP and LTD or depotentiation occur in approximately equal amounts, thus canceling each other in terms of the net effect on the field potential (Miller, 1996). This would produce a field potential that does not differ from the prelearning condition even though synaptic weights have actually changed in the circuit. This possibility must be taken into account before it can be concluded that the failure to find alterations in field potentials in animals that displayed robust spatial learning means that changes in synaptic weight do not occur during learning.

A way of dealing with this problem might be to reset synaptic weights prior to training the animal. This could be done by either saturating the circuit, or the reverse: inducing LTD or depotentiating any LTP that exists in the circuit at the outset. If a change in synaptic weight in either direction can underlie learning, starting from a fully potentiated or a fully depressed condition should not prevent learning. Indeed, as is discussed below, Moser's group has recently shown that saturation of hippocampal LTP does not prevent spatial learning providing the animal knows the behavioral strategies that are required in the task (Otnaess et al., 1999). It is not known what effect depressing synaptic weights in a circuit does to learning.

Using this approach might allow potentiation or depression effects to manifest themselves more clearly in the field potential, because there would be only one possible direction for changes to occur. To date only one study has used the prelearning saturation approach. Xu et al. (1998) found a decrease in saturated hippocampal area CA1 LTP in rats that explored a novel box. The authors saturated LTP prior to the exploration, and found a lasting decrease in the evoked response after the exploration compared to saturated control rats that did not explore. They interpreted this result to mean that inconsequential (baseline) potentiation, presumably occurring as a result of ongoing brain activity before the exploration, was reduced through depotentiation by memory mechanisms in the rat's brain, making way for new potentiation from the learning that occurred during the exploration. This result might be taken as evidence of depotentiation due to learning, but questions remain. Evidence of neither inconsequential baseline potentiation nor of the hypothesized new potentiation was provided. The relation of the depotentiation to conventional LTP or LTD phenomena is not clear, nor is it known whether the depotentiation was dependent on mechanisms involved in laboratory LTD.

Despite these questions, this general approach may be the most fruitful way of fulfilling Morris and Davis's call for the demonstration of natural potentiation due to learning in the intact animal. However, more precise control over what is learned and the timing of the learning would be desirable, because it would clarify the nature of the learned information and make the understanding of what the animal was learning less hypothetical than the Xu et al. study. One way to achieve this would be to use a task in which the behavioral and memory processes are better understood than those involved in exploring a box. Spatial learning in the Morris water maze is such a task. The reasons for this will become clearer in the next section.

The Saturation Strategy

The saturation strategy involves electrically stimulating a brain circuit that has been identified as crucial for a certain form of learning in an attempt to saturate, or use up, all of the available plasticity in the circuit. The animal is then trained in a relevant task and the performance of saturated animals is compared to that of nonsaturated animals. This strategy was first used by McNaughton and colleagues (McNaughton et al., 1986; Castro et al., 1989) to manipulate LTP in a way that might allow causal relations between LTP and learning to be studied. If the saturated animals learned less well than controls, this would be evidence for a causal role for LTP in the learning. Of course, if the saturation strategy works as envisaged to impair learning processes, it would not be usable in the manner described in the previous section with the correlation strategy because it would block learning. However, as will be discussed below, research suggests that it does not block spatial learning.

Early efforts involved saturation of LTP in dentate gyrus, which produced unreliable effects on behavioral learning because the effects of saturation were probably not complete (Moser et al., 1998). With more complete saturation using extensive electrical stimulation applied through multiple electrodes, reliable impairment was recently seen (Moser et al., 1998). However, more recent work has shown that spatial learning can occur with LTP saturated (Otnaess et al., 1999). Whether this can be taken to mean that potentiation effects are not important for learning is not clear since, using the logic discussed in the previous section, learning might have occurred because the saturated synaptic weights were simply being depotentiated during the learning.

The articles on saturation just mentioned and most of the research in the remainder of this chapter used the water maze task with rats, and it would be useful to describe this task in more detail. The Morris water maze task is well suited to the research because it involves robust learning that occurs rapidly and can be analyzed in detail. It also depends on an important natural ability, spatial navigation. The task requires an animal to swim in a pool of water about 1.5 meters in diameter and in so doing learn the location of a small platform hidden just below the surface. The platform cannot be seen, and its location must be learned either in relation to distal cues in the room, or by the self-monitoring of navigation movements. Rats with chronic electrode implants can be trained in this task, which allows comparisons between LTP and behavioral learning in the same animal. The fact that the hippocampus is involved in spatial navigation in rodents made it useful to study hippocampal LTP in this task.

Using their perfected technique of saturation with the water maze task, Moser and colleagues found an impairment in spatial learning in naive rats that was related to the degree of LTP saturation (Moser et al., 1998). However, this task is complex, and successful acquisition requires that at least two main components be learned. First, the rats must learn the strategies needed in the task: how to swim; that the only refuge in the pool was an unseen platform; to swim away from the wall to find the platform; and if they contact the platform, to get onto it. Second, the rats must learn the exact location of the platform with respect to the pool walls and the visual cues in the room. Learning the strategies is a necessary prelude for obtaining information about the location of the platform during spatial training. Normally the two components of the task are learned concurrently, and in normal rats this occurs quickly. However, recent research indicates that in drugged rats it is essential to design water maze experiments differently if interpretable information about spatial learning ability is to be obtained.

The impetus for this approach was Morris's work with nonspatial pretraining, which consisted of swimming experience in the water maze pool that was designed to familiarize the rats with the required behavioral strategies without training them to swim to a specific spatial location in the pool (Morris, 1989). The rats were allowed to have twelve brief swims in the pool, spaced over 3 days, with black curtains drawn around the pool to occlude distal visual cues, and with the hidden platform moved to a new location after each swim. This invariably led to the rats learning to swim very effectively, and learning to use the platform as a refuge. It also reduced the severe stress that occurs in rats that have never swum or used the hidden platform as a refuge (Hölscher, 1999). Additional evidence for this came from our finding that naive rats have extremely high blood levels of corticosterone after an initial swim, but nonspatially pretrained rats have much lower levels that are close to resting levels (Beiko et al., 1998). Thus, there are a number of consequences of nonspatial pretraining, both in training animals to adopt successful behavioral strategies in the pool and in allowing them to have greatly reduced stress responses while in the pool (Hölscher, 1999).

An important aspect of nonspatial pretraining is that while the drug treatments caused sensorimotor disturbances and problems in using appropriate behavioral strategies in naive rats, the same drug treatments did not cause sensorimotor disturbances or strategy impairments in pretrained rats. How could these paradoxical results occur? The pretraining effect is not new. Morris's original study found that nonspatial pretraining nearly eliminated the sensorimotor disturbances caused by the drug (Morris, 1989). Earlier work found very similar effects of prior experience with the specific training environment or situation in rats given a drug and trained in the same environment or situation (Herz, 1959; Steinberg et al.,

1961; DeVietti et al., 1985). All of this emphasizes that (1) knowing the behavioral strategies required in a task is essential for successful acquisition and performance of the task, (2) pretraining experience involves strategy learning that is relevant to the requirements of a particular task, and (3) animals that already know the required task strategies are much less impaired in the task by drugs that markedly impair naive animals, presumably because their nervous systems are altered by the learning that occurs during nonspatial pretraining in a way that allows them to better cope with the neural perturbations that the drugs cause. Thus, it is clear that considerable learning occurs during nonspatial pretraining, and that the learning relates to the general task strategies and not to any specific platform location. Interestingly, our nonspatially pretrained rats were not benefited by nonspatial pretraining in the pool in their ability to walk along a narrow wooden beam while drugged (Cain et al., 1996, 1997; Saucier et al., 1996; Cain, 1997b). They had as much difficulty performing this task as naive controls under drug, which indicates that the nonspatial pretraining effect was specific to a task involving the particular strategies that were learned during the pretraining. It also indicates that the drugs were having their full effect on the central nervous system but that this was shown only in behaviors that were not involved in the nonspatial pretraining.

Getting back to Moser's work, in his original experiment, which had found an impairment in saturated rats, he had used naive rats (Moser et al., 1998). As a consequence of the work with pretraining discussed above, Moser and colleagues decided to use a two-pool water maze protocol with their perfected LTP saturation technique (Otnaess et al., 1999). They first spatially trained rats in one pool to consistently find a hidden platform in a stable location. The rats were unstimulated electrically at this time, and they learned both the required strategies and the platform location readily. The rats then received LTP saturation and were spatially trained to find a hidden platform in a second pool, which was placed in a different room and used different distal cues. The rats were able to learn this spatial task very effectively despite the LTP saturation. This result indicates that LTP saturation does not prevent spatial learning, and it suggests that the water maze impairment in the earlier work with naive rats (Moser et al., 1998) was due to some effect on strategy learning or on behavioral performance in the pool, and not to an impairment of spatial learning per se. Further interpretation is difficult because the electrical stimulation that was given could be expected to produce a variety of physiologic and cellular consequences in addition to the LTP saturation, such as expression of genes, neurotransmitter release, and other consequences, and any of these could be involved in the strategy impairment that the LTP saturation apparently caused.

Thus it appears that LTP saturation may cause a behavioral strategy impairment in the water maze, but not a spatial learning impairment. This result makes the use of LTP saturation in the correlation strategy experiments discussed above feasible. It also emphasizes the need to use pretraining to separate the strategy learning component from the spatial learning component. The need for this approach is also important in the blockade strategy, to be discussed next.

The Blockade Strategy

The goal of the blockade strategy, like that of the saturation strategy, is to impair LTP during behavioral training, typically using pharmacologic manipulation, to see whether animals are prevented from learning the task. A pharmacologic manipulation was first used with the water maze by Sutherland and colleagues (Sutherland et al., 1982), who found that muscarinic cholinergic blockade severely impaired acquisition of the task. The first use of the blockade strategy to evaluate the role of LTP in the water maze was by Morris and colleagues, who pharmacologically blocked NMDA receptors in rats that were being trained in the water maze (Morris et al., 1986). They found that the rats were severely impaired. Morris extended this work by showing that this treatment also impaired rats that had been taught the required behavioral strategies beforehand by nonspatial pretraining (Morris, 1989).

Morris introduced nonspatial pretraining as a control procedure because some of the drugged rats fell off the hidden platform after climbing onto it (Morris, 1989). NMDA receptor antagonists are known to cause muscular incoordination as well as hyperactivity (Hargreaves and Cain, 1992), and Morris's rats were falling off the platform because of the ataxia and hyperactivity the drug caused. It is possible that the motor problems could have contributed to the behavioral impairment that was seen in these rats. As was discussed above, nonspatial pretraining was used to train the rats in the behavioral strategies required in the task before they received the NMDA receptor antagonist and spatial training. This would help ensure that any behavioral difference in performance between drugged and control rats was due to a spatial learning impairment and not an impairment in using the required strategies or in performing the necessary behaviors. Nonspatial pretraining reduced falling off the platform, which supported the idea that it was the blockade of LTP and not sensorimotor disturbances that caused the spatial learning impairment (Morris, 1989).

In this work Morris used implanted minipumps to deliver small quantities of NMDA receptor antagonist into the cerebral ventricle adjacent to the hippocampus over a period of days (Morris et al., 1986; Morris, 1989). In contrast, we used the newly available NMDA receptor antagonists that were capable of crossing the blood-brain barrier, and we administered these by the systemic route of administration to ensure that LTP was blocked throughout the brain. We did this because we were concerned that LTP occurring in regions not adjacent to the ventricles, and thus relatively unaffected by the antagonist, might support learning, and we wanted to prevent this possibility. When the NMDA receptor antagonist was given to naive rats, they were severely impaired in the task (Saucier and Cain, 1995; Cain et al., 1996, 1997; Saucier et al., 1996; Hoh et al., 1999), just as had been reported earlier in the minipump study. We also observed marked sensorimotor disturbances in addition to the impaired navigation. Many of these rats behaved quite maladaptively in the pool, circling the pool repeatedly close to the wall much of the time, and deflecting off the hidden platform when it was contacted, or even swimming over it and off the other side (Saucier and Cain, 1995;

Cain and Saucier, 1996; Cain et al., 1996, 1997; Saucier et al., 1996; Cain, 1997b, 1998; Hoh et al., 1999). Some of these problems may have been caused by the hyperactivity and ataxia that NMDA antagonists produce (Hargreaves and Cain, 1992). These behaviors would be expected to contribute to poor learning scores even if LTP is not involved in the learning, by increasing platform search latency due to the periphery swimming, and by reducing the amount of information that the rats obtained about the platform's location due to the deflections and swimovers.

We next administered the same dose of NMDA receptor antagonist to nonspatially pretrained rats. Their performance of both the previously learned strategies and, more important, their spatial learning ability, was excellent, and was indistinguishable from that of control animals (Saucier and Cain, 1995; Cain et al., 1996, 1997; Saucier et al., 1996; Hoh et al., 1999). This result was found whether the antagonist was administered intraventricularly or systemically, and it occurred with a variety of different NMDA receptor antagonists. Some of the same rats that were trained in the water maze under drug treatment carried implanted electrodes for monitoring hippocampal LTP, which was found to be blocked in both dentate gyrus and area CA1 as a result of the antagonists (Saucier and Cain, 1995; Cain et al., 1997).

The excellent spatial learning by the nonspatially pretrained rats given an NMDA receptor antagonist was a surprising result, especially in view of the severe challenge the large dose of antagonist posed for them. However, it has proven to be a very robust and reliable result, and has been obtained repeatedly in my laboratory by various experimenters. Excellent spatial learning was also obtained by Morris's group in rats with hippocampal LTP blocked, using the two-pool technique that was described above (Bannerman et al., 1995). The rats were spatially trained in one pool, and were then given minipumps containing NMDA receptor antagonist and retrained in a different pool placed in a different room and with a different set of distal cues (Bannerman et al., 1995). Again, the spatial learning of the antagonist-treated rats was as effective as that of controls despite the blockade of NMDA receptor-dependent LTP.

How general is this result? Are nonspatially pretrained rats able to learn a hidden platform location if they are given other drugs that are known to impair performance in the water maze? We attempted to answer this question by giving nonspatially pretrained rats the cholinergic antagonist scopolamine, the benzodiazepine drug diazepam, or ethanol. Given to naive rats, the doses we used produced impairments in the task, as well as marked sensorimotor disturbances. In contrast, nonspatially pretrained rats given the same dose of the same drugs performed as well as controls in every case (Saucier et al., 1996; Beiko et al., 1997; Cain, 1997b; Hoh and Cain, 1997; Finalyson et al., 1998). Again, a systemic route of administration was used, which produced a more widespread distribution of the drugs than would have been the case with delivery to a specific brain structure or into ventricle. The fact that nonspatially pretrained animals performed as well as controls with these challenging drug treatments, which severely impaired naive rats, emphasizes the robustness of the spatial learning that was observed. It also emphasizes the generality of the pretraining effect, and indicates that its effectiveness and value is not limited to treatments involving NMDA receptor antagonism.

To this point, the results showed that rats that know the required behavioral strategies could learn the specific spatial location of the hidden platform with dentate and area CA1 NMDA receptor-dependent LTP blocked. Since it would not be possible for animals to learn the platform's location without knowledge of the appropriate behavioral strategies, the naive rats' spatial learning impairment under drug treatment might be explained by an inability to learn the strategies themselves, which could have resulted from the blockade of LTP. This raised the obvious question whether rats can learn the required behavioral strategies when LTP is blocked, and then make use of the strategies to learn the location of a hidden platform. To answer this question we first trained naive rats in the strategies by giving them nonspatial pretraining in a single session (Hoh et al., 1999). The pretraining was conducted while the rats were under the influence of our standard NMDA receptor antagonist treatment. During the next session we again gave the rats the same drug treatment, followed by three nonspatial pretraining "reminder" trials, followed immediately by conventional spatial training with no curtains around the pool and the hidden platform in a stable position. During a subsequent session we again administered drug, followed by reversal training with the hidden platform in a different position in the pool. In all phases of the experiment the rats were under the influence of the NMDA receptor antagonist, which was confirmed to block hippocampal LTP in both dentate gyrus and area CA1 (Hoh et al., 1999). This experimental design effectively separated the strategy learning phase, the spatial learning phase, and the reversal learning phase, and ensured that NMDA receptor-dependent LTP was blocked during all phases of training.

The results showed that the rats learned all phases of the task just as effectively as controls. They learned the strategies quickly, then made use of them to learn the location of the hidden platform, then learned a new platform location, all with LTP blocked (Hoh et al., 1999). This striking result demonstrated that, while NMDA receptor-dependent LTP might contribute to the learning, neither the learning of the complex behavioral strategies, nor spatial learning, nor reversal learning required NMDA receptor-dependent LTP. The dose of NMDA receptor antagonist that was used appears to have been sufficient to block NMDA receptor-dependent LTP in neocortex, which suggests that the LTP might well have been blocked throughout the entire central nervous system. However, we did not actually confirm that LTP was blocked outside the hippocampal complex.

In sum, we appear to have the beginning of an answer to the main question of interest: What is the role of NMDA receptor-dependent hippocampal LTP in learning the water maze task? Taken together, the results consistently show that animals with NMDA receptor-dependent LTP blocked can learn to navigate as accurately as control animals, provided they are familiar with the behavioral strategies required in the task. The results also show that the strategies themselves can be learned when this form of LTP is blocked. These results are consistent with the finding that rats with hippocampal lesions can acquire the strategies and learn the location of a hidden platform when trained with a visible platform and tested with the platform removed (Whishaw et al., 1995).

Although the results indicate that this form of LTP is not required for these particular forms of learning, they are nevertheless consistent with a nonessential role for LTP in the learning. However, since the animals performed in a manner that was statistically indistinguishable from that of controls, there is nothing in the data to indicate exactly what the role of LTP is. Assuming that LTP contributes in a nonessential way to the learning, this implies that there must be multiple neural mechanisms for establishing the memory trace. Knowing this tells us that it is important to search for additional neural mechanisms of learning.

The Task Difficulty Issue

A brief summary of what our rats treated with a single pharmacologic agent can and cannot do in the water maze might go like this: They can learn the task quite well provided they do not have to learn everything at once.

In water maze studies with six different agents representing widely different pharmacologic actions, in every case we found that naive drugged rats performed poorly, but that nonspatially pretrained rats or rats that received separate, sequential training in the different phases of the task all performed extremely well (Saucier and Cain, 1995; Cain et al., 1996, 1997; Saucier et al., 1996; Beiko et al., 1997; Cain, 1997b, 1998; Hoh and Cain, 1997; Finlayson et al., 1998; Hoh et al., 1999). As was discussed above, other researchers have obtained similar results using different methods (Bannerman et al., 1995; Otnaess et al., 1999). Training the rats in all aspects of the task at once seemed to create a condition with which the experimentally treated rats could not cope adaptively. To this must be added the important factor of stress that accompanies initial training in the water maze, and which is reduced during nonspatial pretraining (Beiko et al., 1998; Hölscher, 1999). It is not clear what the exact events are during the training that result in stress abatement and a concomitant reduction in the blood corticosterone response, but presumably they involve repeated handling and exposure to the general test environment, and this is beneficial for subsequent learning in the environment.

All this suggests that task difficulty and stress factors are important in experiments of this kind. Separating the learning of various components of a complex task such as the water maze might facilitate the learning in experimentally treated animals because each component is less difficult to master by itself, and requires less neural processing and computation than if all of the components are learned together. For a drugged rat the degree of task difficulty and stress involved in a specific task may be a major factor in whether it will be able to deal effectively it. If task difficulty is too great, drug treatment might severely impair acquisition and performance because the processing of information and the generation of appropriate behavioral strategies is impaired by the compromised function of the nervous system due to the drug. If appropriate behavioral strategies are not developed the rat will not be able to learn the location of the hidden platform. An example of the effect of increased task difficulty is contained in a recent report by Morris's group, in which the water maze task was made especially difficult by the use of a large pool and small hidden platform (relative to those used in many laboratories), and the requirement to repeatedly learn new platform locations (i.e., reversals) in a single trial and remember them for a long time (Steele and Morris, 1999). In this case a spatial memory deficit occurred in nonspatially pretrained rats given an NMDA receptor antagonist, where one did not occur with a less difficult version of the task (Bannerman et al., 1995).

Another approach to the task difficulty question made initial use of a large hidden platform that occupied nearly all of the pool, followed in successive training sessions by progressively smaller hidden platforms that "shrank" into a specific quadrant of the pool (Day and Schallert, 1996; Schallert et al., 1999). Schallert and colleagues found that rats given a muscarinic cholinergic antagonist or hippocampal lesions very quickly found the hidden platform when trained in this way. These treatments, when given to naive rats in a conventional water maze training format, consistently produced severe impairments, although nonspatial pretraining completely eliminated the deficit seen in rats given a muscarinic cholinergic antagonist (Saucier et al., 1996; Beiko et al., 1997; Hoh and Cain, 1997), and initial training with a visible platform allowed rats with hippocampal lesions to learn an accurate place response (Whishaw et al., 1995).

The interpretation offered by Day and Schallert of the good performance of their drugged or hippocampally lesioned rats was that the training regimen prevented them from learning behavioral strategies that were incompatible with effective performance in the pool, such as periphery swimming. An additional, nonmutually exclusive interpretation is possible: The initial training circumstances were very easy for the treated rats. When they began swimming they very quickly encountered the platform because it occupied nearly all of the pool. Unless they sank (which the experimenter prevented by rescuing them), they quickly contacted and climbed onto the platform. During the first few sessions they easily learned the required strategies. By the time the hidden platform shrank to the size used in conventional water maze tasks, the treated rats were performing as well as controls. The most parsimonious interpretation seems to be that the remaining brain mechanisms in these rats were fully capable of accurate and effective navigation in the pool, but that this could only be displayed if the rats were trained in a manner that allowed them to learn the required behavioral strategies. This was accomplished by exposing them to initially easy, followed by progressively harder, versions of the task. A similar interpretation can be given to our finding that rats with LTP blocked by an NMDA receptor antagonist very quickly learned the required water maze strategies, and then used them to learn a place response and a subsequent reversal response (Hoh et al., 1999). Separating the task into individual components makes acquiring the components easier and allows the rats' remaining brain mechanisms to master the task components just as quickly as controls do (see Hoh et al., 1999).

What all of these examples have in common is that the treated rats can learn quite effectively provided they do not have to learn everything at once. The need to take into account the issue of task difficulty in research with the water maze, and probably in other tasks used in LTP-learning research, seems inescapable.

The Importance of Behavioral Analysis in LTP-Learning Research

The importance of both nonspatial pretraining and detailed behavioral analysis in the research discussed above seems clear. Based on studies with naive animals by many researchers, we know that administration of any of a variety of pharmacologic treatments is likely to produce an impairment in the water maze task. However, without additional information, the nature of the impairment would be unknown. One possibility is that there might be a specific impairment in spatial learning. Another possibility is an impairment in the ability to acquire the behavioral strategies required in the task. Virtually all tasks used in learning research require that the animal master essential behavioral strategies for coping with the requirements of the task and for acquiring information relevant to successful performance in the task. In the case of the water maze, we have found unambiguous evidence of severe disruptions in strategy acquisition in naive drugged animals in every one of our experiments, as discussed above. The performance of nonspatially pretrained animals was excellent when they were given the same drug treatments.

Still another possibility is that the behavioral impairments result from sensorimotor disturbances caused by the treatments. For example, NMDA receptor antagonists interfere with a large variety of sensory and motor mechanisms including motor coordination, visual and other sensory processing (see Cain, 1997a; Cain et al., 1997), and complex instinctive behaviors such as grooming (Robertson et al., 1999). That is because NMDA receptors are widely distributed in the central nervous system and participate in many sensorimotor mechanisms.

As a further example of the insights that can be obtained from the detailed behavioral analysis approach we have used, I will describe a recent experiment in which we found a specific impairment in spatial learning without an impairment in behavioral strategy use. Some time ago we began administering two different pharmacologic agents in combination to rats tested in the water maze. The combinations that were used were intended to mimic aspects of the neurochemical deficits found in Alzheimer patients. The first such combination was scopolamine, a muscarinic cholinergic antagonist, together with p-chlorophenylalanine, an agent that depletes serotonin (Beiko et al., 1997). This combination of agents severely disrupts normal electroencephalographic activity throughout the entire neocortex, and animals are greatly impaired in a variety of behavioral tasks (Vanderwolf, 1987). Both naive and nonspatially pretrained rats given this combination of treatments were also severely impaired in the water maze (Beiko et al., 1997). We next tried an NMDA receptor antagonist together with either scopolamine or diazepam. Naive rats given either combination of agents were severely impaired in all aspects of performance. They exhibited poor strategy use as well as poor spatial navigation. In contrast, nonspatially pretrained rats given the same treatments exhibited excellent strategy use that was as good as that of controls, but despite this they could not learn where the hidden platform was located (Cain and Ighanian, 1999). They had a highly specific spatial learning impairment that was not due to an inability to make use of the required behavioral strategies. This was the first demonstration of a specific spatial learning impairment due to pharmacologic treatment, in a conventional water maze task in which the required strategies were confirmed to be unimpaired.

Without nonspatial pretraining and a detailed analysis of behavior in the pool, we could not have determined which aspects of the task the animals were impaired in and which ones they could perform well. Nor, in other experiments, could we have adequately evaluated the role of LTP in the different phases of the task.

The long history of research on the neural basis of learning and memory shows how difficult it can be to arrive at firm conclusions regarding unseen, inferred processes inside the brain, such as the establishment of a neural memory trace. Making inferences from locomotion, swimming, and other behaviors to unseen processes in the brain must be done with caution if we are to have confidence in the conclusions. Taking this caution seriously involves according the same degree of effort to the analysis of behavior, through appropriate experimental design and detailed analysis, as is accorded to the study and analysis of the nervous system itself.

The Need for More Data

Based on our results cited above we know that a normal rat with no pretraining acquires water maze strategies quickly and makes use of them to rapidly learn a hidden platform location, usually in ten trials or less. A rat given any single one of a variety of pharmacologic agents displays spatial learning only if it knows the required behavioral strategies, or if it is trained in individual task components in a sequential manner. A rat given two pharmacologic agents together cannot display effective spatial learning, and in some cases is not able to use previously learned behavioral strategies. These results seem to form a crude continuum of increasing behavioral impairment with increasing perturbation of brain mechanisms. The absence of specific links between particular pharmacologic treatments and particular behavioral impairments is striking, and in the context of rather specific recent theories on the neural basis of learning and memory, is also somewhat surprising.

However, the data on which this idea is based are limited, and relate to only one laboratory task. Skepticism about this idea, as with all ideas in science, is in order. What is needed now is additional data from experiments in which task difficulty and experimental treatments are systematically varied and components of the task are fractionated in the way that Morris fractionated the water maze task using nonspatial pretraining. The goal should be to collect needed data to examine further any links that might exist between the function of specific neural mechanisms and specific aspects of learning and memory. Only when there is a comprehensive body of data involving a large variety of experimental treatments and behavioral tasks will we be in a position to make firmer statements about the specificity of neural mechanisms and specific forms of spatial learning and memory. One promising direction to follow is to combine antagonists in an effort to mimic aspects of the neurochemical deficits that occur in Alzheimer disease (Cain and Ighanian, 1999).

Conclusions

The following general conclusions emerge from this research. First, the exact role of NMDA receptor-dependent LTP in spatial learning remains unclear. There is evidence that it plays a necessary role in particularly difficult water maze tasks, but it is not necessary for water maze tasks of conventional difficulty. Whether it contributes in a nonobligatory way in the latter case is unclear. Second, future research with the correlation strategy should make use of some means of resetting synaptic weights prior to training to better reveal any changes in weights caused by behavioral learning. Third, recent research has revealed the underlying complexity of seemingly simple laboratory tasks, such as the water maze. With recently developed experimental approaches, the very complexity of this task becomes an advantage in that the components can be fractionated and studied separately in detail. Nonspatial pretraining to separate the strategy learning phase from the spatial learning phase is a crucial aspect of this research. Together with a detailed analysis of behavior conducted using commercially available digital tracking systems, the array of behavioral tools available for the work is formidable. Perhaps the most general conclusion that can be drawn from the work is the fact that attention to detail in the behavioral aspects of the work is essential for reliable conclusions about mechanisms of spatial learning. Considering the millions of years of evolutionary history represented by the remarkably adaptive behavioral abilities of the average laboratory rat, this conclusion is not surprising. Behavioral neuroscientists are now in a position to take advantage of approaches and technology that should yield the data that are needed to make significant advances in understanding the neural basis of spatial learning and memory.

REFERENCES

Barnes, C.A. (1979). Behavioral deficits associated with senescence: A neurophysiological and behavioral study in the rat. *J. Comp. Physiol. Psychol.* 93: 74–104.

Bannerman, D.M., Good, M.A., Butcher, S.P., Ramsay, M. et al. (1995). Distinct components of spatial learning revealed by prior training and NMDA receptor blockade. *Nature* 378: 182–186.

Beiko, J., and Cain, D.P. (1998). The effect of water maze spatial training on posterior parietal cortex transcallosal evoked potentials in the rat. *Cereb. Cortex* 8: 407–414.

Beiko, J., Candusso, L., and Cain, D.P. (1997). The effect of nonspatial water maze pretraining in rats subjected to serotonin depletion and muscarinic receptor antagonism: A detailed behavioral assessment of spatial performance. *Behav. Brain Res.* 88: 201–211.

Beiko, J., Lander, R., Hampson, E., and Cain, D.P. (1998). Differential corticosterone stress response profiles in male and female rats appears to contribute to sex differences in water maze spatial performance. *Soc. Neurosci. Abstr.* 24: 946.

Bliss, T.V.P., and Lomo, T. (1973). Long-lasting potentiation of synaptic transmission in the dentate area of the anaesthetized rabbit following stimulation of the perforant path. *J. Physiol.* 232: 331–356.

Cain, D.P. (1997a). LTP, NMDA, genes and learning. *Curr. Opin. Neurobiol.* 7: 235–242.

Cain, D.P. (1997b). Prior non-spatial pretraining eliminates sensorimotor disturbances and impairments in water maze learning caused by diazepam. *Psychopharmacology* 130: 313–319.

Cain, D.P. (1998). Testing the NMDA, long-term potentiation, and cholinergic hypotheses of spatial learning. *Neurosci. Biobehav. Rev.* 22: 181–193.

Cain, D.P., and Saucier, D. (1996). The neuroscience of spatial navigation: Focus on behavior yields advances. *Rev. Neurosci.* 7: 215–231.

Cain, D.P., and Ighanian, K. (1999). Combined but not individual antagonism of muscarinic and NMDA receptors causes a spatial learning impairment in non-spatially pretrained rats. *Soc. Neurosci. Abstr.* 25: 253.5.

Cain, D.P., Hargreaves, E.L., Boon, F., and Dennison, Z. (1993). An examination of the relations between hippocampal long-term potentiation, kindling, afterdischarge, and place learning in the water maze. *Hippocampus* 3: 153–164.

Cain, D.P., Hargreaves, E.L., and Boon, F. (1994). Brain temperature- and behavior-related changes in the dentate gyrus field potential during sleep, cold water immersion, radiant heating, and urethane anesthesia. *Brain Res.* 658: 1235–1244.

Cain, D.P., Saucier, D., Hall, J., Hargreaves, E.L. et al. (1996). Detailed behavioral analysis of water maze acquisition under APV or CNQX: Contribution of sensorimotor disturbances to drug-induced acquisition deficits. *Behav. Neurosci.* 110: 86–102.

Cain, D.P., Saucier, D., and Boon, F. (1997). Testing hypotheses of spatial learning: The role of NMDA receptors and NMDA-mediated long term potentiation. *Behav. Brain Res.* 84: 179–193.

Castro, C.A., Silbert, L.H., McNaughton, B.L., and Barnes, C.A. (1989). Recovery of spatial learning deficits after decay of electrically induced synaptic enhancement in the hippocampus. *Nature* 342: 545–548.

Daw, N.W., Stein, P., and Fox, K. (1993). The role of NMDA receptors in information processing. *Ann. Rev. Neurosci.* 16: 207–222.

Day, L.B., and Schallert, T. (1996). Anticholinergic effects on acquisition of place learning in the Morris water task: Spatial mapping deficit or inability to inhibit non-place strategies? *Behav. Neurosci.* 110: 998–1005.

DeVietti, T.L., Pellis, S.M., Pellis, V.C., and Teitelbaum, P. (1985). Previous experience disrupts atropine-induced stereotyped trapping in rats. *Behav. Neurosci.* 99: 1128–1141.

Finlayson, C., Beiko, J., Boon, F., and Cain, D.P. (1998). Ethanol causes water maze impairments in naive but not nonsptailly pretrained rats. *Soc. Neurosci. Abstr.* 24: 688.

Hargreaves, E.L., and Cain, D.P. (1992). Hyperactivity, hyper-reactivity, and sensorimotor deficits induced by low doses of the N-methyl-D-aspartate non competitive channel blocker MK-801. *Behav. Brain Res.* 47: 23–33.

Hargreaves, E.L., Cain, D.P., and Vanderwolf, C.H. (1990). Learning and behavioral-long-term potentiation: Importance of controlling for motor activity. *J. Neurosci.* 10: 1472–1478.

Hebb, D.O. (1949). *The Organization of Behavior. A Neuropsychological Theory.* New York: John Wiley.

Herz, A. (1959). Uber die Wirkung von Scopolamin, Benactyzin, und Atropin auf das Verhalten der Ratte. *Naunyn Schmiedebergs Arch Path Pharmakol* 236: 110–111.

Heynen, A.J., Abraham, W.C., and Bear, M.F. (1996). Bidirectional modification of CA1 synapses in the adult hippocampus in vivo. *Nature* 381: 163–166.

Hoh, T., Beiko, J., Boon, F., and Cain, D.P. (1999). Complex behavioral strategy and reversal learning in the water maze without NMDA receptor-dependent long-term potentiation. *J. Neurosci.* 19: RC2 1–5.

Hoh, T., and Cain, D.P. (1997). Fractionating the nonspatial pretraining effect in the water maze task. *Behav. Neurosci.* 111: 1285–1291.

Hölscher, C. (1999). Stress impairs performance in spatial water maze learning tasks. *Behav. Brain Res.* 100: 225–235.

McEachern, J.C., and Shaw, C.A. (1996). An alternative to the LTP orthodoxy: A plasticity-pathology continuum model. *Brain Res. Rev.* 22: 51–92.

McKernan, M.G., and Shinnick-Gallagher, P. (1997). Fear conditioning induces a lasting potentiation of synaptic currents in vitro. *Nature* 390: 607–661.

McNaughton, B.L., Barnes, C.A., Rao, G., Baldwin, J. et al. (1986). Long-term enhancement of hippocampal synaptic transmission and the acquisition of spatial information. *J. Neurosci.* 6: 563–571.

McNaughton, B.L., and Morris, R.G.M. (1987). Hippocampal synaptic enhancement and information storage within a distributed memory system. *Trends Neurosci.* 10: 408–415.

Miller, K. (1996). Synaptic economics: Competition and cooperation in synaptic plasticity. *Neuron* 17: 371–374.

Morris, R.G.M. (1989). Synapitic plasticity and learning: Selective impairment of learning in rats and blockade of long-term potentiation in vivo by the N-methyl-D-aspartate receptor blocker AP5. *J. Neurosci.* 9: 3040–3057.

Morris, R.G.M., Anderson, E., Lynch, G.S., and Baudry, M. (1986). Selective impairment of learning and blockade of long-term potentiation by an N-methyl-D-aspartate receptor antagonist, AP5. *Nature* 319: 774–776.

Morris, R.G.M., and Davis, M. (1994). The role of NMDA receptors in learning and memory. In L. Collingridge and J.C. Watkins (Eds.), *The NMDA receptor* (2nd ed., pp. 340–375). New York: Oxford University Press.

Moser, E., Mathiesen, J., and Andersen, P. (1993). Association between brain temperature and dentate field potentials in exploring and swimming rats. *Science* 259: 1324–1326.

Moser, E.I., Moser, M.-B., and Andersen, P. (1994). Potentiation of dentate synapses initiated by exploratory learning in rats: Dissociation from brain temperature, motor activity, and arousal. *Learn. Mem.* 1: 55–73.

Moser, E., Krobert, K., Moser, M.-B., and Morris, R.G.M. (1998). Impaired spatial learning after saturation of long-term potentiation. *Science* 281: 2038–2041.

Otnaess, M.K., Brun, V.H., Moser, M.-B., and Moser, E.I. (1999). Pretraining prevents spatial learning impairment following saturation of hippocampal long-term potentiation. *J. Neurosci.*

Robertson, B.J., Boon, F., Cain, D.P., and Vanderwolf, C.H. (1999). Behavioural effects of anti-muscarinic, anti-serotonergic, and anti-NMDA treatments: Hippocampal and neocortical slow wave electrophysiology predict the effects on grooming in the rat. *Brain Res.* 838: 234–240.

Rogan, M.T., Staubli, U., and LeDoux, J. (1997). Fear conditioning induces associative long-term potentation in the amygdala. *Nature* 390: 604–607.

Ruthrich, H., Matthies, H., and Ott, T. (1982). Long-term changes in synaptic excitability of hippocampus cell populations as a result of training. In C. Marsan and H. Matthies (Eds.), *Neural plasticity and memory formation* (pp. 589–594). New York: Raven Press.

Saucier, D., and Cain, D.P. (1995). Spatial learning without NMDA receptor-dependent long-term potentiation. *Nature* 378: 186–189.

Saucier, D., Hargreaves, E.L., Boon, F., Vanderwolf, C.H. et al. (1996). Detailed behavioral analysis of water maze acquisition under systemic NMDA or muscarinic antagonist: Nonspatial pretraining eliminates spatial learning deficits. *Behav. Neurosci.* 110: 103–116.

Schallert, T., Day, L.B., and Weisend, M., and Sutherland, R.J. (1999). Spatial learning by hippocampal rats in the Morris water task. *Soc. Neurosci. Abstr.* 22: 678.

Sharp, P.E., McNaughton, B.L., and Barnes, C.A. (1985). Enhancement of hippocampal field potentials in rats exposed to a novel, complex environment. *Brain Res.* 339: 361–365.

Skelton, R., Scarth, A., Wilkie, D., Miller, J. et al. (1987). Long-term increases in dentate granule cell responsivity accompany operant conditioning. *J. Neurosci.* 7: 3081–3087.

Staubli, U., and Lynch, G. (1990). Stable depression of potentiated synaptic responses in the hippocampus with 1-5 Hz stimulation. *Brain Res.* 513: 113–118.

Steele, R.J., and Morris, R.G.M. (1999). Delay-dependent impairment of a matching-to-place task with chronic and intrahippocampal infusion of the NMDA antagonist D-AP5. *Hippocampus* 9: 118–136.

Steinberg, H., Rushton, R., and Tinson, C. (1961). Modification of the effects of an amphet-amine-barbiturate mixture by the past experience of rats. *Nature* 192: 533–535.

Sutherland, R.J., Whishaw, I.Q., and Regehr, J.C. (1982). Cholinergic receptor blockade impairs spatial localization by use of distal cues in the rat. *J. Comp. Physiol. Psychol.* 96: 563–573.

Vanderwolf, C.H. (1987). Near-total loss of learning and memory as a result of combined cholinergic and serotonergic blockade in the rat. *Behav. Brain Res.* 23: 43–57.

Vanderwolf, C.H., Harvey, G.C., and Leung, L.-W.S. (1987). Transcallosal evoked potentials in relation to behavior in the rat: Effects of atropine, p-chlorophenylalanine, reserpine, scopolamine and trifluoperazine. *Behav. Brain Res.* 25: 31–48.

Weisz, D., Clark, G., Yang, B., Thompson, R. et al. (1982). Activity of the dentate gyrus during NM conditioning in the rabbit. *Adv. Behav. Biol.* 26: 131–145.

Whishaw, I.Q., Cassel, J.-C., and Jarrard, L.E. (1995). Rats with fimbria-fornix lesions display a place response in a swimming pool: A dissociation between getting there and knowing where. *J. Neurosci.* 15: 5779–5788.

Winson, J., and Abzug, C. (1978). Neuronal transmission through hippocampal pathways dependent upon behavior. *J. Neurophysiol.* 41: 716–732.

Xu, L., Anwyl, R., and Rowan, M.J. (1998). Spatial exploration induces a persistent reversal of long-term potentiation in rat hippocampus. *Nature* 394: 891–894.

CHAPTER FOURTEEN

What Studies in Old Rats Tell Us about the Role of LTP in Learning and Memory

Gregory M. Rose and David M. Diamond

SUMMARY

Advanced aging is usually accompanied by declines in cognitive function, particularly in the areas of learning and memory. The presence of these behavioral deficits makes aged animals a good system in which to explore basic tenets of the hypothesis that long-term potentiation (LTP) is important for learning and memory. Here we review the existing literature describing studies of hippocampal LTP in aged rodents. These studies indicate that age-related decrements in LTP are often, but not always, reported; discrepancies between studies appear to be due to the stimulation protocol used or type of LTP being measured. Correlations between hippocampal LTP status and spatial learning ability in individual aged animals support the notion of an LTP/learning relationship, as do the results of interventional studies demonstrating that drug-related behavioral improvements also reduce LTP deficits. However, these promising results need verification and expansion. We conclude that, due to the complexity of the linkage between its physiologic and behavioral functions, the hippocampal system may not be appropriate for validating the hypothesis that LTP is critical for learning and memory. Nevertheless, studies of hippocampal LTP, particularly in aged animals, may provide an excellent framework for approaches to develop therapeutic interventions for age-related cognitive impairments.

Introduction

For many neuroscientists, long-term potentiation (LTP) has become a mantra for describing changes in the brain that are logically part of a memory encoding mechanism. However, problems arise when this idea is expressed as some formal hypothesis, the simplest examples of which are that inducing LTP should produce

Christian Hölscher, editor, *Neuronal Mechanisms of Memory Formation*. © 2001 Cambridge University Press. Printed in the United States of America. All rights reserved.

learning, or that preventing LTP should prevent learning. While some of the contributors to this book may argue otherwise, we feel that neither of these straight-forward-sounding hypotheses has yet been unequivocally shown to be valid. To begin with, it is important to recognize that such broadly stated propositions may not even *be* provable. First, it is not reasonable to expect to demonstrate that inducing LTP causes learning without knowing all the neuronal circuitry involved in the acquisition of the particular behavioral task, and how many of these connections are capable of modification. Second, as will be discussed further later on, preventing LTP to impair learning is only a viable strategy if (1) the blockade of LTP is complete; (2) all routes (relevant receptors and biochemical pathways) of generating LTP are blocked; and (3) learning in the particular task can be achieved only through LTP-dependent circuit alterations. Thus, it is clear that a major reason why we are not yet in a position to precisely define the relationship of LTP to learning is because we still do not understand either phenomenon well enough.

One very important motivation for understanding how learning and memory occur is to potentially gain the ability to correct conditions where impairments in these behaviors are present. The most common prescription for learning and memory dysfunction is simply getting old. Even in the absence of classifiable disease, aged subjects (both animal and human) show declines in their ability to learn and remember new information (e.g., Zyzak et al., 1995; Burke and Mackay, 1997). A hypothesis that predicts a link between LTP and learning would, therefore, have the corollary that LTP should also be impaired in regions of the aged brain that subserve the type of learning involved. A further extension of this hypothesis would be that treatments that somehow improve learning and memory in aged subjects would also improve LTP, and vice versa. Importantly, the use of aging to test the relationship between LTP and learning does not require precise knowledge of how or when LTP occurs. Initially, it is enough to ask simply whether the condition of being able to generate LTP is associated with the condition of being able to learn or remember.

The goals of this chapter are to summarize the current evidence for age-related changes in LTP and to evaluate the relationship between such changes and learning or memory. Then, the results of experiments examining how treatments that improve age-related learning impairments modify LTP will be described. Finally, some criteria for strengthening the learning/LTP relationship will be proposed. We will limit ourselves primarily to a discussion of LTP phenomena in the hippocampus and their potential relevance to hippocampus-dependent cognitive processes (e.g., spatial learning).

The Phenomenon of LTP

At the risk of being redundant in the context of this book, a brief discussion of LTP is in order. At this point, LTP is a phenomenon that has been best characterized using invasive electrophysiologic techniques. LTP was first described as a long-lasting increase in extracellularly recorded field potentials, population spikes, or discharge latencies of single neurons recorded in the hippocampal dentate gyrus in response to stimulation of afferents from the entorhinal cortex in either anesthetized or unanesthetized rabbits (Bliss and Gardner-Medwin, 1973; Bliss and Lomo, 1973). The capacity to generate LTP was subsequently shown to be a property of other hippocampal formation synapses, both *in vivo* and *in vitro* (Alger and Teyler, 1976; Bliss et al., 1983; Teyler and DiScenna, 1987; Zalutsky and Nicoll, 1990; Maren and Baudry, 1995; Voronin et al., 1995; Commins et al., 1998). In addition, LTP can be induced in other brain regions, including neocortical areas (Teyler, 1989; Laroche et al., 1990; del Cerro et al., 1992; Bear and Kirkwood, 1993; Kirkwood and Bear, 1994; Castro Alamancos et al., 1995; Cousens and Otto, 1998; Escobar et al., 1998; Teskey and Valentine, 1998; Trepel and Racine, 1998), the amygdala (Chapman and Bellavance, 1992; Shindou et al., 1993; Maren, 1996; Huang and Kandel, 1998), neostriatum (Calabresi et al., 1997; Charpier and Deniau, 1997), and cerebellum (Salin et al., 1996; D'Angelo et al., 1999).

The focus on LTP as a memory mechanism is based on several parallels between this electrophysiologically observable phenomenon and characteristics of learning and memory, such as rapid onset, long duration, and strengthening with practice (i.e., more stimulation in the case of LTP). A potentially critical bridge for linking LTP with behavior was the discovery that antagonists of NMDA-subtype glutamate receptors blocked LTP induction in hippocampal area CA1 (Collingridge et al., 1983; Harris et al., 1984). This work led to studies showing that NMDA receptor antagonists also impaired learning (Morris et al., 1986; Staubli et al., 1989; Shapiro and Caramanos, 1990). Subsequent work further demonstrated that LTP blockade in the hippocampus and spatial learning impairments were observed in the same dose range (Davis et al., 1992; Hargreaves et al., 1997; Steele and Morris, 1999), strengthening the case for a relationship between the two phenomena. In addition, many other pharmacologic studies have shown that a number of drugs that modulate learning and memory also affect LTP (reviewed by Izquierdo, 1994; Izquierdo and Medina, 1995).

When viewed as a whole, these pharmacologic studies provide a suggestive indication that LTP and learning have something to do with each other. However, other work has shown that considerable spatial learning can take place even when NMDA-receptor-dependent hippocampal LTP seems to be completely blocked (Saucier and Cain, 1995; Hoh et al., 1999). A particular weakness of the approach to using drugs that block LTP as a way of demonstrating the necessity of LTP for learning is that a negative outcome is meaningless unless it can be unequivocally shown that (1) the blockade of LTP induction was complete, and lasted for the entire period during which LTP induction would participate in memory formation; (2) the drug acted in all the brain regions that might be using LTP to encode information necessary to learning the particular task being examined; and (3) that the drug employed prevents all possible forms of LTP from being induced.

Complete, selective antagonism of any physiologic function is very difficult to achieve. Knowledge of the neuronal circuitry underlying most learned behaviors in mammals is far from complete. Finally, there are forms of LTP that clearly do not depend on NMDA-receptor activation (e.g., in the hippocampal mossy fiber system; Harris and Cotman, 1986; Zalutsky and Nicoll, 1990), involving instead a variety of (probably to some extent interrelated) mechanisms including opioids (Derrick et al., 1991; Bramham and Sarvey, 1996; Williams and Johnston, 1996), calcium channels (Turner et al., 1982; Grover and Teyler, 1990; Diana et al., 1995), muscarinic cholinergic receptors (Auerbach and Segal, 1994, 1997), potassium channels (Aniksztejn and Ben Ari, 1991; Hanse and Gustafsson, 1994), or activation of particular second messenger systems (Frey et al., 1993; Matthies and Reymann, 1993; Abel et al., 1997). Thus, the failure of a drug that impairs LTP to prevent learning clearly does not disprove the hypothesis that LTP is necessary for learning. Nevertheless, the struggle to link LTP with learning and memory has had a very positive outcome: It has sharpened neuroscientists' appreciation of the variety of memory subtypes, the range of brain regions that could be involved, and the numerous elements of any learning task that are distinct from the actual learning or recall elements (e.g., stimulus recognition or performance aspects).

An alternative approach to establishing that LTP is part of a learning system has been, instead of trying to prevent LTP induction, to exhaust the capacity of particular systems to generate LTP as part of the learning process. The rationale for these experiments was derived from an early observation about LTP that it, like memory, was of limited capacity. If an LTP-like mechanism was necessary for learning, it seemed reasonable to suggest that completely expressing ("saturating") electrophysiologically demonstrable LTP should result in the subsequent impairment of learning in a task that required long-term plasticity for learning. Initial experiments tested this hypothesis by generating maximal LTP in the dentate gyrus prior to training rats in spatial learning tasks. This work suggested that saturating LTP impaired new learning, but not the retrieval of previously learned information (McNaughton et al., 1986). Further, the ability to learn returned after the LTP had decayed (Castro et al., 1989).

Unfortunately, later studies were unable to replicate these findings (Cain et al., 1993; Jeffery and Morris, 1993; Korol et al., 1993; Sutherland et al., 1993; Barnes et al., 1994), which left the validity of the hypothesis unclear. However, a recent experiment by Moser et al. (1998; Moser and Moser, 1999) provided a potential resolution for the conflicting sets of results. These investigators found that it was, in fact, quite difficult to completely saturate LTP in a given set of (in this case) hippocampal afferents. Further, they found that LTP induction in only a very small component of an afferent pathway was sufficient to permit learning. These results strongly indicate that relatively few synapses needed to be strengthened for an animal to show learning, at least in the simple tasks that are commonly employed. Thus, in the final analysis, the saturation approach suffers from the same limitation as pharmacologic blockade, in that the lack of complete treatment renders a negative result uninterpretable.

Yet another problem in specifying a role for LTP in learning has been the growing recognition that the electrical stimulation used to induce LTP does not bear even superficial similarity to normal afferent activity in the brain regions where plasticity was being recorded. Historically, LTP was induced using long (usually

>500 msec) trains of high frequency (typically 100 to 400 Hz) stimulation. By contrast, patterns of neuronal discharge recorded from the brains of unanesthetized animals indicated that while such discharge frequencies could sometimes be observed, they were never of the requisite duration. With the caveat that electrical stimulation causes more generalized and synchronized activation than is probably ever likely to take place in the brain, some investigators began to explore whether stimuli patterned to more closely mimic normal afferent activity was capable of generating LTP. The first study of this kind was by Douglas (1977), who reported that delivering several short (4 to 10 pulse) bursts of 100 to 400 Hz to perforant path fibers evoked robust LTP in the dentate gyrus. Later, Buszaki and colleagues (Buzsaki et al., 1987; Buzsaki, 1989) presented evidence that intense afferent activation designed to imitate hippocampal sharp waves can induce LTP in CA1.

However, the experiments of this type that have had the greatest impact are those that involved delivering patterns of electrical stimulation designed around hippocampal rhythmical slow activity (RSA), or theta rhythm. Theta rhythm is a prominent component of the hippocampal electroencephalogram (EEG) that is observed only under specific behavioral conditions, including exploration and attending to novel stimuli, and that had long been hypothesized to be linked to cognitive processing. (For a discussion of the characteristics and hypothesized functions of theta rhythm, see Bland, 1986; Vinogradova, 1995; Vertes and Kocsis, 1997; Oddie and Bland, 1998.) In the mid-1980s, three different laboratories published results showing that electrical stimulation patterned to mimic afferent activity at theta rhythm frequencies would induce LTP (Larson et al., 1986; Rose and Dunwiddie, 1986; Greenstein et al., 1988). Such stimulation patterns have since come into common use. Most employ a series of brief bursts (usually five pulses at 100 to 200 Hz) given at a 200-msec interval (so-called theta burst stimulation; TBS). A more threshold pattern consists of a single pulse followed 140 to 200 msec later by a burst of two to ten pulses at 100 to 200 Hz (primed burst stimulation; PB). Direct comparisons using the PB protocol have shown that the same number of stimuli given using theta patterning was both more effective and more efficient in inducing LTP than other methods (Rose and Dunwiddie, 1986; Diamond et al., 1988). Further, long-term plasticity induced by theta-patterned stimulation was found to interact with conventionally induced LTP (i.e., each occludes the other; Diamond et al., 1988), and was also sensitive to NMDA-receptor blockade (Diamond et al., 1988; Larson and Lynch, 1988).

The current consensus is that theta-patterned stimulation and conventional LTP stimulation activate the same plasticity mechanisms. The increased efficacy of theta-patterned stimulation appears to be due to its taking advantage of a naturally occurring window of disinhibition (Pacelli et al., 1989; Davies et al., 1991) that coincides with the rising phase of the theta rhythm cycle (Pavlides et al., 1988; Huerta and Lisman, 1995; Hölscher et al., 1997). In addition, recent work has shown that prolonged delivery of single stimuli at theta rhythm frequency initiates complex spiking in CA1 hippocampal neurons, providing intrinsic "bursts" that are capable of inducing LTP (Thomas et al., 1998). Taken together, the studies linking LTP with theta rhythm have added considerable support to the idea that an LTP-like process could underlie learning. However, the gap between electrical stimulation and natural afferent activity still represents an obstacle to unqualified acceptance of this idea.

It has long been recognized that memories can have different durations. This observation led to the idea that memory processing has different stages, likely involving different brain structures and/or different biochemical mechanisms. In contrast, until fairly recently it was thought that LTP was essentially a unitary process. This discrepancy between LTP and memory was explained in different ways, e.g., that LTP lasted forever, that LTP was a regenerative process, or that information transfer to other brain regions necessary for long-term memory storage took place during the time when LTP was present but decaying. While this issue is still far from being resolved, recent work indicates that LTP itself can consist of different temporal phases. The most developed research in this area has focused on so-called late-stage LTP (reviewed by Huang et al., 1996).

Late-stage LTP can be differentiated from the earlier forms of LTP by its delayed appearance (1 to 3 hours) following very strong electrical stimulation. Late-stage LTP is also distinguished from early-stage LTP in that it requires cyclic AMP (cAMP), activation of cAMP-dependent protein kinase A, and protein synthesis. While electrical stimulation is not very efficient at inducing late-stage LTP, it can be directly evoked in *in vitro* brain slice preparations by analogs of cAMP or dopamine D1/D5 receptor agonists (Frey et al., 1995; Huang and Kandel, 1995). Thus, the identification of late-stage LTP, perhaps one of many types of LTP yet to be characterized (see, for example, Winder et al., 1998), may help to fill the gap between what is expected of a learning/memory process and what the brain has been shown to be able to do.

In summary, discovery of electrophysiologic phenomena of LTP has had a major impact on research into the neurobiologic substrates for learning and memory. Continually increasing knowledge about LTP has helped to deflect emerging criticisms about its appropriateness as a learning/memory mechanisms. Most important, it has not been proven that an LTP-like process is *not* involved in learning and memory. However, neither has it been possible to unequivocally show that LTP is essential for learning or memory. The following sections address the question of whether studies of LTP in aged rodents contribute to the resolution of this issue.

Age-Related Decrements in LTP

Of the thousands of articles that have been published on LTP, relatively few have examined for alterations in LTP during aging. With few exceptions (Baskys et al., 1990; Wu et al., 1991; Garcia and Jaffard, 1993), such studies have been performed in the hippocampal formation. Overall, the results of this work are not consistent. However, individual laboratories usually replicate their own findings, suggesting that differences in experimental methods can significantly influence the results.

Work from the Barnes group has consistently shown no age-related difference in the magnitude of LTP induced by repeated stimulation of entorhinal cortex afferents, although the time course of the decay of the enhanced response was usually faster in aged animals (Barnes, 1979; Barnes and McNaughton, 1985; Davis et al., 1993). Similar results were reported by deToledo-Morrell and colleagues (deToledo-Morrell et al., 1988; Geinisman et al., 1992) and Diana et al. (Diana et al., 1994a, 1994b). In contrast, other laboratories have observed deficits in LTP induction in the dentate gyrus (McGahon et al., 1997; Murray and Lynch, 1998), although only in a subset of animals (Lynch and Voss, 1994; Bergado et al., 1997). A similar inconsistency is present in the literature describing age-related changes in LTP in the commissural/associational inputs to the CA1 pyramidal cells. While some studies have reported a decrement in conventionally induced LTP with aging (Landfield et al., 1978; Tielen et al., 1983; Hori et al., 1992; Deupree et al., 1993), the majority observed no effect (Chang et al., 1991; Deupree et al., 1991, 1993; Moore et al., 1993; Diana et al., 1994a, 1994b; Barnes et al., 1996; Norris et al., 1996; Shankar et al., 1998; Bach et al., 1999).

This mix of results clearly does not provide unqualified support for the idea that impairments in LTP underlie age-related learning and memory problems. More recent studies, however, have consistently shown impairments in the induction of LTP when theta-patterned stimulation was employed (Moore et al., 1993; Rose et al., 1996; Rosenzweig et al., 1997). It has been argued that threshold stimulation protocols promote LTP induction via NMDA-receptor-dependent mechanisms, while stronger stimulation also activates voltage-dependent calcium channels (VDCC) as a route to LTP (Shankar et al., 1998). NMDA-receptor-dependent LTP appears to decline in area CA1 of aged rats, while VDCC-dependent LTP actually increases (Shankar et al., 1998). The net result of these processes can be that no net change in LTP is observed when strong stimulation is used. In addition, an age-related deficit has been shown in LTP induced in CA1 in hippocampal slices by pharmacologic manipulations, for example, transiently elevating calcium concentrations in the medium (Diana et al., 1995) or application of the cholinergic agonist carbachol (Auerbach and Segal, 1997). Finally, it has recently been shown that late-stage LTP is impaired in aged mice (Bach et al., 1999). Taken together, these results suggest that, indeed, deterioration of long-term plasticity mechanisms in the hippocampus could be linked to the cognitive impairments observed in aging. However, they also demonstrate that the traditional approach to studying LTP (e.g., examining for changes induced 30 minutes after a 100-Hz/1-second stimulus train) is not likely to be informative in terms of linking LTP to behavior.

Correlations Between LTP and Learning/Memory in Aged Animals

A better approach to trying to link LTP with learning is to examine both electrophysiology and behavior in the same subjects. Aged rodents are known to be impaired in tests of spatial learning and memory, behaviors in which the hippocampal formation plays a critical role (Moser et al., 1995; Moser and Moser,

1998). Thus, the expectation would be that some aspect of hippocampal LTP should also be compromised in aged animals. Further, it is known that aging does not uniformly affect a given study population; even at advanced ages, when most animals show profound impairments, a small percentage do not. This variability offers a powerful tool for examining the relationship of LTP to learning and memory, because it removes aging per se as a complicating factor. A hypothesis linking LTP to learning and memory predicts that LTP should be weakened in aged animals that are cognitively impaired, but not in those with preserved behavioral function.

Very few studies have directly examined both LTP and cognitive behavior in aged animals, perhaps because of the conflicting data on whether LTP is impaired during aging in the first place. Barnes and McNaughton were the first to show a relationship, reporting a correlation between decay of LTP in the perforant path-dentate connection and retention in their circular platform task (Barnes, 1979; Barnes and McNaughton, 1985). These authors found that the LTP decay rate was more rapid in aged rats, that the decay rate was significantly related to memory performance in both young and aged rats, and that faster decay of LTP was associated with faster forgetting for individual animals. Deupree et al. (1991) reported a similar finding, that persistence of LTP in CA1 of aged rats was significantly correlated with retention in the spatial version of the Morris water maze. Bergado et al. (1997) found that LTP in the dentate gyrus was impaired in a group of aged rats that had spatial learning deficits, but not in aged rats whose performance in the water maze was not significantly different from young animals. Similarly, Davis et al. (1993) found a correlation between the overall amount of perforant pathway LTP in aged rats and spatial learning in the water maze. Diana et al. (1995) found that the amplitude of Ca^{2+}-induced LTP in CA1 was significantly reduced in a group of aged rats that were impaired in water maze learning, but not in aged animals who showed the same level of learning as young rats. Finally, Bach et al. (1999) found that the amplitude of late-stage LTP in CA1 was significantly correlated with learning performance in aged mice.

The results of these studies provide additional tantalizing evidence in favor of a role for LTP in learning. However, the values of correlation coefficients in studies where an analysis of individual animals was performed are generally low (≤ 0.5), suggesting that variability in LTP induction, maintenance, or decay is responsible for only a small part of the differences in behavioral performance. If LTP is critical for learning or memory, why aren't these correlations better? An obvious answer would be that the assessments of LTP or behavioral status, or both, are not very accurate; this variability, combined with what are usually small sample sizes, works against finding relationships between LTP and behavior. However, it is important to recognize that no single brain region is entirely responsible for learning a complex task, as is often implied for the relationship between the hippocampus and spatial learning. It may be that LTP occurs in several brain regions involved in a particular type of learning, so that LTP deficits in several brain regions act additively or synergistically to result in impaired behavior. In this case, assessing LTP at only one site becomes less likely to provide convincing evidence of a role of LTP in behavior. Finally, given the number of seemingly different varieties of LTP, it could be that discovery of the "right" kind of LTP (i.e., that predicts behavioral performance) has yet to be made.

Interventions That Modify LTP or Behavior in Aged Animals

Finding correlations between impairments in some aspect of LTP and learning or memory behavior in aged rodents is a necessary step toward linking the two phenomena. However, in terms of providing convincing evidence that LTP is linked to learning/memory, it would be much more impressive to show that reversing age-related deficits in one process occurs under conditions that also lead to improvement in the other. A considerable amount of experimental work has been directed toward reversing age-related cognitive impairments. While an evaluation of this work is far beyond the scope of this chapter, there have been some consistently positive results (Dubey et al., 1996; Bickford et al., 1997; Eid and Rose, 1999; Rose, 1999).

Unfortunately, there has been very little work examining the effects of aging interventions on both cognition and LTP. There have been some successes reported using pharmacologic treatments to reduce LTP deficits in the dentate gyrus of aged rats (McGahon et al., 1997; Murray and Lynch, 1998), although the effect of these same treatments on behavioral performance was not investigated. A study using mice showed that drugs that reverse an age-related reduction in late-stage LTP also reduce spatial learning deficits (Bach et al., 1999). Finally, it has recently been shown that chronic administration of nerve growth factor (NGF) to learning-impaired aged rats enhanced LTP in both the dentate gyrus (Bergado et al., 1997) and hippocampal area CA1 (Rose et al., 1996); in the latter study, NGF-treated animals were also shown to have improved spatial learning following treatment.

Where Do We Go from Here?

As has been argued eloquently by Jeffery (1997), it may be that LTP and hippocampus-dependent learning and memory are both such multifaceted phenomena that the task of successfully linking them together is essentially impossible. For example, one type or phase of LTP may be responsible for a particular part of the learning or remembering required by a particular task, and only during a particular time period during the performance of the task. However, before conceding defeat, there are still some experiments to be done. The progress of the past several years has demonstrated the existence of more types of LTP to investigate (e.g., Huang et al., 1996), and new work is continually refining knowledge of when and how LTP-like mechanisms might be participating in hippocampally mediated behaviors (e.g., Steele and Morris, 1999). Aged animals that show individually variable impairments in such behaviors continue to offer a good experimental system in which to evaluate possible correlations between LTP and learning or memory. Much more work of this kind is needed, with the initial goal of simply improving the evidence for a relationship between some kind of LTP and distinct facets of learning or memory. Still more useful information will come from applying knowledge gained from mechanistic (e.g., biochemical) studies of the various kinds of LTP to directly modulate the aspects of cognition they are hypothesized to regulate.

In the simplest terms, LTP should be compromised in aged, learning-impaired animals, and pharmacologic treatments that reverse the LTP deficits should also restore their learning ability. The challenge remains to determine which type of LTP and which type of learning, and to have at hand the means for appropriate and selective pharmacologic manipulations.

Conclusion

Studies in aged animals provide suggestive, but by no means conclusive, evidence supporting a role for LTP in learning or memory. Thus, aging studies make the same dismayingly tangential contribution to solving the LTP/learning dilemma that has emerged from work in young animals. We question, as have others, whether the LTP/learning issue can ever be unequivocally resolved, at least for the hippocampus. However, we also wonder whether it needs to be. It could be argued that the primary value of trying to understand the relationship of LTP to learning or memory has been that it has led to a better understanding of the behavioral processes themselves. In our view, aging studies will likely not provide information that decisively defines the relationship between synaptic plasticity and behavior. The value of such work lies in the possibility that studies of LTP processes in aging may guide the development of truly effective treatments for age-related cognitive dysfunction.

REFERENCES

Abel, T., Nguyen, P.V., Barad, M., Deuel, T.A. et al. (1997). Genetic demonstration of a role for PKA in the late phase of LTP and in hippocampus-based long-term memory. *Cell* 88: 615–626.

Alger, B.E., and Teyler, T.J. (1976). Long-term and short-term plasticity in the CA1, CA3, and dentate regions of the rat hippocampal slice. *Brain Res.* 110: 463–480.

Aniksztejn, L., Ben Ari, Y. (1991). Novel form of long-term potentiation produced by a K+ channel blocker in the hippocampus. *Nature* 349: 67–69.

Auerbach, J.M., and Segal, M. (1994). A novel cholinergic induction of long-term potentiation in rat hippocampus. *J. Neurophysiol.* 72: 2034–2040.

Auerbach, J.M., and Segal, M. (1997). Peroxide modulation of slow onset potentiation in rat hippocampus. *J. Neurosci.* 17: 8695–8701.

Bach, M.E., Barad, M., Son, H., Zhuo, M. et al. (1999). Age-related defects in spatial memory are correlated with defects in the late phase of hippocampal long-term potentiation in vitro and are attenuated by drugs that enhance the cAMP signaling pathway. *Proc. Natl. Acad. Sci. USA* 96: 5280–5285.

Barnes, C.A. (1979). Memory deficits associated with senescence: A neurophysiological and behavioral study in the rat. *J. Comp. Physiol. Psychol.* 93: 74–104.

Barnes, C.A., and McNaughton, B.L. (1985). An age comparison of the rates of acquisition and forgetting of spatial information in relation to long-term enhancement of hippocampal synapses. *Behav. Neurosci.* 99: 1040–1048.

Barnes, C.A., Jung, M.W., McNaughton, B.L., Korol, D.L. et al. (1994). LTP saturation and spatial learning disruption: Effects of task variables and saturation levels. *J. Neurosci.* 14: 5793–5806.

Barnes, C.A., Rao, G., and McNaughton, B.L. (1996). Functional integrity of NMDA-dependent LTP induction mechanisms across the lifespan of F-344 rats. *Learn. Mem.* 3: 124–137.

Baskys, A., Reynolds, J.N., and Carlen, P.L. (1990). NMDA depolarizations and long-term potentiation are reduced in the aged rat neocortex. *Brain Res.* 530: 142–146.

Bear, M.F., and Kirkwood, A. (1993). Neocortical long-term potentiation. *Curr. Opin. Neurobiol.* 3: 197–202.

Bergado, J.A., Fernandez, C.I., Gomez Soria, A., and Gonzalez, O. (1997). Chronic intraventricular infusion with NGF improves LTP in old cognitively-impaired rats. *Brain Res.* 770: 1–9.

Bickford, P.C., Adams, C.E., Boyson, S.J., Curella, P. et al. (1997). Long-term treatment of male F344 rats with deprenyl: Assessment of effects on longevity, behavior, and brain function. *Neurobiol. Aging* 18: 309–318.

Bland, B.H. (1986). The physiology and pharmacology of hippocampal formation theta rhythms. *Prog. Neurobiol.* 26: 1–54.

Bliss, T.V.P., and Gardner-Medwin, A.R. (1973). Long-lasting potentiation of synaptic transmission in the dentate area of the unanaesthetized rabbit following stimulation of the perforant path. *J. Physiol.* 232: 357–374.

Bliss, T.V.P., and Lomo, T. (1973). Long-lasting potentiation of synaptic transmission in the dentate area of the anaesthetized rabbit following stimulation of the perforant path. *J. Physiol.* 232: 331–356.

Bliss, T.V.P., Lancaster, B., and Wheal, H.V. (1983). Long-term potentiation in commissural and Schaffer projections to hippocampal CA1 cells: An *in vivo* study in the rat. *J. Physiol.* 341: 617–626.

Bramham, C.R., and Sarvey, J.M. (1996). Endogenous activation of mu and delta-1 opioid receptors is required for long-term potentiation induction in the lateral perforant path: dependence on GABAergic inhibition. *J. Neurosci.* 16: 8123–8131.

Burke, D.M., and Mackay, D.G. (1997). Memory, language, and ageing. *Philos. Trans. R. Soc. London B Biol. Sci.* 352: 1845–1856.

Buzsaki, G. (1989). Two-stage model of memory trace formation: A role for "noisy" brain states. *Neuroscience* 31: 551–570.

Buzsaki, G., Haas, H.L., and Anderson, E.G. (1987). Long-term potentiation induced by physiologically relevant stimulus patterns. *Brain Res.* 435: 331–333.

Cain, D.P., Hargreaves, E.L., Boon, F., and Dennison, Z. (1993). An examination of the relations between hippocampal long-term potentiation, kindling, afterdischarge, and place learning in the water maze [see comments]. *Hippocampus* 3: 153–163.

Calabresi, P., Saiardi, A., Pisani, A., Baik, J.H. et al. (1997). Abnormal synaptic plasticity in the striatum of mice lacking dopamine D2 receptors. *J. Neurosci.* 17: 4536–4544.

Castro Alamancos, M.A., Donoghue, J.P., and Connors, B.W. (1995). Different forms of synaptic plasticity in somatosensory and motor areas of the neocortex. *J. Neurosci.* 15: 5324–5333.

Castro, C.A., Silbert, L.H., McNaughton, B.L., and Barnes, C.A. (1989). Recovery of spatial learning deficits after decay of electrically induced synaptic enhancement in the hippocampus. *Nature* 342: 545–548.

Chang, P.L., Isaacs, K.R., and Greenough, W.T. (1991). Synapse formation occurs in association with the induction of long-term potentiation in two-year-old rat hippocampus in vitro. *Neurobiol. Aging* 12: 517–522.

Chapman, P.F., and Bellavance, L.L. (1992). Induction of long-term potentiation in the basolateral amygdala does not depend on NMDA receptor activation. *Synapse* 11: 310–318.

Charpier, S., and Deniau, J.M. (1997). *In vivo* activity-dependent plasticity at cortico-striatal connections: Evidence for physiological long-term potentiation. *Proc. Natl. Acad. Sci. USA* 94: 7036–7040.

Collingridge, G.L., Kehl, S.J., and McLennan, H. (1983). Excitatory amino acids in synaptic transmission in the Schaffer collateral-commissural pathway of the rat hippocampus. *J. Physiol.* 334: 33–46.

Commins, S., Gigg, J., Anderson, M., and O'Mara, S.M. (1998). The projection from hippocampal area CA1 to the subiculum sustains long-term potentiation. *Neuroreport* 9: 847–850.

Cousens, G., and Otto, T.A. (1998). Induction and transient suppression of long-term potentiation in the peri- and postrhinal cortices following theta-related stimulation of hippocampal field CA1. *Brain Res.* 780: 95–101.

D'Angelo, E., Rossi, P., Armano, S., and Taglietti, V. (1999). Evidence for NMDA and mGlu receptor-dependent long-term potentiation of mossy fiber-granule cell transmission in rat cerebellum. *J. Neurophysiol.* 81: 277–287.

Davies, C.H., Starkey, S.J., Pozza, M.F., and Collingridge, G.L. (1991). GABA$_B$ autoreceptors regulate the induction of LTP. *Nature* 349: 609–611.

Davis, S., Butcher, S.P., and Morris, R.G. (1992). The NMDA receptor antagonist D-2-amino-5-phosphonopentanoate (D-AP5) impairs spatial learning and LTP in vivo at intracerebral concentrations comparable to those that block LTP in vitro. *J. Neurosci.* 12: 21–34.

Davis, S., Markowska, A.L., Wenk, G.L., and Barnes, C.A. (1993). Acetyl-L-carnitine: Behavioral, electrophysiological, and neurochemical effects. *Neurobiol. Aging* 14: 107–115.

del Cerro, S., Jung, M., and Lynch, G. (1992). Benzodiazepines block long-term potentiation in slices of hippocampus and piriform cortex. *Neuroscience* 49: 1–6.

Derrick, B.E., Weinberger, S.B., and Martinez, J.L. Jr. (1991). Opioid receptors are involved in an NMDA receptor-independent mechanism of LTP induction at hippocampal mossy fiber-CA3 synapses. *Brain Res. Bull.* 27: 219–223.

deToledo-Morrell, L., Geinisman, Y., and Morrell, F. (1988). Age-dependent alterations in hippocampal synaptic plasticity: Relation to memory disorders. *Neurobiol. Aging* 9: 581–590.

Deupree, D.L., Turner, D.A., and Watters, C.L. (1991). Spatial performance correlates with *in vitro* potentiation in young and aged Fischer 344 rats. *Brain Res.* 554: 1–9.

Deupree, D.L., Bradley, J., and Turner, D.A. (1993). Age-related alterations in potentiation in the CA1 region in F344 rats. *Neurobiol. Aging* 14: 249–258.

Diamond, D.M., Dunwiddie, T.V., and Rose, G.M. (1988). Characteristics of hippocampal primed burst potentiation *in vitro* and in the awake rat. *J. Neurosci.* 8: 4079–4088.

Diana, G., Domenici, M.R., Loizzo, A., Scotti de Carolis, A. et al. (1994a). Age and strain differences in rat place learning and hippocampal dentate gyrus frequency-potentiation. *Neurosci. Lett.* 171: 113–116.

Diana, G., Scotti de Carolis, A., Frank, C., Domenici, M.R. et al. (1994b). Selective reduction of hippocampal dentate frequency potentiation in aged rats with impaired place learning. *Brain Res. Bull.* 35: 107–111.

Diana, G., Domenici, M.R., Scotti de Carolis, A., Loizzo, A. et al. (1995). Reduced hippocampal CA1 Ca(2+)-induced long-term potentiation is associated with age-dependent impairment of spatial learning. *Brain Res.* 686: 107–110.

Douglas, R.M. (1977). Long lasting synaptic potentiation in the rat dentate gyrus following brief high frequency stimulation. *Brain Res.* 126: 361–365.

Dubey, A., Forster, M.J., Lal, H., and Sohal, R.S. (1996). Effect of age and caloric intake on protein oxidation in different brain regions and on behavioral functions of the mouse. *Arch. Biochem. Biophys.* 333: 189–197.

Eid, C.N. Jr., and Rose, G.M. (1999). Cognition enhancement strategies by ion channel modulation of neurotransmission. *Curr. Pharm. Des.* 5: 345–361.

Escobar, M.L., Alcocer, I., and Chao, V. (1998). The NMDA receptor antagonist CPP impairs conditioned taste aversion and insular cortex long-term potentiation in vivo. *Brain Res.* 812: 246–251.

Frey, U., Huang, Y.-Y., and Kandel, E.R. (1993). Effects of cAMP simulate a late stage of LTP in hippocampal CA1 neurons. *Science* 260: 1661–1664.

Frey, U., Schollmeier, K., Reymann, K.G., and Seidenbecher, T. (1995). Asymptotic hippocampal long-term potentiation in rats does not preclude additional potentiation at later phases. *Neuroscience* 67: 799–807.

Garcia, R., and Jaffard, R. (1993). A comparative study of age-related changes in inhibitory processes and long-term potentiation in the lateral septum of mice. *Brain Res.* 620: 229–236.

Geinisman, Y., de Toledo Morrell, L., Morrell, F., Persina, I.S. et al. (1992). Structural synaptic plasticity associated with the induction of long-term potentiation is preserved in the dentate gyrus of aged rats. *Hippocampus* 2: 445–456.

Greenstein, Y.J., Pavlides, C., and Winson, J. (1988). Long-term potentiation in the dentate gyrus is preferentially induced at a theta rhythm periodicity. *Brain Res.* 438: 331–334.

Grover, L.M., and Teyler, T.J. (1990). Two components of long-term potentiation induced by different patterns of afferent activation. *Nature* 347: 477–479.

Hanse, E., and Gustafsson, B. (1994). TEA elicits two distinct potentiations of synaptic transmission in the CA1 region of the hippocampal slice. *J. Neurosci.* 14: 5028–5034.

Hargreaves, E.L., Cote, D., Shapiro, M.L. (1997). A dose of MK801 previously shown to impair spatial learning in the radial maze attenuates primed burst potentiation in the dentate gyrus of freely moving rats. *Behav. Neurosci.* 111: 35–48.

Harris, E.W., and Cotman, C.W. (1986). Long-term potentiation of guinea pig mossy fiber responses is not blocked by N-methyl D-aspartate antagonists. *Neurosci. Lett.* 70: 132–137.

Harris, E.W., Ganong, A.H., and Cotman, C.W. (1984). Long-term potentiation in the hippocampus involves activation of N-methyl-D-aspartate receptors. *Brain Res.* 323: 132–137.

Hoh, T., Beiko, J., Boon, F., Weiss, S. et al. (1999). Complex behavioral strategy and reversal learning in the water maze without NMDA receptor-dependent long-term potentiation. *J. Neurosci.* 19: RC2.

Hölscher, C., Anwyl, R., and Rowan, M.J. (1997). Stimulation on the positive phase of hippocampal theta rhythm induces long-term potentiation that can be depotentiated by stimulation on the negative phase in area CA1 in vivo. *J. Neurosci.* 17: 6470–6477.

Hori, N., Hirotsu, I., Davis, P.J., and Carpenter, D.O. (1992). Long-term potentiation is lost in aged rats but preserved by calorie restriction. *Neuroreport* 3: 1085–1088.

Huang, Y.Y., and Kandel, E.R. (1995). D1/D5 receptor agonists induce a protein synthesis-dependent late potentiation in the CA1 region of the hippocampus [see comments]. *Proc. Natl. Acad. Sci. USA* 92: 2446–2450.

Huang, Y.Y., and Kandel, E.R. (1998). Postsynaptic induction and PKA-dependent expression of LTP in the lateral amygdala. *Neuron* 21: 169–178.

Huang, Y.-Y., Nguyen, P.V., Abel, T., and Kandel, E.R. (1996). Long-lasting forms of synaptic potentiation in the mammalian hippocampus. *Learn. Mem.* 3: 74–85.

Huerta, P.T., and Lisman, J.E. (1995). Bidirectional synaptic plasticity induced by a single burst during cholinergic theta oscillation in CA1 in vitro. *Neuron* 15: 1053–1063.

Izquierdo, I. (1994). Pharmacological evidence for a role of long-term potentiation in memory. *FASEB J.* 8: 1139–1145.

Izquierdo, I., and Medina, J.H. (1995). Correlation between the pharmacology of long-term potentiation and the pharmacology of memory. *Neurobiol. Learn. Mem.* 63: 19–32.

Jeffery, K.J. (1997). LTP and spatial learning—where to next? *Hippocampus* 7: 95–110.

Jeffery, K.J., and Morris, R.G. (1993). Cumulative long-term potentiation in the rat dentate gyrus correlates with, but does not modify, performance in the water maze [see comments]. *Hippocampus* 3: 133–140.

Kirkwood, A., and Bear, M.F. (1994). Hebbian synapses in visual cortex. *J. Neurosci.* 14: 1634–1645.

Korol, D.L., Abel, T.W., Church, L.T., Barnes, C.A. et al. (1993). Hippocampal synaptic enhancement and spatial learning in the Morris swim task. *Hippocampus* 3: 127–132.

Landfield, P.W., McGaugh, J.L., and Lynch, G. (1978). Impaired synaptic potentiation processes in the hippocampus of aged, memory-deficient rats. *Brain Res.* 150: 85–101.

Laroche, S., Jay, T.M., and Thierry, A.M. (1990). Long-term potentiation in the prefrontal cortex following stimulation of the hippocampal CA1/subicular region. *Neurosci. Lett.* 114: 184–190.

Larson, J., and Lynch, G. (1988). Role of N-methyl-D-aspartate receptors in the induction of synaptic potentiation by burst stimulation patterned after the hippocampal θ-rhythm. *Brain Res.* 441: 111–118.

Larson, J., Wong, D., and Lynch, G. (1986). Patterned stimulation at the theta frequency is optimal for the induction of hippocampal long-term potentiation. *Brain Res.* 368: 347–350.

Lynch, M.A., and Voss, K.L. (1994). Membrane arachidonic acid concentration correlates with age and induction of long-term potentiation in the dentate gyrus in the rat. *Eur. J. Neurosci.* 6: 1008–1014.

Maren, S. (1996). Synaptic transmission and plasticity in the amygdala. An emerging physiology of fear conditioning circuits. *Mol. Neurobiol.* 13: 1–22.

Maren, S., and Baudry, M. (1995). Properties and mechanisms of long-term synaptic plasticity in the mammalian brain: Relationships to learning and memory. *Neurobiol. Learn. Mem.* 63: 1–18.

Matthies, H., and Reymann, K.G. (1993). Protein kinase A inhibitors prevent the maintenance of hippocampal long-term potentiation. *Neuroreport* 4: 712–714.

McGahon, B., Clements, M.P., and Lynch, M.A. (1997). The ability of aged rats to sustain long-term potentiation is restored when the age-related decrease in membrane arachidonic acid concentration is reversed. *Neuroscience* 81: 9–16.

McNaughton, B.L., Barnes, C.A., Rao, G., Baldwin, J. et al. (1986). Long-term enhancement of hippocampal synaptic transmission and the acquisition of spatial information. *J. Neurosci.* 6: 563–571.

Moore, C.I., Browning, M.D., and Rose, G.M. (1993). Hippocampal plasticity induced by primed burst, but not long-term potentiation, stimulation is impaired in area CA1 of aged Fischer 344 rats. *Hippocampus* 3: 57–66.

Morris, R.G.M., Anderson, E., Lynch, G.S., and Baudry, M. (1986). Selective impairment of learning and blockade of long-term potentiation by an N-methyl-D-aspartate receptor antagonist, AP5. *Nature* 319: 774–776.

Moser, M.B., and Moser, E.I. (1998). Distributed encoding and retrieval of spatial memory in the hippocampus. *J. Neurosci.* 18: 7535–7542.

Moser, E.I., and Moser, M.B. (1999). Is learning blocked by saturation of synaptic weights in the hippocampus? *Neurosci. Biobehav. Rev.* 23: 661–672.

Moser, M.-B., Moser, E.I., Forrest, E., Andersen, P. et al. (1995). Spatial learning with a mini-islab in the dorsal hippocampus. *Proc. Natl. Acad. Sci. USA* 92: 9697–9701.

Moser, E.I., Krobert, K.A., Moser, M.B., and Morris, R.G. (1998). Impaired spatial learning after saturation of long-term potentiation. *Science* 281: 2038–2042.

Murray, C.A., and Lynch, M.A. (1998). Dietary supplementation with vitamin E reverses the age-related deficit in long term potentiation in dentate gyrus. *J. Biol. Chem.* 273: 12161–12168.

Norris, C.M., Korol, D.L., and Foster, T.C. (1996). Increased susceptibility to induction of long-term depression and long-term potentiation reversal during aging. *J. Neurosci.* 16: 5382–5392.

Oddie, S.D., and Bland, B.H. (1998). Hippocampal formation theta activity and movement selection. *Neurosci. Biobehav. Rev.* 22: 221–231.

Pacelli, G.J., Su, W., and Kelso, S.R. (1989). Activity-induced depression of synaptic inhibition during LTP-inducing patterned stimulation. *Brain Res.* 486: 26–32.

Pavlides, C., Greenstein, Y.J., Grudman, M., and Winson, J. (1988). Long-term potentiation in the dentate is induced preferentially on the positive phase of θ-rhythm. *Brain Res.* 439: 383–387.

Rose, G.M. (1999). Behavioral effects of neurotrophic factor supplementation in aging. *Age* 22: 1–8.

Rose, G.M., and Dunwiddie, T.V. (1986). Induction of hippocampal long-term potentiation using physiologically patterned stimulation. *Neurosci. Lett.* 69: 244–248.

Rose, G.M., Heman, K.L., and Williams, L.R. (1996). Chronic nerve growth factor administration enhances hippocampal primed burst potentiation in aged, but not young male Fischer 344 rats. *Neurosci. Abstr.* 22: 752.

Rosenzweig, E.S., Rao, G., McNaughton, B.L., and Barnes, C.A. (1997). Role of temporal summation in age-related long-term potentiation-induction deficits. *Hippocampus* 7: 549–558.

Salin, P.A., Malenka, R.C., and Nicoll, R.A. (1996). Cyclic AMP mediates a presynaptic form of LTP at cerebellar parallel fiber synapses. *Neuron* 16: 797–803.

Saucier, D., and Cain, D.P. (1995). Spatial learning without NMDA receptor-dependent long-term potentiation. *Nature* 378: 186–189.

Shankar, S., Teyler, T.J., and Robbins, N. (1998). Aging differentially alters forms of long-term potentiation in rat hippocampal area CA1. *J. Neurophysiol.* 79: 334–341.

Shapiro, M.L., and Caramanos, Z. (1990). NMDA antagonist MK-801 impairs acquisition but not performance of spatial working and reference memory. *Psychobiology* 18: 231–243.

Shindou, T., Watanabe, S., Yamamoto, K., and Nakanishi, H. (1993). NMDA receptor-dependent formation of long-term potentiation in the rat medial amygdala neuron in an in vitro slice preparation. *Brain Res. Bull.* 31: 667–672.

Staubli, U., Thibault, O., DiLorenzo, M., and Lynch, G. (1989). Antagonism of NMDA receptors impairs acquisition but not retention of olfactory memory. *Behav. Neurosci.* 103: 54–60.

Steele, R.J., and Morris, R.G. (1999). Delay-dependent impairment of a matching-to-place task with chronic and intrahippocampal infusion of the NMDA-antagonist D-AP5 [see comments]. *Hippocampus* 9: 118–136.

Sutherland, R.J., Dringenberg, H.C., and Hoesing, J.M. (1993). Induction of long-term potentiation at perforant path dentate synapses does not affect place learning or memory [see comments]. *Hippocampus* 3: 141–147.

Teskey, G.C., and Valentine, P.A. (1998). Post-activation potentiation in the neocortex of awake freely moving rats. *Neurosci. Biobehav. Rev.* 22: 195–207.

Teyler, T.J. (1989). Comparative aspects of hippocampal and neocortical long-term potentiation. *J. Neurosci. Methods* 28: 101–108.

Teyler, T.J., and DiScenna, P. (1987). Long-term potentiation. *Ann. Rev. Neurosci.* 10: 131–161.

Thomas, M.J., Watabe, A.M., Moody, T.D., Makhinson, M. et al. (1998). Postsynaptic complex spike bursting enables the induction of LTP by theta frequency synaptic stimulation. *J. Neurosci.* 18: 7118–7126.

Tielen, A.M., Mollevanger, W.J., Lopes Da Silva, F.H., and Hollander, C.F. (1983). Neuronal plasticity in hippocampal slices of extremely old rats. In W.H. Gispen and J. Traber (Eds.), *Aging of the brain* (pp. 73–84). Amsterdam: Elsevier Science Publishers B.V.

Trepel, C., and Racine, R.J. (1998). Long-term potentiation in the neocortex of the adult, freely moving rat. *Cereb. Cortex.* 8: 719–729.

Turner, R.W., Baimbridge, K.G., and Miller, J.J. (1982). Calcium-induced long-term potentiation in the hippocampus. *Neuroscience* 7: 1411–1416.

Vertes, R.P., and Kocsis, B. (1997). Brainstem-diencephalo-septohippocampal systems controlling the theta rhythm of the hippocampus. *Neuroscience* 81: 893–926.

Vinogradova, O.S. (1995). Expression, control, and probable functional significance of the neuronal theta-rhythm. *Prog. Neurobiol.* 45: 523–583.

Voronin, L., Byzov, A., Kleschevnikov, A., Kozhemyakin, M. et al. (1995). Neurophysiological analysis of long-term potentiation in mammalian brain. *Behav. Brain Res.* 66: 45–52.

Williams, S.H., and Johnston, D. (1996). Actions of endogenous opioids on NMDA receptor-independent long-term potentiation in area CA3 of the hippocampus. *J. Neurosci.* 16: 3652–3660.

Winder, D.G., Mansuy, I.M., Osman, M., Moallem, T.M. et al. (1998). Genetic and pharmacological evidence for a novel, intermediate phase of long-term potentiation suppressed by calcineurin. *Cell* 92: 25–37.

Wu, R.L., McKenna, D.G., and McAfee, D.A. (1991). Age-related changes in the synaptic plasticity of rat superior cervical ganglia. *Brain Res.* 542: 324–329.

Zalutsky, R.A., and Nicoll, R.A. (1990). Comparison of two forms of long-term potentiation in single hippocampal neurons. *Science* 248: 1619–1624.

Zyzak, D.R., Otto, T., Eichenbaum, H., and Gallagher, M. (1995). Cognitive decline associated with normal aging in rats: A neuropsychological approach. *Learn. Mem.* 2: 1–16.

CHAPTER FIFTEEN

Implications of the Neuropsychology of Anxiety for the Functional Role of LTP in the Hippocampus

Neil McNaughton

SUMMARY

Amnesics and hippocampally lesioned animals fail to suppress incorrect information rather than failing to store correct information. There is also strong evidence that anxiolytic drugs act on a behavioral inhibition system involving the hippocampus. This has led to a theory of the neuropsychology of anxiety (Gray and McNaughton, 2000) that has as a corollary, the view that all memories are stored outside the hippocampus. It follows that long-term potentiation (LTP) in the hippocampus cannot be the basis of memory. There is good evidence, however, that LTP is involved in hippocampal function in some way. Our theory would be consistent with hippocampal LTP storing hippocampal-specific data or reprogramming the hippocampal computer. In both cases LTP would be a means of altering the input–output relationships of the hippocampus (and hence indirectly performance on hippocampal-sensitive tasks). If this is true, the hippocampus may often function without the requirement for LTP.

Introduction

In the Introduction to this book, Hölscher notes that the bulk of studies, which see long-term potentiation (LTP) as the substrate for learning and memory, focus on the hippocampus. They manipulate LTP in the hippocampal formation and assess storage of spatial memories. In this chapter I argue that the hippocampus (unlike the cortex or amygdala) does not use LTP to store any type of memory and is not especially concerned with space. Further, I suggest that the hippocampus prevents rather than promotes the formation of connections within the brain. This view derives from a recent update of Gray's (1982) theory of the neuropsychology of anxiety (Gray and McNaughton, 2000). According to this theory, the role of the

Christian Hölscher, editor, *Neuronal Mechanisms of Memory Formation*. © 2001 Cambridge University Press. Printed in the United States of America. All rights reserved.

hippocampus in memory tasks is a special case of a more general nonmemorial resolution of conflicts between incompatible goals. I summarize the key features of the theory for memory tasks and I tentatively suggest that, within the hippocampus, LTP is best seen as more akin to altering the instructions of a computer program than altering the data on which that program operates.

Is Hippocampal LTP a Substrate for Memory?

Lesions of the hippocampal formation appear to produce amnesia and do so even when the damage appears to be restricted to the hippocampus proper (Zola-Morgan et al., 1986). The hippocampal formation is also where LTP was first discovered (Bliss and Lømo, 1973), where it is most often studied, and where it is most easily observed. LTP can occur in pathways that terminate within the hippocampus while not occurring in collaterals of the same neurons that leave the hippocampus (McNaughton and Miller, 1986). LTP can produce structural changes in the hippocampus (see Beardsley, 1999) and there is evidence (see Introduction) that saturation of hippocampal LTP or blocking of hippocampal LTP impairs learning. When we add to these data the fact that LTP has the precise properties of associativity and specificity (see Introduction) required by Hebb's (1949) oft-cited theory of long-term memory formation, it may seem that hippocampal LTP must be the substrate of long-term memory.

While apparently straightforward, this argument does not fit with other facts. LTP occurs outside the hippocampus (see Introduction). Indeed, Hebb originally proposed that long-term memory resulted from synaptic strengthening in areas such as the visual cortex. The best evidence that LTP is the substrate of a specific case of associative learning has been obtained with thalamic input to the amygdala (Le Doux, 1994) not the hippocampus. Extensive LTP of hippocampal synapses (or pharmacologic blockade of hippocampal NMDA receptors) should disrupt hippocampal function whatever its normal function and so is not evidence of a specifically memorial role. It has also been suggested by Graham Goddard (personal communication) that LTP is most easily observed in the hippocampus because it does not occur there naturally; thus hippocampal synapses are less LTP saturated, and so more apparently plastic, than those of areas that do show LTP naturally.

These counterarguments do not disprove the idea that hippocampal LTP is the substrate for memory. But they are of a similar form to the positive arguments and so shift the burden of proof back on those who wish to locate memory in the hippocampus. They suggest that experiments involving saturation of LTP, pharmacologic intervention, or gene knock-outs provide relatively flimsy evidence for a specific memory-storage function.

If one looks beyond the properties of LTP itself, there is a much stronger argument against hippocampal LTP as a substrate for memory. There is evidence that memories are *never* stored in the hippocampus. Rather, it can be argued that they are stored elsewhere in the brain and that the hippocampus is involved in *the prevention of inappropriate storage or recall*. On this view, so-called amnesic patients with hippocampal damage would have instead a catastrophic hyperamnesia

(McNaughton, 1997). This chapter briefly reviews the evidence for this non-memorial view of amnesia. It summarizes a small part of a detailed nonmemorial theory of hippocampal function (see Gray and McNaughton, 2000, for a full version of the arguments and Gray, 1982 for an earlier version of the theory), and it discusses the possible nonmemorial functions of hippocampal LTP.

Do Amnesics Remember Too Little or Too Much?

Memory theories of hippocampal function exclude much data that suggest a role for the hippocampal formation in the inhibition of behavior rather than the production of memory (Gray, 1982; Gray and McNaughton, 1983, 2000). These data show that the theories are incomplete. However, for many theorists this incompleteness is not seen as a serious problem. The "large body of literature on the effects of hippocampal system damage on behaviours that are only indirectly related to learning and memory" is excluded on the grounds that they are "either a consequence of amnesia or an indirect result of disconnections of the limbic system that have non-mnemonic as well as mnemonic effects" (Eichenbaum et al., 1994). While the greater parsimony of our theory should make it preferable, the memory theories of hippocampal function are deeply entrenched in the literature. I will, therefore, consider here only data from specific tests of memory so that the argument remains on the home ground of the memory theories.

It is now clear that hippocampal damage does not eliminate well-established memories. Nor does hippocampal damage impair even the formation of memory in some tasks (see, e.g., Eichenbaum et al., 1994). This has led to postulation of a bewildering variety of types of hippocampal-sensitive versus hippocampal-insensitive memory (Table 15.1). Many of these mutually incompatible views are still current (principally because none *can* explain all the data). This gives us good reason not to explore their minutiae. Rather let us look at two particular results that contrast intact versus impaired function and that suggest that hippocampal damage affects something other than formation of any specific type of memory.

Our first case is the paradigm example of hippocampal involvement in behavioral inhibition in animals – extinction of responding. Hippocampal-lesioned animals (such as rats) can learn and retain over long periods many simple tasks (such as pressing a lever). The intactness of such memories is the basis for the postulation of the hippocampal-insensitive "types" of memory shown in Table 15.1. However, when reinforcement is discontinued, placing the animal in experimental extinction, hippocampal animals are greatly impaired in unlearning the response. Such unlearning (involving, in theory, only weakening of a connection) should be simpler than the original learning. For the bulk of theories it also involves the same "type" of information as the original learning. It is difficult to see, therefore, how the observed hippocampal deficit can be attributed to a failure to form memories.[1] At the purely

---

[1] O'Keefe and Nadel (1978), unlike some more recent theories, solve the problem by postulating *ad hoc* that hippocampal animals use "taxon hypotheses" for the original learning of the task while controls use "locale hypotheses." The taxon hypotheses are as easy to learn as locale hypotheses but are more resistant to extinction. However, it is difficult to see how this hypothesis accounts for, for example, the resistance to extinction of a specific choice in a brightness discrimination.

Table 15.1. Types of Memory That Have Been Postulated to Be Differentially Sensitive to Hippocampal Damage

Hippocampal Sensitive	Hippocampal Insensitive
fact	skill
conscious recollection	skills
conscious	automatic
memory	habit
knowing that	knowing how
representational	dispositional
declarative	procedural
declarative	nondeclarative
explicit	implicit
locale	taxon
cognitive mediation	semantic
episodic	semantic
elaboration	integration
memory with record	memory without record
autobiographical	perceptual
conceptual	perceptual
working	reference
instance	rule
data based	expectancy based
contextual	associative
relational	associative
configural	associative
intermediate	long term

Sources: Hirsh, 1974; Olton, 1978; Squire and Zola-Morgan, 1984; Tulving, 1984; Rawlins, 1985; Kesner and Beers, 1988; Rudy and Sutherland 1989; Miller, 1991; Squire, 1992; Cohen and Eichenbaum, 1993; Baddeley and Wilson, 1994; Shanks and St. John, 1994; Gabrieli, 1995; Robbins, 1996.

observational level the extinction results (and related results with discrimination reversal; Gray and McNaughton, 1983) show, instead, a failure to forget a prepotent memory.

Our second case is of failure of recall in human amnesics. Figure 15.1 shows results obtained by Warrington and Weiskrantz (1978) in a form of verbal "reversal learning." The subjects had first to learn a list of words. Recall of these words was cued with the first three letters of each word. As can be seen, simple acquisition of this list (A in Figure 15.1) was not impaired in amnesics. Thus, despite the use of stimuli that should (for most of the theories in Table 15.1) be hippocampal sensitive there is intact learning and memory. The list of words had the special property that the first three letters were shared by only one other word in English. The subjects were then required to learn a list consisting of these alternate words and then tested with the same set of three-letter recall cues as were used for the first list. Since there are only two possible response alternatives, this is the formal equivalent of reversal learning that, in animals, is impaired by hippocampal

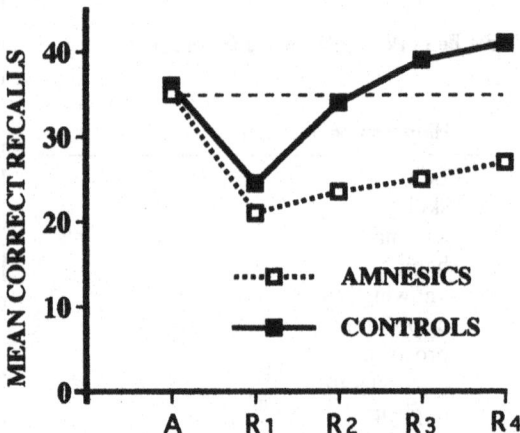

Figure 15.1. Recall of word from a list by amnesics and controls. Recall was cued by the presentation of the first three letters of the word and words (and cues) were chosen so that there were only two possible alternative answers. Controls and amnesics showed similar memory for an initial list of words (A). Controls and amnesics were equally impaired in the initial learning (R₁) of a second list of words consisting of the second of the two possible alternatives and cued by the same three-letter cues as for the list tested in A. Over successive trials on the second "reversal" list (R₂, R₃, R₄), controls, but not amnesics, overcame the effects of interference (intrusion errors from the first list). (Redrawn from Warrington and Weiskrantz, 1978, with permission.)

lesions (Gray and McNaughton, 2000). There was a substantial drop in correct responses on the first reversal trial. This demonstrates an effect of interference (intrusion) from items in the first list on recall of the items in the second list. The fact that this drop was similar in the amnesics and controls shows that amnesics are not more sensitive to interference per se than controls. The important result, for a nonmemorial view of hippocampal function, is that with further training on the second list controls produced recall that was back to the level of the first list by the second reversal trial. Their recall was superior on subsequent trials. In contrast, the amnesics show very little *recovery* from the effects of interference. These data suggest that, in memory experiments, the function of the hippocampus is not to store or recall information (as there is no deficit on trial A or trial R₁). Rather, the function of the hippocampus is to suppress recall of previously stored (or otherwise salient) information that is currently inappropriate (i.e., it is there to resolve conflict between incompatible alternatives).

The Hippocampus and Anxiety

It is easy to propose in one sentence a "new theory of hippocampal function." The literature exemplified by Table 15.1 is full of such theories. However, especially given the sterling example of O'Keefe and Nadel (1978), it is surprising that so few modern theories attempt a detailed, comprehensive account of hippocampal mechanisms consistent with what is known of the anatomy and physiology. We have attempted to provide such an account (Gray and McNaughton, 2000). There is only room here to comment on a few key memory-related features of the theory. Where these seem idiosyncratic, it should be remembered that the database that they explain is much wider than that of memory phenomena – and that their details have been simplified here.

The core of our theory is the proposal that the hippocampus detects conflict between concurrent goals and returns, to goal-processing areas, a signal that increases the valence of the affectively negative associations of each goal while leaving unchanged the affectively positive associations. "Detection of conflict," here, is a computationally simple process (see Figure 15.3). The hippocampus receives input from areas involved in the preprocessing of goal-directed action. Where two or more such inputs are large, and no one of them is clearly greatest, there is concurrent processing of two or more mutually incompatible goals – conflict. The circuitry of the hippocampus continuously compares these inputs to detect this condition. It produces output (detecting conflict) only when at least two inputs are similarly highly active. This sends feedback to the original sources of the input, and this feedback magnifies the effect of affectively negative associations. Thus, in the reversal experiment described in the previous section, we postulate that the hippocampal formation is required for the correct processing of the affectively negative frustration resulting from failure at trial R1 that allows suppression of the incorrect of the two response alternatives over trials R2 to R4.

This focus on affectively negative information (and particularly the effects of fear and frustration) derives from data fundamental to our theory and largely ignored by other theories of hippocampal function. As can be seen from Table 15.2, the behavioral effects of anxiolytic drugs are similar to those of hippocampal lesions. Further, both classical and novel anxiolytic drugs produce common dysfunctions in the control of hippocampal theta activity (McNaughton and Coop, 1991) that are not shared by any nonanxiolytic drugs.[2] They produce this common action through pharmacologically distinct routes. They have no direct pharmacologic actions in common, and they have opposed or nonoverlapping, rather than similar, clinical side effects. They thus share clinical anxiolytic action and a capacity to degrade hippocampal information processing and share very little else. We have also recently demonstrated that changes in the frequency of theta activity produced by specific intrahypothalamic injection of the drugs can have similar behavioral effects to systemic injection (e.g., Pan and McNaughton, 1997; Woodnorth and McNaughton, 1999). We have concluded from this that the septo-hippocampal system mediates significant components of anxiolytic drug action and, hence, that hippocampal function is related to cognitive processing (McNaughton, 1997) fundamental to anxiety.[3]

---

[2] See Section Two of this volume for chapters that discuss the importance of theta activity for hippocampal processing.

[3] There are multiple sites through which the drugs affect hippocampal theta activity and hence *cognitive* aspects of anxiety (see McNaughton and Mason, 1980; McNaughton, 1997). Further, the reduction in *arousal* produced by the drugs is held by us to be mediated by a direct action on the amygdala and not to be mediated in any way by the hippocampus.

Table 15.2 Comparison of the Common Behavioral Effects (ANX) of Novel (NOV) and Classical (CLAS) Anxiolytics with the Common Effects (S/H) of Septal (SEP) and Hippocampal (HIP) Lesions and Lesions of the Amygdala (AMYG) Dorsal Ascending Noradrenergic Bundle (NA), Ascending Serotonergic System (5HT), and Blockade of the Cholinergic System (ACh)

	NOV	CLAS	ANX	S/H	SEP	HIP	AMYG	NA	5HT	ACh
Eating	+	+	+	0	0/+	0	0		+	
Drinking	0	+	0	0	+	0	0		0	0
Responses to aversive stimuli	-	0	0	+/0	+	+/0	-		-	
Aggression		+	+	+/0		-	-		0	-
Escape	0	0	0	0	0	0	0	0	0	-
Reward learning	0	0	0	0	0	0	-	0	0	
Frustration		0	0	0	0	0	-	0		
One-way avoidance	0/-	0	0	0	-	0	-	0		0
Classical aversive conditioning		0	0	0	0/-	0	-			
Conditioned suppression	-	-	-	-	(-)	0	-	-	-	
Conditioned freezing						0	0			
Defensive burying	-		-	0/-	-	0	0	0/-	+	-
Fear potentiated startle	-	-/0	-	0	-	0	-	0/+	-	+
Passive avoidance	+		+	+	+	+	-			+
Two-way avoidance	+		+	+	+	+	-			-
Nonspatial avoidances	-		-	-	-	-	-	0/-	-/0	-
Extinction	-	(-)	0/-	(-)	-	-/0	-	-	0	-
Reversal	-		-		-	+/0/-	-		0	-
Successive discrimination	-	0	0	?	+?	0	-	0		-
Single alternation		0	0	0	0	-	-			
Simultaneous spatial discrimination		0/-	0/-	-	-	-	-			
Spontaneous Alternation	-	0	0	0	-	0	0	0	-/0	
Radial arm maze	+				-	-	0	0	0	-
Water maze				-?	-?	-/+	+	0	-	+
Defecation	-/0	-	-			(-)	0		-	
Rearing	-/0	-	-	(-)	(-)		-/(0)	-	+	0
Social interaction		(-)	(-)	(-)	(-)	(-)	-		0	-
Elevated + maze	-/0	-	-	-	-		0	0		-
Partial reinforcement extinction effect	-/0	-	-	-	-	(-)	0	0	-	0

Source: From Gray and McNaughton (2000), with permission.

The effects of anxiolytic drugs on approach-avoidance conflict are to decrease avoidance while leaving approach intact – and this is true whether the approach and avoidance are learned or innate. It is also fundamental to our analysis that the drugs do not affect fear as such (Blanchard and Blanchard, 1990) but affect only that aspect of avoidance (passive rather than active avoidance) that operates when an animal is approaching threat (i.e., when there is conflict between incompatible goals). Goal conflict (in the form of approach-approach conflict) is often present in delayed matching and similar tasks. Here, the effects of anxiolytic drugs (Tan et al., 1996) are qualitatively if not quantitatively like those of amnesia (Money et al., 1992; see Figure 15.2). In all of these cases we believe that the drugs (and, where this involves hippocampal dysfunction, the pathology of amnesia) impair the capacity of the hippocampal formation to inhibit current (and future) approach to prepotent incorrect goals. The drugs, and hippocampal dysfunction, do not prevent the formation of, or increase the rate of decay of, associative memory traces (see below).

On this theory, hippocampal amnesics will show a deficit only if (1) there is a prepotent goal (learned or innate), the attractiveness of which is similar to or greater than the correct goal; and (2) the intact hippocampus of the control subjects can resolve the conflict. This latter point is important. In the semantic reversal experiment (Figure 15.1), the controls overcame the initial tendency to choose the wrong alternative. If the parameters of the experiment were such that they could not overcome this tendency then we would not predict an amnesic deficit. Conversely, on trial R1 the controls had had no experience of failure and so had

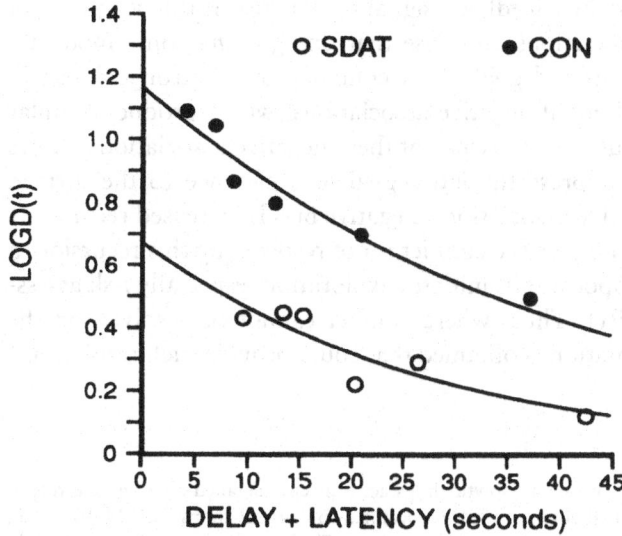

Figure 15.2. An initial deficit in recall with no increase in forgetting in amnesic patients (senile dementia of the Alzheimer type, SDAT) compared to age-matched controls (CON). Recall was assessed using a response-bias-free measure and decay assessed using a simple exponential decay model that across many tasks and species accounts for most of the variance in forgetting (LogD, White, 1985). (From Money et al., 1992, with permission.)

not learned to suppress the previously correct, now incorrect alternative, and so there was no amnesic deficit.

The Role of the Hippocampus in Memory Processing

Since we are rejecting the conventional memory-forming view of the hippocampus, it behooves us to explain the involvement of the hippocampus in memory tasks. The main mechanism we propose for conflict detection and resolution is shown in Figure 15.3. Goal processing areas of the brain receive information about stimuli in the environment (Sa ... Sz), which activate representations that combine these stimuli with available responses into goal representations. Thus the goal G1 represents the possibility of directing a specific response (R1) to Sa – for example, it might represent the possibility of running to eat food at the end of a runway. A change in stimulus (e.g., moving food to a new location) or a change in response type (e.g., replacing food at the end of the runway with water) will change the nature of the goal. Each goal can have positive and negative associations (+ and – in the figure) depending on the outcomes on previous occasions when the response was directed at the stimulus. The tendency to make the response depends on the net sum of these positive and negative associations. The net level of activation of each goal is passed to response programming mechanisms and is copied to the hippocampal formation.

Where only one such goal is activated, or when one goal is much more strongly activated than any other, it will be selected and approached. However, where there is conflict (i.e., more than one goal is highly activated), it is the business of the hippocampal formation to detect this (via comparison of its copies of the goal representations). Detection results in a feedback signal that increases the weighting of any affectively negative associations. Suppose that one goal has only moderate positive associations and a second goal has a combination of stronger positive associations coupled to additional negative associations, which produces similar net input to the hippocampus. The presence of these negative associations allows hippocampal feedback to suppress the latter goal in preference to the former. Where both goals have negative associations, negative bias is increased recursively until a winner emerges.[4] As long as the conflict is not resolved by this recursion, a separate output from the hippocampus initiates exploration (especially risk assessment; Blanchard et al., 1991). Thus, where conflict cannot be resolved on the basis of memory, new information is obtained that could provide such resolution.[5]

[4] In our theory, the theta activity on which anxiolytic drugs act is given a detailed coordinating role in recursive processing in hippocampal-cortical and hippocampal-subcortical loops (see Miller et al., 1995), but the details are not important for the current argument. The recursive processing is similar, in principle, to that proposed for figure-ground separation in models of global stereopsis (Frisby and Mayhew, 1979).

[5] The theory also postulates important roles for serotonergic and noradrenergic inputs to the hippocampus (and actions of anxiolytic drugs on these inputs), which are particularly relevant to processing of novelty and for attentional aspects of hippocampal function – but these can be ignored here.

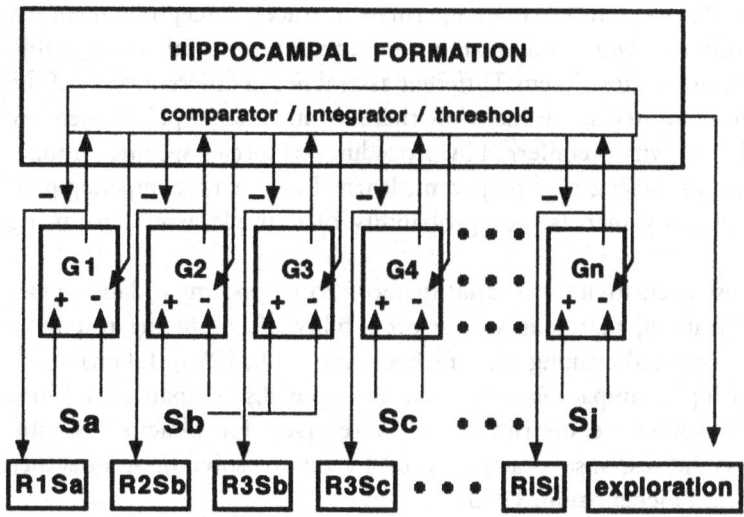

Figure 15.3. A schematic model of the principal information processing carried out by the hippocampal formation according to Gray and McNaughton (2000). Goals (e.g., G1) represent specific combinations of stimulus (e.g., Sa) and response (e.g., R1). They can differ in the stimuli eliciting a response (R3Sb: R3Sc), in the response elicited by a stimulus (R2Sb: R3Sb), or both. Both affectively positive (+) and affectively negative (−) consequences of achieving the goal are fed into the representation and their net sum calculated. This determines both the speed and intensity with which the appropriate action will be performed (if it is allowed to occur). The net sum is also copied to the hippocampus. This produces output only when more than one such input is highly active. The output increases the valence of negative affective input to goal representations and so tends to suppress those with relatively greater negative associations. Such a system could function if the hippocampus had no information about the sources of input and sent a similar feedback signal to all goal-processing areas. However, both the anatomy of the hippocampus and the occurrence of phenomena such as displacement activity have persuaded us to propose tentatively in the current version of our theory that the hippocampus only sends feedback to the most active and conflicting goal representations. This form of circuit is held to be replicated at different levels of the hippocampus with the entorhinal cortex being most important for goal conflicts where the principal difference between the goals is in the cortical representation of the stimuli involved.

"Increase in negative bias" sounds cognitively complex but is achieved by a simple increase in the postsynaptic efficacy of neurons coding aversive events. This increase will not only affect events on the current trial but has the capacity, through LTP or similar processes, to alter the strength of the association retrieved on a subsequent trial.

Memory Processing Outside the Hippocampus

In our view, both the original associations of a goal and alterations in their strength, always occur in cell assemblies *outside* the hippocampal formation. This nonstorage view of the hippocampus results in an essentially unitary view of long-term memory. In a nutshell, we follow Hebb in seeing all memory as being associative (with the exception of working/active memory, which is represented by patterns of electrical activity rather than a permanent trace). Perception, memory, and imaging are different ways of activating the same fundamental cell assembly for any particular informational item. Different assemblies in different parts of the brain represent different items. On this view there is only one "type" of memory and hippocampal sensitivity is conferred by procedure- or species-specific arrangements that increase the strength of prepotent, learned or innate, competing goal representations (i.e., they increase the probability of multiple assemblies being activated).

Thus the supposed sensitivity of spatial memory to hippocampal damage can be eliminated by training that reduces the probability of competing responses being emitted during initial training (e.g., Eichenbaum et al., 1990). Likewise, the normal pattern of hippocampal-insensitive simultaneous discrimination and hippocampal-sensitive successive discrimination is reversed for olfactory stimuli because of the specific response strategies used by rats to solve these olfactory problems (Cohen and Eichenbaum, 1993).

This is not to say that stimulus properties are not important for determining hippocampal sensitivity. In the model of Figure 15.3, goals can be distinguished as much by the stimulus to which a response is directed as by the response itself. Thus, we would argue that the apparent sensitivity of "relational memory" (Cohen and Eichenbaum, 1993) to hippocampal damage results from the problems facing a simple associative network in encoding such stimuli. While the true relation (say A-B-C) is being learned, many competing alternatives with overlapping representations (say C-A-B) are also likely to be strengthened. The hippocampus will be required to suppress these. Similarly, a cue, such as the first letter of a word, will usually activate many competing semantic memories. This will require the hippocampus to suppress all but the correct alternative from the pandemonium. Where (as with the combination of three letter cues with carefully selected words that was used in the experiment of Figure 15.1) the alternatives are limited or easy to separate, the hippocampus is not required.

Does Hippocampal LTP Have a Function?

The model of Figure 15.3 appears to have no use for LTP. It can explain the bulk of the data on the effects of hippocampal lesions in both memorial and non-memorial tests without an apparent need for plasticity of its circuitry. In rejecting a memory-forming role for the hippocampus we must account, therefore, for the widely held belief that LTP is important for hippocampal function.

The first question to ask is whether a role needs to be assigned to LTP at all. If, as suggested by Graham Goddard, LTP does not normally occur in the hippocampus, we can ignore the phenomenon.

There are two reasons for believing that hippocampal LTP has functional consequences under normal conditions. First, there has been some success in demonstrating a functional role for hippocampal LTP in behavior, even when memory as such may not have been implicated (see reviews by Morris and Baker, 1994; Morris et al., 1990; Barnes, 1995; Shors and Matzel, 1997, and the commentaries on the last). Positive results have been much rarer than would be expected if hippocampal LTP were the basis of all memory storage (or even of storage of "hippocampal" types of memory, Table 15.1). Nonetheless, there are enough unequivocal cases to indicate some function for LTP. Second, and more persuasively, the induction rules for LTP imply that it should occur, fairly frequently, under natural conditions in at least some hippocampal terminals. It would be very surprising if this occurrence did not alter function.

The second, and more difficult, question to ask is what the function of LTP might be. Experimental LTP of, for example, the perforant path input to the hippocampus will not only affect the hippocampus, but could also affect (via antidromic invasion of entorhinal cortex) those structures that receive entorhinal collaterals. The LTP-inducing input to the hippocampus will also affect multiple fields synchronously and concurrently in a fashion that will not occur normally. This nonphysiologic patterning is particularly significant for theories that see the hippocampus as containing parallel distributed memory processing systems (e.g., B. McNaughton and Morris, 1987). It is the differentiation in the timing of arrival of inputs that provides such systems with their processing and storage capacity.

Experiments that report that artificial LTP changes behavior must be treated, therefore, with some caution. However, where such changes are observed, the pattern can be illuminating, thus,

> McNaughton et al. (1986) found that bilateral saturation of LTP produced impairments on the Barnes circular platform task, in which animals were given one trial per day on a brightly illuminated white platform ... from which they could escape by finding a dark tunnel located beneath one of 18 peripherally located holes. ... [They] exhibited a pronounced, lasting deficit in the reversal of a previously learned spatial habit, a disruption of initial acquisition of spatial variables when the task was previously learned in a different environment, and disruption of recently stored spatial information. *Saturation produced no effect on performance of a previously learned spatial "working memory" task,* despite the presumed requirement in this task of at least temporary storage of information about which locations had been recently visited. (Korol et al., 1993; my emphasis)

This suggests, as did the semantic reversal experiment considered above, that the hippocampus does not use LTP to store information, but that LTP could have some functional significance when previously learned information needs to be altered.

Further studies (Castro et al., 1989; see *Hippocampus* special issue, 1993, pp. 123–164; Rioux and Robinson, 1995) have attempted to demonstrate effects of LTP saturation on initial acquisition in apparatus such as the water maze. They have obtained very mixed results. Positive effects may require both that saturation is obtained throughout the hippocampus and that specific task parameters have appropriate values (Barnes et al., 1994; see also Barnes, 1995). Given the phenomenon of metaplasticity, that is, the capacity for LTP itself to change (Abraham and Bear, 1996), there is an issue as to how to prove that "saturation" has been achieved. Critically, where impairments have been shown they tend not to involve erasure of preexisting memories.

The current findings, both positive and negative, are inconsistent with storage of detailed memory information by hippocampal LTP. However, there are at least two functions that hippocampal LTP could perform that are consistent with both the occurrence of positive results and their relative infrequency. First is a data-storage–like role (but one specific to hippocampal operation and distinct from what is conventionally termed memory). Second is a program-storage–like role.

■ **Is There a Role for LTP in Hippocampal Data Storage?** In our full theory (Gray and McNaughton, 2000), Figure 15.3 represents a general procedure, the machinery for which is repeated in different parts of the hippocampal formation. In particular, we propose that goal conflicts that are differentiated more by their stimuli than their responses (e.g., pecking a red key as opposed to pecking a green key) will in many cases be processed by interaction of the entorhinal cortex with cortical (and subcortical) areas. In contrast, goal conflicts that are differentiated more by their responses (approach the goal box and eat food, versus move away from the goal box and avoid shock) will in many cases be processed by interaction of the subiculum with subcortical (and cortical) areas. In addition to this, as we have noted, when conflict cannot be resolved by reprocessing aversive information in memory we suppose that the hippocampus commands the assessment of environmental information that can update the aversive status of goals. We also suppose that area CA3 deals with the specific case of novelty where this involves an orienting reflex and where resolution of the conflicting appetitive and aversive aspects of novelty involves habituation of the orienting reflex.

The minutiae of the theory are, therefore, quite complex even though the fundamental idea represented in Figure 15.3 is simple. There are also large gaps in the literature, bridged in our theory by inferences close to speculation. We did not, therefore, explore the possible role of LTP in hippocampal function, as this would have been pure speculation. In the remainder of this chapter, I will discuss general ways hippocampal LTP could have a role in nonmemorial hippocampal processing. However, I will not propose a specific role for it in our theory.

Analysis of single cell firing patterns by Vinogradova (1975; Vinogradova and Brazhnik, 1978) indicates that activity in perforant path input to the hippocampal formation sends a signal equivalent to the command "familiar ignore." This signal cancels the CA3 and CA1 responses that would otherwise be produced by septal input. Vinogradova (personal communication) has shown that if LTP is artificially induced by perforant path stimulation, the hippocampus proper becomes totally unresponsive to natural stimuli that previously elicited a response (see also Miller et al., 1995). Putting these facts together suggests that, in the hippocampus, LTP of extrinsic input need not increase the probability of functional output from principal cells, but rather can decrease it. This is a form of data storage, but not one that maps to conventional memory storage. An interesting consequence, if this pattern of results is typical and if our theory is correct, is that behavioral effects of saturation of perforant path input would be expected most in habituation paradigms (rather than the learning paradigms normally tested). Its predicted effect would be an enhanced habituation of novelty-elicited exploration. Effects in learning paradigms could thus be due to a loss of salience of stimuli.

A relatively nonspecific "attentional" role rather than a specific "memorial" role for hippocampal LTP has also been suggested by Shors and Matzel (1997; see also Chapter 12 in this volume).

■ **Is There a Role for LTP in Hippocampal Program Storage?** Computer analogies of brain function are suspect. However, the fact that the loading of a computer program itself requires a form of data storage does show us that neuronal plasticity could as easily function to alter the way memory (and other information) is processed as to store memories. That this could be a real possibility is shown by neural development. During development, in areas such as the visual cortex, associative plasticity is thought to control the final wiring of the structure (see, e.g., Bear et al., 1996). This plasticity contains, in one sense, a record of the experience that gave rise to it. However, in terms of the psychological processes subserved by the adult brain, the plasticity is better thought of as programming the machine.

The hippocampus has highly recursive connections with the rest of the brain (Miller, 1991) and its internal structure appears to consist of the same basic circuitry repeated in parallel many times. Whatever the function one wishes to attribute to the hippocampus, then, it is highly likely that its processing will need to be fine-tuned, probably on a regular basis. It could need to adjust its processing to reflect changing environmental contingencies. It could need to adjust to changes in the areas with which it is recursively linked. It could need to adjust specific modules within its structure, differentially, to produce a balanced output. Finally, it could need to adjust the longitudinal connections between these modules to maintain balanced operation across modules.

The available evidence suggests that disruption of hippocampal LTP or saturation of hippocampal LTP can affect behavior in tasks, and in the specific variants of those tasks, which are sensitive to hippocampal lesions. However, saturation experiments suggest that quite major disturbances are required in the patterns of strengthening of hippocampal synapses if such disruption is to be produced – and even this may be produced in only some task variants.

This is explicable if the basic circuitry of the hippocampal formation can solve the bulk of the problems required of it and if modification of that circuitry is required only for particularly complex problems or problems of a type that have not been met before.

Certainly, for the circuitry of Figure 15.3, a sudden large change in all of the inputs to the hippocampus would have little effect on its capacity to compare their relative size, provided all inputs started and finished at equivalent levels. One possible function of LTP in such circuitry could be to adjust the threshold for detection of conflict in general or to adjust the specific valence of inputs from one area relative to another. Another possibility is that LTP [and long-term depression (LTD)] occurs in small clusters of neurons fairly frequently but has little functional significance. It may affect larger areas only when a particular set of inputs occurs in the context of a reinforcer (signaled by the release of monoamines). The detailed mechanisms of hippocampal function, their relation to behavior, and the capacity of the mechanisms themselves to change over time are so little known that there is little point in speculating much further. The important point is that for our model of hippocampal function (and by implication for many other models), there is no inherent difficulty in the idea that hippocampal LTP is a functionally significant form of plasticity – but is far from essential for all hippocampal function. It seems most plausible, if you take a nonmemorial view of hippocampal function, that LTP reflects a means of altering "programs" rather than "data." However, for such suggestions to move beyond the realms of pure speculation, many experiments of quite new types will be required.

Conclusions

There is good reason (Gray and McNaughton, 2000) to believe that the hippocampus does not store long-term, intermediate, or short-term memories. Rather, it appears to act to suppress false memories (or previously correct memories) that would interfere with correct recall. It follows that LTP in the hippocampus (as opposed to the amygdala) does not store memories. It could be a form of data storage related to specific local processing within the hippocampus. This is a weaker, more specific case of a more exciting possibility: LTP could represent reprogramming of the hippocampal computer. If this is true it could have considerable significance for the kind of model we build of hippocampal function – and hence for our understanding of the mechanisms that support storage and recall of memories in other parts of the brain.

REFERENCES

Abraham, W.C., and Bear, M.F. (1996). Metaplasticity: The plasticity of synaptic plasticity. *Trends Neurosci.* 19: 126–130.

Baddeley, A., and Wilson, B.A. (1994). When implicit learning fails: Amnesia and the problem of error elimination. *Neuropsychologia* 32: 53–68.

Barnes, C.A. (1995). Involvement of LTP in memory: Are we "searching under the street light"? *Neuron* 15: 751–754.

Barnes, C.A., Jung, M.W., McNaughton, B.L., Korol, D.L. et al. (1994). LTP saturation and spatial learning disruption: Effects of task variables and saturation levels. *J. Neurosci.* 14: 5793–5806.

Bear, M.F., Connors, B.W., and Paradiso, M.A. (1996). *Neuroscience: Exploring the Brain.* Baltimore: Williams & Wilkins.

Beardsley, T. (1999). Getting wired. *Sci. Am.* 280: 19–20.

Blanchard, D.C., and Blanchard, R.J. (1990). Effects of ethanol, benzodiazepines and serotonin compounds on ethopharmacological models of anxiety. In N. McNaughton and G. Andrews (Eds.), *Anxiety* (pp. 188–200). Dunedin: University of Otago Press.

Blanchard, D.C., Blanchard, R.J., and Rodgers, R.J. (1991). Risk assessment and animal models of anxiety. In B. Olovier, J. Mos, and J.L. Slangdon (Eds.), *Animal models in psychopharmacology* (pp. 117–134). Basel: Birkhäuser Verlag.

Bliss, T.V.P., and Lømo, T. (1973). Long-lasting potentiation of synaptic transmission in the dentate area of the anaethetised rabbit following stimulation of the perforant path. *J. Physiol. (London)* 232: 331–356.

Castro, C.A., Silbert, L.H., McNaughton, B.L., and Barnes, C.A. (1989). Recovery of spatial learning deficits after decay of electrically induced synaptic enhancement in the hippocampus. *Nature* 342: 545–548.

Cohen, N.J., and Eichenbaum, H. (1993). *Memory, Amnesia, and the Hippocampal Memory System*. Cambridge, MA: MIT Press.

Eichenbaum, H., Steward, C., and Morris, R.G.M. (1990). Hippocampal representation in place learning. *J. Neurosci.* 10: 3531–3542.

Eichenbaum, H., Otto, T., and Cohen, N.J. (1994). Two functional components of the hippocampal memory system. *Behav. Brain Sci.* 17: 449–518.

Frisby, J.P., and Mayhew, J.E. (1979). Does visual texture discrimination precede binocular fusion? *Perception* 8: 153–156.

Gabrieli, J.D.E. (1995). A systematic view of human memory processes. *J. Int. Neuropsychol. Soc.* 1: 115–118.

Gray, J.A. (1982). *The Neuropsychology of Anxiety: An enquiry in to the Functions of the SeptoHippocampal System*. Oxford: Oxford University Press.

Gray, J.A., and McNaughton, N. (1983). Comparison between the behavioural effects of septal and hippocampal lesions: A review. *Physiol. Behav.* 7: 119–188.

Gray, J.A., and McNaughton, N. (2000). *The Neuropsychology of Anxiety: An Enquiry in to the Functions of the Septo-Hippocampal System*. Oxford: Oxford University Press.

Hebb, D.O. (1949). *The Organization of Behavior*. New York: Wiley-Interscience.

Hirsh, R. (1974). The hippocampus and contextual retrieval of information from memory: A theory. *Behav. Biol.* 12: 421–424.

Kesner, R.P., and Beers, D.R. (1988). Dissociation of data-based and expectancy-based memory following hippocampal lesions in rats. *Behav. Neural Biol.* 50: 46–60.

Korol, D.L., Abel, T.Y., Church, L.T., Barnes, C.A. et al. (1993). Hippocampal synaptic enhancement and spatial learning in the Morris swim task. *Hippocampus* 3: 127–132.

LeDoux, J.E. (1994). Emotion, memory and the brain. *Sci. Am.* 270: 50–59.

McNaughton, N. (1997). Cognitive dysfunction resulting from hippocampal hyperactivity— a possible cause of anxiety disorder. *Pharmacol. Biochem. Behav.* 56: 603–611.

McNaughton, N., and Coop, C.F. (1991). Neurochemically dissimilar anxiolytic drugs have common effects on hippocampal rhythmic slow activity. *Neuropharmacology* 30: 855–863.

McNaughton, N., and Mason, S.T. (1980). The neuropsychology and neuropharmacology of the dorsal ascending noradreneregic bundle—a review. *Prog. Neurobiol.* 14: 157–219.

McNaughton, N., and Miller, J.J. (1986). Collateral specific long term potentiation of the output of field CA3 of the hippocampus of the rat. *Exp. Brain Res.* 62: 250–258.

McNaughton, B.L., and Morris, R.G.M. (1987). Hippocampal synaptic enhancement and information storage within a distributed memory system. *Trends Neurosci.* 10: 408–415.

Miller, C.L., Bickford, P.C., Wiser, A.K., and Rose, G.M. (1995). Long-term potentiation disrupts auditory gating in the rat hippocampus. *J. Neurosci.* 15: 5820–5830.

Miller, R. (1991). *Cortico-Hippocampal Interplay and the Representation of Contexts in the Brain*. Berlin: Springer-Verlag.

Money, E.A., Kirk, R.C., and McNaughton, N. (1992). Alzheimer's dementia produces a loss of discrimination but no increase in rate of memory decay in delayed matching to sample. *Neuropsychologia* 30: 133–145.

Morris, R., and Baker, M. (1984). Does long term potentiation/synaptic enhancement have anything to do with learning and memory? In N. Butters and L.R. Squire (Eds.), *The neuropsychology of memory* (pp. 521–535). New York: Guilford Press.

Morris, R.G.M., Davis, S., and Butcher, S.P. (1990). Hippocampal synaptic plasticity and NMDA receptors: A role in information storage? *Phil. Trans. R. Soc. London [B]* 329: 187–204.

O'Keefe, J., and Nadel, L. (1978). *The Hippocampus as a Cognitive Map*. Oxford: Clarendon Press.

Olton, D.S. (1978). Characteristics of spatial memory. In S.H. Hulse, H. Fowler, and W.K. Honig (Eds.), *Cognitive processes in animal behavior* (pp. 341–373). Hillsdale, NJ: Erlbaum.

Pan, W.X., and McNaughton, N. (1997). The medial supramammillary nucleus, spatial learning and the frequency of hippocampal theta activity. *Brain Res.* 764: 101–108.

Rawlins, J.N.P. (1985). Association across time: The hippocampus as a temporary memory store. *Behav. Brain Sci.* 8: 479–496.

Rioux, G.F., and Robinson, G.B. (1995). Hippocampal long-term potentiation does not affect either discrimination learning or reversal learning of the rabbit nictitating membrane response. *Hippocampus* 5: 165–170.

Robbins, T.W. (1996). Refining the taxonomy of memory. *Science* 273: 1353–1354.

Rudy, J.W., and Sutherland, R.J. (1989). The hippocampal formation is necessary for rats to learn and remember configural discriminations. *Behav. Brain Res.* 34: 97–109.

Shanks, D.R., and St. John, M.F. (1994). Characteristics of dissociable human learning systems. *Behav. Brain Sci.* 17: 367–395.

Shors, T.J., and Matzel, L.D. (1997). Long-term potentiation: What's learning got to do with it? *Behav. Brain Sci.* 20: 597–613.

Squire, L.R. (1992). Declarative and nondeclarative memory: Multiple brain systems supporting learning and memory. *J. Cogn. Neurosci.* 4: 230–243.

Squire, L.R., and Zola-Morgan, S. (1984). The neuropsychology of memory: New links between humans and experimental animals. *Ann. NY Acad. Sci.* 444: 137–149.

Tan, S., Kirk, R.C., Abraham, W.C., and McNaughton, N. (1996). Chlordiazepoxide reduces discriminability but not rate of forgetting in delayed conditional discrimination. *Psychopharmacology (Berlin)* 101: 550–554.

Tulving, E. (1984). Multiple book review of *Elements of Episodic Memory. Behav. Brain Sci.* 7: 223–238.

Vinogradova, O.S. (1975). Functional organization of the limbic system in the process of registration of information: Facts and hypotheses. In R.I. Isaacson and K.H. Pribram (Eds.), *The hippocampus* (Vol. 2, pp. 3–69). New York: Plenum Press.

Vinogradova, O.S., and Brazhnik, P.S. (1978). Neuronal aspects of septo-hippocampal relations. In K. Elliott and J. Whetan (Eds.), *Functions of the septo-hippocampal system.* Ciba Foundation Symposium 58 (New Series) (pp. 145–171). Amsterdam: Elsevier.

Warrington, E.K., and Weiskrantz, L. (1978). Further analysis of the prior learning effect in amnesic patients. *Neuropsychologia* 16: 169–177.

White, K.G. (1985). Characteristics of forgetting functions in delayed matching to sample. *J. Exp. Anal. Behav.* 44: 15–34.

Woodnorth, M., and McNaughton, N. (1999). Anxiolytic action on the supramammillary nucleus reduces theta frequency and increases fixed interval responding. *Soc. Neurosci. Abstr.* 25: 1641.

Zola-Morgan, S., Squire, L.R., and Amaral, D.G. (1986). Human amnesia and the medial temporal region: Enduring memory impairment following a bilateral lesion limited to field CA1 of the hippocampus. *J. Neurosci.* 6: 2950–2967.

CHAPTER SIXTEEN

Differential Effects of Stress on Hippocampal and Amygdaloid LTP

Insight into the Neurobiology of Traumatic Memories

David M. Diamond, Collin R. Park, Michael J. Puls, and Gregory M. Rose

SUMMARY

This chapter begins with a brief discussion of the complexity of the long-term potentiation (LTP)-memory debate. We suggest that the notion of LTP as a unitary "memory encoding device" is too simplistic to survive rigorous experimentation and debate. However, while there are difficulties in making the direct connection between LTP and memory, we have not abandoned the proposition that LTP studies can enhance our understanding of the physiology of memory. The primary focus of this chapter is to incorporate studies on LTP, memory, and stress into a synthesis on the dynamics of emotional memory storage in the hippocampus and amygdala. The work is based on the idea that the induction or blockade of LTP can serve as a "diagnostic" measure of how stress affects information processing by different brain structures. The synthesis provides a novel perspective on why the characteristics of nonemotional memories differ from the pathologically intense, and fragmented, characteristics of traumatic memories.

Introduction

Long-term potentiation (LTP) has long been embraced as a model of memory because its characteristics are consistent with models of synaptic storage mechanisms and it has features in common with learning and memory. Just as memory is a lasting trace formed as a result of a brief experience, LTP is a lasting enhancement of synaptic efficacy produced by brief electrical stimulation. Initially, the field was buoyed by repeated findings of commonalities between LTP and memory. The early work showed, for example, that drugs that blocked hippocampal LTP impaired hippocampal-dependent learning, and that LTP, as with memory, was impaired in old animals. However, the once highly regarded LTP-memory

Christian Hölscher, editor, *Neuronal Mechanisms of Memory Formation.* © 2001 Cambridge University Press. Printed in the United States of America. All rights reserved.

connection has been weakened by a barrage of recent studies that have called into question the viability of LTP as a mechanism of information storage.

LTP's allure as a model of memory, followed by increased skepticism regarding its relevance to information storage, has been reviewed extensively by others and will not be discussed in detail here. In Chapter 14 we focused in detail on the hippocampal LTP-memory debate. Here, we will only briefly address some of the problems in attempting to relate LTP to memory. The primary focus of this chapter is to present a synthesis, based on the proposition that the LTP-memory connection is valid, which attempts to describe how stress affects multiple memory systems. An important feature of this synthesis is that it considers how LTP in areas other than the hippocampus (e.g., the amygdala) could be involved in information storage.

Evaluating the LTP-Memory Debate: An Alternative Approach

In this section we discuss how the LTP-memory controversy has been fueled by our lack of understanding of how different forms of synaptic plasticity map onto different forms of learning and memory. We conclude with an alternative approach that may provide insight into how emotionality affects information storage in the hippocampus and amygdala.

First, the integrity of the hippocampus is necessary for many different forms of learning to occur, including temporal, spatial, olfactory, and fear-related learning (Olton et al., 1979; Becker and Olton, 1981; Meck et al., 1984; Eichenbaum et al., 1989; Zador et al., 1990; Phillips and LeDoux, 1992; Cassaday and Rawlins, 1997). Just as there are different forms of hippocampal-dependent learning, there are also different forms of LTP, such as those that depend on activation of either NMDA or opiate receptors (Derrick et al., 1992; Breindl et al., 1994; Martinez and Derrick, 1996). One source of controversy in the LTP-memory debate has been based on the assumption that a manipulation that affects "LTP" should have the same effect on "memory." However, considering that there are diverse forms of LTP in different subregions of the hippocampus and diverse forms of hippocampal-dependent learning, it would seem unlikely that a manipulation of any one form of LTP (e.g., NMDA- or opiate-mediated LTP) would always produce isomorphic effects on any one form of learning and memory (e.g. spatial learning) and vice versa.

Second, diverse methodologic procedures have been used to study learning and memory, and differences in training procedures may have provided a confounding influence in the LTP-memory debate. For example, the Morris water maze is commonly used to evaluate the hypothesis that pharmacologic treatments that block LTP should also impair spatial learning (Bannerman et al., 1995; Barnes and McNaughton, 1985; Hölscher et al., 1997a-c; Morris et al., 1986, 1989; Saucier and Cain, 1995; Voronin et al., 1995). However, there are a number of variables that can affect an animal's performance in the maze, including the potential confound that the rate of "learning" is influenced by how rapidly animals can acclimate to the stress of the cold water experience (Brandeis et al., 1989; Hölscher

1999). In addition, the Morris maze has routinely been used to study two different forms of memory: reference memory (the escape platform is located in the same place each day) or working memory (the escape platform is located in a different place each day) (Whishaw 1985; Bohbot et al., 1996; Steele and Morris, 1999). The reference/working memory variable is important because the reference memory version of the water maze is less sensitive to modulation by drugs or behavioral manipulations than is the working memory version of the maze (Warren et al., 1991; Steele and Morris, 1999; Diamond et al., 1999). We suggest that a more challenging task, such as the working memory version of the water maze, provides a better means with which to evaluate the role of LTP in memory than does the simpler (i.e., reference memory) version of the Morris maze (Morris and Frey, 1997).

Third, diverse methodologic procedures have been used to induce LTP, including those that have employed physiologically patterned (theta burst or primed burst, PB) stimulation as compared to those that have employed more conventional or "nonpatterned" trains of pulses (Larson and Lynch, 1986; Larson et al., 1986; Rose and Dunwiddie, 1986; Diamond et al., 1988). A comparison of findings from studies employing patterned versus nonpatterned stimulation provides a strong indication that methodologic factors can influence the outcome of studies addressing the LTP-memory connection. Specifically, it has been shown that PB potentiation is more sensitive to modulation by behavioral and pharmacologic influences than is conventional LTP. For example, stress, aging, drugs, hormones, and neuromodulators can all have profound effects on learning, memory, and PB potentiation, but, under some conditions, may have no effect on conventional LTP (Corradetti et al., 1992; Moore et al., 1993; Diamond et al., 1995, 1996a, in press; Bramham et al., 1998; Mesches et al., 1999; Staubli et al., 1999). Thus, differences in how pharmacologic and behavioral manipulations affect LTP versus PB potentiation may have added fuel to the LTP-memory controversy.

Finally, different forms of LTP occur in brain regions other than the hippocampus, including the thalamus (Gerren and Weinberger, 1983), neocortex (Aroniadou and Teyler, 1992; Bear, 1996; Kudoh and Shibuki, 1997), and amygdala (Clugnet and LeDoux, 1990; Chapman and Bellavance, 1992; Maren and Fanselow, 1995; Maren, 1996; McKernan and Shinnick-Gallagher, 1997; Rogan et al., 1997; Li et al., 1998). The conceptual and methodologic quagmire described above for attempts to relate hippocampal LTP to memory applies to these forms of LTP as well, that is, what are the optimal stimulation parameters to induce extrahippocampal plasticity and does LTP in each brain region serve the same memory storage function?

Taken together, the notion that a unitary "LTP" underlies a unitary "memory encoding function" was too simplistic to survive rigorous experimentation and debate. Should we give up on making any attempt at relating LTP to memory? Shors and Matzel (1997) suggested that we abandon the idea that LTP is a memory encoding device in favor of the view that LTP is involved in enhancing attention and sensory processing. The commentaries that followed their provocative article revealed a conspicuous absence of a consensus on how, or even if, LTP is involved in memory. Opinions ranged from Fanselow's supportive view that "LTP is a learning mechanism" (p. 616) to Rudy and Keith's dismissal of the phenomenon, noting that "LTP may have no functional significance" (p. 629). In closing, Shors and Matzel offered the extreme view that "LTP is neither an information-processing device nor a memory mechanism" (p. 613).

Our group favors a retreat to more conservative grounds, rather than completely abandoning the search for an LTP-memory connection. Our perspective can be illustrated with the following scenario. Consider two behavioral conditions: Under condition "A" tetanizing stimulation produces hippocampal LTP and under condition "B" the same stimulation produces no change in response. One interpretation of these two observations is that under condition "A" hippocampal synapses are in a state that makes them more receptive to generating plasticity, and thereby more amenable to storing information, than they are under condition "B." To take this one step further, the findings would also suggest that the hippocampus, in general, may process information more efficiently in condition "A" than in condition "B." This systems-level perspective interprets the successful induction or the blockade of LTP as a diagnostic measure for assessing how an experience affects the information-processing capacity of any given brain structure.

The idea that LTP serves a diagnostic function can be applied to the well-described finding that stress or glucocorticoids can block the induction of hippocampal LTP and PB potentiation. For example, we have shown that PB potentiation was blocked when animals were stressed, and then PB potentiation was not blocked when the same animals, at a different time, were not stressed (Diamond et al., 1994). This work suggests that the capacity for hippocampal synapses to generate plasticity is continuously modulated by an animal's emotional state, that is, under nonemotional conditions the hippocampus functions optimally and under stressful conditions hippocampal processing, as indicated by the blockade of PB potentiation, is impaired (Diamond et al., 1990, 1994, 1998).

If the induction of LTP and PB potentiation can serve as a diagnostic for how emotionality affects hippocampal functioning, then perhaps we can apply the same strategy to assess how emotionality affects LTP in other brain structures, such as the amygdala. This comparative approach may be fruitful because the hippocampus and amygdala both exhibit learning-related synaptic plasticity and are critically involved in emotional memory storage (Phillips and LeDoux, 1992; Kim et al., 1993; Bremner et al., 1995; Grillon et al., 1996; McGaugh et al., 1996; Cahill, 1997). In this chapter we have developed a synthesis that incorporates studies on LTP in the hippocampus and amygdala with cognitive studies on emotion and memory in animals and humans. This synthesis may prove to be useful in understanding how stress, or trauma, produces such complex and long-lasting effects on learning and memory.

Stress and Hippocampal Functioning: Cognitive and Electrophysiologic Studies

A vast amount of research has focused on elucidating the role of the hippocampus in learning and memory. More than four decades of research have shown that the hippocampus is involved in the storage of declarative memories, which is described in human work as the conscious recall of facts and events (Squire and Zola, 1996, 1997; Eichenbaum, 1997). Animal studies have reported complementary observations in that the hippocampus is recognized as being necessary in generating spatiotemporal and contextual representations (O' Keefe and Nadel, 1978; Meck et al., 1984; Alvarez et al., 1994, 1995; Alvarado and Rudy, 1995; Bunsey and Eichenbaum, 1996).

Largely independent of the work on the hippocampus and memory is an extensive literature describing the pivotal role of the hippocampus in the regulation of stress, and in particular, glucocorticoid responses (Knigge and Hays, 1963; Bouille and Bayle, 1973; Ely et al., 1977; Feldman and Conforti, 1979, 1980; Dunn and Orr, 1984; Sapolsky et al., 1985, 1991; Angelucci and Scaccianoce, 1990; Brady et al., 1992). Multiple levels of analysis have converged on the common finding that the hippocampus is involved in the capacity for an organism to inhibit the hypothalamic-pituitary-adrenal axis (HPAA). First, the hippocampus has great sensitivity to stress because it has the highest concentration of receptors for glucocorticoids (corticosterone in rats or cortisol in humans) of any structure in the nervous system (Gerlach and McEwen, 1971; Reul and de Kloet, 1985; McEwen et al., 1994). Second, electrical stimulation of the hippocampus can reduce peripheral levels of glucocorticoids and blocks the development of stress-induced pathology (Henke, 1982, 1989, 1990a; Dunn and Orr,1984). Third, damage to the hippocampus, as can occur in aging, depression, Cushing's disease, or in experimental animal models, is associated with the hypersecretion of glucocorticoids and an exacerbation of stress-induced pathology (Henke, 1990a; Sapolsky et al., 1991; Starkman et al., 1992; Axelson et al., 1993; O'Brien et al., 1996; Herbert, 1998; Lupien et al., 1999). Thus, the integrity of the hippocampus is necessary for an organism to respond effectively to a stressful experience.

These different lines of experimentation indicate that the hippocampus functions to store episodic information and to inhibit the HPAA. Based on these findings, the following sequence of events would be expected to occur during a stressful experience: The onset of a stress or fear-provoking experience would activate the hippocampus, which would induce LTP-like synaptic plasticity. The stress-induced enhancement of synaptic transmission would enable the individual to store information about the experience into long-term memory. Finally, this activation of the hippocampus would aid in homeostasis by returning the hyperaroused HPAA to its baseline state.

The problem with the above scenario is that it does not appear to be an accurate portrayal of how the hippocampus actually responds to increased emotionality. Some hormones in the HPAA that are released at the onset of a stressor, such as epinephrine, adrenocorticotropic hormone (ACTH), and corticotropin releasing factor (CRF), can produce rapid excitatory effects on hippocampal cell activity (Segal, 1976; Aldenhoff et al., 1983; Gold et al., 1984; Siggins et al., 1985; Trifiletti and Pranzatelli, 1992; Abrahám et al., 1996; Smriga et al., 1998). However, an extensive literature has shown that stress levels of glucocorticoids produce a profound and long-lasting inhibitory influence on hippocampal cell activity (Pfaff et al., 1971; Vidal et al., 1986; Rey et al., 1987; Talmi et al., 1992, 1993). Studies have shown that one way in which corticosteroids facilitate hippocampal inhibition is by increasing the magnitude of long-latency inhibitory postsynaptic potentials (Joels and de Kloet, 1989; Joels et al., 1995; Karten et al., 1999). Moreover, corticosterone or stress can potentiate the inhibitory effects of neuromodulatory transmitters, such as serotonin, on hippocampal activity (Joëls and de Kloet, 1992; Joels et al., 1995; Hesen and Joels, 1996). Thus, any transient excitatory effects of stress on the hippocampus produced by the rapid release of epinephrine, CRF, and ACTH are followed by a profound and long-lasting inhibitory influence of corticosterone on hippocampal cell activity.

How does the stress-induced inhibition of hippocampal activity affect synaptic plasticity? A wealth of studies employing a broad range of techniques (behaving, anesthetized, and *in vitro* preparations), stressors (novelty, restraint, shock, predator exposure), and recording measures [plasticity of the population spike and excitatory postsynaptic potential (EPSP)] have consistently shown that stress or elevated levels of corticosterone inhibit the induction of excitatory plasticity (PB potentiation and LTP) and promote the induction of inhibitory plasticity (long-term depression, LTD) (Foy et al., 1987; Shors et al., 1989, 1997; Diamond et al., 1992, 1994; Pavlides et al., 1993, 1996; Diamond and Rose, 1994; Rey et al., 1994; Bodnoff et al., 1995; Garcia et al., 1997a, 1997b; Xu et al., 1997, 1998; Kim and Yoon, 1998; Rowan et al., 1998). We have shown that stress blocks the induction of PB potentiation in behaving rats and in hippocampal slices obtained from rats unavoidably exposed to a predator (Diamond et al., 1990, 1994; Mesches et al., 1999; Figure 16.1). We also found that stress levels of corticosterone reduced the magnitude of PB potentiation, and that animals with the highest levels of corticosterone developed PB depression (a lasting enhancement of inhibition) (Bennett et al., 1991; Diamond et al., 1992). Later research showed that one of the most effective means with which to induce hippocampal synaptic depression *in vivo* is to deliver tetanizing stimulation to animals that are either stressed or have pharmacologically elevated levels of glucocorticoids (Kim et al., 1996; Pavlides et al., 1996; Xu et al., 1997, 1998; Kim and Yoon, 1998).

Because stress blocks the induction of excitatory hippocampal plasticity, stress would also be expected to interfere with hippocampal-dependent forms of learning and memory. Indeed, studies have shown that acute or chronic stress impairs hippocampal-specific learning and memory in rats and in humans (Arbel et al., 1994; Luine et al., 1994; Bodnoff et al., 1995; Conrad et al., 1996; Diamond et al., 1996b; Kirschbaum et al., 1996; Lupien et al., 1997; de Quervain et al., 1998), and that administration of cortisol or dexamethasone, a cortisol agonist, impairs hippocampal-dependent (declarative) memory in humans (Newcomer et al., 1994, 1999; Keenan et al., 1995; Kirschbaum et al., 1996). Our studies have shown that placing rats into a fear-provoking environment selectively impairs hippocampal-dependent (working) memory (Diamond et al., 1996b, 1998, 1999). For example, placing rats in close proximity to a cat, which evokes an intense fear response in the rats, impaired their memory for recently acquired spatial informa-

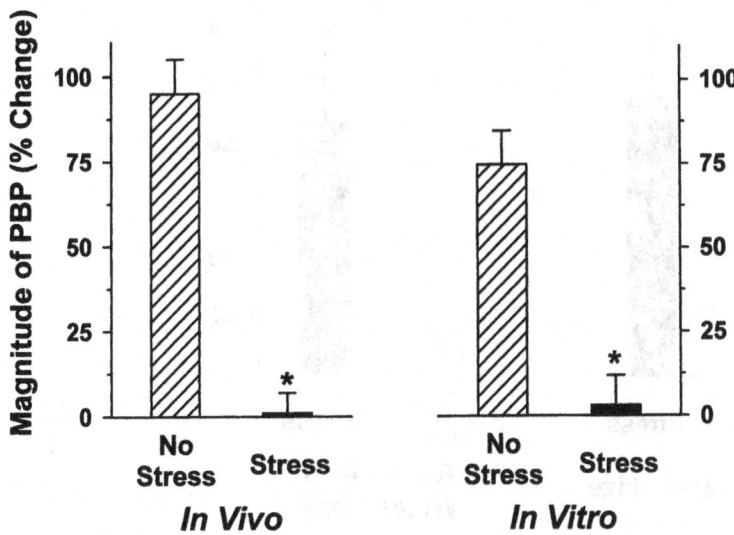

Figure 16.1. Primed burst (PB) potentiation was blocked by stress recorded *in vivo* or *in vitro*. PB stimulation produced a lasting increase in the amplitude of the CA1 population spike when rats were in a familiar environment (no stress), but produced no enhancement of response when the rats were in an unfamiliar (stress) environment. (Left side; from Diamond et al., 1994, with permission.) Similarly, PB potentiation of the CA1 population spike occurred in hippocampal slices obtained from rats in their home cage (no stress), but not from slices obtained from rats that spent 75 minutes in close proximity to a cat (stress) (Right side; from Mesches et al., 1999, with permission.)

tion (locating a hidden platform in a water maze) (Diamond et al., 1999) (Figure 16.2).

Thus, there is great concordance between the electrophysiologic and behavioral studies in that stress or corticosterone amplifies inhibitory synaptic potentials in the hippocampus, blocks the induction of synaptic plasticity, and impairs hippocampal-dependent learning and memory. From this extensive base of research one can draw the conclusion that an increase in emotionality interferes with hippocampal processing, thereby providing a physiologic basis for the well-described observation that emotionality can impair the accuracy of episodic memories (Loftus and Burns, 1982; Kramer et al., 1991; Christianson, 1992b, Bornstein et al., 1998).

Given the consistency of the behavioral and electrophysiologic findings, it is tempting to conclude that the story on stress, memory, and hippocampal function is complete. That is, stress impairs memory because it blocks LTP and suppresses hippocampal functioning. However, there is a piece missing from this conceptual puzzle. While there is an extensive literature demonstrating that heightened emotionality does indeed impair declarative memory, there is also an extensive literature demonstrating that emotionally arousing experiences or administration of hormones, such as epinephrine, ACTH, or even corticosterone, can *enhance* learning and memory (Gold and Van Buskirk, 1975, 1976; McCarty and Gold, 1981;

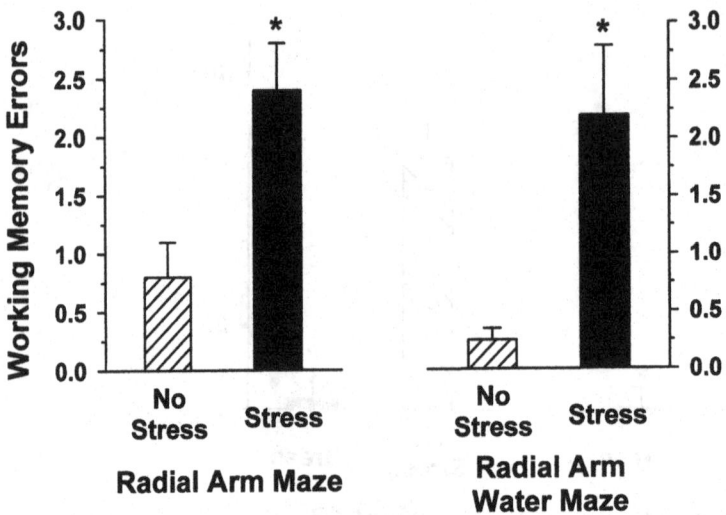

Figure 16.2. Spatial working memory was impaired by stress in two versions of the radial arm maze. In the radial arm maze, rats ate food in four of seven baited arms and then spent a 4-hour delay in their home cages. The graph on the left side shows the number of errors the rats made in the postdelay retention (working memory) test. Rats made significantly more working memory errors when they spent the delay period in an unfamiliar location (stress), than when they spent the delay in a familiar location (no stress). (Data on the left side from Diamond et al., 1996.) In the radial arm water maze rats were trained to find a hidden escape platform located at the end of one of six arms radiating away from an open central area of a water maze. The graph on the right side shows the number of errors the rats made in the post-delay retention (working memory) test. Rats made significantly more working memory errors when they spent the delay period in close proximity to a cat (stress) than when they spent the delay in their home cage (no stress). (Data on the right side from Diamond et al., 1999, with permission.)

Sandi and Rose, 1994; Cahill and McGaugh, 1996; Quirarte et al., 1997; Sandi et al., 1997). Moreover, studies have shown that fear conditioning, which by its nature evokes a substantial stress response, results in the formation of distinct hippocampal-dependent (i.e., contextual) memories of the experience (Phillips and LeDoux, 1992, 1994). Finally, perhaps the greatest levels of arousal and fear that can occur in one's life are generated during traumatic experiences, such as an assault, rape, or wartime combat exposure. These horrific experiences can produce intense declarative/episodic (hippocampal-type) memories that can last for years after the original experience. This pathologically intense stress-induced *enhancement* of memory provides the basis of the symptomatology of posttraumatic stress disorder (PTSD), such as persistent and intrusive memories of the trauma (Grillon et al., 1996).

Addressing how stress affects learning and memory is relatively straightforward if we limit our analysis to the stress-induced impairment of declarative learning and memory. If the hippocampus is unable to generate synaptic plasticity under stressful conditions, then the formation and recall of declarative memories at these times will be impaired. Understanding how heightened emotionality enhances declarative memory, however, is a far greater challenge. If, as so much research indicates, the hippocampus is rendered nonfunctional during emotionally intense experiences, then which neural system(s) encode and store declarative memories of experiences that occur, for example, during trauma? We will address this question in the final section of the chapter.

Stress and Amygdala Functioning: Cognitive and Electrophysiologic Studies

One of the most well-studied areas in the neurobiology of behavior is the involvement of the amygdala in emotional learning. Evidence from a broad range of research has supported the hypothesis that the amygdala is an essential component of the neural circuitry involved in emotional responses, in general, and in attaching emotional significance to learned stimuli (Sarter and Markowitsch, 1985; McGaugh et al., 1990; LeDoux, 1993; Izquierdo and Medina, 1997). Damage to the amygdala in humans and animals results in learning impairments, especially in those tasks that require the subject to make a connection between environmental stimuli and strong emotional responses (Davis, 1992, 1994; Adolphs et al., 1995; LaBar et al., 1995; Bremner et al., 1996; Maren and Fanselow, 1996).

The specific role of the amygdala in memory formation has been a topic of recent debate. Cahill et al. (1999) asserted that the amygdala modulates information storage in other brain areas, but that it does not serve as the site of long-term memory storage. Among the findings they discussed was their observation that pharmacologic activation of the amygdala immediately after training enhanced hippocampal-dependent, and also caudate nucleus-dependent, forms of learning (Packard et al., 1994; Packard and Teather, 1998). Moreover, electrical stimulation of the amygdala increases the magnitude of hippocampal LTP (Henke 1990b, 1992; Ikegaya et al., 1995a, 1995b, 1995c, 1996) and, conversely, animals with amygdala damage have reduced hippocampal LTP (Ikegaya et al., 1996). These findings suggest that amygdala activation enhances the memory-related processing in extra-amygdala brain structures. Cahill and colleagues also pointed out that posttraining inactivation or lesioning of the amygdala does not impair performance on memory (retention) testing (Liang et al., 1982; Packard et al., 1994; Poremba and Gabriel, 1999). These findings provide strong support for their assertion that the amygdala is not the storehouse of emotional memories.

An alternative view of the role of the amygdala in the storage of emotional memories has been proposed by other researchers (Maren, 1996; Armony and LeDoux, 1997). While these investigators recognized that the amygdala modulates the storage of information in other structures, they suggested that information about emotional events can be stored within the amygdala. Their viewpoint has been summarized recently (Fanselow and LeDoux, 1999), and perhaps the most compelling component of their argument is based on a series of anatomic and electrophysiologic studies. First, the amygdala receives highly processed cortical and subcortical sensory input, giving it access to specific information about salient environmental cues (LeDoux et al., 1991; Romanski and LeDoux, 1993;

Doron and LeDoux, 1999). Second, the amygdala receives input from structures, such as the medial geniculate nucleus and auditory cortex, which have been shown to exhibit learning-induced plasticity (Diamond and Weinberger, 1984; LeDoux et al., 1985, 1991; Weinberger and Diamond, 1987; Edeline and Weinberger, 1992; Lennartz and Weinberger, 1992; Bakin et al., 1996; Edeline 1999). Third, amygdala cells develop learning-induced changes in discharge activity (Applegate et al., 1982; Pascoe and Kapp, 1985; Quirk et al., 1995; Rogan and LeDoux, 1996). Moreover, learning-induced changes in amygdala cell activity reflect systematic changes in sensory (auditory) receptive fields (Armony et al., 1995), a phenomenon that has also been characterized in amygdala afferents from the thalamocortical auditory system (Weinberger and Diamond, 1987; Edeline and Weinberger, 1992; Lennartz and Weinberger, 1992; Bakin et al., 1996; Edeline, 1999). Fourth, different forms of LTP occur in the amygdala (Chapman et al., 1990; Clugnet and LeDoux, 1990; Watanabe et al., 1995; Maren and Fanselow, 1995). Finally, fear conditioning results in an LTP-like enhancement of synaptic transmission in the amygdala (Rogan and LeDoux, 1995; McKernan and Shinnick-Gallagher, 1997; Rogan et al., 1997; Garcia et al., 1998a), but not in the hippocampus (Garcia et al., 1998b).

Thus, amygdaloid neurons have access to specific sensory information, exhibit learning-induced plasticity, and express an enhancement of synaptic plasticity during fear-provoking experiences. We suggest that the current debate on whether the amygdala is, or is not, the site of storage of emotional memories reflects our lack of knowledge on where these memories are formed. What has been missing from the debate is an appreciation of the functional significance of amygdaloid LTP and its enhancement by fear conditioning. The findings of learning- and electrically induced synaptic plasticity in the amygdala indicate that, in theory, the amygdala contains the neural substrates involved in the storage of emotional memories.

Qualitative Distinctions between Emotional and Nonemotional Memories

Insight into the locations of the neural substrates of emotional memory storage may be gained by assessing qualitative distinctions between emotional and non-emotional memories. Hippocampal-type memory storage is characterized by a representation of the contextual elements of an experience. This form of processing has been referred to as a "configurational representation" (Alvarado and Rudy, 1995) or "episodic memory binding" (Metcalfe and Jacobs, 1998). Similarly, Cohen and Eichenbaum (1993) concluded that the hippocampus serves to "chunk" or "bind" together the converging processing outcomes reflecting the learning event. Much evidence indicates, therefore, that it is the hippocampus (and the prefrontal cortex; Chiba et al., 1994; McCarthy et al., 1996; Kesner et al., 1996; Arnsten, 1997) that enables accurate episodic memories to be formed by binding together multiple events that co-occur during an experience. This kind of in-depth, context-rich processing appears to occur best under low to intermediate levels of arousal (Metcalfe and Jacobs, 1998).

Empirical work indicates that traumatic memories are qualitatively different from nontraumatic memories. When people have a highly stressful experience, their memories of the experience tend to begin as unbound fragmentary elements that, over time, are woven together in a reconstructive process to emerge as a plausible, but less than veridical, biographical episode (Metcalfe and Jacobs, 1998). This perspective on emotional memories has also been addressed by van der Kolk and Fisler (1995), who reported that immediate recollections of traumatic events are usually disjointed fragments of the sensory components of the experience. In time, people tend to assimilate these fragmented memories into a schema that slowly may become richer in contextual details. However, in the process of reconstructing the episode, posttrauma ideations and experiences become incorporated, or "spliced," into memories of the original events (Neisser, 1997). This reconstruction process, therefore, can lead to memories of emotionally charged events that are a combination of veridical intense and vivid recollections intermixed with equally intense, but potentially inaccurate, fragments (Neisser and Harsch, 1992). In time, the individual may recall the details of the experience with a great sense of certainty, despite the fact that the memory was contaminated by information acquired after the termination of the experience (Neisser and Harsch, 1992; Neisser, 1997).

The paucity of spatiotemporal and contextual details in accounts of trauma is consistent with the idea that hippocampal processing is suppressed during periods of intense stress (Jacobs and Nadel, 1985; Diamond et al., 1990, 1996b; Diamond and Rose, 1994; Armony and LeDoux, 1997; Metcalfe and Jacobs, 1998; Nadel and Jacobs, 1998). Metcalfe and Jacobs (1998) suggested that the stress-induced suppression of hippocampal function is accompanied by heightened processing by the amygdala. This formulation has heuristic value in that it explored anatomic constraints on emotional memory processing. However, their emphasis on dominance by the amygdala memory system in the processing of emotional memories is counter to the point emphasized repeatedly by McGaugh, Cahill, and co-workers that posttraining damage to the amygdala does not impair the recall of emotional memories (McGaugh et al., 1996; Cahill et al., 1999). If the amygdala is not a storehouse of emotional memories, and if the hippocampus is rendered "dysfunctional" by heightened emotionality (Metcalfe and Jacobs, 1998), then where are emotional memories stored?

Emotional Experiences Are Processed by Shifts in Dominance between the Amygdaloid and Hippocampal Memory Systems

In this section we have developed the idea that during a stressful experience, hippocampal processing is suppressed and emotional memories are stored in the amygdala. In the aftermath of the trauma, the hippocampus recovers and constructs a "post hoc" representation of the events that had occurred during the original experience. The source of the information available to the hippocampus is not the experience itself; the hippocampus must access the representation of the experience that was stored in the amygdala. In the following subsections we illustrate this idea in terms of sequential shifts in dominance between the hippocampal versus amygdaloid memory systems. The dynamic shifts between these two memory systems, and its effects on cognitive processing, are divided into three phases: processing that occurs before (Phase 1), during (Phase 2), and then after (Phase 3) a stressful experience occurs.

■ **Phase 1: The Transition From Neutral to Heightened Emotionality.** In our schema, hippocampal processing dominates under emotionally neutral conditions enabling the individual to accomplish complex (e.g., divided attention) tasks effectively and to generate episodic memories replete with spatiotemporal and contextual details. This form of processing allows for great breadth and depth of storage, but the information is transiently maintained in a working memory buffer that is susceptible to disruption by emotionality.

With the onset of a stressful experience, there would be a shift in dominance of memory systems from the hippocampus to the amygdala, which would result in impaired access to information stored in the hippocampal working memory buffer. Studies have shown that humans and animals exhibit retrograde amnesia for information that was acquired soon before an increase in emotionality occurred. For example, we (Diamond et al., 1996b, 1999) and de Quervain et al. (1998) have shown that rats are impaired at remembering spatial (hippocampal-dependent) information that they had acquired before they had the stressful experience. Similarly, people exhibit retrograde amnesia for declarative information they had acquired soon before being stressed or in response to being administered glucocorticoids (Loftus and Burns, 1982; Newcomer et al., 1994, 1999; Keenan et al., 1995; Kirschbaum et al., 1996). Thus, through the inconsistent and heterogeneous findings in the stress-memory literature, one consistency emerges in that the transition from a neutral to an emotional state results in impaired recall of information that had been acquired before the increase in emotionality occurred.

Electrophysiologic studies indicate that stress or exposure to a novel environment suppresses the induction of synaptic plasticity in the hippocampus and can reverse (or depotentiate) previously induced LTP. More specifically, stress or elevated glucocorticoids suppress excitatory synaptic plasticity (PB potentiation or LTP) and enhance inhibitory plasticity (LTD) (Foy et al., 1987; Shors et al., 1989, 1997; Diamond et al., 1992, 1994; Pavlides et al., 1993; Diamond and Rose, 1994; Rey et al., 1994; Bodnoff et al., 1995; Pavlides et al., 1996; Garcia et al., 1997a, 1997b; Xu et al., 1997, 1998; Kim and Yoon 1998). The suppression of excitatory plasticity and the enhancement of inhibitory plasticity in the hippocampus may provide the basis for the commonly described observation of stress-induced retrograde amnesia for recently acquired declarative information.

■ **Phase 2: Amygdala-Dominated Memory Processing During Emotional Experiences.** Earlier in this chapter we reviewed an extensive literature indicating that heightened emotionality impairs the induction and maintenance of hippocampal synaptic plasticity, and enhances the induction of amygdaloid synaptic plasticity. For example, increased emotionality or novelty blocks hippocampal PB potentiation and LTP, and enhances inhibitory plasticity (LTD). Conversely, fear conditioning enhances the induction of LTP in the amygdala, but blocks LTP in the hippocampus. These physiologic studies support our hypothesis that during emotionally charged experiences there is a shift in dominance from hippocampal to amygdaloid memory systems.

The arousal-induced shift in processing from one brain system to another should be expressed as a systematic change in aspects of cognition with high arousal. As Reisberg and Heuer (1992) pointed out, increased emotionality shifts one's "informational priorities" … such that an emotional event "will serve to rivet one's attention on the central action, effectively leading … to narrowed attention." (p. 279). More than 40 years ago Easterbrook (1959) proposed that emotionally charged experiences lead to a reduction in the range of cues to which an individual is sensitive. Thus, at high levels of arousal the narrowing of attention would provide for highly efficient processing of singular cues occurring during an emotional event. For example, the commonly cited "weapon focus" phenomenon illustrates the finding that witnesses to a crime involving a weapon appear to divert their attentional resources to the weapon to the exclusion of all other cues (Koss et al., 1995; Safer et al., 1998). This process is adaptive in the sense that the subset of cues producing the increased emotional response will receive greater attentional resources than irrelevant cues. However, in the process, increased arousal draws attention away from abstractions and contextual details of the environment (Weltman and Egstrom, 1966; Wachtel, 1968; Burke et al., 1992).

We propose that it is the transition in dominance from hippocampal to amygdaloid processing that produces the narrowing of attention with heightened arousal. As synaptic plasticity in the hippocampus is being suppressed by arousal, amygdaloid plasticity is functioning optimally to generate a representation of a limited set of the cues that occur during an emotional event. Thus, the pervasive descriptions of the fragmented and singular focus of traumatic memories, such as the intense disjointed memory of a weapon thrust into a victim's face (weapon focus), would be stored at the time of the experience by synaptic plasticity within the amygdala.

Finally, if the amygdala, alone, can store emotional memories, then arousal should enhance memory formation in people with hippocampal, but not amygdala, damage. Two studies have provided observations consistent with this hypothesis. Hamann and co-workers (Hamann et al., 1997a, 1997b) presented a sequence of neutral and emotionally evocative slides to people. Control subjects tested under these conditions exhibited enhanced recall for slides that generated an emotional response. The authors found that amnesics with bilateral damage to the hippocampus and related structures exhibited an enhancement of declarative memory for the arousing slides. By contrast, people with amygdala damage showed no enhancement of memory for the arousing slides. Thus, the arousal-induced enhancement of memory may be mediated, in part, by information storage mechanisms located within the amygdala.

■ **Phase 3: Hippocampal Functioning Recovers Following the Termination of the Experience.** In the aftermath of an emotional experience, hippocampal (and related neocortical) storage capabilities would slowly recover. Electrophysiologic studies have provided insight into the duration of the hippocampal recovery period. We have found that PB potentiation was blocked in behaving rats 75 minutes (Mesches et al., 1999) and 4 hours (Diamond et al., 1990, 1994) after they were placed in a stress-provoking environment. Others have extended this analysis to show that hippocampal plasticity is suppressed for up to 48 hours after the termination of a stressful event (Garcia et al., 1997a; Shors et al., 1997a). Thus, the electrophysiologic studies would suggest that the hippocampus is impaired at storing information for up to 2 days after the termination of a stressful event.

What would be the consequences of the hippocampus going "off-line" during an emotional experience, and then having a "recovery of function" up to 2 days later? Since the hippocampus was not functioning optimally at the time of the original experience, during the recovery period it would need to access the representation of the experience that was stored in the amygdala. However, the information stored by the amygdala may be limited to isolated stimulus elements, rather than a composite representation of the entire experience. The amygdala, therefore, applies a filter at the first stage of emotional memory storage that will determine the elements of the original experience that will be made available to the hippocampus as it generates a "post hoc" representation of the original experience.

The hypothesis that the amygdala can transfer information to other brain memory storage systems is admittedly speculative, but is indirectly supported by electrophysiologic studies. Numerous studies have shown that there is a two-way interaction between the hippocampus and amygdala: Stimulation of either structure can enhance LTP in the other structure (Henke 1990a, 1990b, 1992; Maren and Fanselow, 1995; Ikegaya et al., 1996; Akirav and Richter-Levin, 1999, in press). These studies suggest that the amygdala is functionally connected to the hippocampus, and may interact with hippocampal storage capacity after the termination of an emotional experience.

Our emphasis on the necessary role of the amygdala in the first stage of emotional memory formation, and the subsequent transfer of that representation to the hippocampus, leads to a general prediction. The reconstructed memory should be susceptible to modulation by postlearning experiences and hormonal fluctuations as the transfer process is occurring. The influence of postlearning (i.e., post-training) experiences on the veracity of memories was first addressed 100 years ago by Mueller and Pilzecker (1900). These early investigators noted that memory traces are initially fragile and subsequently become more resistant to disruption by postlearning influences. Subsequent work has thoroughly described the memory consolidation process, and specifically, the role of the amygdala in determining the characteristics of memory consolidation (McGaugh and Cahill, 1997). We suggest that one of the reasons why new, and especially emotional, memories are so susceptible to modulation by posttraining influences is that memories of the experience are a composite of sequentially formed representations that begin in the amygdala and then later come to be represented in the hippocampus.

Finally, numerous studies have shown that the hippocampus is necessary for the retrieval of recently acquired information, but it is not the exclusive site of long-term memory storage (Squire and Zola, 1996, 1997; Eichenbaum, 1997; Anagnostaras et al., 1999). In time, therefore, the hippocampal (and possibly amygdaloid) representations of the emotional experience, with their errors, spliced in components, and fragmented records, would serve as the reference source for the construction of additional (i.e., neocortical) representations of the experience. The hypothesis that there are multiple representations of intense emotional experiences in different brain memory systems may be relevant toward understanding why memories of traumatic events are often intrusive and resistant to extinction.

In closing, comments by Christianson (1992a) are relevant to the thesis we have developed here. He noted that "certain characteristics of emotional events are perceived and retained in an automatic fashion. Thus, it is possible that emotional events are perceived by a preattentive mechanism ... which does not involve consciously controlled processes ... which interact with ... more sophisticated memory mechanisms." We have suggested that the source of the activated preattentive process, as well as the site of preliminary emotional memory storage, is the amygdala. In the aftermath of an emotional experience, the recovery of function by the hippocampus with its "more sophisticated memory mechanisms" subserves the process of filling in memory gaps and provides a means with which the memories of the emotional events can be transferred into long-term storage.

REFERENCES

Abrahám, I., Juhász, G., Kékesi, K.A., and Kovács, K.J. (1996). Effect of intrahippocampal dexamethasone on the levels of amino acid transmitters and neuronal excitability. *Brain Res.* 733: 56–63.

Adolphs, R., Tranel, D., Damasio, H., and Damasio, A.R. (1995). Fear and the human amygdala. *J. Neurosci.* 15: 5879–5891.

Akirav, I., and Richter-Levin, G. (1999). Priming stimulation in the basolateral amygdala modulates synaptic plasticity in the rat dentate gyrus. *Neurosci. Lett.* 270: 83–86.

Akirav, I., and Richter-Levin, G. (in press). Biphasic modulation of hippocampal plasticity by behavioral stress and basolateral amygdala stimulation in the rat. *J. Neurosci.*

Aldenhoff, J.B., Gruol, D.L., Rivier, J., Vale, W. et al. (1983). Corticotropin releasing factor decreases postburst hyperpolarizations and excites hippocampal neurons. *Science* 221: 875–877.

Alvarado, M.C., and Rudy, J.W. (1995). Comparison of "configural" discrimination problems: Implications for understanding the role of the hippocampal formation in learning and memory. *Psychobiology.* 23: 178–184.

Alvarez, P., Zola-Morgan, S., and Squire, L.R. (1994). The animal model of human amnesia: Long-term memory impaired and short-term memory intact. *Proc. Nat. Acad. Sci. USA* 91: 5637–5641.

Alvarez, P., Zola-Morgan, S., and Squire, L.R. (1995). Damage limited to the hippocampal region produces long-lasting memory impairment in monkeys. *J. Neurosci.* 15: 3796–3807.

Anagnostaras, S.G., Maren, S., and Fanselow, M.S. (1999). Temporally graded retrograde amnesia of contextual fear after hippocampal damage in rats: Within-subjects examination. *J. Neurosci.* 19: 1106–1114.

Angelucci, L., and Scaccianoce, S. (1990). Mechanisms in the control of stress responsiveness. *Ann. Ist. Super. Sanita.* 26: 75–78.

Applegate, C.D., Frysinger, R.C., Kapp, B.S., and Gallagher, M. (1982). Multiple unit activity recorded from amygdala central nucleus during Pavlovian heart rate conditioning in rabbit. *Brain Res.* 238: 457–462.

Arbel, I., Kadar, T., Silbermann, M., and Levy, A. (1994). The effects of long-term corticosterone administration on hippocampal morphology and cognitive performance of middle-aged rats. *Brain Res.* 657: 227–235.

Armony, J.L., and LeDoux, J.E. (1997). How the brain processes emotional information. *Ann. NY Acad. Sci.* 821: 259–270.

Armony, J.L., Servan-Schreiber, D., Cohen, J.D., and LeDoux, J.E. (1995). An anatomically constrained neural network model of fear conditioning. *Behav. Neurosci.* 109: 246–257.

Arnsten, A.F. (1997). Catecholamine regulation of the prefrontal cortex. *J. Psychopharmacol.* 11: 151–162.

Aroniadou, V.A., and Teyler, T.J. (1992). Induction of NMDA receptor-independent long-term potentiation (LTP) in visual cortex of adult rats. *Brain Res.* 584: 169–173.

Axelson, D.A., Doraiswamy, P.M., McDonald, W.M., Boyko, O.B. et al. (1993). Hypercortisolemia and hippocampal changes in depression. *Psychiatr. Res.* 47: 163–173.

Bakin, J.S., South, D.A., and Weinberger, N.M. (1996). Induction of receptive field plasticity in the auditory cortex of the guinea pig during instrumental avoidance conditioning. *Behav. Neurosci.* 110: 905–913.

Bannerman, D.M., Good, M.A., Butcher, S.P., Ramsay, M. et al. (1995). Distinct components of spatial learning revealed by prior training and NMDA receptor blockade. *Nature* 378: 182–186.

Barnes, C.A. (1990). Effects of aging on the dynamics of information processing and synaptic weight changes in the mammalian hippocampus. *Prog. Brain Res.* 86: 89–104.

Barnes, C.A., and McNaughton, B.L. (1985). An age comparison of the rates of acquisition and forgetting of spatial information in relation to long-term enhancement of hippocampal synapses. *Behav. Neurosci.* 99: 1040–1048.

Bear, M.F. (1996). A synaptic basis for memory storage in the cerebral cortex. *Proc. Natl. Acad. Sci. USA* 93: 13453–13459.

Becker, J.T., and Olton, D.S. (1981). Cognitive mapping and hippocampal system function. *Neuropsychologia* 19: 733–744.

Bennett, M.C., Diamond, D.M., Fleshner, M., and Rose, G.M. (1991). Serum corticosterone level predicts the magnitude of hippocampal primed burst potentiation and depression in urethane-anesthetized rats. *Psychobiology* 19: 301–307.

Bodnoff, S.R., Humphreys, A.G., Lehman, J.C., Diamond, D.M. et al. (1995). Enduring effects of chronic corticosterone treatment on spatial learning, synaptic plasticity, and hippocampal neuropathology in young and mid-aged rats. *J. Neurosci.* 15: 61–69.

Bohbot, V., Otahal, P., Liu, Z., Nadel, L. et al. (1996). Electroconvulsive shock and lidocaine reveal rapid consolidation of spatial working memory in the water maze. *Proc. Nat. Acad. Sci. USA* 93: 4016–4019.

Bornstein, B.H., Liebel, L.M., and Scarberry, N.C. (1998). Repeated testing in eyewitness memory: A means to improve recall of a negative emotional event. *Appl. Cogn. Psychol.* 12: 119–131.

Bouille, C., and Bayle, J.D. (1973). Effects of limbic stimulations or lesions on basal and stress-induced hypothalamic-pituitary-adrenocortical activity in the pigeon. *Neuroendocrinology* 13: 264–277.

Brady, L.S., Lynn, A.B., Whitfield, H.J. Jr., Kim, H. et al. (1992). Intrahippocampal colchicine alters hypothalamic corticotropin- releasing hormone and hippocampal steroid receptor mRNA in rat brain. *Neuroendocrinology* 55: 121–133.

Bramham, C.R., Southard, T., Ahlers, S.T., and Sarvey, J.M. (1998). Acute cold stress leading to elevated corticosterone neither enhances synaptic efficacy nor impairs LTP in the dentate gyrus of freely moving rats. *Brain Res.* 789: 245–255.

Brandeis, R., Brandys, Y., and Yehuda, S. (1989). The use of the Morris water maze in the study of memory and learning. *Int. J. Neurosci.* 48: 29–69.

Breindl, A., Derrick, B.E., Rodriguez, S.B., and Martinez, J.L., Jr. (1994). Opioid receptor-dependent long-term potentiation at the lateral perforant path-CA3 synapse in rat hippocampus. *Brain Res. Bull.* 33: 17–24.

Bremner, J.D., Krystal, J.H., Southwick, S.M., and Charney, D.S. (1995). Functional neuroanatomical correlates of the effects of stress on memory. *J. Traum. Stress* 8: 527–553.

Bremner, J.D., Krystal, J.H., Charney, D.S., and Southwick, S.M. (1996). Neural mechanisms in dissociative amnesia for childhood abuse: Relevance to the current controversy surrounding the "false memory syndrome". *Am. J. Psychiatr.* 153: 71–82.

Bunsey, M., and Eichenbaum, H. (1996). Conservation of hippocampal memory function in rats and humans. *Nature* 379: 255–257.

Burke, A., Heuer, F., and Reisberg, D. (1992). Remembering emotional events. *Memory Cogn.* 20: 277–290.

Cahill, L. (1997). The neurobiology of emotionally influenced memory. Implications for understanding traumatic memory. *Ann. NY Acad. Sci.* 821: 238–246.

Cahill, L., and McGaugh, J.L. (1996). Modulation of memory storage. *Curr. Opin. Neurobiol.* 6: 237–242.

Cahill, L., Weinberger, N.M., Roozendaal, B., and McGaugh, J.L. (1999). Is the amygdala a locus of conditioned fear? Some questions and caveats. *Neuron* 23: 227–228.

Cassaday, H.J., and Rawlins, J.N. (1997). The hippocampus, objects, and their contexts. *Behav. Neurosci.* 111: 1228–1244.

Chapman, P.F., and Bellavance, L.L. (1992). Induction of long-term potentiation in the basolateral amygdala does not depend on NMDA receptor activation. *Synapse* 11: 310–318.

Chapman, P.F., Kairiss, E.W., Keenan, C.L., and Brown, T.H. (1990). Long-term synaptic potentiation in the amygdala. *Synapse* 6: 271–278.

Chiba, A.A., Kesner, R.P., and Reynolds, A.M. (1994). Memory for spatial location as a function of temporal lag in rats: Role of hippocampus and medial prefrontal cortex. *Behav. Neural Biol.* 61: 123–131.

Christianson, S.A. (1992a). Do flashbulb memories differ from other types of memories? In E Winograd and U. Neisser (Eds.), *Affect and accuracy in recall: Studies of "flashbulb" memories* (pp. 191–211). New York: Cambridge University Press.

Christianson, S.A. (1992b). Emotional-stress and eyewitness memory—a critical-review. *Psycho. Bull.* 112: 284–309.

Clugnet, M.C., and LeDoux, J.E. (1990). Synaptic plasticity in fear conditioning circuits: Induction of LTP in the lateral nucleus of the amygdala by stimulation of the medial geniculate body. *J. Neurosci.* 10: 2818–2824.

Cohen, N.J., and Eichenbaum, H. (1993). *Memory, Amnesia, and the Hippocampal System.* Cambridge, MA: MIT Press.

Conrad, C.D., Galea, L.A.M., Kuroda, Y., and McEwen, B.S. (1996). Chronic stress impairs rat spatial memory on the Y maze, and this effect is blocked by tianeptine pretreatment. *Behav. Neurosci.* 110: 1321–1334.

Corradetti, R., Ballerini, L., Pugliese, A.M., and Pepeu, G. (1992). Serotonin blocks the long-term potentiation induced by primed burst stimulation in the CA1 region of rat hippocampal slices. *Neuroscience* 46: 511–518.

Davis, M. (1992). The role of the amygdala in fear and anxiety. *Ann. Rev. Neurosci.* 15: 353–375.

Davis, M. (1994). The role of the amygdala in emotional learning. *Int. Rev. Neurobiol.* 36: 225–266.

de Quervain, D.J., Roozendaal, B., and McGaugh, J.L. (1998). Stress and glucocorticoids impair retrieval of long-term spatial memory. *Nature* 394: 787–790.

Derrick, B.E., Rodriguez, S.B., Lieberman, D.N., and Martinez, J.L., Jr. (1992). Mu opioid receptors are associated with the induction of hippocampal mossy fiber long-term potentiation. *J. Pharmacol. Exp. Ther.* 263: 725–733.

Diamond, D.M., and Rose, G.M. (1994). Stress impairs LTP and hippocampal-dependent memory. *Ann. NY Acad. Sci.* 746: 411–414.

Diamond, D.M., and Weinberger, N.M. (1984). Physiological plasticity of single neurons in auditory cortex of the cat during acquisition of the pupillary conditioned response: II. Secondary field (AII). *Behav. Neurosci.* 98: 189–210.

Diamond, D.M., Dunwiddie, T.V., and Rose, G.M. (1988). Characteristics of hippocampal primed burst potentiation in vitro and in the awake rat. *J. Neurosci.* 8: 4079–4088.

Diamond, D.M., Bennett, M.C., Stevens, K.E., Wilson, R.L. et al. (1990). Exposure to a novel environment interferes with the induction of hippocampal primed burst potentiation. *Psychobiology* 18: 273–281.

Diamond, D.M., Bennett, M.C., Fleshner, M., and Rose, G.M. (1992). Inverted-U relationship between the level of peripheral corticosterone and the magnitude of hippocampal primed burst potentiation. *Hippocampus* 2: 421–430.

Diamond, D.M., Fleshner, M., and Rose, G.M. (1994). Psychological stress repeatedly blocks hippocampal primed burst potentiation in behaving rats. *Behav. Brain Res.* 62: 1–9.

Diamond, D.M., Branch, B.J., Fleshner, M., and Rose, G.M. (1995). Effects of dehydroepiandrosterone sulfate and stress on hippocampal electrophysiological plasticity. *Ann. NY Acad. Sci.* 774: 304–307.

Diamond, D.M., Branch, B.J., and Fleshner, M. (1996a). The neurosteroid dehydroepiandrosterone sulfate (DHEAS) enhances hippocampal primed burst, but not long-term, potentiation. *Neurosci. Lett.* 202: 204–208.

Diamond, D.M., Fleshner, M., Ingersoll, N., and Rose, G.M. (1996b). Psychological stress impairs spatial working memory: Relevance to electrophysiological studies of hippocampal function. *Behavi. Neurosci.* 110: 661–672.

Diamond, D.M., Ingersoll, N., Branch, B.J., Mesches, M.H. et al. (1998). Stress impairs cognitive and electrophysiological measures of hippocampal function. In A. Levy, E. Grauer, D. Ben-Nathan, and E.R. de Kloet (Eds.), *New frontiers in stress research: Modulation of brain function* (pp. 117–126). Amsterdam: Harwood Academic.

Diamond, D.M., Park, C.R., Heman, K.L., and Rose, G.M. (1999). Exposure to a predator impairs spatial working memory in the radial arm water maze. *Hippocampus* 9: 542–552.

Diamond, D.M., Fleshner, M., and Rose, G.M. (in press). The enhancement of hippocampal primed burst potentiation by dehydroepiandrosterone sulfate (DHEAS) is blocked by psychological stress. *Stress.*

Doron, N.N., and LeDoux, J.E. (1999). Organization of projections to the lateral amygdala from auditory and visual areas of the thalamus in the rat. *J. Comp Neurol.* 412: 383–409.

Dunn, J.D., and Orr, S.E. (1984). Differential plasma corticosterone responses to hippocampal stimulation. *Exp. Brain Res.* 54: 1–6.

Easterbrook, J.A. (1959). The effect of emotion on the utilisation and the organisation of behavior. *Psychol. Rev.* 66: 183–201.

Edeline, J.M. (1999). Learning-induced physiological plasticity in the thalamo-cortical sensory systems: A critical evaluation of receptive field plasticity, map changes and their potential mechanisms. *Prog. Neurobiol.* 57: 165–224.

Edeline, J.M., and Weinberger, N.M. (1992). Associative retuning in the thalamic source of input to the amygdala and auditory cortex: Receptive field plasticity in the medial division of the medial geniculate body. *Behav. Neurosci.* 106: 81–105.

Eichenbaum, H. (1997). Declarative memory: Insights from cognitive neurobiology. *Annu. Rev. Psychol.* 48: 547–572.

Eichenbaum, H., Mathews, P., and Cohen, N.J. (1989). Further studies of hippocampal representation during odor discrimination learning. *Behav. Neurosci.* 103: 1207–1216.

Ely, D.L., Greene, E.G., and Henry, J.P. (1977). Effects of hippocampal lesion on cardiovascular, adrenocortical and behavioral response patterns in mice. *Physiol. Behav.* 18: 1075–1083.

Fanselow, M.S., and LeDoux, J.E. (1999). Why we think plasticity underlying Pavlovian fear conditioning occurs in the basolateral amygdala. *Neuron* 23: 229–232.

Feldman, S., and Conforti, N. (1979). Effect of dorsal hippocampectomy or fimbria section on adrenocortical responses in rats. *Isr. J. Med. Sci.* 15: 539–541.

Feldman, S., and Conforti, N. (1980). Participation of the dorsal hippocampus in the glucocorticoid feedback effect on adrenocortical activity. *Neuroendocrinology* 30: 52–55.

Foy, M.R., Stanton, M.E. Levine, S., and Thompson, R.F. (1987). Behavioral stress impairs long-term potentiation in rodent hippocampus. *Behav. Neural Biol.* 48: 138–149.

Garcia, R., Musleh, W., Tocco, G., Thompson, R.F. et al. (1997a). Time-dependent blockade of STP and LTP in hippocampal slices following acute stress in mice. *Neurosci. Lett.* 233: 41–44.

Garcia, R., Vouimba, R.M., and Jaffard, R. (1997b). Contextual conditioned fear blocks the induction but not the maintenance of lateral septal LTP in behaving mice. *J. Neurophysiol.* 78: 76–81.

Garcia, R., Paquereau, J., Vouimba, R.M., and Jaffard, R. (1998a). Footshock stress but not contextual fear conditioning induces long-term enhancement of auditory-evoked potentials in the basolateral amygdala of the freely behaving rat. *Eur. J. Neurosci.* 10: 457–463.

Garcia, R., Tocco, G., Baudry, M., and Thompson, R.F. (1998b). Exposure to a conditioned aversive environment interferes with long-term potentiation induction in the fimbria-CA3 pathway. *Neuroscience* 82: 139–145.

Gerlach, J.L., and McEwen, B.S. (1971). Rat brain binds adrenal steroid hormone: Radioautography of hippocampus with corticosterone. *Science* 175: 1133–1136.

Gerren, R.A., and Weinberger, N.M. (1983). Long term potentiation in the magnocellular medial geniculate nucleus of the anesthetized cat. *Brain Res.* 265: 138–142.

Gold, P.E., and Van Buskirk, R.B. (1975). Facilitation of time-dependent memory processes with posttrial epinephrine injections. *Behav. Biol.* 13: 145–153.

Gold, P.E., and van Buskirk, R. (1976). Enhancement and impairment of memory processes with posttrial injections of adrenocorticotropic hormone. *Behav. Biol.* 16: 387–400.

Gold, P.E., Delanoy, R.L., and Merrin, J. (1984). Modulation of long-term potentiation by peripherally administered amphetamine and epinephrine. *Brain. Res.* 305: 103–107.

Grillon, C., Southwick, S.M., and Charney, D.S. (1996). The psychobiological basis of post-traumatic stress disorder. *Mol. Psychiatr.* 1: 278–297.

Hamann, S.B., Cahill, L., McGaugh, J.L., and Squire, L.R. (1997a). Intact enhancement of declarative memory for emotional material in amnesia. *Learn. Mem.* 4: 301–309.

Hamann, S.B., Cahill, L., and Squire, L.R. (1997b). Emotional perception and memory in amnesia. *Neuropsychology* 11: 104–113.

Henke, P.G. (1982). The telencephalic limbic system and experimental gastric pathology: A review. *Neurosci. Biobehav. Rev.* 6: 381–390.

Henke, P.G. (1989). Synaptic efficacy in the entorhinal-dentate pathway and stress ulcers in rats. *Neurosci. Lett.* 107: 110–113.

Henke, P.G. (1990a). Hippocampal pathway to the amygdala and stress ulcer development. *Brain Res. Bull.* 25: 691–695.

Henke, P.G. (1990b). Potentiation of inputs from the posterolateral amygdala to the dentate gyrus and resistance to stress ulcers formation in rats. *Physiol. Behav.* 48: 659–664.

Henke, P.G. (1992). Naloxone-sensitive potentiation at granule cell synapses in the ventral dentate gyrus and stress ulcers. *Physiol. Behav.* 51: 823–826.

Herbert, J. (1998). Neurosteroids, brain damage, and mental illness. *Exp. Gerontol.* 33: 713–727.

Hesen, W., and Joels, M. (1996). Modulation of 5HT1A responsiveness in CA1 pyramidal neurons by in vivo activation of corticosteroid receptors. *J. Neuroendocrinol.* 8: 433–438.

Hölscher, C. (1997). Long-term potentiation: A good model for learning and memory? *Prog. Neuropsychopharmacol. Biol. Psychiatr.* 21: 47–68.

Hölscher, C. (1999). Stress impairs performance in spatial water maze learning tasks. *Behav. Brain Res.* 100: 225–235.

Hölscher, C., Anwyl, R., and Rowan, M. (1997a). Block of HFS-induced LTP in the dentate gyrus by 1S,3S-ACPD: Further evidence against LTP as a model for learning. *NeuroReport* 8: 451–454.

Hölscher, C., McGlinchey, L, Anwyl, R., and Rowan, M.J. (1997b). HFS-induced long-term potentiation and LFS-induced depotentiation in area CA1 of the hippocampus are not good models for learning. *Psychopharmacology* 130: 174–182.

Hölscher, C., Anwyl, R., and Rowan, M.J. (1997c). Block of theta-burst-induced long-term potentiation by (1S,3S)-1-aminocyclopentane-1,3-dicarboxylic acid: Further evidence against long-term potentiation as a model for learning. *Neuroscience* 81: 17–22.

Hölscher, C., McGlinchey, L., and Rowan, M.J. (1996). L-AP4 (L-(+)-2-amino-4-phospho-nobutyric acid) induced impairment of spatial learning in the rat is antagonized by MAP4 ((S)-2-amino-2-methyl-4-phosphonobutanoic acid). *Behav. Brain Res.* 81: 69–79.

Ikegaya, Y., Abe, K., Saito, H., and Nishiyama, N. (1995a). Medial amygdala enhances synaptic transmission and synaptic plasticity in the dentate gyrus of rats in vivo. *J. Neurophysiol.* 74: 2201–2203.

Ikegaya, Y., Saito, H., and Abe, K. (1995b). Amygdala N-methyl-D-aspartate receptors participate in the induction of long-term potentiation in the dentate gyrus in vivo. *Neurosci. Lett.* 192: 193–196.

Ikegaya, Y., Saito, H., and Abe, K. (1995c). High-frequency stimulation of the basolateral amygdala facilitates the induction of long-term potentiation in the dentate gyrus in vivo. *Neurosc. Res.* 22: 203–207.

Ikegaya, Y., Saito, H., and Abe, K. (1996). The basomedial and basolateral amygdaloid nuclei contribute to the induction of long-term potentiation in the dentate gyrus in vivo. *Eur. J. Neurosci.* 8: 1833–1839.

Izquierdo, I., and Medina, J.H. (1997). Memory formation: The sequence of biochemical events in the hippocampus and its connection to activity in other brain structures. *Neurobiol. Learn. Mem.* 68: 285–316.

Jacobs, W.J., and Nadel, L. (1985). Stress-induced recovery of fears and phobias. *Psych. Rev.* 92: 512–531.

Joels, M., and de Kloet, E.R. (1989). Effects of glucocorticoids and norepinephrine on the excitability in the hippocampus. *Science* 245: 1502–1505.

Joëls, M., and de Kloet, E.R. (1992). Coordinative mineralocorticoid and glucocorticoid receptor-mediated control of responses of serotonin in rat hippocampus. *Neuroendocrinology* 55: 344–350.

Joels, M., Hesen, W., and de Kloet, E.R. (1995). Long-term control of neuronal excitability by corticosteroid hormones. *J. Steroid Biochem. Mol. Biol.* 53: 315–323.

Karten, Y.J.G., Slagter, E., and Joels, M. (1999). Effect of long-term elevated corticosteroid levels on field responses to synaptic stimulation, in the rat CA1 hippocampal area. *Neurosci. Lett.* 265: 41–44.

Keenan, P.A., Jacobson, M.W., Soleymani, R.M., and Newcomer, J.W. (1995). Commonly used therapeutic doses of glucocorticoids impair explicit memory. *Ann. NY Acad. Sci.* 761: 400–402.

Kesner, R.P., Hunt, M.E., Williams, J.M., and Long, J.M. (1996). Prefrontal cortex and working memory for spatial response, spatial location, and visual object information in the rat. *Cereb. Cortex* 6: 311–318.

Kim, J.J., and Yoon, K.S. (1998). Stress: Metaplastic effects in the hippocampus. *Trends Neurosci.* 21: 505–509.

Kim, J.J., Rison, R.A., and Fanselow, M.S. (1993). Effects of amygdala, hippocampus, and periaqueductal gray lesions on short- and long-term contextual fear. *Behav. Neurosci.* 107: 1093–1098.

Kim, J.J., Foy, M.R., and Thompson, R.F. (1996). Behavioral stress modifies hippocampal plasticity through N-methyl-D-aspartate receptor activation. *Proc. Natl. Acad. Sci. USA* 93: 4750–4753.

Kirschbaum, C., Wolf, O.T., May, M., Wippich, W. et al. (1996). Stress- and treatment-induced elevations of cortisol levels associated with impaired declarative memory in healthy adults. *Life Sci.* 58: 1475–1483.

Knigge, K.M., and Hays, M. (1963). Evidence of inhibitive role of hippocampus in neural regulation of ACTH release. *Proc. Soc. Exp. Biol. Med.* 114: 67–69.

Koss, M.P., Tromp, S., and Tharan, M. (1995). Traumatic memories—empirical foundations, forensic and clinical implications. *Clin. Psychol. Sci. Pract.* 2: 111–132.

Kramer, T.H., Buckhout, R., Fox, P., Widman, E. et al. (1991). Effects of stress on recall. *Appl. Cogn. Psychol.* 5: 483–488.

Kudoh, M., and Shibuki, K. (1997). Comparison of long-term potentiation between the auditory and visual cortices. *Acta Otolaryngol. (Stockh.)* 532: 109–111.

LaBar, K.S., LeDoux, J.E., Spencer, D.D., and Phelps, E.A. (1995). Impaired fear conditioning following unilateral temporal lobectomy in humans. *J. Neurosci.* 15: 6846–6855.

Larson, J., and Lynch, G. (1986). Induction of synaptic potentiation in hippocampus by patterned stimulation involves two events. *Science* 232: 985–988.

Larson, J., Wong, D., and Lynch, G. (1986). Patterned stimulation at the theta frequency is optimal for the induction of hippocampal long-term potentiation. *Brain Res.* 368: 347–350.

LeDoux, J.E. (1993). Emotional memory: In search of systems and synapses. *Ann. NY Acad. Sci.* 702: 149–157.

LeDoux, J.E., Sakaguchi, A., Iwata, J., and Reis, D.J. (1985). Auditory emotional memories: Establishment by projections from the medial geniculate nucleus to the posterior neostriatum and/or dorsal amygdala. *Ann. NY Acad. Sci.* 444: 463–464.

LeDoux, J.E., Farb, C.R., and Romanski, L.M. (1991). Overlapping projections to the amygdala and striatum from auditory processing areas of the thalamus and cortex. *Neurosci. Lett.* 134: 139–144.

Lennartz, R.C., and Weinberger, N.M. (1992). Frequency-specific receptive field plasticity in the medial geniculate body induced by Pavlovian fear conditioning is expressed in the anesthetized brain. *Behav. Neurosci.* 106: 484–497.

Li, H., Weiss, S.R., Chuang, D.M., Post, R.M. et al. (1998). Bidirectional synaptic plasticity in the rat basolateral amygdala: Characterization of an activity-dependent switch sensitive to the presynaptic metabotropic glutamate receptor antagonist 2S-alpha-ethylglutamic acid. *J. Neurosci.* 18: 1662–1670.

Liang, K.C., McGaugh, J.L., Martinez, J.L. Jr., Jensen, R.A. et al. (1982). Post-training amygdaloid lesions impair retention of an inhibitory avoidance response. *Behav. Brain Res.* 4: 237–249.

Loftus, E.F., and Burns, T.E. (1982). Mental shock can produce retrograde amnesia. *Mem. Cogn.* 10: 318–323.

Luine, V., Villegas, M., Martinez, C., and McEwen, B.S. (1994). Repeated stress causes reversible impairments of spatial memory performance. *Brain Res.* 639: 167–170.

Lupien, S.J., Gaudreau, S., Tchiteya, B.M., Maheu, F. et al. (1997). Stress-induced declarative memory impairment healthy elderly subjects: Relationship to cortisol reactivity. *J. Clin. Endocrinol. Metab.* 82: 2070–2075.

Lupien, S.J., Nair, N.P.V., Briere, S., Maheu, F. et al. (1999). Increased cortisol levels and impaired cognition in human aging: Implication for depression and dementia in later life. *Rev. Neurosci.* 10: 117–139.

Maren, S. (1996). Synaptic transmission and plasticity in the amygdala. An emerging physiology of fear conditioning circuits. *Mol. Neurobiol.* 13: 1–22.

Maren, S., and Fanselow, M.S. (1995). Synaptic plasticity in the basolateral amygdala induced by hippocampal formation stimulation in vivo. *J. Neurosci.* 15: 7548–7564.

Maren, S., and Fanselow, M.S. (1996). The amygdala and fear conditioning: Has the nut been cracked? *Neuron* 16: 237–240.

Martinez, J.L., Jr., and Derrick, B.E. (1996). Long-term potentiation and learning. *Annu. Rev. Psychol.* 47: 173–203.

McCarthy, G., Puce, A., Constable, R.T., Krystal, J.H. et al. (1996). Activation of human prefrontal cortex during spatial and nonspatial working memory tasks measured by functional MRI. *Cereb. Cortex* 6: 600–611.

McCarty, R., and Gold, P.E. (1981). Plasma catecholamines: Effects of footshock level and hormonal modulators of memory storage. *Horm. Behav.* 15: 168–182.

McEwen, B.S., Cameron, H., Chao, H.M., Gould, E. et al. (1994). Resolving a mystery: Progress in understanding the function of adrenal steroid receptors in hippocampus. *Prog. Brain Res.* 100: 149–155.

McGaugh, J.L., and Cahill, L. (1997). Interaction of neuromodulatory systems in modulating memory storage. *Behav. Brain Res.* 83: 31–38.

McGaugh, J.L., Introini-Collison, I.B., Nagahara, A.H., Cahill, L. et al. (1990). Involvement of the amygdaloid complex in neuromodulatory influences on memory storage. *Neurosci. Biobehav. Rev.* 14: 425–431.

McGaugh, J.L., Cahill, L., and Roozendaal, B. (1996). Involvement of the amygdala in memory storage: Interaction with other brain systems. *Proc. Natl. Acad. Sci. USA* 93: 13508–13514.

McKernan, M.G., and Shinnick-Gallagher, P. (1997). Fear conditioning induces a lasting potentiation of synaptic currents in vitro [see comments]. *Nature* 390: 607–611.

Meck, W.H., Church, R.M., and Olton, D.S. (1984). Hippocampus, time, and memory. *Behav. Neurosci.* 98: 3–22.

Mesches, M.H., Fleshner, M., Heman, K.L., Rose, G.M. et al. (1999). Exposing rats to a predator blocks primed burst potentiation in the hippocampus in vitro. *J. Neurosci.* 19 (RC18): 1–5.

Metcalfe, J., and Jacobs, W.J. (1998). Emotional memory: The effects of stress on "cool" and "hot" memory systems. *Psychcol. Learn. Motiv.* 38: 187–222.

Moore, C.I., Browning, M.D., and Rose, G.M. (1993). Hippocampal plasticity induced by primed burst, but not long-term potentiation, stimulation is impaired in area CA1 of aged Fischer 344 rats. *Hippocampus* 3: 57–66.

Morris, R.G. (1989). Synaptic plasticity and learning: Selective impairment of learning rats and blockade of long-term potentiation in vivo by the N-methyl-D-aspartate receptor antagonist AP5. *J. Neurosci.* 9: 3040–3057.

Morris, R.G., and Frey, U. (1997). Hippocampal synaptic plasticity: Role in spatial learning or the automatic recording of attended experience? *Philos. Trans. R. Soc. London Ser. B Biol. Sci.* 352: 1489–1503.

Morris, R.G., Anderson, E., Lynch, G.S., and Baudry, M. (1986). Selective impairment of learning and blockade of long-term potentiation by an N-methyl-D-aspartate receptor antagonist, AP5. *Nature* 319: 774–776.

Mueller, G.E., and Pilzecker, A. (1900). Experimentelle Beiträge zur Lehre vom Gedächtniss. *Z. Psychol.* 1: 1–288.

Nadel, L., and Jacobs, W.J. (1998). Traumatic memory is special. *Curr. Direct. Psychol. Sci.* 7: 154–157.

Neisser, U. (1997). The ecological study of memory. *Philos. Trans. R. Soc. London B Biol. Sci.* 352: 1697–1701.

Neisser, U., and Harsch, N. (1992). Phantom flashbulbs: False recollections of hearing the news about Challenger. In E. Winograd and U. Neisser, (Eds.), *Affect and accuracy in recall: Studies of flashbulb memories* (pp. 9–31). New York: Cambridge University Press.

Newcomer, J.W., Craft, S., Hershey, T., Askins, K. et al. (1994). Glucocorticoid-induced impairment in declarative memory performance in adult humans. *J. Neurosci.* 14: 2047–2053.

Newcomer, J.W., Selke, G., Melson, A.K., Hershey, T. et al. (1999). Decreased memory performance in healthy humans induced by stress-level cortisol treatment. *Arch. Gen. Psychiatr.* 56: 527–533.

O'Brien, J.T., Ames, D., Schweitzer, I., Colman, P. et al. (1996). Clinical and magnetic resonance imaging correlates of hypothalamic-pituitary-adrenal axis function in depression and Alzheimer's disease. *Br. J. Psychiatr.* 168: 679–687.

O'Keefe, J., and Nadel, L. (1978). *The Hippocampus as a Cognitive Map*. Oxford: Oxford University Press.

Olton, D.S., Becker, J.T., and Handelmann, G.E. (1979). Hippocampus, space, and memory. *Behav. Brain Sci.* 2: 313–365.

Packard, M.G., and Teather, L.A. (1998). Amygdala modulation of multiple memory systems: Hippocampus and caudate- putamen. *Neurobiol. Learn. Mem.* 69: 163–203.

Packard, M.G., Cahill, L., and McGaugh, J.L. (1994). Amygdala modulation of hippocampal-dependent and caudate nucleus-dependent memory processes. *Proc. Natl. Acad. Sci. USA* 91: 8477–8481.

Pascoe, J.P., and Kapp, B.S. (1985). Electrophysiological characteristics of amygdaloid central nucleus neurons during Pavlovian fear conditioning in the rabbit. *Behav. Brain Res.* 16: 117–133.

Pavlides, C., Watanabe, Y., and McEwen, B.S. (1993). Effects of glucocorticoids on hippocampal long-term potentiation. *Hippocampus* 3: 183–192.

Pavlides, C., Ogawa, S., Kimura, A., and McEwen, B.S. (1996). Role of adrenal steroid mineralocorticoid and glucocorticoid receptors in long-term potentiation in the CA1 field of hippocampal slices. *Brain Res.* 738: 229–235.

Pfaff, D.W., Silva, M.T.A., and Weiss, J.M. (1971). Telemetered recording of hormone effects on hippocampal neurons. *Science* 172: 394–395.

Phillips, R.G., and LeDoux, J.E. (1992). Differential contribution of amygdala and hippocampus to cued and contextual fear conditioning. *Behav. Neurosci.* 106: 274–285.

Phillips, R.G., and LeDoux, J.E. (1994). Lesions of the dorsal hippocampal formation interfere with background but not foreground contextual fear conditioning. *Learn. Mem.* 1: 34–44.

Poremba, A., and Gabriel, M. (1999). Amygdala neurons mediate acquisition but not maintenance of instrumental avoidance behavior in rabbits. *J. Neurosci.* 19: 9635–9641.

Quirarte, G.L., Roozendaal, B., and McGaugh, J.L. (1997). Glucocorticoid enhancement of memory storage involves noradrenergic activation in the basolateral amygdala. *Proc. Natl. Acad. Sci. USA* 94: 14048–14053.

Quirk, G.J., Repa, C., and LeDoux, J.E. (1995). Fear conditioning enhances short-latency auditory responses of lateral amygdala neurons: Parallel recordings in the freely behaving rat. *Neuron* 15: 1029–1039.

Reisberg, D., and Heuer, F. (1992). Remembering the details of emotional events. In E. Winograd and U. Neisser (Eds.), *Affect and accuracy in recall: Studies of "flashbulb" memories.* (pp. 162–190). New York: Cambridge University Press.

Reul, J.M., and de Kloet, E.R. (1985). Two receptor systems for corticosterone in rat brain: Microdistribution and differential occupation. *Endocrinology* 117: 2505–2511.

Rey, M., Carlier, E., and Soumireu-Mourat, B. (1987). Effects of corticosterone on hippocampal slice electrophysiology in normal and adrenalectomized BALB/c mice. *Neuroendocrinology* 46: 424–429.

Rey, M., Carlier, E., Talmi, M., and Soumireu-Mourat, B. (1994). Corticosterone effects on long-term potentiation in mouse hippocampal slices. *Neuroendocrinology* 60: 36–41.

Rogan, M.T., and LeDoux, J.E. (1995). LTP is accompanied by commensurate enhancement of auditory-evoked responses in a fear conditioning circuit. *Neuron* 15: 127–136.

Rogan, M.T., and LeDoux, J.E. (1996). Emotion: Systems, cells, synaptic plasticity. *Cell* 85: 469–475.

Rogan, M.T., Staubli, U.V., and LeDoux, J.E. (1997). Fear conditioning induces associative long-term potentiation in the amygdala. *Nature* 390: 604–607.

Romanski, L.M., and LeDoux, J.E. (1993). Information cascade from primary auditory cortex to the amygdala: Corticocortical and corticoamygdaloid projections of temporal cortex in the rat. *Cereb. Cortex* 3: 515–532.

Rose, G.M., and Dunwiddie, T.V. (1986). Induction of hippocampal long-term potentiation using physiologically patterned stimulation. *Neurosci. Lett.* 69: 244–248.

Rowan, M.J., Anwyl, R., and Xu, L. (1998). Stress and long-term synaptic depression. *Mol. Psychiatr.* 3: 472–474.

Safer, M.A., Christianson, S.A., Autry, M.W., and Osterlund, K. (1998). Tunnel memory for traumatic events. *Appl. Cogn. Psychol.* 12: 99–117.

Sandi, C., and Rose, S.P.R. (1994). Corticosterone enhances long-term retention in one-day-old chicks trained in a weak passive avoidance learning paradigm. *Brain Res.* 647: 106–112.

Sandi, C., Loscertales, M., and Guaza, C. (1997). Experience-dependent facilitating effect of corticosterone on spatial memory formation in the water maze. *Eur. J. Neurosci.* 9: 637–642.

Sapolsky, R.M., Meaney, M.J., and McEwen, B.S. (1985). The development of the glucocorticoid receptor system in the rat limbic brain. III. Negative-feedback regulation. *Brain Res.* 350: 169–173.

Sapolsky, R.M., Zola-Morgan, S., and Squire, L.R. (1991). Inhibition of glucocorticoid secretion by the hippocampal formation in the primate. *J. Neurosci.* 11: 3695–3704.

Sarter, M., and Markowitsch, H.J. (1985). Involvement of the amygdala in learning and memory: A critical review, with emphasis on anatomical relations. *Behav. Neurosci.* 99: 342–380.

Saucier, D., and Cain, D.P. (1995). Spatial learning without NMDA receptor-dependent long-term potentiation. *Nature* 378: 186–189.

Segal, M. (1976). Interactions of ACTH and norepinephrine on the activity of rat hippocampal cells. *Neuropharmacology* 15: 329–333.

Shors, T.J., and Matzel, L.D. (1997). Long-term potentiation: What's learning got to do with it? *Behav. Brain Sci.* 20: 597–614.

Shors, T.J., Seib, T.B., Levine, S., and Thompson, R.F. (1989). Inescapable versus escapable shock modulates long-term potentiation in the rat hippocampus. *Science* 244: 224–226.

Shors, T.J., Gallegos, R.A., and Breindl, A. (1997). Transient and persistent consequences of acute stress on long-term potentiation (LTP), synaptic efficacy, theta rhythms and bursts in area CA1 of the hippocampus. *Synapse* 26: 209–217.

Siggins, G.R., Gruol, D., Aldenhoff, J., and Pittman, Q. (1985). Electrophysiological actions of corticotropin-releasing factor in the central nervous system. *Fed. Proc.* 44: 237–242.

Smriga, M., Nishiyama, N., and Saito, H. (1998). Mineralocorticoid receptor-mediated enhancement of neuronal excitability and synaptic plasticity in the dentate gyrus in vivo is dependent on the beta-adrenergic activity. *J. Neurosci. Res.* 51: 593–601.

Squire, L.R., and Zola, S.M. (1996). Structure and function of declarative and nondeclarative memory systems. *Proc. Natl. Acad. Sci. USA* 93: 13515–13522.

Squire, L.R., and Zola, S.M. (1997). Amnesia, memory and brain systems. *Philos. Trans. R. Soc. London [Biol.]* 352: 1663–1673.

Starkman, M.N., Gebarski, S.S., Berent, S., and Schteingart, D.E. (1992). Hippocampal formation volume, memory dysfunction, and cortisol levels in patients with Cushing's syndrome. *Biol. Psychiatr.* 32: 756–765.

Staubli, U., Scafidi, J., and Chun, D. (1999). GABAB receptor antagonism: Facilitatory effects on memory parallel those on LTP induced by TBS but not HFS. *J. Neurosci.* 19: 4609–4615.

Steele, R.J., and Morris, R.G.M. (1999). Delay-dependent impairment of a matching-to-place task with chronic and intrahippocampal infusion of the NMDA-antagonist D-AP5. *Hippocampus* 9: 118–136.

Talmi, M., Carlier, E., Rey, M., and Soumireu-Mourat, B. (1992). Modulation of the in vitro electrophysiological effect of corticosterone by extracellular calcium in the hippocampus. *Neuroendocrinology* 55: 257–263.

Talmi, M., Carlier, E., and Soumireu-Mourat, B. (1993). Similar effects of aging and corticosterone treatment on mouse hippocampal function. *Neurobiology Aging* 14: 239–244.

Trifiletti, R.R., and Pranzatelli, M.R. (1992). ACTH binds to [3H]MK-801-labelled rat hippocampal NMDA receptors. *Eur. J. Pharmacol. Mol. Pharmacol.* 226: 377–379.

Vidal, C., Jordan, W., and Zieglgansberger, W. (1986). Corticosterone reduces the excitability of hippocampal pyramidal cells in vitro. *Brain Res.* 383: 54–59.

Voronin, L., Byzov, A., Kleschevnikov, A., Kozhemyakin, M. et al. (1995). Neurophysiological analysis of long-term potentiation in mammalian brain. *Behav. Brain Res.* 66: 45–52.

van der Kolk, B.A. and Fisler, R. (1994). Dissociation and the fragmentary nature of traumatic memories: Overview and exploratory study. *J. Traumatic Stress.* 8: 525.

Wachtel, P.L. (1968). Anxiety, attention, and coping with threat. *J. Abnorm. Psychol.* 73: 137–143.

Warren, D.A., Castro, C.A., Rudy, J.W., and Maier, S.F. (1991). No spatial learning impairment following exposure to inescapable shock. *Psychobiology* 19: 127–134.

Watanabe, Y., Ikegaya, Y., Saito, H., and Abe, K. (1995). Roles of GABAA, NMDA and muscarinic receptors in induction of long-term potentiation in the medial and lateral amygdala in vitro. *Neurosci. Res.* 21: 317–322.

Weinberger, N.M., and Diamond, D.M. (1987). Physiological plasticity in auditory cortex: Rapid induction by learning. *Prog. Neurobiol.* 29: 1–55.

Weltman, G., and Egstrom, G.H. (1966). Perceptual narrowing in novice divers. *Hum. Factors* 8: 499–506.

Whishaw, I.Q. (1985). Formation of a place learning-set by the rat: A new paradigm for neurobehavioral studies. *Physiol. Behav.* 35: 139–143.

Xu, L., Anwyl, R., and Rowan, M.J. (1997). Behavioural stress facilitates the induction of long-term depression in the hippocampus. *Nature* 387: 497–500.

Xu, L., Hölscher, C., Anwyl, R., and Rowan, M.J. (1998). Glucocorticoid receptor and protein/RNA synthesis-dependent mechanisms underlie the control of synaptic plasticity by stress. *Proc. Natl. Acad. Sci. USA* 95: 3204–3208.

Zador, A., Koch, C., and Brown, T.H. (1990). Biophysical model of a Hebbian synapse. *Proc. Natl. Acad. Sci. USA* 87: 6718–6722.

Transgenic Mice as Tools to Unravel the Mechanisms of Memory Formation

CHAPTER SEVENTEEN

In Vivo Recording of Single Hippocampal Place Cells in Behaving Transgenic Mice

Yoon H. Cho and Howard B. Eichenbaum

SUMMARY

In order to draw a closer connection between spatial memory and hippocampal long-term potentiation (LTP), the activity of a place cell that fires selectively when an animal is located in a certain area of a maze was examined in freely behaving knock-out mice that exhibit spatial learning deficit and altered hippocampal plasticity. This approach seeks to examine the effects of altered synaptic plasticity on the information coding mechanism by characterizing firing properties of certain hippocampal neurons directly underlying perception and memory. Available recording data indicated that synaptic plasticity in the hippocampus is not an essential mechanism for the formation of place selective firing of hippocampal pyramidal neurons, but is important for fine tuning and stabilizing its neural activity across time.

Together with genetic, pharmacologic, and in vitro electrophysiologic studies, this type of approach should allow us to examine whether experimental manipulations that block LTP change the capacity of neurons to process critical sensory stimuli and to code relevant cues into memory, and thus should provide a unique and promising avenue in bringing further insight into the cellular and physiologic mechanisms underlying learning and memory.

Introduction

A major focus of neuroscience research, and the central topic of this volume, is the identification of cellular and molecular plasticity mechanisms that mediate memory. Most studies aimed at this goal involve attempts to relate physiologic or molecular indices of neural plasticity to behavioral performance in learning and memory tests. This general strategy underlies a broad range of experiments, such

Christian Hölscher, editor, *Neuronal Mechanisms of Memory Formation.* © 2001 Cambridge University Press. Printed in the United States of America. All rights reserved.

as efforts to correlate changes in synaptic efficacy with learning, or efforts to block learning by "saturation" of synaptic efficacy, as well as attempts to influence learning and memory performance by pharmacologic or genetic manipulations that affect the molecular cascade of events that mediate forms of neural plasticity (for a review, see Eichenbaum, 1996). Each of these approaches has offered support for the view that lasting changes in synaptic efficacy (long-term potentiation, LTP) and memory share common mechanisms. At the same time, however, findings from some of these studies have also indicated that making a direct leap from the level of synaptic physiology to the level of memory performance is fraught with pitfalls and gaps for making a compelling case for the connection between LTP and memory. The present chapter considers a different and complementary approach, focused at the level of neural activity patterns that are presumably altered by synaptic plasticity and that underlie behavioral performance. This approach seeks to characterize the firing properties of neurons in brain areas that are critical for memory, and to determine the effects of altered cellular plasticity on neural firing patterns related to perception and memory. These studies can examine whether experimental manipulations that block LTP change the capacity of neurons to process critical sensory stimuli, and whether these manipulations alter the coding of relevant cues into memory. Thus, these studies can provide a unique insight into whether drugs and genetic manipulations that affect memory performance do so by compromising information "processing" or by blocking information "storage".

This chapter reviews recent studies that have characterized the firing patterns of neurons in the hippocampus of behaving animals in which the capacity for inducing LTP has been compromised. Experiments using a variety of techniques in several vertebrate species have consistently revealed that the hippocampus and related brain structures play a key role in spatial memory (lesions: Morris et al., 1982; Jarrard, 1993; Cho et al, 1999; unit recording: O'Keefe and Dostrovsky, 1971; functional brain imaging: Maguire et al., 1998). Correspondingly, the activity of the CA1 and CA3 pyramidal neurons (place cells) in rats and in monkeys encode an animal's position in space as indicated by selective firing when the animal is located in a particular area of an environment and that is sometimes independent of the animal's ongoing behavior. The finding of location selective activity of hippocampal neurons has been taken as evidence in support of the hypothesis that the hippocampus is important for representation of environments (O'Keefe and Nadel, 1978), and a reflection of the kind of general memory processing performed by the hippocampus (Eichenbaum et al., 1999).

In addition to place-related neuronal activity, hippocampal circuitry has long been a focus of active research with respect to synaptic plasticity and related electrophysiologic phenomena, among which the best known is that mediated via N-methyl-D-asparate receptors (NMDAR). Experimental findings from pharmacologic studies have attributed an important role for hippocampal NMDAR-dependent plasticity in spatial navigation capability in rodents (Morris et al., 1986). In addition, neurogenetic studies have recently contributed to this endeavor by enabling greater specificity for identifying the precise molecular and cellular mechanisms involved in these forms of synaptic plasticity. In an attempt to draw a closer connection between spatial memory and NMDAR-dependent hippocampal LTP, the spatial coding mechanism reflected within place cell activity has recently been assessed in "knock-out" (KO) mutant mice that exhibit altered NMDAR-dependent synaptic plasticity and impaired spatial learning. Three studies have so far been performed using single unit recording techniques in freely behaving transgenic mice that carry a bundle of microelectrodes implanted into the dorsal hippocampus. This technique constitutes an adaptation of procedures commonly used in rats. The present chapter is intended, first, to summarize the data obtained in our laboratory (Cho et al., 1998) using these techniques and, second, to compare the data with those obtained in other laboratories (McHugh et al., 1996; Rotenberg et al., 1996).

Place Cells in CaMKIIt286a and CREB Knock-Out Mice

We have recorded extracellular action potentials via multichannel microelectrodes using a tetrode configuration (Wilson and McNaughton, 1993). Custom-made microdrive arrays containing four 25-μm Formvar-coated nichrome wires were permanently implanted using dental cement to the skull bone. The electrodes were initially located in the cortex above the right hippocampus. After recovery from the implantation surgery, hippocampal complex-spike cell activity was screened daily while mice explored a four-arm radial maze to retrieve small pieces of sweetened cereal scattered over the surface of the maze. Recordings were taken following the isolation of one or more place cells, the subpopulation of hippocampal complex-spike cells that exhibit location-specific activity. These cells typically exhibited at least one "place field," an area of the maze associated with increased spike activity.

When considering important features of the place cells, the influence of environmental sensory cues has been extensively investigated in a series of landmark recording studies performed by Muller and Kubie (1987) and Muller et al. (1987). These studies have demonstrated that location selective activity can be controlled by a single predominant visual cue. However, under most conditions an environment contains multiple visual, auditory, and other sensory cues and the locations of most place fields are not determined by any single (distal) cue in the environment, but rather by a combination of stimulus features. Thus most cells fire in only one place (or a few places) because the particular stimulus combination (or combinations) occur at that place in the environment. Only radical changes in the layout of the environment are capable of disrupting the location-specific firing of the cells (Best and White, 1998).

Furthermore, previous recording studies have demonstrated that disconnection of the hippocampus from its cortical or subcortical associates reduces the precision of the place cell activity, and affects the nature of the external stimuli that influence field location. More precisely, the locations of the place fields become more influenced by local (intramaze) cues than distal (extramaze) cues under these conditions (Miller and Best, 1980; Best and White, 1998), indicating a shift in the predominant use of information encoded by the hippocampus from external to internal maze cues. These findings support the long-standing view that the hippocampus is important for a memory when behavior depends on the use of the relational properties of the distant but not local cues. Therefore, we were particularly interested in evaluating the nature of stimuli of different kinds that are incorporated into spatial representations in KO mice lacking hippocampal plasticity. In particular, we anticipated that place cells of KO mice would be more tuned to local cues rather than distal cues because of the lack of synaptic plasticity.

The radial maze we used for recording contained a large set of controlled stimuli including local cues consisting of a distinctive surface on each maze arm and distal cues composed of distinct three-dimensional objects on a curtain surrounding the maze. Animals were initially familiarized with the maze for approximately 1 to 2 weeks, then recordings were taken for a 5 to 10 minute baseline (BS1) trial in which all distal and local cues were in their usual configuration. Immediately following the initial baseline trial, the same cells were recorded during a double rotation (DR) trial in which the distal cues and local cues were rotated in opposite directions. The DR trial was followed by the second baseline (BS2) trial where the cues were returned to their original configuration. Between these trials the mice were placed in a deep round plastic bucket. During each trial the mice were encouraged to visit all four arms at least three times to ensure exploration of the entire maze (see Figure 17.1 for recording protocol). The experimenter entered and exited the maze enclosure using a single entry point to provide animals with a consistent laboratory reference frame.

During the DR trial we rotated the four local cues 90° clockwise and the four distal cues 90° counterclockwise without altering the relative position of the cues

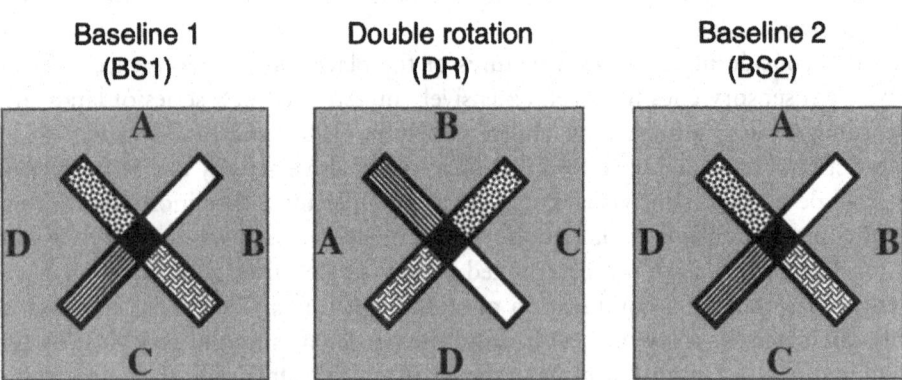

Figure 17.1. Recording protocol: A schematic diagram showing the recording apparatus that contains four distal cues hung on inner walls of the curtain surrounding the four-arm maze (A, B, C, and D), and four local cues placed on the surface of each of the four arms (different patterns). After recording for a 10 to 15 minute baseline trial (BS1), the environmental cues were rearranged during a probe recording trial called double rotation trial (DR) such that the four distal cues were rotated 90° in clockwise direction, whereas the four local cues were rotated 90° in counterclockwise direction without changing the relative position among the four local and distal cue sets. The recording ended with an additional baseline trial (BS2) during which the initial cue configuration was reinstated.

within the local and distal cue sets. If a cell was controlled solely by the distal cues, the spatial firing pattern would be expected to rotate into alignment with those cues. Conversely, in cells controlled by the local cues the activity would be expected to rotate with that cue set. In rats, place cells recorded in a similar context are preferentially controlled by distal cues, thus we predicted a similar trend in wild-type mice (Shapiro et al., 1997; Tanila et al., 1997). Conversely, we expected that hippocampal cells from KO mice would be preferentially controlled by single local cues, corresponding to the impairment in their spatial navigation ability.

One type of KO mouse examined in our study involves an alteration in the activity of CaMKII, an enzyme known to be important for induction of LTP (see Figure 17.2). Previous studies have shown that a null mutation of the alpha subunit of this enzyme produces a deficiency in the induction of CA1-LTP and in spatial learning and memory performance, with somewhat less severe deficits in nonspatial learning (Silva et al., 1992a, 1992b). Because CaMKII can undergo autophosphorylation, resulting in CaM-independent activity that is putatively critical to enduring LTP and long-term memory (Lisman and Goldring, 1988), we used a strain of mouse (CaMKIIt286a mouse) that had undergone genetic manipulation that prevents CaMKII from autophosphorylation (Giese et al., 1998). A second type of KO mouse investigated was a line of mouse (CREB mouse) in which the alpha and delta subunits of cAMP responsive element binding protein (CREB) are inactivated

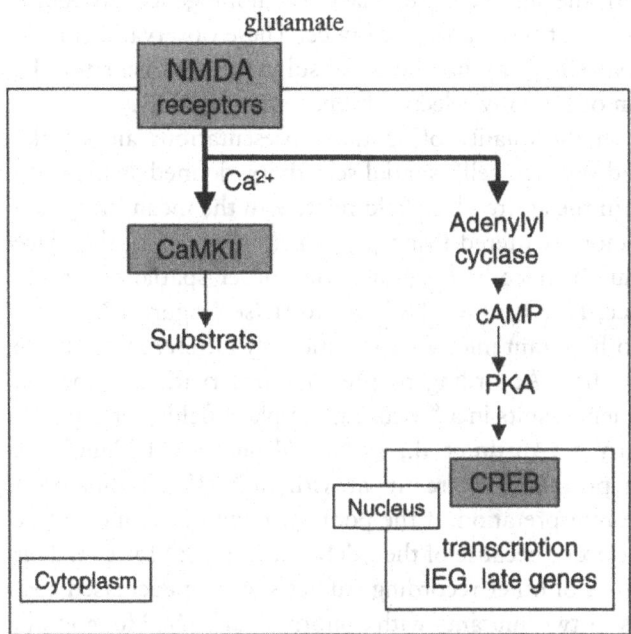

Figure 17.2. Schematic drawing of the molecular cascade involved in NMDA receptor-dependent LTP. The molecules indicated in shaded boxes have been specifically targeted in knock-out studies, investigating the changes induced in the place cell firing properties in mice.

(see Figure 17.2). CREB is a transcription factor regulated by the cAMP signaling pathway and that is known to be important for the late phase of LTP. We specifically selected these mutant mice because they differ substantially in the relative severity of their defects in synaptic plasticity and learning. CaMKII mice are severely impaired in spatial learning as well as in NMDAR-dependent LTP in the CA1 region of the hippocampus (Giese et al., 1998). In contrast, CREB mutants have reduced LTP and mild spatial learning deficits (Bourtchuladze et al., 1994). Consequently, we expected to find more profound abnormalities in the spatial representations of CaMKIIt286a mice than in CREB mice.

We identified complex-spike cells as well as theta cells in the CA1 and CA3 regions of the hippocampus of both types of KO mutant and wild-type mice. The electrophysiologic characteristics of these cells were similar to those described in rats by Ranck (1973). A considerable proportion of hippocampal cells in both wild-type and mutant mice exhibited increased firing rates in limited proportions of the maze. In this study we identified place cells as neurons that exhibited an average firing rate within a continuous area of at least 9.5 cm² at least twofold higher than the cell's overall mean firing rate. Some cells had more than one distinct area of increased firing that met this criterion, and each of these areas was considered a separate place field. Using these criteria place fields were identified in approximately one-half of the hippocampal neurons from wild-type mice, as well as from both strains of mutant mice, indicating that the particular genetic mutations did not modify the incidence of place cells either in CaMKIIt286a or in CREB mice. In addition, as can be seen in the distribution of geometric centers of the place fields (Figure 17.3), the surface of the maze was homogeneously represented by place cells from each of these groups of mice. These observations indicate that intact hippocampal LTP may not be an absolute requirement for the development and expression of spatially selective hippocampal activity.

An analysis performed on the quality of spatial representations among the experimental groups focused on each cell's spatial selectivity, defined as the ratio of the mean firing rate within the entire place field relative to the mean firing rate elsewhere. As reflected by more scattered firing patterns (Figure 17.4), the place cells from both types of mutant mice had significantly poorer spatial selectivity than those of wild-type mice, $F(2, 126) = 7.835$, $p < .001$ (see Figure 17.5), and the selectivities of cells in both mutant mice were significantly different from those of wild-type cells (all $ps < .05$). According to previous observations, repeated exposure to a new environment results in a "focusing" of place fields, reflected by an increase in spatial selectivity (Austin et al., 1990; Wilson and McNaughton, 1993). This phenomenon is prevented by treatment with an NMDAR antagonist (Kentros et al., 1998). One interpretation of the poor selectivity in mutant place cells is that focusing did not occur because of their deficient capacity for LTP. This view is consistent with reports of other recording studies showing decreased spatial selectivity of place cells in two mutants with abnormal LTP (McHugh et al., 1996; Rotenberg et al., 1996).

Additional analyses were aimed at several parameters of the firing patterns of place cells (Table 17.1). The overall mean firing rate, defined as the total number of spikes divided by total time spent in the maze, did not differ significantly

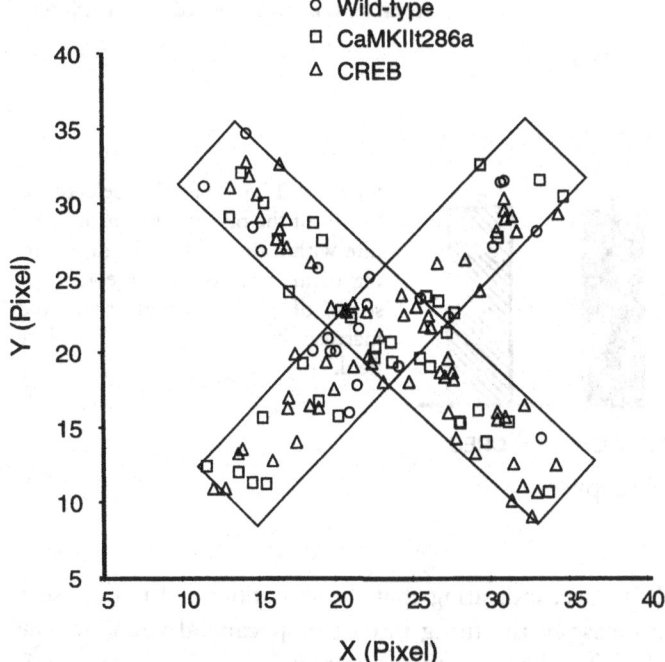

Figure 17.3. Place field centers. Centers of place fields of all place cells recorded during the BS1 trial for wild-type, CaMKIIt286a, and CREB mice, but represented on the same plan. Note that field centers were randomly distributed for place cells from each of the three groups of mice, suggesting that each location of the maze was equally represented by place cells from these mice.

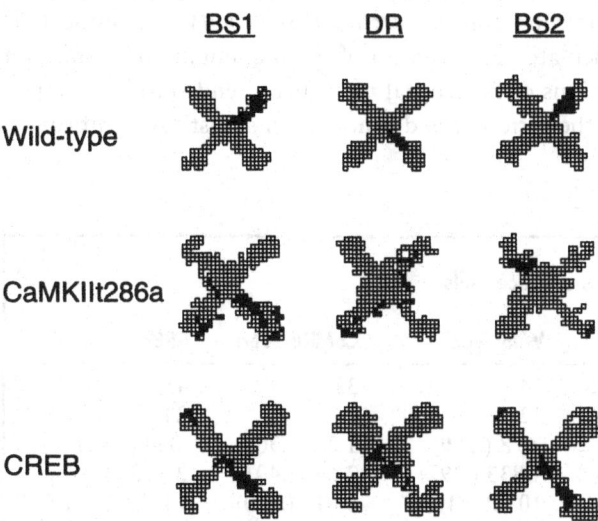

Figure 17.4. Typical examples of place cell firing from wild-type, CaMKIIt286a mice. Empty pixels indicate locations visited at least three times by animals without cell activity, and black pixels indicate local activity rates that are at least twofold higher than the cell's overall firing rate. The place field of the wild-type cell followed rotated local cues in the DR trial, and returned to the original location in the BS2 trial. In the CaMKIIt286a cell, spatially localized firing in BS1 was unstable, that is, it changed loci unpredictably across subsequent trials. In the CREB cell, multiple place fields developed in the BS1 trial were degraded in the DR trial, but were restored in the BS2 trial. (Adapted from Cho et al., 1998, with permission.)

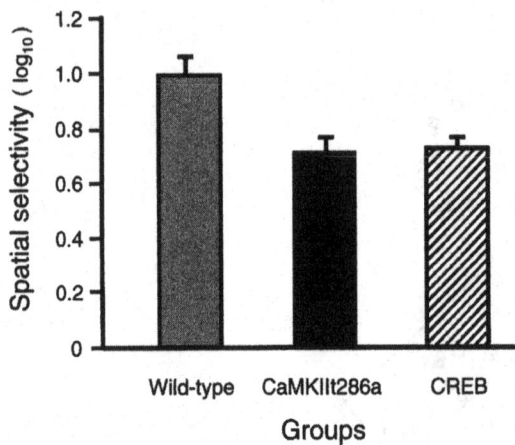

Figure 17.5. Spatial selectivity. Log10 of the ratio of the mean firing rate within the field to the mean firing of all rates outside the field. A score of 1.0 indicates a tenfold increase in firing inside the place field.

between wild-type and KO mice, indicating that the mutations did not cause a nonspecific increase or decrease in the firing rate of hippocampal neurons. The average size of place fields differed among the groups, $F(2, 47) = 2.978$, $p < .05$. Post hoc analyses indicated that cells in CREB mice, but not in CaMKIIt286a mice, significantly differed from those in wild-type mice ($p < .05$). There also was a tendency toward an increased number of fields in both types of mutants, but this effect was not significant.

Finally, when animals traverse a linear apparatus, such as a linear track, place cells only fire, or fire more frequently when the animal runs in only one of the two opposing directions, a phenomenon called *directional selectivity*. We found that the directional selectivity, calculated as the ratio of the maximum and minimum firing rates across eight directions of horizontal movement, tended to be lower in both mutant place cells, but the differences did not reach statistical significance, $F(2, 126) = 2.457$, $p = .08$.

Table 17.1. Firing Properties of Place Cells

	Wild-Type	CaMKIIt286a	CREB
Number of complex spike cells	24	32	45
Number of place cells	12	14	24
Mean firing rate[a]	.678 (.189)	1.239 (.304)	.844 (.161)
Number of fields/cell	1.833 (.297)	2.643 (.401)	2.917 (.345)
Place field size (pixels)	10.091 (1.147)	8.811 (.910)	11.129 (1.185)
Infield firing rate[b]	4.342 (.467)	6.337 (.776)*†	3.607 (.265)

* Significantly different (Newman-Keuls tests, $p < .05$) from wild-type cells and † from CREB[αΔ–] cells.
[a] Total number of spikes divided by total time spent in the maze.
[b] Mean firing rates for pixels within the place fields.
Numbers in parentheses indicate standard errors.

During the DR condition, place cells identified in both mutant and wild-type mice responded to cue manipulation in one of five ways: The place fields of some cells rotated with the local cues. Others rotated with the distal cues. Yet others remained fixed despite the cue rotations. Each of these types was categorized as maintaining aspects of the "old" spatial representation. In addition, some cells changed their responses in some way not explained by a cue rotation, and instead indicated a new spatial firing pattern. Another group of cells showed a cessation of their spatial firing pattern, probably indicating that they were originally under the control of some configuration of the local, distal, and fixed cues that was disrupted by the double rotation of cues. The cells having these responses to the cue alterations were classified as having "new" representations.

As summarized in Figure 17.6, in wild-type mice, two-thirds of place cells maintained their initial place field shapes with the largest proportion following the local cues. Indeed, 35 percent of place fields from wild-type mice followed the local cues and did not respond to the distal cues, even though the cells came under the control of the distal cues when the local cues were removed. This indicates that the predominance of the local cues is not a consequence of poor distance vision in mice. These data are surprising when compared to data obtained from recording studies in rats (Shapiro et al., 1997). In that study distal cues predominated in control over the place fields, suggesting that a distinction between place cell properties in the two rodent species might be related to other differences in

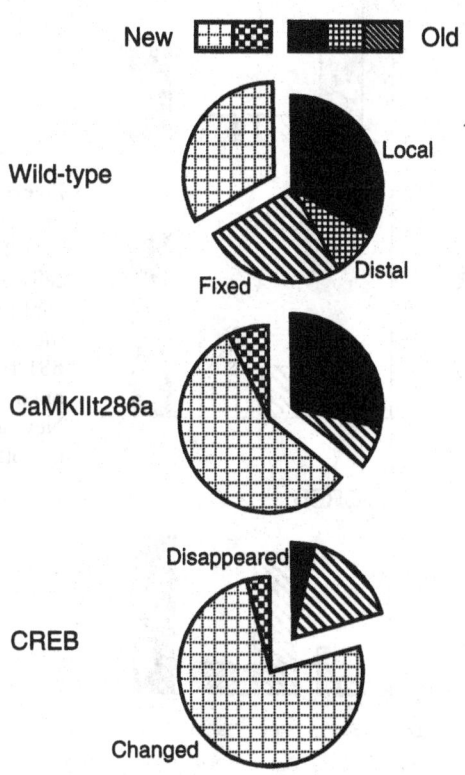

Figure 17.6. Proportions of place cells showing different patterns of response to the cue manipulation in the DR trial. Cells maintaining place fields developed in the BS1 trial (Same) include those that remained fixed in the same maze arm (Fixed) or rotated with the local (Local) or distal (Distal) cues. Cells considered to have different representations (New) include those whose place fields changed location inconsistent with a simple rotation (Changed), and those in which the place field disappeared (Disappeared) altogether. (Adapted from Cho et al., 1998, with permission.)

general behavior patterns and learning performances of rats and mice when tested for maze learning or classical conditioning (Whishaw and Tomie, 1996; Cho et al., 1999). The remaining cells from wild-type mice developed new place fields, but no cells lost their spatial firing altogether. In contrast, in both types of KO mice only a minority of cells maintained their initial place fields in the DR trial. In addition no cells from either of the mutant mice followed the distal cues after this manipulation. Conversely, the majority of cells in the mutant mice developed new place fields and some cells in each type of mutant mice lost spatial selectivity altogether. These findings indicate that, by comparison to cells from wild-type mice, a few hippocampal cells in both types of mutants were under the control of specific sets of local or fixed cues and control by distal cues was entirely absent.

An additional analysis of the responses of place cells during the DR and BS2 trials further clarified the nature of cues controlling these place cells and the stability of the spatial representations in the mutant mice. This analysis focused on comparisons of the responses of cells to the DR and BS2 manipulations, characterizing each cell into one of four patterns of response on these two test trials (Figure 17.7). Some cells maintained their place field representation in the same or rotated

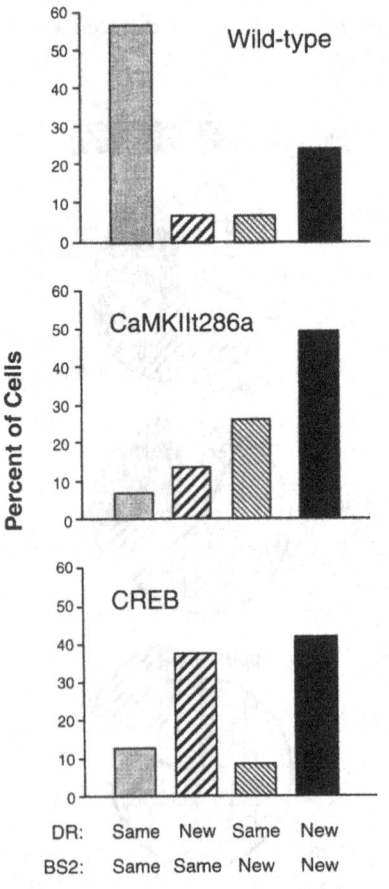

Figure 17.7. Distribution of four types of response of place cells in wild-type, CaMKIIt286a, and CREB mice in DR and BS2 trials. Same-Same are cells that developed new representations in the DR trial but recovered their original representations in the BS2 trial. Same-New are cells that retained the BS1 trial representation in the DR trial but developed a new representation in the BS2 trial. New-New are cells that developed new representations in both the DR and BS2 trials. (Adapted from Cho et al., 1998, with permission.)

location on both test trials (old-old), whereas others developed a new representation by changing shape or disappearing in the DR trial but then recovered the initial representation during the BS2 trial (new-old). Other cells maintained the initial form of the place field in the DR trial, but changed to a new representation in the BS2 trial (old-new), or changed representations during both test trials (new-new).

Comparison of the patterns of same and new responses across all three testing sessions showed that the distributions differed among the three groups, $(X^2(6)=18.489)$, $p < .01$, and those for both the CaMKIIt286a and CREB cells significantly differed from that of wild-type cells ($p < .05$). In wild-type mice, the majority of cells maintained their initial spatial representations on both test trials (old-old). By contrast, only a minor proportion of the cells in CaMKIIt286a mice and CREB mice maintained their spatial representation across these tests, confirming the finding that cells from both KO mice are less likely to be controlled by specific subsets of the stimuli that were present throughout these test trials. However, this finding is not entirely attributable to an overall instability of place fields in either of the mutants. A substantial proportion of cells in CREB mice exhibited new place fields during the DR trial but restored their initial fields during the BS2 trial (new-old). This finding indicates that CREB mice have some preserved stability when re-placed in a familiar environment, and suggests that the new place fields observed during the DR trial were a consequence of their initial representation of a novel combination of local, distal, and fixed cues, and an inability to recognize a familiar subset of controlling cues put in a novel configuration. A substantial proportion of place cells in CaMKIIt286a mice exhibited a different pattern. These cells maintained their place representations during the DR trial, but subsequently switched to a new spatial representation during the BS2 trial (old-new). This finding suggests that these cells were able to only briefly maintain a representation of a subset of the local, distal, or fixed cues, but subsequently lost that representation. Moreover, the largest proportion of cells in both KO mice developed new spatial firing patterns during both the DR and BS2 trials (new-new), suggesting a common general instability of their spatial representations superimposed on other differences between the two mutant strains.

Comparison with Other Data

To date, in addition to the above experiment, two other studies have examined the firing properties of place cells in mutant mice. Rotenberg et al. (1996) examined a line of transgenic mice that expresses, in the hippocampus, a form of CaMKII that was rendered Ca^{2+}-independent by a Thr-Asp mutation at position 286 (CaMKIIasp286; Mayford et al., 1995). These mice exhibit normal LTP at 100 Hz, but impaired LTP following 5 to 10 Hz stimulation – the frequency of the hippocampal theta rhythm (Mayford et al., 1995). This specific defect in LTP is correlated with a severe spatial memory deficit in a Barnes circular maze in which mice had to find a hole leading to a darkened escape tunnel, but not in a cued version of the task where the location of the whole is indicated by a visual cue (Bach et al., 1995). McHugh et al. (1996) recorded from a line of KO mice that carried a gene deletion of the subtype I of NMDAR in the restricted CA1 field of the hippocampus (CA1-NMDA). These KO mice lack NMDAR-mediated synaptic currents and LTP in the CA1 Schaffer collateral pathway, and exhibit impaired spatial memory but normal nonspatial learning in the Morris water maze. A summary of the available *in vitro* electrophysiologic and behavioral phenotypes, as well as place cell data from these mice, is presented in Table 17.2, and will be discussed in detail below.

Our comparison of the data across all three of the studies on place cells in mutant mice indicated several similarities and differences in the effects of the genetic manipulations. First, substantial and equivalent proportions of cells recorded from both CaMKIIt286a and CREB mice fired in a place-specific manner in our study, as also observed in CA1-NMDA mice (McHugh et al., 1996). However, the proportion of the place cells among the recorded hippocampal complex-spike cells was found to be significantly diminished in CaMKIIasp286 mice. It is not known why CaMKIIasp286 exhibited a decreased number of the place cells, whereas CaMKIIt286a, in which genetic mutations focused on the same molecular locus, did not (but see below). However, the results of these recording studies could be taken to suggest that normal hippocampal LTP in CA1 Schaffer collateral may not be an absolute requirement for the development and expression of spatially specific hippocampal activity.

Second, the major measure of place cell spatial tuning [variously defined as spatial coherence (Rotenberg et al., 1996), spatial specificity (McHugh et al., 1996), or spatial selectivity (Cho et al., 1998)], was significantly diminished in the mutant mice used in all three experiments. This observation could be related to a familiarization technique, used in all three experiments, in which animals were made highly familiar with the environment before any place cell recording took place. Several studies on place cells indicate that the extent to which the animal has prior experience with the recording apparatus influences whether the place cells either change the firing patterns when the environment is modified ("remap") or reproduce and refine the same spatial firing pattern, reflecting successful recognition of the environment (stability and focusing). In particular, focusing of place fields, reflected by an increase in spatial selectivity with experience, is known to be blocked by NMDAR antagonists (Austin et al., 1990). The combined findings of these studies suggest that focusing is absent in the KO mutant mice due to their deficient capacity for LTP.

Third, the size of place fields was larger and more diffuse in both CA1-NMDA and CaMKIIasp286 mice, whereas normal place field sizes were observed in both CREB and CaMKIIt286a mice. These differences may be explained by the different criteria used to define place cells in these studies. Rotenberg et al. (1996) reported that place cells from wild-type mice exhibited somewhat larger place fields, a finding that was related to their relatively high average firing rate. This conclusion was based on a calculation of spatial coherence, a measure that is insensitive to the absolute firing rate of the place cells. They considered a cell to be

Table 17.2. Summary of Place Cell Recording Data Obtained with Four Different Mutant Mice

Phenotype	CaMKIIasp286 (Rotenberg et al., 1996)	CA1-NMDAR1 (McHugh et al., 1996)	CREB (Cho et al., 1998)	CaMKIIt286a (Cho et al., 1998)
	Gen. background C57bl6/SJL[a]	CBA-C57bl/sv	sv129/C57bl6	sv129/C57bl6
Spatial learning				
Spatial	sev imp[b]	mod imp[c]	mod imp[d]	sev imp[e]
Nonspatial	normal	normal	normal	trans imp
In vitro electrophysiology in CA1				
Induction	imp (theta Hz)	imp (100 Hz–1 s)	mod imp	imp (100 Hz–1 s)
Maintenance	–	–	imp	–
STP	–	imp	normal	imp
LTD	increased	normal	increased	normal
Place cell recording in CA1				
Apparatus	cylinder	L-shape track	radial maze	radial maze
Repeated record	yes/familiar	yes/familiar	yes/familiar	yes/familiar
# complex cells	52 (26 from wt)[f]	198 (112)	45 (24)	32 (24)
# place cells	16 (15)	74 (56)	24 (12)	14 (12)
% place cells	31% (58%)*	37 (49)	53 (50)	44 (50)
Recording wires	single wires	tetrode	tetrode	tetrode
Mean firing rate	0.52 Hz (1.46)*	2.31 (2.11)	0.84 (0.68)	1.24 (0.68)
Peak firing rate	16.1 Hz (27.2)*	–	3.60 (4.34)	6.34 (4.34)
# fields/cell	–	increased	2.92 (1.83)	2.64 (1.83)
Field size[g]	410 (251)*	140.3 (106)*	11.13 (10.09)	8.81 (10.09)
Criterion[h]	>0.26 (coherence)	firing rate > 1 Hz	2 × gmr[i]	2 × gmr
Field size in cm^2	1049 (642.56)	561.2 (424)	62.55 (56.71)	49.48 (56.71)
Coherence	low*	–	–	–
Spat. specificity	–	imp	–	–
Spat. selectivity	–	–	imp*	imp*
Stability	low (–1 hr)*	normal (–1 hr)	normal (10–15 min)	imp
Directionality	–	imp	mod imp	mod imp

Abbreviations: imp, impaired; sev imp, severely impaired; mod imp, moderately impaired; trans imp, transiently impaired; gmr, grand mean rate.

* Significantly different from their wild-type litermates.

[a] Mayford et al. (1995).

[b] Bach et al. (1995).

[c] Tsien et al. (1996).

[d] Bourtchuladze et al. (1994).

[e] Giese et al. (1998).

[f] Data in parentheses hereafter are those from the wild-type mice.

[g] Units are pixels.

[h] Statistical criterion used for a given complex-spike cell to be considered as a place cell.

[i] gmr (grand mean rate) calculated by the number of spikes for the session divided by time(s).

a place cell if its spatial coherence was greater than 0.26. Based on this criterion, the average coherence of all classified place cells was 0.62 for wild-type mice and 0.42 for the mutant mice, resulting in a significant difference between the wild-type and transgenic place cells. In contrast, McHugh et al. (1996) based their analyses on absolute firing rate; they considered a place field to include all the pixels having firing rates higher than 1 Hz. Their analysis revealed a slightly increased size of the place fields in the mutant mice as compared to their littermate wild-type mice. In the Cho et al. (1998) study, the heterogeneity of the firing rate of individual place cells was taken into consideration, such that place fields included all pixels with firing rates twice the average firing rate (total number of spikes / total time in seconds for the given recording session). In this study, CREB and CaMKIIt286a place cells showed equivalent size of place fields compared to those of wild-type place cells. An increase of the place field size in CREB and CaMKIIt286a, as well as a decrease in CaMKIIasp286 mice, might have been found if the method used by McHugh et al. was applied, leading to different conclusions. It will become increasingly more important to employ uniform statistical analyses for direct comparison among different lines of mice used in different laboratories.

Fourth, different patterns of responses emerged in the tests for place field stability. The place cells in the CA1 region of the CA1-NMDA mice had place fields that were stable for at least 1 hour. In contrast, CaMKIIasp286 mice have place cells that showed significantly deteriorated place cell stability over the period of 1 to 2 hours, as evidenced by diminished similarity measures from a cross-correlational analysis for pairs of separate recording sessions. In our study, the majority of the place cells from the CaMKIIt286a, but not the place cells from CREB mice, were unstable following a probe (DR) trial in which a change in the environmental cue configuration was performed to test the capacity of the cells to remap in slightly altered environment. The severity of the defect in the stability in the two different lines of mutant mice used in our experiment closely matched with the differing severity of deficits in spatial learning ability. Collectively, these findings suggest that NMDAR-dependent plasticity in the CA1 region of the hippocampus may play an important role in place cell stability, which probably underlies the capacity to retrieve previously established spatial representations.

Fifth, the place cells from CA1-NMDA mice had significantly impaired directionality when recording took place in a linear track, producing some erroneous firing even when the animal moves in the "wrong" direction. In our experiment, the place cells from the CaMKIIt286a and CREB mice also showed signs of diminished directional selectivity, and this tendency was greater when the recording was made in an environment where all four local cues were removed from the maze arms in an additional recording session (unpublished observation). These findings suggest that the extent to which animal's movement is integrated into the spatial representation is lower in the mutant mice. An examination of movement and directional properties of mutant place cells could provide substantial insights into how spatial information and representation of behavioral actions are integrated by synaptic plasticity.

Molecular Components Underlying Place Cell Activity

Further insights can be derived by comparing the findings across these studies from the perspective of the locus of molecular disruption at the site of NMDAR activation or at the site of subsequent influx of Ca^{2+} into the postsynaptic densities (see Figure 17.2). CaMKII occupies an important step in the molecular cascade involved in synaptic plasticity, and especially in LTP. Furthermore, a particularly interesting property of CaMKII is its ability to maintain activity by autophosphorylation even after the intracellular concentration of Ca^{2+} has returned to basal levels. This biochemical characteristic of the kinase led Lisman and Goldring (1988) to suggest that CaMKII might act as a molecular switch for the long-term maintenance of the activity necessary for memory storage throughout the neural circuit involved.

Two of the place cell recording studies involved different mutations of CaMKII function. Rotenberg et al. (1996) recorded from a line of transgenic mice, CaMKIIasp286, expressing a constitutively active (i.e., independently of the intracellular calcium concentration) form of the CaMKII. In contrast, Cho et al. (1998) performed recordings from a line of mice in which the same enzyme had been rendered permanently dependent on the intracellular Ca^{2+} as a result of the point mutation (threonine at position 286 mutated to alanine) preventing the enzyme from turning into the autophosphorylated state. A comparison of these two different mutant mice provides potentially useful information toward an understanding of the functional involvement of the different biochemical process associated with this kinase: (1) Place cells from both lines of mice developed some degree of place-specific activity although their spatial signal-to-noise ratio, as well as the stability of the place fields, was significantly diminished as compared to cells from their wild-type littermates. (2) There was a diminished number of place cells in transgenic mice, but no such change was found in the mice with point mutations. (3) An increased size in the place fields was found in transgenic mice but not in point mutant mice. The comparisons of electrophysiologic properties suggest that transgenic mice have more severe place cell defects than point mutant mice. However, the *in vitro* physiologic and behavioral phenotypes of these mice indicate the opposite pattern of results: The point mutants have more severe deficits than transgenic mice in both the capacity to induce LTP and to learn the spatial memory task. This paradox highlights the complexity of the molecular and biochemical mechanisms involved in information processing by the target neural network, and calls for further studies involving a variety of experimental techniques to bring better insights into this issue.

Another interesting comparison involves the effects of blocking activation of NMDAR either by genetic manipulation (McHugh et al., 1996) or by pharmacologic treatment using a competitive NMDAR antagonist CPP [3-(2-carboxypiperazin-4-yl)propyl-1-phosphonic acid] (Kentros et al., 1998). The global pharmacologic blockade of NMDAR in all brain areas (by intraperitoneal injections) in adult rats produced approximately the same pattern of results of genetic deletion of NMDAR, confirming a main conclusion of

McHugh et al. (1996) that NMDAR must be available for place cells to be normal. Furthermore, NMDAR blockade prevented the place fields formed in a new environment from being stable across recording sessions, even though the place fields are normally established in this condition. These data suggest that the NMDAR-dependent plasticity is not required for the maintenance of the old place fields, but is necessary for the long-term maintenance of newly formed fields under NMDAR blockade, an issue that may not have been properly addressed in previous studies using KO mice. Because the pharmacologic approach lacks the regional and molecular specificity offered by gene targeting, it would be desirable to use new lines of mutant mice in which molecules important for NMDAR function could be selectively and reversibly inactivated during key stages of learning or retrieval performance in adult animals.

LTP and Place Cells

Consistent with the patterns of electrical stimulation that have been identified as being optimal for producing LTP (Larson et al., 1986; Rose and Dunwiddie, 1986), some studies have investigated the frequency of endogenous hippocampal rhythmic slow wave activity (theta rhythm) and the related bursting patterns of complex-spike cells (Otto et al., 1991; Hölscher et al., 1997; Thomas et al., 1998; Dobruntz and Stevens, 1999). In addition, some firing properties of hippocampal place cells have been explained from the perspective of LTP-like phenomenon. For example, when rats repeatedly traverse a route in the same direction, the sizes of CA1 place fields increase rapidly and their centers of mass shift backward. This is presumed to reflect increased presynaptic activity to drive earlier firing of the postsynaptic cell, a phenomenon called *asymmetric expansion* (Mehta et al., 1997). These changes were predicted and explained by models incorporating NMDAR-mediated, temporally asymmetric, Hebbian LTP in the recurrent collateral of CA3 of the hippocampus (Tsodyks et al., 1996). Further experiments showed that this phenomenon is absent in aged animals in which an impaired synaptic plasticity related to glutamatergic dysfunction was observed (Shen et al., 1997), as well as in rats treated with CPP, an NMDAR blocker (Mehta and McNaughton, 1997), suggesting that the phenomenon is NMDAR-dependent. In addition, the phase of hippocampal location-specific firing relative to the theta rhythm advances gradually as the rat traverses the cells' place field under the same recording conditions, a phenomenon called *theta precession* (O'Keefe and Reece, 1993). Both of these phenomena appear as an animal's experience with a given environment increases, thus sharing similar features with experience-dependent LTP.

Together with evidence for a decrease in correlated cell firing in CA1-NMDA mice, revealing an altered property of synchronized firing among pairs of cells sharing the same fields (McHugh et al., 1996), these electrophysiologic data provide significant insights into a possible link between LTP and *in vivo* electrophysiology observable as a consequence of behavior. These observations also inspire testable hypotheses that could be verified using unit recording techniques in behaving KO mice with altered plasticity. The information that could be obtained from this type of study should tell us more about the nature and functional significance of interactions among a variety of physiologic phenomena in the hippocampus capable of supporting memory coding and storage, and may inform us about the extent to which synaptic plasticity in the hippocampus constitutes a functional memory mechanism.

Future Directions and Conclusion

Considerable behavioral and electrophysiologic data have provided evidence for an important functional role of the hippocampus in declarative or episodic memory for a broad range of learning materials (Hampson and Deadwyler, 1998; Eichenbaum et al., 1999). One recent recording study that supports such a point of view involved recording hippocampal complex-spike cells while rats are performing an odor recognition memory task in a spatial environment. In this task the particular odor, but not the spatial contingency, is the relevant information for memory performance (Wood et al., 1999). The study showed that the activity of many hippocampal neurons was related consistently to perceptual, behavioral, or cognitive events, regardless of the location where these events occurred, indicating that nonspatial elements are fundamental components of the hippocampal memory representations (Eichenbaum, 1997; Eichenbaum et al., 1999).

In addition, available pharmacologic data have demonstrated that the blockade of NMDAR prevents nonspatial learning (for example, in spontaneous alternation, Walker and Gold, 1994; in an operant DRL task, Tonkiss et al., 1988; in nonspatial working memory, Lyford et al., 1993; in contextual conditioning, Good and Bannerman, 1997; and in olfactory discrimination, Staubli et al., 1989). Recording from transgenic mice performing such nonspatial memory tasks should provide us with information about the nature of the coding mechanisms that are altered by the blockade of LTP, thus enabling a broader characterization of the involvement of hippocampal plasticity in memory coding.

In addition, *in vivo* unit recording could be used to characterize the memory coding properties in transgenic mouse models of neurodegenerative diseases, such as Alzheimer's disease, in which a severe and progressive recent memory deficit constitutes a major cognitive symptom. Knowledge provided by this approach should help us validate specific transgenic lines as the animal models for therapeutic strategies, as well as help us understand how memory is organized in both normal and pathologic brains.

REFERENCES

Austin, K., Fortin, W.J., and Shapiro, M.L. (1990). Place fields are altered by NMDA antagonist MK-801 during spatial learning. *Soc. Neurosci. Abstr.* 16: 263.
Bach, M.E., Hawkins, R.D., Osman, M., Kandel, E.R. et al. (1995). Impairment of spatial but not contextual memory in CaMKII mutant mice with a selective loss of hippocampal LTP in the range of the theta frequency. *Cell* 81: 905–915.

Best, P.J., and White, A.M. (1998). Hippocampal cellular activity: A brief history of space. *Proc. Natl. Acad. Sci.* 95: 2717–2719.

Bourtchuladze, R., Frenguelli, B., Blendy, J., Cioffi, D. et al. (1994). Deficient long-term memory in mice with a targeted mutation of the cAMP-responsive element-binding protein. *Cell* 9: 59–68.

Cho, Y.H., Giese, K.P., Tanila, H., Silva, A.J. et al. (1998). Abnormal hippocampal spatial representations in αCaMKII^{T286A} and CREB$^{α\Delta-}$ mice. *Science* 279: 867–869.

Cho, Y.H., Friedman, E., and Silva, A.J. (1999). Ibotenate lesions of the hippocampus impair spatial learning but not contextual fear conditioning in mice. *Behav. Brain Res.* 98: 77–87.

Dobruntz, L.E., and Stevens, C.F. (1999). Response of hippocampal synapses to natural stimulation patterns. *Neuron* 22: 157–166.

Eichenbaum, H. (1996). Learning from LTP: A comment on recent attempts to identify cellular and molecular mechanisms of memory. *Learn. Mem.* 3: 61–73.

Eichenbaum, H. (1997). Declarative memory: Insights from cognitive neurobiology. *Ann. Rev. Psychol.* 48: 547–572.

Eichenbaum, H., Dudchenko, P., Wood, E., Shapiro, M. et al. (1999). The hippocampus, memory, and place cells: Is it spatial memory or a memory space? *Neuron* 23: 209–226.

Giese, K.P., Fedorov, N., Filipkowski, R.K., and Silva, A.J. (1998). Autophosphorylation of the α calcium-calmodulin-kinase II is required for LTP and learning. *Science* 279: 870–873.

Good, M., and Bannerman, D. (1997). Differential effects of ibotenic acid lesions of the hippocampus and blockage of N-methyl-D-asparate receptor-dependent long-term potentiation on contexual processing in rats. *Behav. Neurosci.* 111: 1171–1183.

Hampson, R.E., and Deadwyler, S.A. (1998). LTP and LTD and the encoding of memory in small ensembles of hippocampal neurons. In M. Baudry and J.L. Davis (Eds.), *Long-term potentiation* (pp. 199–214). Cambridge, MA: MIT Press.

Hölscher, C., Anwly, R., and Rowan, M.J. (1997). Stimulation on the positive phase of hippocampal theta rhythm induces LTP that can be depotentiated by stimulation on the negative phase in area CA1 *in vivo*. *J. Neurosci.* 15: 6470–6477.

Jarrard, L.E. (1993). On the role of the hippocampus in learning and memory in the rat. *Behav. Neural Biol.* 60: 9–26.

Kentros, C., Hargreaves, E., Hawkins, R.D., Kandel, E.R. et al. (1998). Abolition of long-term stability of new hippocampal place cell maps by NMDA receptor blockade. *Science* 280: 2121–2126.

Larson, J., Wong, D., and Lynch, G. (1986). Patterned stimulation at the theta frequency is optimal for the induction of hippocampal LTP. *Brain Res.* 368: 347–350.

Lisman, J.E., and Goldring, M.A. (1988). Feasibility of long-term stage of graded information by the Ca^{++} calmodulin-dependent protein kinase molecules of the postsynaptic density. *Proc. Natl. Acad. Sci. USA.* 85: 5320–5324.

Lyford, G.L., Gutnikov, S.A., Clark, A.M., and Rawlins, J.N. (1993). Determinants of non-spatial working memory deficits in rats given intraventricular infusions of the NMDA antagonist AP5. *Neuropsychologia* 31: 1079–1098.

Maguire, E.A., Burgess, N., Donnett, J.F., Franckowiak, R.S.J. et al. (1998). Knowing where, and getting there: A human navigation network. *Science* 280: 921–924.

Mayford, M., Wang, L., Kandel, E.R., and O'Dell, T.J. (1995). CaMKII regulated the frequency-response function of hippocampal synapses for the production of both LTD and LTP. *Cell* 81: 81–94.

McHugh, T.J., Blum, K.I., Tsien, T.Z., Tonegawa, S. et al. (1996). Impaired hippocampal representation of space in CA1-specific NMDAR1 knockout mice. *Cell* 87: 1339–1349.

Mehta, M.R., and McNaughton, B.L. (1997). Lack of experience-dependent place field expansion in dentate gyrus and NMDAR dependence of the effect in CA1. *Soc. Neurosci. Abstr.* 23: 505.

Mehta, M.R., Barnes, C.A., and McNaughton, B.L. (1997). Experience-dependent, asymmetric expansion of hippocampal place fields. *PNAS* 94: 918–8921.

Miller, V.M., and Best, P.J. (1980). Spatial correlates of hippocampal unit activity are altered by lesions of the fornix and entorhinal cortex. *Brain Res.* 194: 311–323.

Morris, R.G., Garrud, P., Rawlins, J.N., and O'Keefe, J. (1982). Place navigation impaired in rats with hippocampal lesions. *Nature* 297: 681–683.

Morris, R.G.M., Anderson, E., Lynch, G.S., and Baudry, M. (1986). Selective impairment of learning and blockade of long term potentiation by an N-methyl-D-aspartate receptor antagonist, AP5. *Nature* 319: 774–776.

Muller, R.U., and Kubie, J.L. (1987). The effects of changes in the environment on the spatial firing of hippocampal complex-spike. *J. Neurosci.* 7: 1951–1968.

Muller, R.U., Kubie, J.L., and Ranck, J.B. Jr. (1987). Spatial firing patterns of hippocampal complex-spike cells in a fixed environment. *J. Neurosci.* 7: 1935–1950.

O'Keefe, J., and Dostrovsky, J. (1971). The hippocampus as a spatial map: Preliminary evidence from unit activity in the freely-moving rat. *Brain Res.* 34: 171–175.

O'Keefe, J., and Nadel, L. (1978). *The hippocampus as a Cognitive Map.* Oxford: Oxford University Press.

O'Keefe, J., and Reece, M.L. (1993). Phase relationship between hippocampal place units and the EEG theta rhythm. *Hippocampus* 3: 317–330.

Otto, T., Eichenbaum, H., Wiener, S.I., and Wible, C.G. (1991). Learning-related patterns of CA1 spike trains parallel stimulation parameters optimal for inducing hippocampal long term potentiation. *Hippocampus* 1: 181–192.

Ranck, J.B. (1973). Studies on single neurons in dorsal hippocampal formation and septum in unrestrained rats. Part I. Behavioral correlates and firing repertoires. *Exp. Neurol.* 41: 461–531.

Rose, G.M., and Dunwiddie, T.V. (1986). Induction of hippocampal LTP using physiologically patterned stimulation. *Neurosci. Lett.* 69: 244–248.

Rotenberg, A., Mayford, M., Hawkins, R.D., Kandel, E.R. et al. (1996). Mice expressing activated CaMKII lack low frequency LTP and do not form stable place cells region of the hippocampus. *Cell* 87: 1351–1361.

Shapiro, M., Tanila, H., and Eichenbaum, H. (1997). Cues that hippocampal place cells encode: Dynamic and hierarchical representation of local and distal stimuli. *Hippocampus* 7: 624–642.

Shen, J., Barnes, C., McNaughton, B.L., Skagg, W.E. et al. (1997). The effect of aging on experience-dependent plasticity of hippocampal place cells. *J. Neurosci.* 17: 6769–6782.

Silva, A.J., Stevens, C.F., Tonegawa, S., and Wang, T. (1992a). Deficient hippocampal LTP in α-calcium-calmodulin kinase II mutant mice. *Science* 257: 201–206.

Silva, A.J., Paylor, C.F.R., Wehner, J.W., and Tonegawa, S. (1992b). Impaired spatial learning in α-calcium-calmodulin kinase II mutant mice. *Science* 257: 206–211.

Staubli, U., Thibault, O., DiLorenzo, M., and Lynch, G. (1989). Antagonism of NMDA receptors impairs acquisition but not retention of olfactory memory. *Behav. Neurosci.* 103: 54–60.

Tanila, H.P., Sipila, P., Shapiro, M., and Eichenbaum, H. (1997). Brain aging: Changes in the nature of information coding by the hippocampus. *J. Neurosci.* 17: 555–566.

Thomas, M.J., Watabe, A.M., Moody, T.D., Makhinson, M. et al. (1998). Postsynaptic complex spike bursting enables the induction of LTP by theta frequency synaptic stimulation. *J. Neurosci.* 15: 7118–7126.

Tonkiss, J., Morris, R.G., and Rawlins, J.N. (1988). Intra-ventricular infusion of the NMDA antagonist AP5 impairs performance on a non-spatial operant DRL task in the rat. *Exp. Brain Res.* 73: 181–188.

Tsien, J.Z., Huerta, J., and Tonegawa, S. (1996). The essential role of hippocampal CA1 NMDA receptor-dependent synaptic plasticity in spatial memory. *Cell* 87: 1327–1338.

Tsodyks, M.V., Skaggs, W.E., Sejnowski, T.J., and McNaughton, B.L. (1996). Population dynamics and theta rhythm phase precession of hippocampal place cell firing: A spiking neuron model. *Hippocampus* 6: 271–280.

Walker, D.L., and Gold, P.E. (1994). Intrahippocampal administration of both the D- and L-isomers of AP5 disrupts spontaneous alteration behavior and evoked potentials. *Behav. Neural Biol.* 62: 151–162.

Whishaw, I.Q., and Tomie, J.A. (1996). Of mice and mazes: Similarities between mice and rats on dry land but not water mazes. *Physiol. Behav.* 60: 1191–1197.

Wilson, M.A., and McNaughton, B.L. (1993). Dynamics of the hippocampal ensemble code for space. *Science* 261: 1055–1058.

Wood, E.R., Dudchenko, P.A., and Eichenbaum, H. (1999). The global record of memory in hippocampal neuronal activity. *Nature* 397: 613–616.

CHAPTER EIGHTEEN

Understanding Synaptic Plasticity and Learning through Genetically Modified Animals

Paul F. Chapman

SUMMARY

Long-term potentiation (LTP) remains the most attractive model for learning-related plasticity. Of course, we must always test alternative hypotheses and be prepared to abandon those that no longer fit the existing data or provide predictive validity. Nonetheless, the LTP hypothesis for learning and memory has so much more data behind it than any alternative, I believe we are justified in continuing to test it rigorously using all available methods.

Among the most useful methods are those that involve direct manipulation of genes to disrupt LTP and learning. The use of genetic mutations to study learning and memory has a long history, but within the past decade its use has increased dramatically, driven by the development of techniques for targeted gene manipulation in mammals. Although these techniques are still essentially lesions, they have nonetheless increased the range of experiments that can be used to test the hypothesis that some forms of LTP underlie some forms of learning.

Introduction: A Brief History of Gene Manipulation in Long-Term Potentiation, Learning, and Memory

The intentional manipulation of genes has been going on for as long as humans have bred domesticated animals to select desirable physical or behavioral characteristics (Darwin, 1859). In the laboratory, this process dates back at least to Tryon (1934), who bred successive generations of rats on the basis of their performance in a complex maze. After several generations, there was nearly complete separation of performance in the maze, with "maze-dull" rats making significantly fewer errors than "maze-bright" ones. Even at this early date it was clear that breeding could select for sets of genes that influence performance on cognitive tasks, although it was equally clear that many factors (e.g., adaptation, attention, motivation) were being selected together.

Another major advance came with the development of efficient behavioral tests for the fruit fly *Drosophila*, which permitted the screening of large numbers of mutant subjects. Because the fly genome is relatively accessible and the reproductive cycle is quite short, generating large numbers of *Drosophila* with mutations introduced randomly (e.g., by exposure to chemical mutagens or X-rays) is relatively easy. The more difficult aspect of this approach is devising and applying appropriate behavioral (and physiologic) screens so that interesting mutational effects can be identified. Moreover, once mutants have been identified, it is also necessary to isolate the mutated gene. Nonetheless, this "forward genetic" approach has yielded critically important insights into which processes may be required for learning and memory. Many of the findings from *Drosophila* (e.g., the importance of the adenylyl cyclase/cAMP/protein kinase A pathway) have subsequently been supported by evidence obtained from rodents.

The late 1970s and early 1980s saw a significant increase in the number of spontaneous or randomly mutated mice. As their names (e.g., *reeler, weaver, staggerer, sprawler, shiverer, wobbler, tottering*) suggest, these mice were mostly identified on the basis of impaired motor function, in many cases involving abnormalities in either cerebellar development or myelination. In spite of being identified as motor control mutants, however, many of these mice had additional phenotypic features that were more cognitive or emotional [e.g., *nervous*, a Purkinje cell mutant that also responded abnormally to benzodiazepines (Skolnick et al., 1979)].

As informative as spontaneous mutations are, they have not made a major contribution to the long-term potentiation (LTP) literature at this point. The time between successive generations of mice and rats is relatively long, and the difficulty involved in conducting comprehensive behavioral screens for learning and memory means that it is impractical to rely on this approach. For the vast majority of experiments that are relevant to LTP, learning, and memory, the mutations have been introduced deliberately by one of several established methods.

Methods of Assessing Nervous System Function

Before describing the techniques that have been used to manipulate the genome and study the central nervous system (CNS), it is important to place these techniques in perspective. In any attempt to identify the function of a molecule, brain region, or physiologic process, there will be a limited number of experimental approaches that can be applied. Moreover, confidently ascribing a function to any process or structure will require convergent information from these different approaches. In essence, there are only three: One can activate the structure and assess the resulting functions, one can inactivate the structure and assess the changes in function compared to normal controls, or one can examine the patterns of activation that occur naturally, and correlate them with ongoing function.

Whether the experimenter uses pharmacologic, molecular, or electrophysiologic manipulations to achieve these ends, the fundamental principles will remain the same.

Inactivating

Perhaps the most common way to assess any CNS function is to inactivate it. The systematic use of lesion dates back at least to Karl Lashley, who discovered its advantages but is perhaps more famous for cataloguing its frustrations (Lashley, 1950). The advantage is the possibility of gaining the most direct (and dramatic) insight into the role any structure plays. Removing or inactivating the amygdala, for example, can abolish fear conditioning (e.g., Hitchcock and Davis, 1986), normally extremely robust in rodents. Blocking NMDA receptors in the amygdala achieves the same end by "lesioning" pharmacologically some process that appears to be critical for the acquisition, maintenance, or even performance of the conditioned fear response (Miserendino et al., 1990). Fear conditioning can also be abolished by genetic lesion, for example, the targeted deletion of the gene for RasGRF (Brambilla et al., 1997). Thus, although different techniques are applied, and different specific structures affected, the logic behind all three of these experiments is the same.

It is equally important to realize that mechanical, pharmacologic, and genetic lesions all share the same shortcomings. Inactivation can be a relatively crude tool, and it is difficult to know with any lesion technique whether the observed functional differences result directly from the experimental manipulation, or indirectly through some compensatory mechanism or secondary damage. Most ablations will damage fibers of passage as well as the intended structure. In other cases, the removal of important signals from the lesioned structure can change the levels of neurotransmitters or gene expression in structures efferent to the target. In a similar manner, deletion of the genes for the a and d isoforms of cAMP-responsive element binding (CREB) causes compensatory changes in the expression of bCREB (Blendy et al, 1996), which does not invalidate the results of experiments on adCREB-deleted mice (Bourtchuladze et al., 1994), but rather emphasizes the need to analyze *all* forms of lesions for unintended knock-on effects. The body of evidence gained from lesion studies is enormous; in the synaptic plasticity field alone nearly everything known about the induction and maintenance of LTP comes from pharmacologic or genetic lesions.

Activating

It is also desirable to assess the results of activating a structure, or increasing the concentration or activity of a specific molecule. If a particular neuronal circuit plays a role in a learned behavior, the activation of the structures in that circuit should reproduce, or at least affect, the behavior. If a gene is implicated in the onset of a disease, then the expression of that gene product should (and in many cases does) produce symptoms of that disease. On the other hand, it is unlikely in all but a few pathologic conditions that one could experimentally activate a brain structure or gene product in exactly the same way the brain does during normal physiologic function. Once again, this technique may give us insight, but cannot by itself give us answers.

Correlating

Because both activation and inactivation impose abnormal conditions on the brain, we can never be certain that processes or structures that have been affected by either of those two approaches would normally contribute to the phenomena we wish to explain. To complement those approaches, it is desirable to observe physiologic, biochemical, or molecular processes that correlate with the behavior in question. For example, recording of firing patterns of individual neurons during exploration (see Chapter 17) or specific behavioral tasks (Berger et al., 1976; Quirk et al., 1997) can give insight into the contributions different brain structures or processes might have in those behaviors. In a similar way, monitoring patterns of gene expression during learning or LTP (see Chapter 19) can help refine our understanding of which biochemical or molecular processes might be engaged by a particular type of plasticity or learning. This approach is limited, as any correlative approach would be, by the impossibility of establishing causality. Thus, our understanding of the conditions under which immediate early genes (IEGs) are activated is growing rapidly, but is not matched by our understanding of their function because it is technically feasible to observe them, but difficult to activate or inactivate them.

Available Techniques

Random Mutagenesis

Mutations to the genome happen without any intervention; the theory of evolution is based on this principle. Waiting for species to evolve is impractical for laboratory experimentation, however, as most of us do not have hundreds of thousands of years to wait. Fortunately, the rate of mutagenesis can be enhanced by X-rays, for example, or the delivery of known chemical agents. In this so-called forward genetic technique, mutations are produced at random and, if passed to offspring, can be identified by their phenotypic effects. It is theoretically possible, for instance, to create random mutations in mice or rats, then screen large numbers of them on simple learning and memory tests (e.g., T-maze alternation, fear conditioning, avoidance learning). Those that demonstrated deficits on one or more of these tasks could then be tested for LTP and/or on a broader range of behavioral tasks, while molecular cloning techniques were used to search for the nature of the actual mutation. In practice, this would be rather difficult to do, both because the number of rodents that must be screened would be prohibitive and because it would be difficult to imagine the behavioral screen that would unequivocally identify a "learning mutant." On the other hand, this technique has been applied with great success to *Drosophila* (see Dubnau and Tully, 1998, for a recent review) where screening of thousands of mutants is possible. It has also proven useful in the identification of circadian rhythm-related clock genes in mammals (Wilsbacher and Takahashi, 1998), probably because the behavioral screens are relatively straightforward.

Transgenes

It is often desirable to examine the effects of introducing a specific gene into a developing animal. In some cases, these genes will be identical to exogenous genes, but for one reason or another the experimenter wishes to examine the effects of overproducing the gene product. More often, the so-called transgene is a mutation of an existing gene that is intended to regulate or compete with an endogenous gene. In many cases the gene is implicated in a disease affecting the nervous system, and may be mutated at a known locus related to the human disease. Finally, transgenic techniques are becoming used increasingly as aids to visualizing plasticity, rather than preventing it; in these cases histologic markers such as β-galactosidase or green fluorescent protein (GFP) are introduced under the control of promoters that are sensitive to LTP-inducing stimulation.

Overexpression

The most logically straightforward way to use transgenes is to overproduce a protein that appears to be essential for the function of interest. By introducing one or more exogenous copies of the gene that codes for that protein, thereby increasing its concentration, one is essentially engaged in an activation-type experiment. How will plasticity and/or learning be affected by producing a superabundant amount of any particular protein? There are numerous examples of how this technique is applied to studying LTP and learning, including glutamate receptors (e.g., Okabe et al., 1998; Feldmeyer et al., 1999; Tang et al., 1999), cell adhesion molecules (e.g., Luthi et al., 1996), tyrosine kinases (e.g., Lu et al., 1999), and serine/threonine kinases (e.g., Mayford et al., 1995, described in detail in section 5.1.2). In some instances, overexpression will essentially constitute activation. For example, the overexpression of NR2B or NR2D subunits of the NMDA receptor appears to be able to augment the normal NMDA-receptor mediated calcium influx in cultured hippocampal neurons, while at the same time enhancing both LTP and performance on several learning tasks that involve hippocampal function (Okabe et al., 1998; Tang et al., 1999). In other cases, however, a protein that might normally contribute to plasticity can produce the opposite effect when expressed ectopically (Lüthi et al., 1996; Feldmeyer et al., 1999).

■ **Disease-Related.** Medical genetics has become increasingly successful at identifying genetic mutations or allelic variations that cause (or contribute to) neurologic disease. Once these genes have been identified and cloned they can be introduced into mice or rats, on the theory that expression of the abnormal protein that results from many of these mutations (e.g., amyloid precursor protein or presenilin in Alzheimer's or huntingtin in Huntington's) will produce similar symptoms to those that arise in the human disease. In fact, neurodegenerative disorders are particularly attractive to model, as they offer a straightforward pathologic yardstick against which to measure the effect of the transgene. Thus, for example, disruption of hippocampal function or synaptic plasticity have been reported in models of motor neuron disease in which Cu/Zn superoxide dismutase is overexpressed (Barkats et al., 1993; Gahtan et al., 1998), of mental retardation using overexpression of S100 (Gerlai et al., 1994; Gerlai and Roder 1995; Roder et al., 1996), or of acquired immunodeficiency syndrome (AIDS) dementia using the viral coat protein gp 120 (Krucker et al., 1998).

Although they are primarily interesting as models of the human disease, these transgenic animals can also offer insight into some the basic properties of neuronal function. An example considered in greater detail below is the overexpression of mutant amyloid precursor protein (APP), which not only produces some of the major pathologic features of Alzheimer's disease (Hsiao et al., 1996; Chapman et al., 1999) but also interferes with hippocampal LTP.

■ **Dominant Negative/Regulatory.** It is also possible to use transgene overexpression as a means of inactivating cellular processes. If the expressed transgene is a protein that either regulates or suppresses the expression of another protein, the effect can be the same as a lesion or a pharmacologic antagonist. For example, Abel et al. (1997) overexpressed the regulatory subunit of cAMP-dependent protein kinase (PKA), thus effectively limiting PKA activity. The effect was an impairment of long-lasting LTP. De Zeeuw et al. (1998) expressed an inhibitor of protein kinase C (PKC) in Purkinje cells, where PKC is thought to mediate long-term depression (LTD). They found not only that LTP was blocked in parallel fiber-Purkinje cell synapses, but that adaptation of the vestibulo-ocular reflex, thought to depend on LTD in cerebellar cortex, was also compromised.

Activity Markers

Gene manipulation can be used to identify neurons on either an anatomic or physiologic basis. Transgenic animals can produce marker proteins under the control of regionally expressed or activity-dependent promoters. The result is to make the expression of the marker selective to cells of a particular type (e.g., GABAergic neurons, Purkinje cells), or to those that have been activated by experience, including LTP. An example is the work by Storm and colleagues (Impey et al., 1996, 1998), in which they placed the lacZ gene under the control of the CREB promoter. Following either the induction of late-phase (protein synthesis dependent) LTP (Impey et al., 1996) or Pavlovian fear conditioning (Impey et al., 1998) and X-gal treatment of hippocampal slices, β-galactosidase staining was seen in hippocampal pyramidal neurons, suggesting that CREB activation is normally associated with learning and LTP induction. In the future, this technology will no doubt be expanded so that other types of behavior (e.g., motor learning, drug self-administration) can be correlated with expression of a variety of genes.

Inducible Transgenes

One of the principal concerns about transgenic techniques is that they can alter development in unpredictable ways. If a gene is overexpressed from the earliest developmental stages, then it has the opportunity to affect normal development in a number of ways. First, expression of the transgenic protein at the wrong stage might adversely affect neural development. Second, the expressed transgene might interfere with the function of a different protein that is critical for normal development. Finally, the existence of high levels of the transgenically expressed protein might initiate compensatory changes in other systems that would lead to abnormal function. Recent developments in the design of transgenes, however, have offered a solution to this particular problem. By placing the expression of the transgene under the control of prokaryotic promoters that are sensitive to exogenously applied substances, the transgene expression becomes inducible (Furth et al., 1994). Thus, a transgene introduced into the genome by standard techniques will remain inactive until the animal carrying the transgene is given a specific drug (e.g., tetracycline) or, alternately, is expressed until the administered substance turns it off. There are still important caveats to the use of transgene expression, and care must be taken that phenotype effects do not result from insertional effects (i.e., the transgene disrupting the function of another gene), from background strain interactions, and so forth. Nonetheless, inducible transgenes represent a significant refinement of the technique and will prove to be particularly useful with dominant-negative constructs.

Knock-Out

Perhaps the most interest (and controversy) has been generated by experiments involving targeted gene deletion, or "knock-out." In this technique, specific genes are disrupted (typically by the insertion of a neomycin resistance gene somewhere in a coding region) in embryonic stem cells, which are then used to create mice that are deficient in that particular gene. The first examples of the application of this technique to LTP came from Silva et al. (1992a,b) and Grant et al. (1992) who knocked out the gene for α-calcium/calmodulin-dependent protein kinase II (αCaMKII) and *fyn* tyrosine kinase, respectively.

The αCaMKII and *fyn* knock-outs represent some of the best and some of the most concerning aspects of the knock-out technique. In each case, pharmacologic experiments had demonstrated that "lesioning" either CaMKII (Malenka et al., 1989) or a rather broad spectrum of tyrosine kinases (O'Dell et al., 1991) could block LTP induction without affecting expression. In the case of CaMKII, the inhibitors were highly selective (e.g., Kelly et al., 1988) but available in only small quantity and had to be administered intracellularly via the recording pipette (Malenka et al., 1989). The inhibitors that O'Dell and colleagues used were available in larger quantity and could be bath applied, but could not distinguish among a variety of nonreceptor tyrosine kinases.

Both knock-outs, in contrast, entirely eliminated a specific enzyme from the brains of mice that could then be used to test both synaptic plasticity and learning in parallel. As discussed in detail below, αCaMKII knock-outs have consistently demonstrated the utility of the technique, including the ability to test a broad range of physiologic and behaviural phenomena and the possibility of testing specific hypotheses about CaMKII function (Silva et al., 1992a, 1992b). Similarly, the *fyn* knockouts introduced a new and growing field examining the role of protein-protein interactions in neuronal plasticity (Grant et al., 1992).

On the other hand, the αCaMKII knock-outs spared βCaMKII (Silva et al., 1992a), and the degree to which this gene could compensate for the missing isoform is difficult to assess. In the case of the *fyn* tyrosine kinase knock-out, gross anatomic differences were apparent in the dentate gyrus, and these might have suggested that LTP reduction does not entirely explain the observed learning deficits. Subsequent work has addressed this issue, however, and Kojima et al. (1997) demonstrated that turning on an inducible (tet-on) *fyn* transgene could rescue normal LTP and learning, even though gross anatomic abnormalities persisted.

Conditional Knock-Out

The standard knock-out technique comes with two sets of potential problems. The first set, introduced above, concerns the interpretation of functional changes in a nervous system that might have developed abnormally. The second problem is a more pragmatic one; some gene mutations are lethal. This second problem is a subset of the first; normal expression of the gene is required for early development, for example, or for some sensory or motor reflex that is crucial to early survival (e.g., suckling). In either case, the knock-out would be more practical, and possibly more interpretable, if it were able to gain the same temporal and spatial control that traditional lesions offer. Thus, the development of both region-specific and experimenter-inducible knock-out has been a high priority.

■ **Region-Specific.** The ability to control the onset or location of gene knock-outs can be gained by combining the knock-out and transgenic expression techniques. In the most commonly used version of the region-specific knockout, the gene of interest (e.g., the NR1 subunit of the NMDA receptor; Tsien et al., 1996) is flanked by the bacterial gene loxP (thus, "floxed"). In the presence of the cre-recombinase enzyme, any DNA physically located between two loxP sites is excised, so that combining cre-recombinase expression in the same cell with the floxed gene will delete that gene. However, expression of the floxed gene will be normal in cells that do not contain cre-recombinase. The trick is to produce a line of mice transgenic for cre-recombinase, in which the transgene is expressed only in a region of interest (e.g., hippocampal CA1). Then, unlike the traditional knock-out in which all cells would function without the gene of interest, only the selected gene in those selected cells in which the cre-recombinase transgene is expressed would be knocked out.

Tsien et al. (1996) used this technique to test mice in which NR1 knock-outs were restricted to CA1 as a result of serendipitously restricted expression of cre-recombinase (under the control of the αCaMKII promoter) in a single line of mice. The mice were given a thorough going-over, being tested for LTP, several learning tasks, and the formation of place cell firing in the hippocampus, all of which supported the contention that NMDA receptors are required for all these functions. By implication, the authors suggest that LTP is also a major player in learning and memory.

■ **Inducible.** In theory, the introduction of inducible knock-outs should simply involve combining the existing cre-loxP technology with that of inducible transgene expression. Thus, a cre-recombinase transgenic mouse in which the transgene is under the control of the tetracycline transactivator is mated to a mouse with a floxed gene of interest. The offspring then carry cre-recombinase in a selected region or cell type that also has a floxed gene, but the enzyme is not produced, and the gene is not deleted, until the mice are treated with a tetracycline analogue. In practice, this technique has proven promising, but problematic, since the currently available regulators of transgene activation (e.g., tet-on or tet-off) can be "leaky," meaning that they express at very low levels when in the inactivated state (Kellendonk et al., 1999). This can be tolerated in a straight transgenic experiment, but if cre recombination events happen even at a relatively low rate over time, the effect could be a significant loss of the target gene in the adult, before the experimenter intended to induce the knock-out. Nonetheless, this technique will doubtless be refined in the near future, and region-specific, inducible knock-outs will be available as needed.

Gene Knock-Out Versus Traditional Lesions

Genetic engineering in general (and gene knock-out in particular) has many proponents in the field of neuroscience (Takahashi et al., 1994; Tonegawa et al., 1995; Wehner et al., 1996), but is also capable of inspiring fear and loathing (e.g., Routtenberg, 1996). The apprehension about the potential pitfalls of gene knock-out are strongest when the technique is applied to analyses of behavior. Certainly, it is important when using knock-outs to be concerned about issues such as developmental abnormalities, compensation, and irreversibility, but it is equally important to realize that knock-outs are no more or less than another kind of lesion, beset by fundamentally the same confounds, but providing essential information about the mechanisms of learning and memory. One of the great strengths of the molecular genetic revolution in neuroscience has been the ability to test the physiologic, biochemical, and behavioral effects of a single manipulation. While this has been possible for some time using pharmacologic means (e.g., Morris et al., 1986), the approach is not universally applicable. The pharmacologic lesion can only be used with drugs that can be administered systemically and can either cross neuronal cell membranes easily or be effective without entering the cell. The compounds must be available in sufficient quantity to be used over the long time periods sometimes required for adequate behavioral testing, and finally, they must be specific enough to allow the experimenter to conclude with some confidence that the physiologic and/or behavioral consequences of drug application were due to its effect on the target molecule. On the other hand, targeted disruption of gene function through deletion of the gene is specific, restricted to the cells in which the gene would normally have been expressed, and, as the technology develops, conditional on various induction factors under the experimenter's control.

Case Studies

A multitude of articles have been published demonstrating that a particular knock-out or transgene has a profound (or subtle) effect on LTP and/or learning, and more are certain to be produced all along. Have they helped us address any of the serious questions we set out to answer? I have chosen two case studies to illustrate the field: αCaMKII, which has been knocked out, added as a transgene, and knocked in with a single point mutation, and APP, which has been added as a transgene in various mutated forms to create a mouse model of Alzheimer's disease.

CaMKII

CaMKII made a very logical place to begin knocking out genes that could be involved in learning and memory. LTP induction was already known to depend on calcium influx (Lynch et al., 1983; Malenka et al., 1988), CaMKII was known to be a major constituent of the postsynaptic density (Kelly et al., 1984) as well as being present in high concentration in the presynaptic terminal, and pharmacologic experiments had shown that blocking CaM kinase activity with either broad-spectrum kinase inhibitors (Malinow et al., 1988) or specific peptide blockers (Malenka et al., 1989) could prevent LTP induction. Moreover, an influential hypothesis put forward by Kennedy (Miller and Kennedy, 1986) and by Lisman (Lisman and Goldring, 1988) suggested that CaMKII could function as a "switch" that turned on long-lasting LTP. They based this hypothesis on the observation that once activated CaMKII can phosphorylate itself and, having done so, would no longer require calcium for its activation. This switch would make CaMKII fit the induction requirements of LTP nicely, as the maintenance of LTP can be impaired by blocking constitutive kinase activity (Malinow et al., 1988), even though the calcium influx that triggers LTP induction is transient. Genetic manipulation, then, could be used for the first time to test a hypothesis about the mechanisms of LTP, and possibly learning.

■ **Targeted Gene Deletion.** There has probably been more intensive investigation, using a wider range of techniques, for the αCaMKII gene than any other believed to be involved in LTP and learning. Genetic manipulation of this target began with the knock-outs by Silva et al. (1992a, 1992b) and continued with standard and inducible transgenes carrying point mutations. More recently, Giese et al. (1998) created a knock-in mouse with a specific mutation that renders the protein incapable of becoming calcium independent, thus testing the switch hypothesis.

■ **Null Mutation.** In 1992, Silva and colleagues reported the results of a series of experiments on mice with null mutations to (i.e., total elimination of) the αCaMKII gene. The isoform is enriched in forebrain (Lin et al., 1987), and is typically not expressed until about 2 weeks after birth. This means that even the conventional knock-out should have no effect on early development or structures that have not been strongly implicated in "declarative" memory.

The results generally supported the hypothesis that αCaMKII plays an important role in plasticity, learning, and memory (Silva et al., 1992a, 1992b). Approximately 90 percent of slices and individual neurons showed no LTP at all following standard tetanic stimulation (either 100 Hz for 1 second for extracellular recordings or pairing of low-frequency stimulation with direct postsynaptic depolarization for whole-cell recordings). In addition, the original findings indicated impairment in paired-pulse facilitation, suggesting that short-term as well as long-term plasticity might be affected by αCaMKII knockout. Indeed, later experiments indicated that both homozygous mutants (with both αCaMKII alleles deleted) and heterozygous mutants (one deleted, one normal, and approximately 50 percent endogenous protein levels) showed decreased paired-pulse facilitation and enhanced posttetanic potentiation, even in the presence of NMDA antagonists (Chapman et al., 1995).

The behavioral analysis of the αCaMKII knockouts used two tests that are now standard for mutants believed to affect hippocampal processing: spatial reference memory in the water maze and fear conditioning. The αCaMKII null mutants showed profound deficit on both these tasks, indicating an inability to learn at least some tasks dependent on hippocampus and amygdala. In addition to these more commonly used tasks, Glazewski et al. (1996) determined the effects of αCaMKII null mutations on plasticity in somatosensory cortex following whisker deprivation and found that the expected reorganization did not occur in homozygous mutants. Similarly, Gordon et al. (1996) tested the rather narrow strip of binocular visual cortex in mice, and found that monocular deprivation generally failed to produce shifts in ocular dominance columns in αCaMKII null mutants (although not in every case), in accordance with the results from somatosensory cortex. Several issues remained unresolved after these initial studies, however: What was the relative contribution of deficits in short-term plasticity to the behavioral abnormalities? Is there upregulation of βCaMKII in response to deletion and if so, can this account for the 10 percent of homozygotes that show normal synaptic plasticity? And finally, does this support the switch hypothesis? This last question could not be answered with the null mutation, since there was no αCaMKII available in either the calcium-dependent or independent state.

■ **Single Point Mutation.** In order to become calcium independent, CaMKII must phosphorylate itself at a specific residue, the threonine at position 286 (T286). Giese et al. (1998) took advantage of this by creating a knock-in mouse – one in which the αCaMKII gene inserted by homologous recombination was neither missing nor truncated, but carried a single point mutation that changed the T286 to an alanine. The T286A mice had no foreign material (i.e., neomycin resistance cassette) inserted in the genome, and had calcium-dependent CaMKII activity that was equivalent to the wild-type littermate mice used as controls. These mice, then, could address the switch hypothesis directly: Is it CaM kinase per se that is required for LTP induction, or is it *calcium-independent* CaM kinase?

The answer, apparently, is that calcium-independent CaM kinase is essential. The LTP data presented by Giese et al. (1998) indicate that enhanced synaptic transmission is completely eliminated by the T286A mutation. On the other hand, short-term plasticity is apparently not affected, nor is LTD, an observation made by Giese et al. in slices from young mice and recently confirmed in adults by Krezel et al. (1999). Behaviorally, the results were essentially identical to those of the null mutant, where the same tests were performed. Additionally, Cho et al. (1998) tested the ability of hippocampal neurons in T286A mice to form stable place fields, a physiologic measure of hippocampal network function. They found that the point mutants did form place fields, but that they were less spatially selective than controls, an observation consistent with that of McHugh et al. (1996) in NMDAR1-deficient mice. Moreover, in the T286A mice, the place fields were less stable over time, suggesting that fine-tuning and plasticity of hippocampal place fields depends on autophosphorylated αCaMKII, and possibly on LTP.

Thus, the more specific T286A point mutations confirmed the findings of the αCaMKII null mutations, and extended them by answering additional questions. Short-term plasticity is apparently normal in the T286A mice, suggesting that long-term plasticity is more important, at least for the behavioral measurements that have been made to this point. Similarly, the lack of effect on LTD suggests that synaptic depression without potentiation will not support any of a variety of spatial and nonspatial learning tasks (but see Migaud et al., 1998, which demonstrates the effects of abnormal LTD on learning and memory when accompanied by enhanced LTP). What is most apparent from the T286A mice is that synapses in CA1 cannot support either LTP or learning when αCaMKII is unable to become calcium-independent.

■ **Transgene Expression.** If inactivating the αCaMKII gene (or its ability to autophosphorylate) blocks LTP and learning, what would happen if αCaMKII were overexpressed? One possible outcome is that an abundance of autophosphorylated CaMKII will lead to either an enhancement (either increased magnitude or reduced threshold) of LTP. Alternately, LTP might become saturated (before the experimenter has an opportunity to measure it), thus resulting in an apparent reduction of potentiation. Moreover, the behavioral consequences of either of these outcomes would be difficult to predict, but potentially very informative about the relationship between synaptic plasticity and learning. To test these hypotheses, Mayford and colleagues conducted a series of experiments in which they overexpressed, using either constitutively active or inducible transgenes, a persistently autophosphorylated form of αCaMKII.

Constitutive. In these studies, several lines of mice transgenic for a constitutively active form of αCaMKII (in which the aspartate was substituted for threonine at the 286 amino acid position) were tested for their ability to support LTP and LTD (Mayford et al., 1995), to learn several behavioral tasks that are disrupted by lesion of the hippocampus or amygdala (Bach et al., 1995) and to generate stable place fields in the hippocampal CA1 region (Rotenberg et al., 1996). The results suggested that shifting the balance between calcium-dependent and calcium-independent CaMKII has no effect on LTP when induced with high-frequency tetanic stimulation, but decreases the probability of LTP induction at lower frequencies (1 to 10 Hz). Stimuli in this frequency range normally produce LTD in juvenile mice, while producing modest LTP in adults. In contrast, the αCaMKII-aspartate mice showed LTD under these conditions, suggesting that balance of plasticity at physiologically relevant activation frequencies is altered by providing an overabundance of calcium-independent CaMKII (Mayford et al., 1995).

The effects on synaptic plasticity were accompanied by changes in both systems physiology and behavior. αCaMKII-aspartate mice were unable to form stable hippocampal place fields (Rotenberg et al., 1996). Fewer fields were formed, and when formed they were less spatially well defined and less stable over repeated introductions to the same apparatus. Moreover, the alterations in stimulus-induced plasticity are accompanied by abnormal spatial learning in the Barnes maze (Bach et al., 1995), although curiously, not in fear conditioning. This latter result suggests that there may be different mechanisms for the plasticity supporting two different forms of learning, even if they have some common anatomic substrates.

Inducible. An obvious concern about the results of the initial transgene studies is that they resulted from a developmental response to increased availability of calcium-independent CaMKII. If true, this would limit our ability to interpret physiologic or behavioral deficits as revealing the normal function of αCaMKII, or of LTP. Mayford et al. (1996) addressed this problem by creating lines of mice that express the αCaMKII-aspartate transgene conditionally. The αCaMKII promoter was combined with the tetracycline transactivator system so that administration of doxycycline could turn off transgene expression. If αCaMKII expression (which is normally not significant until the second postnatal week) causes permanent developmental deficits, turning off the transgene in adulthood would have no effect on the phenotype. Instead, Mayford et al. (1996) found that normal behavior and electrophysiology were restored in mice when the αCaMKII-aspartate transgene was inactivated. This provides significant support for the hypothesis that αCaMKII acts directly as a mediator of use-dependent synaptic plasticity and learning.

Amyloid Precursor Protein

The αCaMKII experiments, both knock-out and transgene, are examples of the "reverse genetic" approach, in which specific genes are mutated and the effects of the mutations on behavior and physiology are assessed. Typically, the target genes are chosen because of suspected role in LTP based on pharmacologic evidence, or because of biochemical or structural interaction with other molecules thought to be involved in LTP. This is still the most commonly used approach in genetically based LTP research. Recently, however, with the advent of more and more rodent models of human neurologic disease, we are finding examples of genetics that are neither strictly "forward" nor "reverse." In this "sideways" genetics, the modified genes are chosen and not mutated randomly, but their interactions with other "LTP molecules" is unknown. At the same time, there is no explicit behavioral screen that can be used to define whether the gene has had an effect. What we do know is that the gene is (somehow) related to a human disease, the characteristics of which may be relatively poorly understood.

Alzheimer's disease (AD) is relatively well understood in humans in terms of neuropathologic features, while the underlying causes remain unknown, but hotly debated. The several gene mutations that have been associated with AD have implicated the β-amyloid protein, one of several pathologic species that are elevated in AD brains. What is not understood, however, is how the mutations lead to elevated concentrations of β-amyloid, and whether elevated β-amyloid concentrations or deposition of insoluble β-amyloid throughout the forebrain are responsible for some or all of the cognitive impairments observed in human AD. Moreover, we do not know what the normal function of amyloid or amyloid-like molecules is, or how they might interact with other key players in cell signaling or synaptic plasticity. On the other hand, what we learn from careful examination of neuropathology, behavior, and LTP in these mice might inform us about normal molecular signaling pathways used in synaptic plasticity and learning.

The strategy in this case is to introduce the mutant gene, then test the resulting animals against any objective criteria that can be obtained. In the case of AD, the logical starting point is with neuropathology, where murine tissue is sufficiently similar to human that the model should carry significant features of the disease. Once the validity of the model has been established to that point, the next step is to evaluate the phenotype where the relationship of the model to the human disorder will be less straightforward; in this case, that will be abnormal behavior. Finally, a useful model will make predictions about the causes of the disease and its less obvious symptoms.

Several different transgenic mouse models of AD have been created to date (see Seabrook and Rosahl, 1999, for a comprehensive review). Some labs have opted to overexpress APP itself (e.g., Games et al., 1995; Hsiao et al., 1995, 1996; Sturchler-Pierat et al., 1997) on the grounds that almost all AD patients have amyloid pathology, even if very few AD patients are known to have mutations to the APP gene. Others have added mutant presenilin-1 (e.g., Duff et al., 1996), which produces AD symptoms in a manner that is not yet well understood but that represents the majority of cases of familial early-onset AD. In general, more (and more severe) symptoms are seen in the APP transgenic mice than in presenilin transgenic mice, although some of the effects on neuronal plasticity are quite different from those seen in APP-overexpressing mice (e.g., Parent et al., 1999). Even among the APP-overexpressing mutants, the different lines vary in the nature of the transgene construct (cDNA versus minigene), APP isoform (695, 715, 770), the specific AD-related mutations within the transgene, as well as the promoter used to drive expression. The pathologic results from these lines are remarkably consistent, but behavioral (and to a lesser extent, physiologic) results have highlighted the difficulty in extending the phenotype beyond what is easily identified and quantified.

Although several lines of APP transgenic mice have been created and described, I will focus on the Tg2576 line (Hsiao et al., 1996). This mouse has been tested on a range of behavioral tasks (Hsiao et al., 1996; Chapman et al., 1999). It has also been well characterized for pathologic (Hsiao et al., 1996; Irizarry et al., 1997) and electrophysiologic changes resulting from a combination of transgene expression and age. Results that are now accumulating for Tg2576 and other APP mutant mice (Larson et al., 1999) suggest a common pattern of age-related deficits that could contribute to our understanding of both AD and LTP.

■ **Neuropathology.** The Tg2576 line of mice demonstrate a set of age-dependent neuropathologic features, some of which re-create AD quite closely. The concentration of β-amyloid in brain increases exponentially with age (Hsiao et al., 1996). From approximately 7 to 10 months onward, the amyloid is deposited in insoluble plaques that, like the dense-core plaques of human AD, bind to Congo red, and are stained by thioflavin-S, indicating a β-pleated sheet configuration (Hsiao et al., 1996). On the other hand, they do not demonstrate significant neuronal loss in CA1 (Irizarry et al., 1997). Although there are neuropil changes in the aged transgenics, there is also no overt formation of intracellular neurofibrillary tangles. There is still no consensus about whether there is any synapse loss, but if there is it is almost certainly less severe than that seen in AD brains. What is significant about this list is that it establishes that transgenic expression of an AD-related protein can produce major AD symptoms that are essentially identical to the human disease, while at the same time allow the model to assess the importance of those features in producing behavioral symptoms relative to other pathologic features that are absent.

■ **Behavior.** Tg2576 mice have been run through a variety of behavioral tests, focusing on learning and memory. The initial reports (Hsiao et al., 1996) were on performance on two tasks sensitive to hippocampal lesions: spontaneous alternation in the Y-maze and swimming to a fixed, hidden platform in the water maze. In both cases, aged (older than 10 months old) Tg2576 mice were significantly impaired relative to both littermate controls and to young transgenics. The impairment in the reference memory (hidden platform) water maze was evident in both the escape latencies and the number of platform crossings on a 60-second probe trial, although controls for swimming speed and thigmotaxis indicated no significant differences.

Aged Tg2576 mice also showed significant deficits in finding and swimming to a visible platform in the same pool. This task is typically regarded as a purely sensory and motor control, so the age-dependent impaired performance of the mice raises questions about their general state of health and CNS function (Routtenberg, 1997). When run through an extensive neurologic examination including assessment of righting reflex, hanging time on wire and dowel, walking on incline, running on a rotarod, pupillary reflexes, and pinna reflex, aged Tg2576 mice showed no impairment (Chapman et al., 1999). This suggests that sensory and motor function are not grossly abnormal, but also points to a general principle in the behavioral testing of genetically modified animals. Although you may intend to create a mutation limited to the hippocampus, and you may test hippocampal function as if your manipulation affected only the hippocampus, you must recognize that you might have affected other parts of the CNS that will also affect performance on behavioral tasks. This is especially relevant in modeling neurodegenerative diseases, as we know from human AD that pathology extends well beyond the hippocampus, and that the dementia that characterizes AD consists of more than specific deficits in learning and memory. One of the major goals for the field of LTP and learning should be a more complete characterization of the mechanisms and functions of synaptic plasticity across brain regions and systems.

More recently, we have found that spatial memory is also impaired in an age-dependent manner when Tg2576 mice are tested in a T-maze (Chapman et al., 1999). On the forced-choice alternation task, the mice are motivated by an appetitive reward (sucrose-water), while the motor demands are considerably less than in the water maze and response time is not a factor in accurate performance. The mice are forced to turn in one direction on the first trial of each pair, and on the second trial are rewarded for turning in the opposite direction. This requires spatial memory (for where they were rewarded on the first trial) and working memory (they must remember the previous forced-choice trial, but not any more remote trials). Two- to 5-month-old Tg2576 mice are unimpaired in acquisition of this task, and do not appear to be abnormally sensitive to the introduction of delays between the forced-choice and free-choice trials (unpublished observations). On the other hand, 15-month-old Tg2576 mice are significantly impaired in task acquisition even with no delay. The timing of this deficit appears to coincide with dramatic increases in brain β-amyloid concentration, and the deposition of amyloid into plaques, particularly in the dentate gyrus and entorhinal cortex (Chapman et al., 1999).

■ **Electrophysiology.** If the LTP hypothesis of learning has any validity, it is reasonable to predict that diseases that affect learning and memory should also have an effect on synaptic plasticity. Although neurodegenerative diseases such as Alzheimer's and Huntington's are associated with significant cell loss, it is not clear whether this is the sole cause of dementia, a contributing factor, or merely epiphenomenal. On the other hand, if there is loss of normal synaptic communication, or of synaptic plasticity, then learning and memory could be compromised in the absence of significant cell loss.

We tested this hypothesis by attempting to induce LTP in the hippocampus of Tg2576 mice at different ages, ranging from 2 to 15 months (Chapman et al., 1999). The experiments were conducted in CA1 and in dentate gyrus of hippocampal slices, and in the dentate gyrus of anesthetized mice *in vivo*. In each case, baseline synaptic transmission was measured by recording extracellular field potentials to low-frequency afferent stimulation across a range of stimulus intensities, and using these responses to generate input/output curves. In no case did these reveal significant differences in the field excitatorg postsynaptic potential (EPSP), in either CA1 or the dentate gyrus. Furthermore, paired-pulse facilitation, taken as a measure of short-term plasticity, was not different in Tg2576 mice than their littermate controls at any age.

High-frequency stimulation, however, did reveal significant differences between aged, transgenic Tg2576 mice and their littermate controls. LTP induction was normal in the dentate gyrus and CA1 of slices taken from adult (less than 8 months old) Tg2576 mice, and of aged nontransgenic controls. LTP was significantly reduced in CA1 of slices taken from aged transgenic mice, and was essentially absent in the dentate gyrus, both *in vitro* and *in vivo* (Chapman et al., 1999). LTP of the population spike, measured in the dentate gyrus *in vivo*, was also impaired in aged (greater than 12 months old) Tg2576 mice when compared to their littermates, although it was significantly enhanced over baseline (Jones et al., 1998).

The hippocampal slices in which the LTP experiments were conducted came from mice that had previously been tested in the T-maze. This enabled us to make a correlation between performance on the working memory task and LTP in both the dentate and CA1. The correlation between percentage of correct choices over the last 2 days of T-maze training and LTP 60 minutes after tetanus was significant in both CA1 (0.6) and dentate (0.8). This correlation cannot prove that a common pathology produced LTP deficits and memory deficits in the T-maze, although that is an attractive explanation. It is most likely that some consequence of overexpressing mutant amyloid precursor protein has affected basic mechanisms of synaptic plasticity, some of which will contribute to LTP while others, perhaps, will not. Whatever these mechanisms are, and whichever brain regions they affect, they do appear to have a significant negative effect on both LTP and the ability to learn and remember.

Conclusion

The Advantages of Using Gene Manipulations

The ability to manipulate genes has already provided the opportunity to conduct broad-ranging, integrative studies of physiology and behavior that were not possible just a short time ago. Examinations of the effects of αCaMKII knock-outs and overexpressing transgenes in LTP and LTD, in learning and memory, in place cell physiology, and in experience-dependent plasticity in the visual and somatosensory cortex have defined the role of this enzyme more clearly than perhaps any other molecule. Moreover, having once created these tools (αCaMKII null mutations and point mutations, wild-type, mutant, and inducible transgenes) they will be available to future researchers as long as there are questions left to ask about this enzyme and plasticity, and about neuronal plasticity and behavior.

In a similar manner, gene manipulation has led directly to animal models that can re-create important aspects of human CNS disease. These models can share a common etiology with the human disease when mutations to human genes are tightly linked to disease onset (e.g., familial AD, Huntington's) and the mutations can be reproduced in rodents. Where these diseases involve abnormal learning and memory, they can also become useful tools for exploring the relationship between synaptic plasticity and behavioral plasticity.

The Limitations of Using Gene Manipulations

For the most part, experiments using gene manipulations have the same limitation as other lesion (i.e., inactivation) studies. Systems are not static, so the removal of one will have consequences for others that are not easily measured. Compensation and unintended damage are problems whether the lesions are mechanical, neurotoxic, pharmacologic, or genetic, but they are perhaps more serious with traditional genetic lesions, since there is less spatial and temporal control. These are problems that will be reduced by the further development of gene manipulation techniques, allowing region-specific, inducible, and possibly reversible gene inactivation.

An additional set of practical problems with gene manipulation is related to the relative difficulty of the procedure. Although more and more laboratories are performing gene manipulation, and institutions are setting up dedicated facilities for transgenesis and gene knock-out, it is still more time-consuming and expensive to create a mouse with a targeted mutation than it is to apply a drug or a neurotoxic lesion. For this reason, it is imperative that researchers consider the use of all available techniques as they ask specific questions about the molecular and anatomic bases of learning and memory.

What We Have Learned (and Could Still Learn) about LTP and Learning through Gene Manipulation

Experiments conducted on genetically modified mice have revealed many cases in which LTP and learning appear to rely on the same mechanisms. Deletion of genes for receptors (e.g., Tsien et al., 1996), protein kinases (e.g., Grant et al., 1992; Giese et al., 1998), second messengers and adapter molecules (e.g., Brambilla et al., 1997; Migaud et al., 1998), and transcription factors (e.g., Bourtchuladze et al., 1994) have all demonstrated some degree of disruption of LTP and learning. Moreover, most of this evidence has been collected with first-generation knock-out techniques, which have (to some degree) been confounded by the possibility of nonspecific changes ranging from compensation by other molecules to embryonic lethality. The next generations of gene-targeting techniques will allow even more precise interpretations of an even greater range of gene manipulations.

There are other cases in which learning and LTP appear to be dissociated. These results should challenge us to think more carefully about the relationship between behavioral plasticity and synaptic plasticity, but are not cause to dismiss the hypothesis that LTP and learning are related. The case of Ras-GRF may be instructive; in one Ras-GRF knockout (Brambilla et al., 1997), hippocampal synaptic plasticity was normal, but LTP in the basolateral amygdala was compromised, along with emotional learning. Had the experimenters only tested LTP in CA1, the conclusion might have been very different. For every knock-out in which LTP appears to be blocked but learning spared, we must ask whether the appropriate form of LTP has been examined, in the appropriate brain region. For every knock-out in which LTP appears to be spared while learning is impaired, we must ask whether other LTP is compromised in other structures that are critical to that form of learning, and whether LTP is induced normally under all physiologically relevant conditions.

Conversely, can we conclude that gene deletion or mutation that produces an LTP deficit proves that that gene product is specifically involved in plasticity? Probably not. It may be the case that plasticity is a function of neurons in robust health, and that the more specific mechanisms are simply compromised by loss of normal cell function (e.g., membrane integrity, energy metabolism). To use a crude analogy, the basic tests of synaptic function used as baseline measures (e.g., input/output curves, paired pulse facilitation) may be asking neurons to walk; on the basis of normal walking we are assuming they should be able to run a marathon. Therefore, some knock-outs are likely to block LTP and learning by affecting specific mechanisms, while others may more generally compromise cell function in a way that is not immediately apparent through testing of baseline responses.

Much of the apparent contradiction between the effects of gene deletion (or pharmacologic blockade, for that matter) on LTP and learning can be attributed to attempts to treat both as unitary phenomena. Definitions of LTP will vary from person to person, but what all the definitions have in common is that they describe a phenomenon, and not a precise mechanism or biochemical pathway. For example, LTP of Schaffer collateral synapses in CA1 and mossy fiber synapses in CA3 are similar phenomena (brief, high-frequency stimulation produces long-lasting increases in synaptic responses), but appear to rely on very different mechanisms. When we block CA1 LTP, we have probably not blocked mossy fiber CA3 LTP. What about LTP in amygdala, neocortex, striatum, or cerebellum? How many of these will be spared by specific gene deletion, and what might they contribute to associative, spatial, emotional, episodic, or working memory? Therefore, when we ask the question "is LTP the mechanism of learning?" we must be careful to define which form of learning we mean, and which form of LTP. With appropriately defined questions, we can begin to catalogue various contributions of systems of genes to the plasticity in systems of neurons that support learning and memory.

REFERENCES

Abel, T., Nguyen, P.V., Barad, M., Deuel, T. A. et al. (1997). Genetic demonstration of a role for PKA in the late phase of LTP and in hippocampal-based long-term memory. *Cell* 88: 615–626.

Bach, M.E., Hawkins, R.D., Osman, M., Kandel, E.R. et al. (1995). Impairment of spatial but not contextual memory in CaMKII mutant mice with a selective loss of hippocampal LTP in the range of the theta frequency. *Cell* 81: 905–915.

Barkats, M., Bertholet, J.Y., Venault, P., Ceballospicot, I. et al. (1993). Hippocampal mossy fiber changes in mice transgenic for the human copper-zinc superoxide dismutase gene. *Neurosci. Lett.* 160: 24–28.

Berger, T.W., Alger, B., and Thompson, R.F. (1976). Neuronal substrate of classical conditioning in the hippocampus. *Science* 192: 483–485.

Blendy, J.A., Kaestner, K.H., Schmid, W., Gass, P. et al. (1996). Targeting of the CREB gene leads to up-regulation of a novel CREB mRNA isoform. *EMBO J.* 15: 1098–1106.

Bourtchuladze, R., Frenguelli, B., Blendy, J., Cioffi, D. et al. (1994). Deficient long-term memory in mice with a targeted mutation of the cAMP-responsive element-binding protein. *Cell* 79: 59–68.

Brambilla, R., Gnesutta, N., Minichiello, L., White, G.L. et al. (1997). A role for the RAS signalling pathway in synaptic transmission and long-term memory. *Nature* 390: 281–286.

Chapman, P.F., Frenguelli, B., Chen, C., Smith, A. et al. (1995). The α-calcium-calmodulin kinase II: A bi-directional modulator of pre-synaptic plasticity. *Neuron* 14: 591–597.

Chapman, P.F., White, G.L., Jones, M.W., Marshall, V.J. et al. (1999). Impaired synaptic plasticity and learning in aged APP transgenic mice. *Nat. Neurosci.* 2: 271–276.

Cho, Y.H., Giese, K.P., Tanila, H., Silva, A.J. et al. (1998). Abnormal hippocampal spatial representations in αCaMKII^{T286A} and CREB$^{\alpha\Delta-}$ mice. *Science* 279: 867–869.

Darwin, C. (1859). *On the Origin of Species by Means of Natural Selection, or the Preservation of Favoured Races in the Struggle for Life.* London: Murray.

De Zeeuw, C.I., Hansel, C., Bian, F., Koekkoek, S.K. et al. (1998). Expression of a protein kinase C inhibitor in Purkinje cells blocks cerebellar LTD and adaptation of the vestibulo-ocular reflex. *Neuron* 20: 495–508.

Dubnau, J., and Tully, T. (1998). Gene discovery in Drosophila: New insights for learning and memory. *Annu. Rev. Neurosci.* 21: 407–444.

Duff, K., Eckman, C., Zehr, C., Yu, X. et al. (1996). Increased amyloid-beta 42(43) in brains of mice expressing presenilin 1. *Nature* 383: 710–713.

Feldmeyer, D., Kask, K., Brusa, R., Kornau, H.C. et al. (1999). Neurological dysfunctions in mice expressing different levels of the Q/R site-unedited AMPAR subunit GluR-B. *Nat. Neurosci.* 2: 57–64.

Furth, P.A., St Onge, L., Boger, H., Gruss, P. et al. (1994). Temporal control of gene expression in transgenic mice by a tetracycline-responsive promoter. *Proc. Natl. Acad. Sci. USA* 91: 9302–9306.

Gahtan, E., Auerbach, J.M., Groner, Y., and Segal, M. (1998). Reversible impairment of long term potentiation in transgenic Cu/Zn SOD mice. *Eur. J. Neurosci.* 10: 538–544.

Games, D., Adams, D., Alessandrini, R., Barbour, R. et al. (1995). Alzheimer-type neuropathology in transgenic mice overexpressing V717F β-amyloid precursor protein. *Nature* 373: 523–527.

Gerlai, R., Marks, A., and Roder, J. (1994). T maze spontaneous alternation rate is decreased in S100 beta transgenic mice. *Behav. Neurosci.* 108: 100–106.

Gerlai, R., and Roder, J. (1995). Abnormal exploratory behavior in transgenic mice carrying multiple copies of the human gene for S100 beta. *J. Psychiatr. Neurosci.* 20: 105–112.

Giese, K.P., Federov, N.B., Filipkowski, R.K., and Silva, A.J. (1998). Autophosphorylation at threonine 286 of the a calcium-calmodulin-kinase II in LTP and learning. *Science* 279: 870.

Glazewski, S., Chen, C.M., Silva, A., and Fox, K. (1996). Requirement for alpha CaMKII in experience dependent plasticity of the barrel cortex. *Science* 272: 421–423.

Gordon, J.A., Cioffi, D., Silva, A.J., and Stryker, M.P. (1996). Deficient plasticity in the primary visual cortex of alpha-calcium/calmodulin-dependent protein kinase II mutant mice. *Neuron* 17: 491–499.

Grant, S.G.N., Odell, T.J., Karl, K.A., Stein, P.L. et al. (1992). Impaired long-term potentiation, spatial learning, and hippocampal development in fyn mutant mice. *Science* 258: 1903–1910.

Hitchcock, J., and Davis, M. (1986). Lesions of the amygdala, but not of the cerebellum or red nucleus, block conditioned fear as measured with the potentiated startle paradigm. *Behav. Neurosci.* 100: 11–22.

Hsiao, K.K., Borchelt, D.R., Olson, K., Johannsdottir, R. et al. (1995). Age-related CNS disorder and early death in transgenic FVB/N mice overexpressing Alzheimer amyloid precursor proteins. *Neuron* 15: 1203–1218.

Hsiao, K.K., Chapman, P.F., Nilsen, S., Eckman, C. et al. (1996). Correlative memory deficits, Aβ elevation and amyloid plaques in transgenic mice. *Science* 274: 99–102.

Impey, S., Mark, M., Villacres, E.C., Poser, S. et al. (1996). Induction of CRE mediated gene expression by stimuli that generate long-lasting LTP in area CA1 of the hippocampus. *Neuron* 16: 973–982.

Impey, S., Smith, D.M., Obrietan, K., Donahue, R. et al. (1998). Stimulation of cAMP response element (CRE)-mediated transcription during contextual learning. *Nat. Neurosci.* 1: 595–601.

Irizarry, M.C., McNamara, M., Fedorchak, K., Hsiao, K.K. et al. (1997). APPSw transgenic mice develop age-related Aβ deposits and neuropil abnormalities, but no neuronal loss in CA1. *J. Neuropathol. Exp. Neurol.* 56: 965–973.

Jones, M.W., Bliss, T.V.P., Hsiao, K.K., and Chapman, P.F. (1998). Age-dependent deficits in spatial memory and hippocampal LTP in vivo in APP transgenic mice. *Soc. Neurosci. Abstr.* 24.

Kellendonk, C., Tronche, F., Casanova, E., Anlag, K. et al. (1999). Inducible site-specific recombination in the brain. *J. Mol. Biol.* 285: 175–182.

Kelly, P.T., McGuinness, T.L., and Greengard, P. (1984). Evidence that the major postsynaptic density protein is a component of a Ca2+/calmodulin-dependent protein kinase. *Proc. Natl. Acad. Sci. USA* 81: 945–949.

Kelly, P.T., Weinberger, R.P., and Waxham, M.N. (1988). Active site-directed inhibition of Ca2+/calmodulin-dependent protein kinase type II by a bifunctional calmodulin-binding peptide. *Proc. Natl. Acad. Sci. USA* 85: 4991–4995.

Kojima, N., Wang, J., Mansuy, I.M., Grant, S.G. et al. (1997). Rescuing impairment of long term potentiation in fyn deficient mice by introducing Fyn transgene. *Proc. Natl. Acad. Sci. USA* 94: 4761–4765.

Krezel, W., Giese, K.P., Silva, A.J., and Chapman, P.F. (1999). Long-term depression is unimpaired in hippocampus of adult αCaMKIIT286A mice. *Soc. Neurosci. Abstr.* 25.

Krucker, T., Toggas, S.M., Mucke, L., and Siggins, G.R. (1998). Transgenic mice with cerebral expression of human immunodeficiency virus type-1 coat protein gp120 show divergent changes in short- and long-term potentiation in CA1 hippocampus. *Neuroscience* 83: 691–700.

Larson, J., Lynch, G., Games, D., and Seubert, P. (1999). Alterations in synaptic transmission and long term potentiation in hippocampal slices from young and aged PDAPP mice. *Brain Res.* 840: 23–35.

Lashley, K.S. (1950). In search of the engram. *Soc. Exp. Biol. Symp.* 4: 454–482.

Lin, C.R., Kapiloff, M.S., Durgerian, S., Tatemoto, K. et al. (1987). Molecular cloning of a brain-specific calcium/calmodulin-dependent protein kinase. *Proc. Natl. Acad. Sci. USA* 84: 5962–5966.

Lisman, J.E., and Goldring, M.A. (1988). Feasibility of long-term storage of graded information by the Ca2+/calmodulin-dependent protein kinase molecules of the postsynaptic density. *Proc. Natl. Acad. Sci. USA* 85: 5320–5324.

Lu, Y.F., Kojima, N., Tomizawa, K., Moriwaki, A. et al. (1999). Enhanced synaptic transmission and reduced threshold for LTP induction in fyn-transgenic mice. *Eur. J. Neurosci.* 11: 75–82.

Luthi, A., Mohajeri, H., Schachner, M., and Laurent, J.P. (1996). Reduction of hippocampal long term potentiation in transgenic mice ectopically expressing the neural cell adhesion molecule L1 in astrocytes. *J. Neurosci. Res.* 46: 1–6.

Lynch, G., Larson, J., Kelso, S., Barrionuevo, G. et al. (1983). Intracellular injections of EGTA block the induction of hippocampal long-term potentiation. *Nature* 305: 719–721.

Malenka, R.C., Kauer, J.A., Zucker, R.S., and Nicoll, R.A. (1988). Postsynaptic calcium is sufficient for potentiation of hippocampal synaptic transmission. *Science* 242: 81–84.

Malenka, R.C., Kauer, J.A., Perkel, D.J., Mauk, M.D. et al. (1989). An essential role for post-synaptic calmodulin and protein kinase activity in long-term potentiation. *Nature* 340: 554–557.

Malinow, R., Madison, D.V., and Tsien, R.W. (1988). Persistent protein kinase activity underlying long-term potentiation. *Nature* 335: 820–824.

Mayford, M., Wang, J., Kandel, E.R., and O'Dell, T.J. (1995). CaMKII regulates the frequency response function of hippocampal synapses for the production of both LTD and LTP. *Cell* 81: 891–904.

Mayford, M., Bach, M.E., Huang, Y.Y., Wang, L. et al. (1996). Control of memory formation through regulated expression of a CaMKII transgene. *Science* 274: 1678–1683.

McHugh, T.J., Blum, K.I., Tsien, J.Z., Tonegawa, S. et al. (1996). Impaired hippocampal representation of space in CA1 specific NMDAR1. *Cell* 87: 1339–1349.

Migaud, M., Charlesworth, P., Dempster, M., Webster, L.C. et al. (1998). Enhanced long-term potentiation and impaired learning in mice with mutant postsynaptic density-95 protein. *Nature* 396: 433–439.

Miller, S.G., and Kennedy, M.B. (1986). Regulation of brain type II Ca2+/calmodulin-dependent protein kinase by autophosphorylation: A Ca2+–triggered molecular switch. *Cell* 44: 861–870.

Miserendino, M.J.D., Sananes, C.B., Melia, K.R., and Davis, M. (1990). Blocking of acquisition but not expression of conditioned fear-potentiated startle by NMDA antagonists in the amygdala. *Nature* 345: 716–718.

Morris, R.G.M., Anderson, E., Lynch, G.S., and Baudry, M. (1986). Selective impairment of learning and blockade of long-term potentiation by an N-methyl-D-aspartate receptor antagonist, AP5. *Nature* 319: 774–776.

O'Dell, T.J., Kandel, E.R., and Grant, S.G.N. (1991). Long-term potentiation in the hippocampus is blocked by tyrosine kinase inhibitors. *Nature* 353: 558–560.

Okabe, S., Collin, C., Auerbach, J.M., Meiri, N. et al. (1998). Hippocampal synaptic plasticity in mice overexpressing an embryonic subunit of the NMDA receptor. *J. Neurosci.* 18: 4177–4188.

Parent, A., Linden, D.J., Sisodia, S.S., and Borchelt, D.R. (1999). Synaptic transmission and hippocampal long-term potentiation in transgenic mice expressing FAD-linked presenilin 1. *Neurobiol. Dis.* 6: 56–62.

Quirk, G.J., Armony, J.L., and LeDoux, J.E. (1997). Fear conditioning enhances different temporal components of tone-evoked spike trains in auditory cortex and lateral amygdala. *Neuron* 19: 613–624.

Roder, J.K., Roder, J.C., and Gerlai, R. (1996). Conspecific exploration in the T maze: Abnormalities in S100 beta transgenic mice. *Physiol. Behav.* 60: 31–36.

Rotenberg, A., Mayford, M., Hawkins, R.D., Kandel, E.R. et al. (1996). Mice expressing activated CaMKII lack low frequency LTP and do not form stable place cells in the CA1 region of the hippocampus. *Cell* 87: 1351–1361.

Routtenberg, A. (1996). Reverse piedpiperase: Is the knockout mouse leading neuroscientists to a watery end? *Trends Neurosci.* 19: 471–472.

Routtenberg, A. (1997). Measuring memory in a mouse model of Alzheimer's disease. *Science* 277: 339–341.

Seabrook, G.R., and Rosahl, T.W. (1999). Transgenic animals relevant to Alzheimer's disease. *Neuropharmacology* 38: 1–17.

Silva, A.J., Stevens, C.F., Tonegawa, S., and Wang, Y. (1992a). Deficient hippocampal long-term potentiation in α-calcium-calmodulin kinase II mutant mice. *Science* 257: 201–206.

Silva, A.J., Paylor, R., Wehner, J.M., and Tonegawa, S. (1992b). Impaired spatial learning in α-calcium calmodulin kinase II mutant mice. *Science* 257: 206–211.

Skolnick, P., Syapin, P.J., Paugh, B.A., and Paul, S.M. (1979). Reduction in benzodiazepine receptors associated with Purkinje cell degeneration in 'nervous' mutant mice. *Nature* 277: 397–399.

Sturchler-Pierrat, C., Abramowski, D., Duke, M., Wiederhold, K.H. et al. (1997). Two amyloid precursor protein transgenic mouse models with Alzheimer disease-like pathology. *Proc. Natl. Acad. Sci. USA* 94: 13287–13292.

Takahashi, J.S., Pinto, L.H., and Vitaterna, M.H. (1994). Forward and reverse genetic approaches to behavior in the mouse. *Science* 264: 1724–1733.

Tang, Y.-P., Shimizu, E., Dube, G.R., Rampon, C. et al. (1999). Genetic enhancement of learning and memory in mice. *Nature* 401: 63–69.

Tonegawa, S., Li, Y., Erzurumlu, R.S., Jhaveri, S. et al. (1995). The gene knockout technology for the analysis of learning and memory, and neural development. *Prog. Brain Res.* 105: 3–14.

Tryon, R.C. (1934). Individual differences. In F.A. Moss (Ed.), *Comparative psychology*. (pp. 409–448). New York: Prentice-Hall.

Tsien, J.Z., Huerta, P.T., and Tonegawa, S. (1996). The essential role of hippocampal CA1 NMDA receptor dependent synaptic. *Cell* 87: 1327–1338.

Tsien, J.Z., Chen, D.F., Gerber, D., Tom, C. et al. (1996). Subregion and cell type restricted gene knockout in mouse brain. *Cell* 87: 1317–1326.

Wehner, J.M., Bowers, B.J., and Paylor, R. (1996). The use of null mutant mice to study complex learning and memory processes. *Behav. Genet.* 26: 301–312.

Wilsbacher, L.D., and Takahashi, J.S. (1998). Circadian rhythms: Molecular basis of the clock. *Curr. Opin. Genet. Dev.* 8: 595–602.

CHAPTER NINETEEN

What Gene Activation Can Tell Us about Synaptic Plasticity and the Mechanisms Underlying the Encoding of the Memory Trace

Sabrina Davis and Serge Laroche

SUMMARY

For almost a century we have been attempting to test the notion that information is stored in the brain as changes in the efficacy of synaptic connections on those neurons that are activated during learning. Since the discovery of long-term potentiation (LTP) in 1973, we have learned a great deal about the mechanisms underlying activity-dependent synaptic modification. To date, LTP is currently accepted as the most viable model of the type of modifications that would occur to process information and store the memory trace. Although over the past 25 years or so there has been a great deal of empirical data that allude to the possibility that this form of synaptic plasticity may well be one of the crucial mechanisms underlying learning and memory, we are still lacking definitive answers. We now know that LTP is the output of a series of biochemical and molecular events that in all likelihood results in a form of modification of neural networks. In this review we describe how the advances in molecular biology give us the tools to both investigate the mechanisms of synaptic plasticity and to apply these to investigations of the underlying mechanisms in learning and the formation of memories that have until now eluded us.

Introduction

One of the major concepts in our understanding of how memories are laid down in the brain lies in the notion that they (the memories) are encoded as spatiotemporal patterns of activity in cell networks, and not at the single cell level. An underlying principle is that the encoding and the storage of memory would therefore require some form of dynamic modification that is driven by the interaction between cells within these networks. Both of these ideas were first conceptualized

---

in the theoretical postulates of Donald Hebb in 1949 in his seminal work *The Organisation of Behavior*. Here, he hypothesized that the memory trace is laid down by the development of cell assemblies where synaptic knobs (sic), which appear during learning, develop with neural activity and represent a lowered synaptic resistance. This gave rise to two important contemporary concepts within the neuroscience field of learning and memory. The first is that synaptic plasticity or synaptic strengthening serves as a potential mechanism underlying the memory trace. The second, by the implication than more that one input is required to induce increased efficacy in the firing of a cell, is the notion that coactivation of converging input fibers serves as a mechanism of associative memory. Elaboration of these prescient ideas of Hebb has led to a physiologic model of synaptic plasticity, long-term potentiation (LTP) (Bliss and Lømo, 1973) and the development of formal theories of associative memory within distributed networks, of which Marr's influential theory utilized known anatomic circuitry in an organized network that incorporated activity-dependent modifiable synapses (Marr, 1971).

Since its original discovery, when Bliss and Lømo stated (1973), "Whether or not the intact animal makes use in real life of a property which has been revealed by synchronous, repetitive volley to a population of fibres the normal rate and pattern of activity along which are unknown, is another matter," LTP has become the most viable model of the type of synaptic modification that may occur during learning, to lay down a representation of the memory trace. Following the discovery of LTP, a great many experimental studies have been carried out in an attempt to draw causal links between LTP and the mechanisms necessary for encoding information during learning. As we are made acutely aware of in the introductory chapter, definitive empirical support for synaptic plasticity modeled by LTP being a mechanism of memory processing is still lacking. For each piece of evidence that lends some support to the theory, there is likely to be equally strong evidence to suggest the contrary. The field of research reached a veritable stalemate some years ago when so-called cornerstones of research that supported the hypothesis were unable to be replicated (Cain et al., 1993; Jeffery and Morris, 1993; Korol et al., 1993) or were contradicted (Moser et al., 1993; Saucier and Cain, 1995; Cain et al., 1996) and the outcome was an increasing skepticism about whether LTP can be considered a neural substrate for learning and memory (see, for example, Shors and Matzel, 1997). Despite the growing skepticism, we believe that the advances made in molecular biology have given us the tools and the resources to reconceptualize how the mechanisms underlying LTP may be reconciled with the type of neural activity necessary and sufficient for establishing memory traces in the brain.

Is There Behavioral Evidence for a Role of LTP in Learning and Memory?

The behavioral experiments that have been carried out to test whether LTP does constitute a neural substrate for learning and memory have, in general, been based on testing whether LTP was sufficient and necessary for learning at an electrophysiologic level. In general four main approaches have been adopted to test this hypothesis. The first, developed by Morris and colleagues, used the NMDA receptor, a critical trigger for the induction of LTP, to demonstrate the relationship between LTP and learning and memory. Using the NMDA receptor antagonist, AP5, they showed that it both blocked LTP and induced a deficit in spatial learning (Morris et al., 1986). More to the point, they showed a dose-dependent inverse relationship between learning and LTP, where the greater the concentration of AP5, the greater the deficit in learning and the smaller the magnitude of potentiation in the dentate gyrus after tetanic stimulation (Morris et al., 1990; Davis et al., 1992). Using a purely electrophysiologic approach McNaughton and colleagues (1986) showed that by repeatedly tetanizing the perforant path they could, by inducing LTP and saturating the dentate gyrus synapses to prevent further potentiation prior to learning, prevent rats from learning a hippocampal-dependent spatial task. They further showed that improvement in learning correlated with the rate of decay of LTP to baseline levels (Castro et al., 1989). These findings formed a cornerstone for the notion that LTP *is* one possible synaptic mechanism underlying the acquisition of learning certain tasks. The third approach adopted the standpoint that if LTP was a mechanism underlying the establishment or stabilization of the memory trace then one would expect to see a similar form of potentiation during learning that one observes following the induction of LTP. Recordings of the evoked response in the dentate gyrus during exploration (Sharp et al., 1989; Green et al., 1990) or during classical conditioning (Doyère et al., 1995) showed an increase in the excitatory postsynaptic potential (EPSP) with a concomitant decrease in the population spike amplitude, which lasted for approximately 30 minutes after cessation of the exploratory behavior or the learning session. Finally, the fourth approach has been to identify changes in biochemical and cellular activity that occur following the induction of LTP and testing whether similar changes occur after learning. Empirical evidence has shown that some of the biochemical changes that occur after learning in a parallel manner to those observed after the induction of LTP are an increase in glutamate release in the hippocampus (Laroche et al., 1987; Richter-Levin et al., 1995), second messenger activity such as IP3 turnover (Nicoletti et al., 1988; Laroche et al., 1990a), cAMP activation (Tully, 1991), and phosphorylation and translocation of kinases such as PKC (see Noguès, 1997) and CaMKII (Zhao et al., 1999).

Taken together these four approaches provide compelling evidence that an LTP-type mechanism may in fact play an important role in activity-dependent modification necessary and sufficient for laying down memory traces. However, since the original publication of the results from experiments using the first three strategies, none have been sucessfully replicated. Numerous studies testing the effect of the NMDA receptor antagonist on learning have suggested that in all likelihood much of the impairment in learning is due to some form of sensorimotor disturbance or hyperactivity (Leung and Desborough, 1988; Keith and Ruddy, 1990; Sillito et al., 1990; Cain et al., 1996), thereby disputing the role of the NMDA receptor in learning and by implication that of LTP. Importantly, Morris and colleagues (Bannerman et al., 1995) in an attempt to address the role of the NMDA receptor at a purely cognitive level, tested rats in one water maze before introducing AP5 into the brain and then tested whether rats could learn the same task in a new environment. Under these conditions there was no impairment in learning and neither was there any effect on sensorimotor activity. This allays the notion that the deficit is essentially a sensorimotor one, and in addition suggests that what the rats learned in the first water maze was sufficient for them to establish a memory trace for one spatial environment where they could "abstract" from that, to learn the spatial layout of a second environment, possibly by using another strategy. It further suggests that the role of the NMDA receptor in learning is in the very early phases and very brief, an effect that is commensurate with its role in LTP.

With the strategy using saturation of the synapses, five laboratories, including the original group, failed to replicate these findings. That saturation of all the synapses along the entire septotemporal axis of the dentate gyrus was not able to be replicated is not in itself surprising. As stated by Bliss and Richter-Levin (1993) in a commentary about these experiments "the surprise is not that the experiments cannot be replicated but that the original experiment worked as well as it did." It must be noted, however, that in a subsequent experiment carried out by Moser and colleagues (1998), they did in fact show that in conjunction with a lesion to the hippocampus (which alone was not sufficient to induce a deficit in learning) saturation of the remaining tissue did result in impaired learning. The most damning of all, perhaps, was the discovery that the natural potentiation of the EPSP during exploration was shown to be due to an increase in brain temperature induced by muscular effort (Moser et al., 1993). However, from their own results, Moser and Andersen (1994) later showed that of the total amount of potentiation that was induced, 8 to 12 percent could actually be attributed to a potential learning induced change, as was shown to be the case in associative learning by Doyère et al. (1995).

The inability to adequately replicate these previous findings and to show a causal link between LTP and any form of learning has been the driving force behind the skepticism that has developed about the natural role of LTP. The most obvious and simple interpretation is that LTP has nothing to do with learning and memory, but this would seem a premature standpoint to take at the present time. Given our understanding of how and where memories are constructed within the brain, how we would expect neural substrate of learning and memory to behave, and what we realistically believe LTP to be, it is glaringly obvious that the experimental approaches that have been taken, though conceptually sound, were analogous to taking a "sledge hammer approach." To take one example, the magnitude of change required within a population of cells, where we are measuring the field response electrophysiologically, would more than likely put it within the range of being pathologic. If, as we believe, the memory trace is encoded within a distributed network of cells, then the necessary approach to take would be to search for more discrete changes that are induced by LTP within a network of interconnected cells, to assess whether these changes also occur during learning. In fact, the only strategy that has stood the test of time has been the fourth strategy, looking for biochemical/molecular correlates. Although it has taken a more indirect and correlational approach, experiments showing parallels in learning and LTP with changes in the cellular milieu have not fallen into dispute as have the other strategies. As will be described below, this approach has been extended to testing LTP and learning in mice with deletions of genes encoding proteins known to play an important role in different phases of LTP.

What We Know and Believe about the Encoding of Memories

After nearly a century of theoretical ruminations and experimental research about how memories are encoded and stored in the brain, our current understanding has evolved with the use of more sophisticated tools and the adoption of a multidisciplinary approach. With the use of selective lesions in conjunction with cerebral imaging of the brain and physiological recordings at multiple sites, it has become increasingly clear that there are specific regions of the brain that are activated during different types of learning and during different stages of learning and remembering. In parallel, formalized theories of how and where memory traces are represented in the brain have used known anatomic circuitry and real-time mathematical algorithms, based on the properties of cellular activity, to make computer simulations of brain activity and predict how it may function to process information.

In general, there are several major concepts about how we believe information to be processed in the brain to form memory traces. At the neurobiological level, we believe information is encoded in the brain as spatiotemporal patterns of activity within distributed networks and a memory trace may have more than one representation, and be localized in more than one brain region or circuit. For example, fundamental information of a sensory modality impinge on sensory regions in the cortex such as the visual, auditory, and motor cortices and are then fed via their anatomic connections in a convergent manner to other brain regions such as the hippocampus, amygdala, striatum, and multimodal areas of the cortex. In essence, it suggests that even a simple memory event may be encoded under different contents, such as an explicit and an implicit representation. Depending on the demand of the task at hand, either one may be independently activated to control behavior. It explains why, for example, in the face of selective damage to certain regions in the brain, learning and memory can still take place (albeit not always at its optimal level) or why there is an increase in cellular activity recorded in the hippocampus during a classical conditioning task in rodents but lesions to the hippocampus do not result in a deficit in learning the task (Laroche et al., 1995).

On another level we must also consider that information acquired during a particular type of learning depends on many attributes and subprocesses such as emotional state, level of arousal, and selective attention, that would not strictly fall into the category of learning. Embedded in these notions is a time component dividing the processing level between acquisition and retention of information, and the later recall, or memory of it. Temporally graded amnesia observed in patients with temporal lobe damage is one example of this time component and suggests that there is continuous reorganization of memory traces. Given the complexities associated with what we believe the representation(s) of the memory trace to be, it is no wonder that there has been great variability in the results where LTP has been manipulated to test its role as a mechanism encoding information necessary for learning. It suggests the need for coupling techniques that can image the circuitry involved with those to determine what discrete changes may be responsible for reorganizing the network.

What Do We Expect a Neural Mechanism of Learning and Memory to Consist of?

In terms of a mechanism that would be necessary for encoding and/or stabilizing a memory trace, one would expect it to be dynamically modifiable and enduring. By this we mean that the system would be modified by certain patterns of activity within a specific temporal window and that this modification will endure. However, whether this modification would endure indefinitely is not currently known. It has been shown experimentally that rats and mice display changes after learning or when reared in an enriched environment, but the duration of the changes is not known (Lowndes and Stewart, 1994; Moser et al., 1994, 1997; Rusakov et al., 1997). As memories are lost or fade over time, where only the salient features are remembered, one may suspect that not all modification will remain, but that the effect of reorganizing the network keeps the most salient features of a memory and depending on the input that is activated may result in different levels of recalling a particular incident that we have experienced. There are two other characteristics that a learning network would require. The first is that it is associative in nature in order to accommodate higher cognitive processing of information (the binding problem), where, for example, when we remember where we were on a particular day we also remember what we were doing. The other would be the need for a threshold of activity within the network before modification could be induced to prevent overload and essential saturation of plasticity. Implicit in the notion of preventing saturation of the system would be the need for a concomitant mechanism that would act in a downregulatory manner to maintain a certain level of balance of activity within the network. It has been suggested that homosynaptic long-term depression (LTD) of the synapses (Dudek and Bear, 1992) or heterosynaptic depression where potentiation of specific synapses also results in depression of others (Lynch et al., 1977) may well serve as a mechanism to keep this balance. To date, however, empirical evidence is still lacking.

In summary, some form of activity-dependent modification would need to occur throughout a network of distributed cells that act together to encode one or more representations of a memory trace at different hierarchical levels. Once the memory trace or traces have been established, recall of an event or some particular memory would require only partial activation of the network.

What Is Known about LTP and What New Information Is on the Horizon

Hebb's notion of "plasticity" became feasible at the physiologic level when, in 1973, Bliss and Lømo discovered an enduring form of cellular excitability in one of the major input pathways to the hippocampus. They showed, following a brief, high-frequency burst of stimulation to this pathway, that an increase in efficacy of synaptic transmission or strength, resulting in increased activity of the cell population, occurs and this exceeded the duration of the burst of stimulation by many hours. It suggested that some form of synaptic modification or strengthening must have occurred to allow the cells to continue firing at a much higher rate than previously, and was reminiscent of Hebb's growth process within a cell assembly. Since then, a great deal of research has been carried out to characterize this phenomenon and determine whether it does possess the properties that would be necessary and sufficient for encoding and storage of the memory trace.

In general, LTP has been shown to possess these properties: It is associative in nature, as it requires simultaneous activity of the pre- and postsynapse, but in addition it has been shown that activation of a weak input can be potentiated if there is stronger, concomitant activation of a separate but converging input (Levy and Steward, 1979). This is reminiscent of associative learning where one inert stimulus coupled with an effective stimulus can result in a behavioral response induced by the inert stimulus alone after learning. It displays cooperativity, as activation of a minimum number of converging fibers is necessary to induce LTP (McNaughton et al., 1978), suggesting that a threshold is required and is in keeping with the activation of the NMDA receptor, which is crucial for the induction of LTP in many pathways. It is enduring and has been shown to last for as long as many days or even weeks in the freely moving rat (Barnes, 1979; Doyère and Leroche, 1992). Although it was originally believed that input specificity demonstrated that only those synapses that were activated during the tetanus would be capable of supporting potentiation at their synapses (Andersen et al., 1977), it has subsequently been shown that inactivated synapses that are within the range of 70 μm will show potentiation (Engert and Bonhoeffer, 1997).

Cellular and Molecular Mechanisms of LTP

■ **The Initiation Process.** Presynaptically, the most important phenomenon is an increase in transmitter release, although whether this is due to the number of quanta released or the size of the quanta is still debatable. Sustained release of transmitter is believed to require an increase in intracellular calcium and also an increase in the efficacy of the presynaptic proteins involved in exocytosis (Bliss et al., 1986; Südhof, 1995).

Postsynaptically, the induction phase of most forms of LTP is critically dependent on the activation of the glutamatergic ionophore linked NMDA receptor (Collingridge et al., 1983), which is voltage dependent (Engberg et al., 1979). These receptors remain inactive until the postsynaptic membrane is sufficiently depolarized to relieve a magnesium blockade of the channel. This restrictive mechanism is characteristic of the need for cooperativity and associativity of fiber inputs that are required to induce sufficient depolarization of the membrane and activate the receptor and its associated channel. Following the displacement of magnesium from the channel there is a rapid influx of calcium to the intracellular milieu and this calcium signal is amplified locally by an increase in IP3-sensitive calcium from intracellular stores. Certain subtypes of the metabotropic receptor may also contribute to the increase in intracellular calcium as they are coupled to G-proteins that also interact with the IP3 system. Following this short-term potentiation, LTP is generally described as having an early and a late phase.

■ **Early Phase of LTP and the Potential Underlying Mechanisms.** Different second messenger systems activate different kinases, such as PKC, CaMKII, PKA, and MAP kinase and this occurs rapidly and transiently after the induction of LTP. Their activation appears to be important for either maintaining activation at the synapse or conveying the signal generated by receptors at the cell surface to nucleus to activate genes and transcription factors and also to activate the trafficking of genes that encode these proteins to locations at the synapse. For example, activation of PKA and PKC leads to their translocation from the cytosol to the synaptic membrane, whereas CaMKII, which is located at the membrane and is activated by calcium transients, is capable of autophosphorylation once the calcium transient has stopped. PKC is also able to continue phosphorylation when its upstream effectors DAG or arachidonic acid are no longer active by a mechanism of proteolysis (Inoue et al., 1977; Huang and Huang, 1986). More recently an increase in the concentration of alpha-CaMKII in the dendrites of postsynaptic neurons has been observed after the induction of LTP (Ouyang et al., 1999). As there is polyribosomal machinery at the dendrites (Steward and Levy, 1982) it has been suggested that the increase in alpha-CaMKII that occurs locally at the dendrites may also contribute to a mechanism for input specificity.

All three kinases have been shown to phosphorylate either AMPA and/or NMDA receptors or receptor subunits (Roche et al., 1996; Cavalho et al., 1999; Leonard et al., 1999). MAP kinase, on the other hand, seems to be involved primarily with transducing the signal from the cell surface to the nucleus as it has been observed in both dendrites and the cell bodies (Fiore et al., 1993), where one of its prime target is activation of the transcription factor, CREB (Xing et al., 1996; Impey et al., 1998). One important feature of the kinases is that although activated by different second messenger systems, there appears to be abundant cross-talk between them. For example, it has been shown that there are links between the PKA and PKC cascades (Sugito et al., 1997) and between PKC and CaMKII (Dash et al., 1991). In terms of cross-talk, perhaps the most important cascade pathway is the MAP kinase. It is linked upstream to the tyrosine-type receptors and its downstream targets are CREB (Xing et al., 1996; Impey et al., 1998) and Elk-1 (Whitmarsh and Davis, 1996). Both PKA and PKC interact with MAP kinase, which subsequently leads to the phosphorylation of CREB (Roberson et al., 1999), and suggests that, as these three kinases are activated by a range of upstream receptor types (NMDA, DA, mGluR, muscarinic acetylcholine receptors, and β-adrenergic receptors) and converge on the MAP kinase pathway to phosphorylate CREB, MAP kinase may act as a "gate" to translate short-term potentiation into LTP. CREB, however, is not the only downstream transcription factor target of MAP kinase. It has been shown recently that Elk-1 is also phosphorylated after the induction of LTP in the dentate gyrus (Davis et al., 2000).

Thus the kinases act as transient intermediaries between the signal at the cell surface and the downstream expression of transcription factors. It seems that they play a role in maintaining the potentiation of the synapse and signaling the activation of genetic machinery.

■ **Synthesis of New Proteins in the Longer Phases of LTP.** The synthesis of new proteins that are a necessary mechanism for the longer-lasting phases of LTP seem to occur between 3 and 6 hours after the induction of LTP. Experiments using protein synthesis inhibitors have shown that if the synthesis of proteins is blocked, then the longer-lasting phases of LTP are not maintained and the response starts to decline to basal levels between 1 and 3 hours after induction of LTP (Krug et al., 1984; Stanton and Sarvey, 1984), suggesting that the synthesis of new proteins may be a mechanism in which LTP can be consolidated (Nguyen et al., 1994). As most proteins are produced in the cell bodies and transported to the dendrites it suggests that the maintenance phase of LTP would be postsynaptically mediated. It has been shown that (1) local injections of protein synthesis inhibitors into the dentate gyrus block the late phase of LTP, but not injections into the entorhinal cortex (Otani et al., 1989), and (2) isolating the apical dendrites of CA1 from the cell bodies results in a decay of LTP that resembles that induced by protein synthesis inhibitors (Frey et al., 1989). Although the synthesis of new proteins seems to be a necessary function of the maintenance of late LTP, the proteins that would constitute this mechanism are not known to date. One potential candidate is PKMzeta, a constitutively active fragment of a specific PKC isoform (Osten et al., 1996).

More recently, Frey and Morris (1997) showed that a tetanus to induce long-lasting LTP, delivered to one pathway, could potentiate another, nearby pathway that only received a tetanus to induce short-lasting LTP. This potentiation of the other pathway was only possible if the second pathway was weakly tetanized within a 90-minute time window, the time in which de novo protein synthesis occurs. Week tetanus to the pathway before the strongly tetanized pathway or 2 hours after did not result in potentiation of the weakly tetanized pathway. It suggests that the synthesis of new proteins, presumably in the cell body, triggered by the strongly tetanized pathway was also sequestered by the weakly tetanized pathway. By implication, it further suggests that during the early phases of LTP, a "tag" is transiently set at activated synapses that would serve as a mechanism to signal where the proteins are to be delivered. This suggests a mechanism whereby an insignificant event may become important through association with a more salient event as is observed in associative learning.

■ **Activation of the Genetic Machinery During the Late Phase of LTP.** The immediate early genes (IEGs) are a necessary requisite for the longer-lasting phases. These genes are rapidly and transiently activated and need no protein synthesis to be activated (see Hughes and Dragunow, 1995, for review). The gene products of the IEGs, once translated, can regulate the transcription of target genes. Empirical evidence using different stimulating parameters has shown that those patterns of stimulation that induce short-lasting potentiation only do not show upregulation of the IEGs, whereas those patterns of stimulation that induce lasting LTP do show an increase in the expression of IEGs (Dragunow et al., 1989; Wisden et al., 1990; Abraham et al., 1992; Richardson et al., 1992). This has led to the suggestion that activation of the genetic machinery, starting with the IEGs, is the molecular basis of the longer-lasting phases of LTP. To date there are at least fifty known IEGs. Those that are activated after the induction of LTP, at least in the hippocampus, and that have best been characterized are *zif-268, c-fos,* members of the *jun* family, and more recently *arc* and *homer.* Importantly, they show a differential distribution in cells, where *zif-268, c-fos,* and the juns are located in the cell body (see Hughs and Dragunow, 1995) and *arc* and *homer* are strictly dendritic (Lyford et al., 1995; Brakeman et al., 1997).

Although phosphorylated kinases and transcription factors activate the IEGs, it is not known whether there is specificity between kinases and IEGs or whether in general all kinases and transcription factors can activate all IEGs, and whether there may be some functional difference between unclear and dendritically located IEGs. Some clues come from the type of sites located on the regulatory elements of the IEGs. For example, *zif268* has four SRE regulatory elements and one CRE element in the promotor region, whereas *c-fos* has one of each. The downstream transcriptional targets of MAP kinase are Elk-1, which binds SRE complexes, and CREB, which binds CRE complexes, and it has been shown that LTP induction in the dentate gyrus leads to a correlated hyperphosphorylation of MAP kinase, Elk-1, and CREB and an upregulation of *zif-268* mRNA. These are all blocked when MEK, an upstream effector of MAP kinase, is inhibited with SL327 (Davis et al., 2000), and suggests that both transcription factors play a role in the activation of *zif-268.* Whether one is more important than the other to date is not known. Activation of nuclear IEGs usually lasts no longer than 60 minutes after the induction of LTP; dendritic IEGs such as *arc* and *homer* can last for as long as 3 hours. As the first step in the activation of the genetic machinery, the IEGs in turn activate second order genes, although to date it is not known which genes are the downstream targets of the IEGs. In a series of experiments, Laroche and colleagues have examined the induction of different genes at different time points after the induction of LTP in the dentate gyrus in the rat *in vivo.* They have shown, interestingly, that there is a particular temporal profile of expression of the several genes investigated. Knowing that the immediate early genes are expressed very shortly after the induction of LTP, they showed that following the increased IEG expression, there is upregulation of genes encoding the kinases, γPKC and αCaMKII. The overexpression of the genes encoding these two kinases is observed in the granule cell bodies approximately 2 hours after the induction of LTP and return to basal levels 24 hours later. At this time point (24 hours post-LTP) there is an increase in the expression of MAPK and an increase in αCaMKII mRNA in

the proximal and distal dendrites that persists for approximately 48 hours
(Thomas et al., 1994a), suggesting that there is trafficking of mRNA to the local
site of potentiation and may contribute to mechanisms underlying input specificity. It has recently been observed in the aged rat that shows decremental LTP
that the gene encoding αCaMKII is not upregulated in the granule cell bodies, but
it is upregulated in the dendrites to the same if not a greater level as that of young
rats (personal observation).

At approximately 2 hours following the induction of LTP in the dentate gyrus
there is an upregulation of the message encoding specific presynaptic proteins,
syntaxin 1B and synapsin I, which persists for at least 5 hours. This increase is
observed throughout the septotemporal axis of the dentate gyrus with syntaxin
1B, but is largely restricted to the dorsal hippocampus with synapsin I (Hicks et
al., 1997). The importance of the upregulation of these two proteins is that the
upregulation of the message is observed postsynaptically in the cell bodies of the
dentate gyrus granule cells. As presynaptic proteins that are implicated in exocytosis and the release of transmitter (Südhof, 1995), it suggests that they may be
targeting synapses downstream of the granules cells at the mossy fiber synaptic
inputs to CA3. In fact, it was also observed with immunocytochemistry that there
appeared to be an increase in the level of protein at these synapses. Further data
confirmed a significant increase in syntaxin 1B in the mossy fiber terminals in correlation with an increase in the capacity for the release of glutamate at the same
synapses (Helme-Guizon et al., 1998). The point these data make together is that
this type of mechanism may underlie the propagation of plasticity through a network of cells, and thus constitutes a mechanism that is important for the encoding
of a memory trace.

Contrary to the argument presented by Shors and Matzel (1997), who suggested that downstream activation of a gene from the site of synaptic modification
is an example of the lack of input specificity, this is exactly the type of mechanism
required for modifying the synapses within a neural network necessary to encode
the memory trace during learning. It is not a matter of lack of input specificity
because this does not suggest that local genetic modifications are not also occurring at the stimulated synapses, as we know that this occurs. It suggests that
potentiated synapses have the capacity to transfer modifiable changes downstream from its site of activation, and in fact a form of transsynaptic modification
has been observed electrophysiologically in the trisynaptic loop in the hippocampus (Yeckel and Berger, 1990).

At much longer time points in the order of 2 to 4 days there is an increase in the
subunits and subtypes of glutamatergic receptors. The NR1 and NR2B subunits
of the NMDA receptor are upregulated 2 days after induction of LTP (Thomas et
al., 1994b) and at 4 days after the induction of LTP there is an upregulation of
genes encoding subtypes of the metabotropic receptors (Thomas et al., 1996).

What exactly this temporal pattern showing waves of gene activity that occur
at different times after the induction of LTP tells us, we cannot say at the present.
Their activation can lead to several types of reorganization of neural networks
based on alterations in the shape of dendritic spines and synapses (see Edwards,

1995), the conversion of silent synapses to active ones (Isaac et al., 1995), and the formation of new synaptic contacts.

Do the Properties of LTP Live Up to Our Expectations of a Neural Substrate of Learning?

On a theoretical level, LTP does live up to our expectations of a neural mechanism necessary and sufficient to encode the memory trace(s). The reason for the lack of a coherent body of empirical evidence to support this notion comes largely from our assumptions that we will observe, using electrophysiologic measurement, similar types of change in the population response that one observes after the induction of LTP. This notion in itself is not feasible given that in the model of electrically induced LTP, there is massive stimulation of a limited number of cells, and if as we believe the memory trace is laid down in multiple distributed networks of connected cells, it is impossible to believe (1) that we could observe this magnitude of effect with one recording electrode, (2) that saturating the synapses (even if all synapses were saturated) the memory trace could not be encoded via other circuits even if at a less optimal level, and (c) that blocking the NMDA receptor, given the wide range of effects it has been shown to be implicated in, will induce more than a deficit in learning. In addition, given its role in the initial induction phases of LTP, it is likely to play a role in only the initial acquisition phases of learning. When we measure LTP, it is the "output" or the overt observation of a series of discontiguous biochemical and molecular changes that occur in response to a tetanus and lead to some final reorganization of the network. If one considers that LTP is the sum total of numerous discrete events, and if we expect learning-induced changes in synaptic weights to occur in a distributed network of cells, then under no circumstance can we imagine that we can measure these changes electrophysiologically given the technology we have at the present time.

With the more recent advances that have been made in cellular and molecular biology, both in terms of the discovery of the function of many genes and proteins and in the advances in the technology for examining their activity, we are more likely to be in a position for drawing parallels between LTP as we understand it electrophysiologically and test whether it is a mechanism necessary and sufficient for learning. Probably the most important information that has come out of the research into the cellular and molecular function of proteins and genes has been to establish mechanisms that are important for different phases of LTP: early LTP, which does not require the synthesis of new proteins or the activation of genes, and the late phase of LTP, which is dependent on protein synthesis and gene activation. By implication, it suggests that these events act in serial manner, but at the same time there appear to be parallel pathways that are activated to induce the same overall effect, albeit through different means. In addition, there seems to be a temporal overlap in the activation of different mechanisms underlying the different phases of LTP. For example, as more than one cascade of kinase activity occurs in response to LTP induction, it suggests that a certain level of parallel processing occurs at this level of activation downstream of the initial induction of

LTP. As activation of each of the pathways leads to gene activation individually and by interaction with other pathways, it suggests that either parallel activity is necessary as a "backup" or "failsafe" means for activating the genetic machinery or there is a "dosage" effect where the activation of more pathways results in the activation of more genes.

Are Cellular and Molecular Mechanisms Activated by LTP Also Activated During Learning?

There is a vast literature on the role of kinases and the synthesis of new proteins in different aspects of learning. If one considers the empirical research carried out in mammals alone, both kinases and the synthesis of new proteins appear to be implicated in many different types of learning. These include rapidly learned associative tasks such as eyeblink conditioning, fear conditioning, passive avoidance, and the early phases of more complex tasks such as spatial learning. Reviewing the literature seems to suggest that the kinase PKC seems to be implicated in the acquisition phase of learning. For example, PKC translocates to the membrane in CA1 of the hippocampus during eyeblink conditioning (Banks et al., 1988), during the early phases of acquisition of spatial learning task in the hippocampus, but not the later phases (Douma et al., 1998), and also appears to correlate with the amount of learning (i.e., the better the learner the more PKC) (Colombo et al., 1997). Moreover, injections of PKC inhibitors block acquisition and not retrieval of learning in conditioned taste aversion (Sacchetti and Bielavska, 1998). In contrast, the pattern of activation of CaMKII suggests it is involved in the early consolidation of learning. For example, there is an increase in phospho CaMKII in the hippocampus 2 hours after learning cued and context fear conditioning (Atkins et al., 1998), and when blocked immediately after training can cause amnesia for retention of passive avoidance (Wolfman et al., 1994).

MAP kinase and PKA, however, seem to be required for consolidation of information necessary for establishing memories. For example MAPK/ERK is hyperphosphorylated after fear conditioning or after several trials of learning a spatial navigation task, and blocking MAPK/ERK activity by inhibiting the upstream kinase MEK results in deficits in retention of the tasks but the actual acquisition phase is not affected (Atkins et al., 1998; Blum et al., 1999). In a similar manner, pharmacologic inhibition of PKA activity can inhibit the consolidation of aversive learning (Bernabeu et al., 1997) or contextual and auditory fear conditioning (Bourtchouladze et al., 1998; Schafe et al., 1999), whereas activation of PKA can facilitate and improve memory (Barad et al., 1998).

In addition, it has been suggested that there is regional specificity of the activation of these kinases. For example, the activation of MAP kinase during spatial learning is restricted to the dorsal hippocampus and not the ventral hippocampus (Blum et al., 1999), which is in keeping with lesion data showing that the ventral hippocampus is not necessary for spatial learning (Moser et al., 1995).

Given the known action of these kinases, where, for example, it is known that PKC and CaMKII are located at the synapse and are capable of autophosphorylation, it does not seem impossible to consider that this form of activity may constitute an underlying "online" activity that may occur during the acquisition or early phases of learning. In contrast, for MAP kinase at least, it is known to translocate from the dendrites to the nucleus upon phosphorylation, where it is believed to activate IEGs that are necessary for the longer phases of LTP. It would thus be plausible to suggest that this transition may well be important for triggering the mechanisms that underlie consolidation of information necessary for the establishment of memories.

Experimental data indicating that the synthesis of new proteins is required for the consolidation of information necessary to establish memories have been shown in several different species and learning tasks (see Davis and Squire, 1984; Matthies, 1989, for review). Although much of the data suggest that synthesis of new proteins occurs about the time of the training (Barraco and Stettner, 1976; Davis and Squire, 1984; Abel et al., 1997; Meira and Rosenblum, 1998), others have also shown that there is a second window in which new proteins are synthesized and that this is between 3 and 6 hours after learning (Grechsch and Matthies, 1980; Freeman et al., 1995; Chew et al., 1996). Bourtchouladze and colleagues (1998), using contextual fear conditioning, showed two important points about the consolidation of information. The first was that if strong training was given there was only the first phase of consolidation, but if weak training was given there were two periods of consolidation. The second was that the first period of consolidation with strong training was highly sensitive to protein synthesis inhibition and only mildly sensitive to inhibition of PKA, but with the weak training both periods were equally affected by inhibition of protein synthesis and PKA. It suggests that different levels of training require different consolidation periods and that different mechanisms have a varying degree of input.

As it has been demonstrated that the consolidation of memory requires de novo synthesis of proteins, the implication follows that there is also a requirement for activation of the genetic machinery to translate new proteins. To date there is not a vast amount of research showing whether genes are specifically regulated during learning, the bulk of the evidence concentrating on the IEGs. Much of the research has reported changes in expression of c-fos in learning tasks such as imprinting, passive avoidance, visual discrimination in the chick and discrimination learning, conditioning tasks including odor and aversive conditioning, spatial alternation, and spatial learning in the rat. Other immediate early genes such as zif-268, fos-B, jun-B, crem, and c-jun have also been shown to be upregulated in different regions of the brain during different forms of learning (see Tischmeyer and Grimm, 1999, for review). However, as pointed out by Tischmeyer and Grimm, much of the expression of the IEGs is not restricted to learning per se. Many of the genes and in particular c-fos are extremely sensitive to stress and sensory stimulation. The upregulation of these genes does not seem to be restricted to a specific phase of learning either, showing regulation during the acquisition phase and recall. Thus, at present, it seems difficult to know exactly whether the IEGs play a role in specific types of learning or different phases of learning.

More recently, experiments using antisense to specific genes have shown, for example, that c-jun antisense impairs performance in rats learning a brightness discrimination task (Tischmeyer et al., 1994), whereas antisense to c-fos impairs retention of the brightness discrimination task (Tischmeyer et al., 1997). The authors suggests that *c-jun* may be implicated in neuronal function during learning whereas *c-fos* may be implicated in mechanisms underlying memory formation. Other studies using c-fos antisense in conditioned taste aversion (Lamprecht and Dudai, 1996; Swank et al., 1996) or passive avoidance (Mileusnic et al., 1996) suggest that suppression of transient activation of Fos during learning leads to an inability to form long-term memories. It is known that certain IEGs are activated by many types of sensory stimulation that are not strictly related to learning. However, it is easy to imagine that the many stimuli present in the early phases of learning would trigger enough IEG activation that would in turn lead to activation of second-order genes, linked to the mechanisms involved in the learning processes.

It is not known to date what these second-order genes are, and there is not a huge amount of literature showing upregulation of genes encoding different proteins. As an example of second-order genes that may be activated during learning, in our own research, we have taken clues from the temporal expression of genes encoding kinases, presynaptic proteins, and receptors that were observed at different times after the induction of LTP, to test whether they may be implicated in learning. We have shown that the gene encoding the presynaptic protein, syntaxin 1B, is upregulated in different regions of the brain, depending on the learning task. When rats were on the brink of learning a spatial working memory task the increase in syntaxin was observed in the dentate gyrus and CA3 and CA1 of the hippocampus, whereas after learning a spatial reference memory task the increase in syntaxin was observed primarily in the prelimbic region of the prefrontal cortex, but also in the accumbens (Davis et al. 1996). More important, the increase in these regions was largely restricted to a window of performance where rats had reached between 75 and 100 percent of their maximum learning ability and not during the early phases of learning or with overtraining (Davis et al., 1998). Although it suggests a dissociation between the structures based on the type of learning, we also found that there was some form of interaction between the hippocampus and the prefrontal cortex during the reference memory task, because after the reference memory task, we found a correlation in the increased levels of syntaxin 1B mRNA between the hippocampus and the prefrontal cortex.

Reports in the literature have, in general, suggested that the hippocampus is implicated in spatial learning and the prefrontal cortex in working memory. However, both theoretical implications and empirical evidence suggest that hippocampal and neocortical networks form a unique functional memory system in which a critical role for the hippocampus has been suggested as directing and organizing cortical representations (Wickelgren, 1979; Teyler and Discenna, 1986; Damasio, 1989; Squire and Alverez, 1995). In addition, it is known that the prelimbic region of the prefrontal cortex receives monosynaptic input from the hippocampus (Jay and Witter, 1991), which supports NMDA receptor-dependent LTP (Laroche et al., 1990b), and given the role that we have suggested syntaxin 1B may play in transsynaptic plasticity, it may well play a role in the transfer of information in the hippocampocortical networks. We suggest that the repeated firing of interconnected cells during learning is stabilized progessively via a mechanism of transsynaptic plasticity, acting to configure a specific distributed memory trace within these circuits.

Et alors, the Knock-Out: What Can It Tell Us?

Since the development of gene deletion technology in the late 1980s, many mutant mice have been developed to test the role of specific proteins in learning and LTP. Some of these, and we name but a few, range from receptor subunit or subtype deletions, kinases such as CaMKII, PKC, and PKA, the transcription factor CREB, presynaptic proteins such as Rab3A, synapsin, phosphatases, and many other proteins including Thy-1, fyn, FRM, ApoE, the amyloid precursor protein, prion protein, BDNF, and so on (see Brandon et al., 1995; Sanes and Lichtman, 1998, for review). In general, the learning experiments have implicated some form of associative learning attributed to hippocampal function, such as spatial learning in the water maze, or contextual fear conditioning, and LTP has been measured in the hippocampal slice, either in CA3 or CA1. Many of these knock-out studies have shown a correlated deficit in hippocampal-dependent learning and a representative modification in LTP, mainly in the CA1 region (Silva et al., 1992a, 1992b; Grant et al., 1992; Aiba et al., 1994; Bourtcheladze et al., 1994; Sakimura et al., 1995; Giese et al., 1998). Other studies, however, have shown a dissociation between the effect in learning and LTP either where there was a reduction or blockade of LTP with no detectable deficit in learning (Huang et al., 1995; Nosten-Bertrand et al., 1996; Montkowski and Holsboer, 1997; Schurmans et al., 1997) or normal LTP and a learning deficit (Bach et al., 1995). Others showed facilitation of LTP coupled with impairment in learning (Jia et al., 1996; Migaud et al., 1998).

Although the experiments showing a dissociation between LTP and learning may lend support to the arguments that LTP does not constitute a mechanism underlying the establishment of the memory trace, there are obvious arguments associated with the experimental procedures that would explain these dissociations. One obvious caveat of measuring LTP in a single area of the brain is that we may risk missing the critical region or subregion involved. A related problem is that of developmental compensation. In the first-generation mutant mice, the gene is deleted at birth and this could easily result in compensatory upregulation of other spliced isoforms or, as in the case of kinases, activation of different signal transduction pathways that activate downstream targets alone or by interaction between pathways may compensate for a missing gene. Thus it is possible that if a single kinase is inactivated the effect can be mediated by those remaining intact, or if LTP is altered in a single pathway the effect could be mediated by bypassing the altered circuit.

The results from these first-generation gene mutations have led to refinements in both the gene mutating technology and also in the experimental approaches to test these mice. From a technological point, the second-generation mutations have produced conditional and region-specific mutations. The conditional knock-out resolve the potential problems associated with developmental compensation and allow within-subject comparisons in learning ability to be made. For example, in an NMDAR1 knockout mouse that is targeted to the CA1 region of the hippocampus, there was impairment in LTP, whereas it was normal in the dentate gyrus. There was also an impairment in spatial learning and there was instability in CA1 place fields (McHugh et al., 1996; Tsien et al., 1996; see Wilson and Tonegawa, 1997). In a CaMKII conditional knock-out, when the gene was knocked out specifically in the hippocampus, there was a deficit in spatial learning and LTP, whereas when knocked out in the amygdala there was impairment in fear conditioning (Mayford et al., 1996).

The technical development of these two types of mutant mice eliminates the problems associated with specificity and developmental compensation, but at the same time our experimental procedures and approaches have become more refined. For example, the development of techniques to record from cells in the freely moving mouse has led to the ability to record place cells in the NMDA1 mutant mouse when coupled with LTP and learning (Wilson and Tonegawa, 1997). This strengthens the arguments that suggest a functional role of the NMDA receptor as a mechanism of synaptic plasticity necessary for learning. Moreover, using the complementary strategy, a transgenic mouse overexpressing the NR2B subunit of the NMDA receptor was developed because it has been shown that when this subunit is coupled with the NR1 subunit there are longer EPSPs (Monyer et al., 1994). This mouse did show facilitated LTP and enhanced learning was observed in several tasks (Tang et al., 1999). This is reminiscent of previous studies showing that stimulation of the reticular formation facilitates both LTP and learning in a correlated manner (Bloch and Laroche, 1985; Laroche et al., 1995)

A further example of how, by modifying our experimental approach, we are able to resolve some of the early dissociations between LTP and learning in these mice is shown with a Thy-1 knock-out mouse. This mouse displayed normal spatial learning, and LTP was blocked in the dentate gyrus, except in the disinhibited state (Nosten-Bertrand et al., 1996). In a subsequent experiment using the freely moving Thy-1 mouse, LTP could be induced in the dentate gyrus, although substantially reduced when compared with wild-type littermates (Errington et al., 1997). This residual level of plasticity in conjunction with normal plasticity may well be sufficient for the mice to learn. Other examples where LTP is different in the slice compared with the *in vivo* preparation, or by rescuing LTP in the dentate gyrus slice by blocking the GABAergic system, have been shown in an mGluR1 mutant mouse (Bordi et al., 1997) and a calretinin mutant mouse (Schurmans et al., 1997). These types of differences may go some way to explain the variability in the results and certain dissociations between LTP and learning that have been shown in different types of mutant mice.

Does the Hypothesis That LTP Constitutes a Mechanism of Synaptic Plasticity Necessary for Learning and Memory Hold up?

For the moment the hypothesis must stand, if only because it cannot be proven wrong. There are still no definitive experiments that have shown a causal link between synaptic plasticity and learning. It seems, however, that on the one hand we have the technical advances to start to dissect out the mechanisms of synaptic plasticity and manipulate them to rigorously test the importance of their individual roles in establishing the memory trace. On the other hand, we have to deal with the ever-evolving theories of what type of memories are encoded in specific regions of the brain, and in particular the hippocampus, the brain region most accessible for testing these mechanisms.

To test the hypothesis, we must start to address, on a mechanistic level, the fact that LTP is the output of many discrete cellular and molecular events that act at some levels in concert with a certain degree of parallelism, but mainly occur in a serial manner, where each major step needs a level of completion before the next step begins, to mediate the different phases of LTP that we now know to exist. We do not, however, know exactly what these different stages of LTP mean in terms of learning, whether they do translate to different phases of learning or different types of learning, or whether, in fact, they are necessary and sufficient for learning. In addition, we must also address the questions of whether this type of mechanism occurs in all types of learning and in brain regions that are implicated in learning, or whether there is some level of specificity.

At the behavioral level, we must contend with the lack of consensus about which circuits and brain structures are involved in different forms of learning. If one considers the hippocampus only, over the past 30 years or so there have been many theories of how the hippocampus is involved in learning and memory, all of which differ with the exception that there appears to be agreement that it processes some form of associative memory. However, we still do not know exactly what information it processes, whether it stores the information permanently, or whether the memory trace for specific events is eventually stored in circuits outside of the hippocampus, but that the hippocampus has access to, for recall of memories. Given the complexities of the events occuring at the cellular and molecular level and this basic lack of knowledge of the details of how information may be encoded, it is not surprising that there is huge variability in the empirical data. We believe, however, that as the techniques become more refined for investigating the potential mechanisms underlying the formation of the memory trace, then the theories will evolve to incorporate this new information and in turn, new and more precise predictions can be made and experimentally tested.

Thus, it would seem that the potential mechanisms are largely in place to be studied. Because measuring the synaptic responses has proven difficult in the past, we need to consider refining these existing techniques so that we have the potential, for example, to measure synaptic transmission at a minimal number of synapses, to make multiple recordings in different parts of a neural circuit, to test whether modified patterns of activity can alter the formation of, for example, place cells, and whether this in turn modifies behavior. The development in techniques from molecular biology allows us (e.g., using *in situ* hybridization) to map the circuits that express a specific mechanism of plasticity during or after learning and at the same time to study the molecular mechanisms of memory. The gene deletion technology, and in particular the second-generation mutants, allow us to confirm the importance of these genes in learning and help to specify more precisely in which aspect of learning they may be involved. In addition, tools for manipulating the system, in the form of antisense oligoneucleotides, adenoviral vectors to block gene expression, or a rescue strategy for gene deletions with pharmacologic or "sense" manipulation, will allow us to decipher exactly what role these genes may have in learning. Thus, what we believe a genomic approach, coupled with behavioral and neurophysiologic approaches, can tell us about synaptic plasticity and the mechanisms underlying the encoding of the memory trace is (1) whether LTP constitutes a viable model of the type of modification that is necessary and sufficient for learning, (2) where the mechanisms are activated in the brain, depending on the task at hand, and (3) what specific process of learning and memory these mechanisms serve. As difficult as the task is, it will help formalize our concepts of learning and memory, giving us a more concise understanding of how the mechanisms of learning operate, and may well open new avenues for the development of therapeutic strategies.

REFERENCES

Abel, T., Nguyen, P., Barad, M., Deuel, T. et al. (1997). Genetic demonstration of a role for PKA in the late phase of LTP in the hippocampus-based long-term memory. *Cell* 88: 615–626.

Abraham, W.C., Dragunow, M., and Tate, W.P. (1992). The role of the immediate early genes in the stabilisation of long-term potentiation. *Mol. Neurobiol.* 5: 297–314.

Aiba, A., Chen, C., Herrup, K., Rosenmund, C. et al. (1994). Reduced hippocampal long-term potentiation and context-specific deficit in associative learning in mGluR1 mutant mice. *Cell* 79: 365–375.

Andersen, P., Sunberg, S.H., Sveen, O., and Wigstom, H. (1977). Specific long-lasting potentiation of synaptic transmission in hippocampal slice. *Nature* 266: 736–737.

Atkins, C.M., Selcher, J.C., Petraitis, J.J., Trzaskos, J.M. et al. (1998). The MAPK cascade is required for mammalian associative learning. *Nat. Neurosci.* 1: 602–609.

Bach, M.E., Hawkins, R.D., Osmn, M., Kandel, E.R. et al. (1995). Impairment of spatial but not contextual memory in CaMKII mutant mice with a selective loss of hippocampal LTP in the range of the theta frequency. *Cell* 81: 905–915.

Banks, B., deWeer, A., Kuzirian, A.M., Rasmussen, H. et al. (1988). Classical conditioning induces long-term translocation of protein kinase C in rabbit hippocampal CA1 cells. *Proc. Natl. Acad. Sci. USA* 85: 1988–1992.

Bannerman, D.M., Good, M.A., Butcher, S.P., Ramsay, M. et al. (1995). Distinct components of spatial learning revealed by prior training and NMDA receptor blockade. *Nature* 378: 182–186.

Barad, M., Bourtchouladze, R., Winder, D.G., Golan, H. et al. (1998). Rolipram, a type IV-specific phosphodiesterase inhibitor, facilitates the establishment of long-lasting long-term potentiation and improves memory. *Proc. Natl. Acad. Sci. USA* 95: 15020–15025.

Barnes, C.A. (1979). Memory deficits associated with senescence: A neuro biolophysiological and behavioral study in the rat. *J. Comp. Physiol. Psychol.* 93: 74–104.

Barraco, R.A., and Stettner, L.J. (1976). Antibiotics and memory. *Psychol. Bull.* 83: 242–302.

Bernabeu, R., Bevilaqua, L., Ardenghi, P., Bromberg, E. et al. (1997). Involvement of hippocampal cAMP/cAMP-dependent protein kinase signaling pathways in a late memory consolidation phase of aversively motivated learning in rats. *Proc. Natl. Acad. Sci. USA* 94: 7041–7046.

Bliss, T.V.P., and Lømo, T. (1973). Long-lasting potentiation of synaptic transmission in the dentate area of the anaesthetised rabbit following stimulation of the perforant path. *J. Physiol. (London)* 232: 331–356.

Bliss, T.V.P., and Richter-Levin, G. (1993). Spatial learning and the saturation of long-term potentiation. *Hippocampus* 3: 123–126.

Bliss, T.V.P., Douglas, R.M., Errington, M.L., and Lynch, M.A. (1986). Correlation between long-term potentiation and release of endogenous amino acids from dentate gyrus of anaesthetised rats. *J. Physiol.* 377: 391–408.

Bloch, V., and Laroche, S. (1985). Enhancement of long-term potentiation n the rat dentate gyrus by post-trial stimulation of the reticular formation. *J. Physiol. (London)* 360: 215–231.

Blum, S., Moore, A.N., Adams, F., and Dash, P.K. (1999). A mitogen-activated protein kinase cascade in the CA1/CA2 subfield of the dorsal hippocampus is essential for long-term spatial learning. *J. Neurosci.* 19: 3535–3544.

Bordi, F., Reggiani, A., and Conquet, F. (1997). Regulation of synaptic plasticity by mGluR1 studied in vivo in mGluR1 mutant mice. *Brain Res.* 76: 121–126.

Bourtchuladze, R., Frenguelli, B., Blendy, J., Cioffi, D. et al. (1994). Deficient long-term memory in mice with a target mutation of the cAMP-responsive element-binding protein. *Cell* 79: 59–68.

Bourtchouladze, R., Abel, T., Berman, N., Gordon, R. et al. (1998). Different training procedures recruit either one or two critical periods for contextual memory consolidation, each of which requires protein synthesis and PKA. *Learn. Mem.* 5: 365–374.

Brakeman, P.R., Lanahan, A.A., O'Brien, R., Roche, K. et al. (1997). Homer: A protein that selectively binds metabotropic glutamate receptors. *Nature* 386: 284–288.

Brandon, E.P., Idzerda, R.L., and McKnight, G.S. (1995). Targeting the mouse genome: A compendium of knockouts. *Curr. Biol.* 5: 1–27.

Cain, D.P., Hargreaves, E.L., Boon, F., and Dennison, Z. (1993). An examination of the relations between hippocampal long-term potentiation, kindling, afterdischarge and place learning in the water maze. *Hippocampus* 3: 153–163.

Cain, D.P., Saucier, D., Hall, J., Hargreaves, E.L. et al. (1996). Detailed behavioural analysis of water maze acquisition under APV or CNQX: Contribution of sensorimotor disturbances to drug-induced acquisition deficits. *Behav. Neurosci.* 110: 86–102.

Castro, C.A., Silbert, L.H., McNaughton, B.L., and Barnes, C.A. (1989). Recovery of spatial learning deficits after decay of electrically induced synaptic enhancement in the hippocampus. *Nature* 342: 545–548.

Cavalho, A.L., Kameyama, K., and Huganir, R.L. (1999). Characterisation of phosphorylation sites on the glutamate receptor 4 subunit of the AMPA receptors. *J. Neurosci.* 19: 4748–4754.

Chew, S., Vicario, D., and Nottebohm, F. (1996). Quantal duration of auditory memories. *Science* 274: 1909–1914.

Collingridge, G.L., Kehl, S.J., and McLennan, H. (1983). Excitatory amino acid in synaptic transmission in the schaffer collateral-commissural pathway of the rat hippocampus. *J. Physiol. (London)* 334: 33–46.

Colombo, P.J., Wetse, W.C., and Gallagher, M. (1997). Spatial memory is related to hippocampal subcellular concentrations of calcium-dependent protein kinase C isoforms in young and aged rats. *Proc. Natl. Acad. Sci. USA* 94: 14195–14199.

Damasio, A.R. (1989). Time-locked multiregional retroactivation: A system-level proposal for the neural substrates of recall and recognition. *Cognition* 33: 25–62.

Dash, P.K., Karl, A.K., Colicos, M.A., Pywes, R. et al. (1991). cAMP response element-binding protein is activated by Ca2+/calmodulin- as well as cAMP-dependent protein kinase. *Proc. Natl. Acad. Sci. USA* 88: 5061–5065.

Davis, H.P., and Squire, L.R. (1984). Protein synthesis and memory: A review. *Psychol. Bull.* 96: 518–559.

Davis, S., Butcher, S.P., and Morris, R.G.M. (1992). The NMDA receptor antagonist D-2-amino-5-phosphonopentanoate (D-AP5) impairs spatial learning and LTP in vivo at intracerebral concentrations comparable to those that block LTP in vitro. *J. Neurosci.* 12: 21–34.

Davis, S., Rodger, J., Hicks, A., Mallet, J. et al. (1996). Brain structure and task specific increase in the expression of the gene encoding syntaxin 1B during learning in the rat: A potential molecular marker for learning-induced synaptic plasticity in neural networks. *Eur. J. Neurosci.* 8: 2068–2074.

Davis, S., Rodger, J., Stéphan, A., Hicks, A. et al. (1998). Increase in syntaxin 1B mRNA in hippocampal and cortical circuits during spatial learning reflects a mechanism of trans-synaptic plasticity involved in establishing a memory trace. *Learn. Mem.* 5: 375–390.

Davis, S., Vanhoutte, P., Pagès, P., Caboche, P., and Laroche, S. (2000). The MAPh/ERK cascade targets ELK-1 to control LTP-dependent gene expression in the dentategyous in vivo *J. Neurosci.* (in press)

Douma, B.R., Van der Zee, E.A., and Luiten, P.G. (1998). Translocation of protein kinase C occurs during the early phase of acquisition of food rewarded spatial learning. *Behav. Neurosci.* 112: 496–501.

Doyère, V., and Laroche, S. (1992). Linear relationship between the maintenance of hippocampal long-term potentiation and retention of an associative memory. *Hippocampus* 2: 39–48.

Doyère, V., Rédini-Del Negro, C., Dutrieux, G., Le Floch, G. et al. (1995). Potentiation or depression of synaptic efficacy in the dentate gyrus is determined by the relationship between the conditioned and unconditioned stimulus in a classical conditioning paradigm in rats. *Behav. Brain Res.* 70: 15–29.

Dragunow, M., Abraham, W.C., Goulding, M., Mason, S.E. et al. (1989). Long-term potentiation and the induction of c-fos mRNA and proteins in the dentate gyrus of the unanesthetised rat. *Neurosci. Lett.* 101: 274–280.

Dudek, S.M., and Bear, M.F. (1992). Homosynaptic long-term depression and effects of N-methyl-D-aspartate receptor blockade. *Proc. Natl. Acad. Sci. USA* 89: 4363–4367.

Edwards, F.A. (1995). LTP—a structural model to explain the inconsistencies. *Trends Neurosci.* 18: 250–255.

Engberg, I., Flatman, J.A., and Lambert, J.D.C. (1979). The actions of excitatory amino acids on motor neurons in the feline spinal cord. *J. Physiol.* 288: 227–261.

Engert, F., and Bonhoeffer, T. (1997). Synaptic specificity of long-term potentiation breaks down at short distances. *Nature* 388: 279–284.

Errington, M.L., Bliss, T.V.P., Morris, R.J., Laroche, S. et al. (1997). Long-term potentiation in awake mutant mice. *Nature* 387: 666–667.

Fiore, R.S., Bayer, V.E., Pelech, S.L., Posada, J. et al. (1993). p42 mitogen-activated protein kinase in brain: Prominent localisation in neuronal cell bodies and dendrites. *Neuroscience* 55: 463–472.

Freeman, F., Rose, S.P., and Scholey, A. (1995). Two time windows of anisomycin-induced amnesia for passive avoidance training in the day-old chick. *Neurobiol. Learn. Mem.* 63: 291–295.

Frey, U., and Morris, R.G.M. (1997). Synaptic tagging and long-term potentiation. *Nature* 385: 533–536.

Frey, U., Krug, M., Brodemann, R., Reymann, K. et al. (1989). Long-term potentiation induced in dendrites separated from rat's CA1 pyramidal somata does not establish a late phase. *Neurosci. Lett.* 97: 135–139.

Giese, K.P., Fedorov, N.B., Filipowski, R.K., and Silva, A.J. (1998). Autophosphorylation at Thr[286] of the calcium-calmodulin kinase II in LTP and learning. *Science* 279: 870–873.

Grant, S.G.N., O'Dell, T.J., Karl, K.A., Stein, P.L. et al. (1992). Impaired long-term potentiation, spatial learning and hippocampal development in fyn mutant mice. *Science* 258: 1903–1910.

Grechsch, G., and Matthies, H. (1980). Two sensitive periods for the amnesic effect of anisomycin. *Pharmacol. Biochem. Behav.* 12: 663–665.

Green, E.J., McNaughton, B.L., and Barnes, C.A. (1990). Exploration-dependent modulation of evoked responses in fascia dentata: Dissociation of motor, EEG, and sensory factors, and evidence for a synaptic efficacy change. *J. Neurosci.* 10: 1455–1471.

Hebb, D.O. (1949). *The Organization of Behavior.* New York: John Wiley and Sons.

Helme-Guizon, A., Davis, S. Israel, M., Lesbats, B. et al. (1998). Increase in syntaxin 1B and glutamate release in mossy fibre terminals following the induction of LTP in the dentate gyrus: A candidate molecular mechanism underlying transsynaptic plasticity. *Eur. J. Neurosci.* 10: 2231–2237.

Hicks, A., Davis, S., Rodger, J., Helme-Guizon, A. et al. (1997). Synapsin I and syntaxin 1B: Key elements in the control of neurotransmitter release are regulated by neuronal activation and long-term potentiation in vivo. *Neuroscience* 79: 329–340.

Huang, K.P., and Huang, F.L. (1986). Conversion of protein kinase C from a Ca^{2+}-dependent to an independent form of phorol ester-binding protein by digestion with trypsin. *Biochem. Biophys. Res. Commun.* 139: 320–326.

Huang, Y-Y., Kandel, E.R., Varshavsky, L., Brandon, E.P. et al. (1995). A genetic test of the effects of mutations in PKA on mossy fibre LTP and its relation to spatial and contextual learning. *Cell* 83: 1211–1222.

Hughes, P., and Dragunow, M. (1995). Induction of immediate-early genes and the control of neurotransmitter-regulated gene expression within the nervous system. *Pharmacol. Rev.* 47: 133–178.

Impey, S., Obrietan, K., Wong, S.T., Poser, S. et al. (1998). Cross talk between ERK and PKA is required for Ca2+ stimulation of CREB-dependent transcription and ERK nuclear translocation. *Neuron* 21: 869–883.

Inoue, M., Kishimoto, A., Takai, Y., and Nishizuka, Y. (1977). Studies on a cyclic nucleotide-independent protein kinase and its proenzyme in mammalian tissues. II. Proenzyme and its activation by calcium-dependent protease from rat brain. *J. Biol. Chem.* 252: 7610–7616.

Isaac, J.T.R., Nicoll, R.A., and Malenka, R.A. (1995). Evidence for silent synapses: Implications for the expression of LTP. *Neuron* 15: 427–434.

Jay, T.M., and Witter, M.P. (1991). Distribution of the hippocampal CA1 and subicular efferents in the prefrontal cortex of the rat: A study using anerograde transports of *Phaseolus vulgaris* leucoagglutinin. *J. Comp. Neurol.* 313: 574–586.

Jeffery, K.J., and Morris, R.G.M. (1993). Cumulative long-term potentiation in the rat dentate gyrus correlates with, but does not modify performance in the water maze. *Hippocampus* 3: 133–140.

Jia, Z., Agopyan, N., Miu, P., Xiong, Z. et al. (1996). Enhanced LTP in mice deficient in the AMPA receptor GluR2. *Neuron* 17: 945–956.

Keith, J.R., and Ruddy, J.W. (1990). Why NMDA-receptor-dependent potentiation may not be a mechanism of learning and memory: Reappraisal of the NMDA-receptor blockade strategy. *Psychobiology* 18: 251–257.

Korol, D.L., Abel, T.W., Church, L.T., Barnes, C.A. et al. (1993). Hippocampal synaptic enhancement and spatial learning in the Morris swim task. *Hippocampus* 3: 127–132.

Krug, M., Lossner, B., and Ott, T. (1984). Anisomycin blocks the late phase of long-term potentiation in the dentate gyrus of freely moving rats. *Brain Res. Bull.* 13: 39–42.

Lamprecht, R., and Dudai, Y. (1996). Transient expression of c-Fos in rat amygdala during training is required for encoding conditioned taste aversion memory. *Learn. Mem.* 3: 31–41.

Laroche, S., Errington, M.L., Lynch, M.A., and Bliss, T.V.P. (1987). Increase in [³H] gluta-mate release from slices of dentate gyrus and hippocampus following classical conditioning in the rat. *Behav. Brain Res.* 25: 23–29.

Laroche, S., Rédini-Del Negro, C., Clemments, M.P., and Lynch, M.A. (1990a). Long-term activation of phophoinositide turnover associated with increased release of amino acids in the dentate gyrus and hippocampus following classical conditioning in the rat. *Eur. J. Neurosci.* 2: 534–543.

Laroche, S., Jay, T.M., and Thierry, A-M. (1990b). Long-term potentiation in th prefrontal cortex following stimulation of the hippocampal CA1/subicular region. *Neurosci. Lett.* 114: 184–190.

Laroche, S., Doyère, V., Rédini-Del Negro, C., and Burette, F. (1995). Neural mechanisms of associative memory: Role of long-term potentiation. In J.L. McGraugh, N.M. Weinberger, and G. Synch (Eds.), *Brain and memory: Modulation and mediation of neuroplasticity* (pp 277–302). New York: Oxford University Press.

Leonard, A.S., Lim, I.A., Hemsworth, D.E., Horne, M.C. et al. (1999). Calcium/calmodulin-dependent protein kinase II is associated with the N-methyl-D-aspartate receptor. *Proc. Natl. Acad. Sci.* 96: 3239–3244.

Leung, L.W., and Desborough, K.A. (1988). APV, an N-methyl-d-aspartate receptor antago-nist, blocks the hippocampal theta rhythm in behaving rats. *Brain Res.* 463: 148–152.

Levy, W.B., and Steward, O. (1979). Synapses as associative memory elements in the hip-pocampal formation. *Brain Res.* 175: 233–245.

Lowndes, M., and Stewart, M.G. (1994). Dendritic spine density in the lobus parolfactorius of the domestic chick is increased 24h after one-trial passive avoidance training. *Brain Res.* 654: 129–136.

Lyford, G.L., Yamagata, K., Kaufmann, W.E., Barnes, C.A. et al. (1995). Arc, a growth factor and activity-regulated gene, encodes a novel cytoskeleton-associated protein that is enriched in neuronal dendrites. *Neuron* 14: 433–445.

Lynch, G.L., Dunwiddie, T., and Gribkoff, V. (1977). Heterosynaptic depression: A post synaptic correlate of long-term potentiation. *Nature* 266: 737–739.

McHugh, T.J., Blum, K.I., Tsien, J.Z., Tonegawa, S. et al. (1996). Impaired hippocampal rep-resentation of space in CA1-specific NMDA1 knockout mice. *Cell* 87: 1339–1349.

McNaughton, B.L., Douglas, R.M., and Goddard, G.V. (1978). Synaptic enhancement in fas-cia dentata: Cooperativity among coactive afferents. *Brain Res.* 157: 277–293.

McNaughton, B.L., Barnes, C.A., Rao, G., Baldwin, J. et al. (1986). Long-term enhancement of hippocampal synaptic transmission and the acquisition of spatial information. *J. Neurosci.* 6: 563–571.

Marr, D. (1971). Simple memory. A theory for archicortex. *Phil. Trans. R. Soc. B.* 262: 23–81.

Matthies, H. (1989). In search of cellular mechanisms of memory. *Prog. Neurobiol.* 32: 277–349.

Mayford, M., Bach, M.E., Huang, Y-Y., Wang, L. et al. (1996). Control of memory formation through regulated expression of a CaMKII transgene. *Science* 274: 1678–1683.

Meira, N., and Rosenblum, K. (1998). Lateral ventricule injection of the protein synthesis inhibitor anisomycin impairs long-term memory in a spatial memory task. *Brain Res.* 789: 48–55.

Migaud M., Charlesworth P., Dempster M., Webster L.C. et al. (1998). Enhanced long-term potentiation and impaired learning in mice with mutant postsynaptic density-95 protein. *Nature* 396: 433–439.

Mileusnic, R., Ahokhin, K., and Rose, S.P.R. (1996). Antisense oligo deoxynucleotides to c-fos are amnestic for passive avoidance in the chick. *Neuroreport* 7: 1269–1272.

Monkowski, A., and Holsboer, F. (1997). Intact spatial learning and memory in transgenic mice with reduced BDNF. *Neuroreport* 8: 779–782.

Monyer, H., Burnashev, N., Laurie, D., Sakmann, B. et al. (1994). Developmental and regional expression in the rat brain and functional properties of four NMDA receptors. *Neuron* 12: 529–540.

Morris, R.G.M., Andersen, E., Lynch, G.S., and Baudry, M. (1986). Selective impairment of learning and blockade of long-term potentiation by an N-methyl-D-aspartate receptor antagonist, AP5. *Nature* 319: 774–776.

Morris, R.G.M., Davis, S., and Butcher, S.P. (1990). Hippocampal synaptic plasticity and NMDA receptors: A role in information storage? *Phil. Trans. R. Soc. London B* 329: 178–204.

Moser, E.I., and Andersen, P. (1994). Conserved spatial learning in cooled rats in spite of slowing of dentate field potentials. *J. Neurosci.* 14: 4458–4466.

Moser, E., Mathiesen, I., and Andersen, P. (1993). Association between brain temperature and dentate field potentials in exploring and swimming rats. *Science* 259: 1324–1326.

Moser, M.B., Trommald, M., and Andersen, P. (1994). An increase in dendritic spine density on hippocampal CA1 pyramidal cells following spatial learning in adult rats suggests the formation of new synapses. *Proc. Natl. Acad. Sci. USA* 91: 12673–12675.

Moser, M.B., Moser, E.I., Forrest, E., Andersen, P. et al. (1995). Spatial learning with a min-islab in the dorsal hippocampus. *Proc. Natl. Acad. Sci. USA* 92: 9697–9701.

Moser, M.B., Trommald, M., Egeland, T., and Andersen, P. (1997). Spatial training in a complex environment and isolation alter the spine distribution differently in rat CA1 pyramidal cells. *J. Comp. Neurol.* 380: 373–381.

Moser, E.I., Krobert, K.A., Moser, M.B., and Morris, R.G. (1998). Impaired spatial learning after saturation of long-term potentiation. *Science* 281: 2038–2042.

Nguyen, P.V., Abel, T., and Kandel, E.R. (1994). Requirement of a critical period of transcription for induction of a late phase of LTP. *Science* 265: 1104–1107.

Nicoletti, F., Valerio, C., Pellegrino, C., Drago, F. et al. (1988). Spatial learning potentiates the stimulation of phosphoinositides hydrolysis by excitatory amino acids in rat hippocampal slices. *J. Neurochem.* 51: 725–729.

Noguès, X. (1997). Protein kinase C, learning and memory: A circular determinism between physiology and behaviour. *Prog. Neuropsychopharmacol. Biol. Psychiat.* 21: 507–529.

Nosten-Bertrand, M., Errington, M.L., Murphy, K.P.S.J., Tokugawa, Y. et al. (1996). Spatial learning is unaffected by a selective impairment of LTP in Thy-1 mutant mice. *Nature* 379: 826–829.

Osten, P., Valsamis, L., Harris, A., and Sacktor, T.C. (1996). Protein synthesis-dependent formation of protein kinase Mzeta in long-term potentiation. *J. Neurosci.* 16: 2444–2451.

Otani, S., Marshal, C.J., Tate, W.P., Goddard, G.V. et al. (1989). Maintenance of long-term potentiation in rat dentate gyrus requires protein synthesis but not messenger RNA synthesis immediately post-tetanization. *Neuroscience* 28: 519–526.

Ouyang, Y., Rosenstein, A., Kreiman, G., Schuman, E.M. et al. (1999). Tetanic stimulation leads to increased accumulation of Ca^{2+}/calmodulin-dependent protein kinase II via dendritic protein synthesis in hippocampal neurons. *J. Neurosci.* 19: 7823–7833.

Richardson, C.L., Tate, W.P., Mason, S.E., Lawlor, P.A. et al. (1992). Correlation between the induction of an immediate early gene, *zif268*, and long-term potentiation in the dentate gyrus. *Brain Res.* 580: 147–154.

Richter-Levin, G., Canevari, L., and Bliss, T.V.P. (1995). Long-term potentiation and glutamate release in the dentate gyrus: Links to spatial learning. *Behav. Brain Res.* 66: 37–40.

Roberson, E.D., English, J.D., Adams, J.P., Selcher, J.C. et al. (1999). The mitogen-activated protein kinase cascade couples PKA and PKC to cAMP response element binding protein phosphorylation in area CA1 of hippocampus. *J. Neurosci.* 19: 4337–4348.

Roche, K.W., O'Brien, R.J., Mammen, A.L., Bernhardt, J. et al. (1996). Characterization of multiple phosphorylation sites on the AMPA receptor GluR1 subunit. *Neuron* 16: 1179–1188.

Rusakov, D.A., Stewart, M.G., and Korogod, S.M. (1997). Branching of active dendritic spines as a mechanism for controlling synaptic efficacy. *Neuroscience* 75: 315–323.

Sacchetti, B., and Bielavska, E. (1998). Chelerythrine, a specific PKC inhibitor, blocks acquisition but not consolidation and retrieval of conditioned taste aversion in rat. *Brain Res.* 799: 84–90.

Sakimura, K., Kutsuwada, T., Ito, I., Manabe, T. et al. (1995). Reduced hippocampal LTP and spatial learning in mice lacking NMDA receptor ε1 subunit. *Nature* 373: 151–155.

Sanes, J.R., and Lichtman, J.W. (1998). Can molecules explain long-term potentiation. *Nat. Neurosci.* 2: 597–604.

Saucier, D., and Cain, D.P. (1995). Spatial learning without NMDA receptor-dependent long-term potentiation. *Nature* 378: 186–189.

Schafe, G.E., Nadel, N.V., Sullivan, G.M., Harris, A. et al. (1999). Memory consolidation for contextual and auditory fear conditioning is dependent on protein synthesis, PKA, and MAP kinase. *Learn. Mem.* 6: 97–110.

Schurnams, S., Schiffmann, S.N., Gurden, H., Lemaire, M. et al. (1997). Impaired long-term potentiation induction in the dentate gyrus of calretinin-deficient mice. *Proc. Natl. Acad. Sci. USA* 94: 10415–10420.

Sharp, P.E., McNaughton, B.L., and Barnes, C.A. (1989). Exploration dependent modulation of evoked responses in fascia dentata: Fundamental observations and time course. *Psychobiology* 17: 257–269.

Shors, T.J., and Matzel, L.D. (1997). Long-term potentiation. What's learning got to do with it? *Behav. Brain Sci.* 20: 597–655.

Sillito, A.M., Murphy, P.C., Salt, T.E., and Moody, C.I. (1990). Dependence of retinogeniculate transmission in cat on NMDA receptor. *J. Neurophysiol.* 63: 347–355.

Silva, A.J., Stevens, C.F., Tonegawa, S., and Wang, Y. (1992a). Deficient hippocampal long-term potentiation in α-calcium-calmodulin kinase II mutant mice. *Science* 257: 201–206.

Silva, A.J., Paylor, R., Wehner, J.M., and Tonegawa, S. (1992b). Impaired spatial learning in α-calcium-calmodulin kinase II mutant mice. *Science* 257: 206–211.

Squire, L.R., and Alvarez, P. (1995). Retrograde amnesia and memory consolidation: A neurobiological perspective. *Curr. Opin. Neurobiol.* 5: 169–177.

Stanton, P.K., and Sarvey, J.M. (1984). Blockade of long-term potentiation in rat hippocampal CA1 region by inhibitors of protein synthesis. *J. Neurosci.* 4: 3080–3088.

Steward, O., and Levy, W.B. (1982). Preferential localisation of polyribosomes under the base of dendritic spines in granule cells of the dentate gyrus. *J. Neurosci.* 2: 284–291.

Südhof, T. (1995). The synaptic vesicle cycle: A cascade of protein-protein interactions. *Nature* 375: 646–653.

Sugito, S., Baxter, D.A., and Byrne, J.H. (1997). Modulation of a cAMP/protein kinase A cascade by protein kinase C in sensory neurons of Aplysia. *J. Neurosci.* 17: 7237–7244.

Swank, M.W., Ellis, A.E., and Cochran, B.N. (1996). c-Fos antisense blocks acquisition and extinction of conditioned taste aversion in mice. *Neuroreport* 7: 1866–1870.

Tang, Y.P., Shimizu, E., Dube, G.R., Rampon, C. et al. (1999). Genetic enhancement of learning and memory in mice. *Nature* 401: 63–69.

Teyler, T.J., and Discenna, P. (1984). The hippocampal memory indexing theory. *Behav. Neurosci.* 100: 147–154.

Thomas, K.L., Laroche, S., Errington, M.L., Bliss, T.V.P. et al. (1994a). Spatial and temporal changes in signal transduction pathways during LTP. *Neuron* 13: 737–745.

Thomas, K.L., Davis, S., Laroche, S., and Hunt, S.P. (1994b). Regulation of the expression of NR1 NMDA glutamate receptor subunits during hippocampal LTP. *Neuroreport* 6: 119–123.

Thomas, K.L., Davis, S., Hunt, S.P., and Laroche, S. (1996). Alterations in the expression of specific glutamate receptor subunits following hippocampal LTP in vivo. *Learn. Mem.* 3: 197–208.

Tischmeyer, W., and Grimm, R. (1999). Activation of immediate early genes and memory formation. *Cell. Mol. Life Sci.* 55: 564–574.

Tischmeyer, W., Grimm, R., Schichnick, H., Brysch, W. et al. (1994). Sequence-specific impairment of learning by c-jun antisense oligo nucleotides. *Neuroreport* 5: 1501–1504.

Tischmeyer, W., Grimm, R., Lohmann, K., Schicknick, H. et al. (1997). Suppression of immediate early gene expression by intracerebrally applied antisense oligonucleotides impairs mechanisms of learning and memory. In A. Tellken and J. Korf (Eds.), *Neurochemistry: Cellular, molecular and clinical aspects* (pp. 1117–1121). New York: Plenum.

Tsein, J.Z., Huerta, P.T., and Tonegawa, S. (1996). The essential role of hippocampal CA1 NMDA receptor-dependent synpatic plasticity in spatial memory. *Cell* 87: 1327–1338.

Tully, T. (1991). Genetic dissociation of learning and memory in Drosophila melanogaster. In J. Madden (Ed.), *Neurobiology of learning, emotion, and affect* (pp. 30–66). New York: Raven Press.

Whitmarsh, A.J., and Davis, R.J. (1996). Transcription factor AP-1 regulation by mitogen-activated protein kinase signal transduction pathways. *J. Mol. Med.* 74: 589–607.

Wickelgren, W.A. (1979). Chunking and consolidation: A theoretical synthesis of semantic networks configuring in conditioning, S R versus cognitive learning, normal forgetting, the amnesic syndrome and the hippocampal arousal system. *Psychol. Rev.* 86: 44–60.

Wilson, M.A., and Tonegawa, S. (1997). Synaptic plasticity, place cells and spatial memory: Study with second generation knockouts. *Trends Neurosci.* 20: 102–106.

Wisden, W., Errington, M.L., Williams, S., Dunnet, S.B. et al. (1990). Differential expression of immediate early genes in the hippocampus and spinal cord. *Neuron* 4: 603–614.

Wolfman, C., Fin, C., Dias, M., Bianchin, M. et al. (1994). Intrahippocampal or intraamygdala infusion of KN62, a specific inhibitor of calcium/calmodulin-dependent protein kinase II, causes retrograde amnesia. *Behav. Neural. Biol.* 61: 203–205.

Xing, J., Ginty, D.D., and Greenberg, M.E. (1996). Coupling of RAS-MAPK pathway to gene activation by RSK2, a growth factor-regulated CREB kinase. *Science* 273: 959–963.

Yeckel, M.F., and Berger, T.W. (1990). Feedforward excitation of the hippocampus by afferents from the entorhinal cortex: Redefinition of the role of the trisynaptic pathway. *Proc. Natl. Acad. Sci. USA.* 87: 5832–5836.

Zhao, W., Lawen, A., and Ng, K.T. (1999). Changes in phosphorylation of Ca2+/calmodulin-dependent protein kinase II (CaMKII) in processing of short-term and long-term memories after passive avoidance learning. *J. Neurosci Res.* 55: 557–568.

Conclusions and Future Targets

Christian Hölscher and Gal Richter-Levin

Overview of the Different Chapters

The opinions expressed in the different chapters show a great variety and span the entire range from researchers who believe that long-term potentiation (LTP) is not a model of learning at all and could be an artifact (chapters by McEachern and Shaw, McNaughton, and Matzel and Shors) to those who do not see any problems with the concept of LTP as a model for learning mechanisms (Abraham, Cho and Eichenbaum, and Rogan et al.). Most authors, however, voice a more diversified opinion and suggest a "revised and improved" model of LTP and memory formation that tries to integrate our increased knowledge of how neurons communicate in living brains. Such a model could account for discrepancies observed between LTP inducibility and learning abilities that have been published so far.

Persisting with LTP As a Model for Learning and Memory Formation

While not discussing the lack of correlations between LTP inducibility and learning abilities in numerous publications, Abraham suggests in Chapter 1 that LTP [and long-term depression (LTD)] is still a useful model and the dominating theory for mechanisms of memory formation. He notes that LTP is not homogeneously expressed in areas of the brain. LTP in the dentate gyrus is usually detrimental, whereas CA1 LTP tends to be robust and nondetrimental. LTP in the cortex is difficult to induce but appears to be very stable once it has been induced. To him, these data indicate that genuine differences exist that might reflect different roles in different areas for LTP as a process of memory formation. The differences in LTP inducibility can be traced to differences in the expression of ion channels, receptor densities, and biochemical intracellular signaling processes. However, behavioral studies have shown that the hippocampus does not seem to

We are indebted to Dr. Timothy VP Bliss, NIMH, UK, for his advice, suggestions and inspiration.

store long-term memory despite the durability of CA1 LTP. It is feasible that LTP is part of a more dynamic mechanism that shifts synaptic weights, and that depotentiation of LTP as well as LTD could be of vital importance. It has been suggested that the overall synaptic weights of the network might not change over time, while individual synapses could be upregulated for a limited period of time. Such a network model could explain the rapid development of place cell fields and the rapid changes of place fields in new environments.

Abraham concludes that further research in the durability of LTP in various brain areas is required before more detailed models can be constructed that might stand the test of time.

Rogan and coauthors also support the theory of LTP as a model for memory formation, in particular for memory of fear conditioning tasks that might be stored in the amygdala. They remind us that previous research has shown that synaptic modulation is the basis for the learning of the gill withdrawal reflex in Aplysia. LTP in the hippocampus was discovered afterward, and considered to be the prime mechanism for memory formation in the brain. However, we still have no clear idea how memory forms in the hippocampus. Also, LTP requires a depolarization of pre- and postsynaptic sites within a short time window, while learning of spatial tasks usually requires several hours to days. The flow of information in the hippocampus is also not known in detail.

Fear conditioning is better understood in terms of the circuitry involved in the flow of information through the structures. Following sensory input projections suggests a number of synapses that could be candidates for modulation during the learning of fear conditioning tasks. The connection from auditory processing nuclei in the thalamus to the lateral nucleus of the amygdala (LA) seems to play a crucial role. In freely moving rats, field excitatory postsynaptic potentials (EPSPs) recorded in the LA increased after fear conditioning. *In vitro* studies showed that this type of LTP is dependent on postsynaptic calcium and that it is NMDA-receptor independent. Additionally, in order to induce LTP, pre- and postsynaptic sites have to be activated simultaneously. The data suggest that although it is not clear what role LTP might play in the hippocampus, LTP in the thalamic-amygdala projection is the basis for learning of fear conditioning tasks.

Maren also supports these views in his chapter. He states that LTP plays a role in fear conditioning, a Pavlovian task for emotional learning. Although LTP might not be involved in spatial learning because such learning is a complex and distributed type of learning, LTP might well be the underlying principle for fear conditioning learning. He also notes that learning of a spatial water maze task is not blocked by NMDA receptor antagonists, but fear conditioning learning is. Therefore, NMDA receptors in the amygdala should play a crucial role in learning, and perhaps NMDA-dependent LTP does also. This concept is supported by the observation that knock-out mice strains that do not exhibit LTP in the amygdala were impaired in learning contextual fear conditioning tasks. In addition, recent studies showed that field EPSPs were increased after learning of fear conditioning tasks. Maren concludes from this that it is likely that LTP plays some role in learning of this task.

Rolls explores in Chapter 10 how the mechanism of synaptic LTP (and LTD) could be implemented in neuronal networks during the formation of memories.

The brain has the architecture that suggests neuronal network types of data processing and storage. For example, in a simple Pavlovian conditioning task, two stimuli (unconditioned and conditioned) are associated. Areas of the brain in which pattern associators may be present include the amygdala and orbitofrontal cortex. The suggested process by which the network can associate and store information follows Hebb's rule: An unconditioned stimulus pattern is received through unmodifiable synapses to produce or force firing of the output neurons. The conditioned stimulus is received through modifiable synapses to the dendrites of the output neurons. The synapses are modifiable in such a way that if there is presynaptic firing on an input axon paired during learning with postsynaptic activity on neurons then the strength or weight between that axon and the dendrite increases (associative LTP).

After learning, presenting the pattern on the input axons will activate the dendrite through the strengthened synapses. If the cue or conditioned stimulus pattern is similar to that learned, then there will be some activation of the postsynaptic neuron produced by each of the firing axons afferent to a synapse strengthened by the previous learning. In this way, only the correct output neurons are strongly activated, and the unconditioned stimulus is effectively recalled. The recall is best when only strong activation of the postsynaptic neuron produces firing.

This model can be extended to include non-Hebbian synaptic changes, such as LTD. In the event that pre- and postsynaptic firing is nonsynchronous, homosynaptic and heterosynaptic LTD could be induced. This process increases the signal-to-noise ratio and reduces wrong connections/associations. Without homosynaptic LTD neurons would be increasingly activated by input as synaptic efficacy becomes upregulated. Heterosynaptic LTD effectively allows gradual overwriting of old memories (forgetting). If sparse (distributed) input patterns are used, then many more patterns can be stored than with "rich" (fully distributed orthogonal) input patterns.

Rolls concludes that even if LTP and LTD are not involved in learning, another type of very similar synapse-specific modification of synaptic strength would be needed in the brain to implement memory and perceptual learning in the ways described here. In different brain regions the duration of LTP may be different according to the role the brain area plays in memory formation. For example, long-term semantic memory might be stored in the cerebral cortex, while episodic memory in the hippocampus may be stored only for a short time and might be constantly overwritten by processes involving LTD. Short-term memory also would require a reversible form of synaptic upregulation.

Such a graded scale of LTP persistence is similar to the concept developed by Abraham (Chapter 1).

Chapman agrees with other authors that LTP is still a theory worth pursuing. He makes the point that gene deletion or genetic manipulation is a particularly promising method for analyzing biochemical processes that are crucial for synaptic plasticity. There are numerous technical approaches of how to address this problem. Individual genes can be targeted and either inactivated (knock-out) or can be overexpressed (e.g., by inserting additional copies of the gene into the genome, or by inactivating cellular regulation of the expression of the gene). Furthermore, new genes can be inserted into a genome that have not existed in that particular genome before. Although it is possible to correlate learning, LTP, and transgenic manipulations of specific genes, there are drawbacks and limitations. For example, redundancy exists for a number of crucial biochemical pathways. Deleting a single gene might be compensated for. However, transgenic techniques offer unique possibilities and opportunities that we can use to investigate synaptic plasticity in learning animals.

In second-generation transgenic techniques, transgenes can be inserted into specific areas only, or can be activated on demand after maturation of the animal. This way we might be able to reduce the technical limitations that present gene-targeting techniques incorporate. More detailed questions can be asked about the role of brain areas or of individual molecules in the process of synaptic plasticity.

Davis and Laroche acknowledge that the theory of LTP as a memory model is under considerable debate at the moment. Some previous experimental results that seemed to support the theory turned out not to be reproducible. One explanation for a mismatch between LTP inducibility and learning is the concept that memory can be localized in more than one brain region or circuit. This could explain why damage to the hippocampus, or blocking of LTP in one brain area, does not completely block the abilities of animals to learn tasks. Additionally, brain areas might play a role in memory formation only for a certain time period, which explains the graded retrograde amnesia in humans after temporal lobe damage.

In agreement with Chapman, Davis and Laroche conclude that transgenic mouse models that have defined genetic alterations can be useful tools to investigate what roles certain types of enzymes of receptors play in neuronal plasticity. Although some publications report a good correlation between LTP and learning abilities, other results do not show any such correlation at all. More recent studies with selective transgenic constructs limited to defined areas, however, show a very good fit between learning abilities and LTP induction.

The authors conclude that the hypothesis of LTP cannot be proven or disproven, but novel techniques will allow us to ask more selective questions that will shed more light on the question.

Cho and Eichenbaum also investigate the phenomenon of place cells in the rat hippocampus. Their experiments show that the hippocampus appears to be crucial in the use of external cues for orientation. Rats impaired in hippocampal functions do not use external cues but rather local, more simple cues. They show that various gene deletion constructs in mice did not show impairments in place field development. However, the spatial selectivity of place fields was poorer than in wild-type animals. When rotating visual cues in a task, control mice did not change two-thirds of their place fields. In knock-out mice, only a minority of place fields remained in the original location. Therefore, Cho and Eichenbaum agree with Jeffery that perhaps LTP-like processes are important for the development of place fields and space cell properties. Place fields are established quickly yet can be retained for a long time. LTP could be the mechanism that makes this happen. Because single-cell recording does not monitor synaptic activity it will require different techniques to study that question.

LTP Is Not Memory at All

Although the authors of the chapters discussed so far all agreed that LTP is a mechanism well worth studying, other authors did not agree with this concept and find that perhaps the concept of LTP has been misleading us.

McEachern and Shaw find that LTP is a dogma that still has not been proven. The problem of finding out what LTP really might model is compounded by the fact that experimental parameters vary immensely among laboratories. A jungle of contradictory results in the literature makes it impossible to draw conclusions.

There are a number of arguments against the concept that LTP is the mechanism for memory formation, for example, that input specificity is not always observed in LTP, and that LTP is not really permanent. More problematic is that the criteria that would let us conclude whether LTP is a model for memory or not are rather loose. Sometimes LTP fulfills the criteria and sometimes not, but then explanations are found for the contradicting results and no consequences appear to be drawn. In addition, LTP occurs during quite unphysiologic processes such as anoxia and during drug addiction. A theory of LTP as a memory mechanism would have to be broad enough to account for these effects. One has to consider alternative roles for LTP. LTP might be a process that is not a "yes or no" mechanism but LTP expression might be found to be on a ranging scale that spans from small increases of synaptic transmission to extreme changes resembling epilepsy and seizures (the plasticity-pathology continuum).

McNaughton also is not convinced that LTP is a model for learning processes. Damage to the hippocampal formation does not interfere with the retrieval of established memory, making it unlikely that memory is actually stored in the hippocampus. Therefore, studying memory processes in the hippocampus will not bear fruit. McNaughton suggests that the function of the hippocampus is to detect negative associations, associations of conflict. It plays a role in the induction of fear and anxiety. Anxiolytic drugs have similar effects in a range of tasks as hippocampectomy. Spatial learning impairments after damage to the hippocampus can be explained by the inability of the rat to eliminate false associations during learning. Memory is not stored in the hippocampus, but LTP-like processes could be used to alter learned programs that are located outside of the hippocampus. McNaughton concludes that LTP is not the physiologic basis of memory.

Matzel and Shors do not accept the concept that LTP is a good model for learning and memory mechanisms, in particular for associative memory formation as seen after Pavlovian conditioning. The authors describe in detail what requirements a model that tries to explain the mechanisms of associative learning would have to meet. They come to the conclusion that existing models have considerable flaws. For example, facilitated acquisition after extinction of a response is considered such a fundamental feature of associative learning that the failure to predict it is considered an intolerable shortcoming of eminent models of associative learning.

Experiments have demonstrated that following extinction of a conditioned fear response, mere exposure of rats to the shock that had previously served as the unconditioned stimulus (US) during initial conditioning is sufficient to reinstate an animal's fear of the nominally extinguished conditioned stimulus (CS). However, if the CS were trained in Context A and extinguished in a distinct context referred to as "B," the CS will elicit a reaction similar to its preextinction conditioned response if subsequently tested in Context A or in a novel location, Context C. Thus the same CS may elicit wildly different responses depending only on where it is tested. Such complex properties of a seemingly simple conditioning task show that the animals learn much more complex associations with environmental cues than expected.

The authors argue that a simple upregulation of synaptic responses within the circuit of reflex induction or modulation cannot account for such complex memories. The authors further believe that neuronal network models cannot model such complex learning of seemingly simple tasks either. In short, the neural network that underlies a conditioned response based on the induction of associative LTP is in essence the description of the modification of reflex arcs (i.e., motor pathways). Despite its appeal and simplicity, this description of a hypothetical neural network for the generation of conditioned responses fails at several levels. Most important, the conditioned response to a CS does not necessarily resemble the response to the US, and in fact may take a form that is "opposite" to that evoked by the US. As a further complication, the response to a CS may often reflect a compendium of behaviors that represent the interaction of that particular CS with the specific US that it predicts. The authors conclude that neuronal network models are not flexible enough to account for the observed learning behaviors.

The authors continue with a list of properties of LTP that do not make it a likely candidate for an associative memory mechanism. For example, the expression of synaptic potentiation following high-frequency stimulation (HFS) is slow to develop, typically requiring several seconds if not minutes to reach asymptotic levels. Yet classically conditioned responses can be observed "immediately."

Other points of concern are the inherently decremental nature of LTP and the facilitation of LTP induction by massed stimulation, a phenomenon not observed after massed training, that would seem to exclude LTP from serious consideration as an associative memory mechanism. In addition, the authors feel that two principal problems follow from our continued focus on LTP as a memory storage mechanism. One is that we have limited our ability to recognize other functional roles that LTP may play within the nervous system. Given that synapses throughout the mammalian brain undergo potentiation using protocols similar to those that induce LTP, it is quite reasonable to assume that synaptic facilitation does play *some* role in the induction or expression of memories, for instance, as a gain control device that influences the rate of learning. The second and perhaps more dangerous consequence of the continued focus on LTP as a memory device is that we might ignore other potential candidates that could underlie memory mechanisms.

LTP Could Be a Memory Process, But There Is More to the Picture Than Meets the Eye

The authors of the chapters mentioned so far discussed the virtues and shortfalls of LTP as a mechanism for memory formation. The chapters discussed below look at the network properties that are found in living brains. These properties establish the framework under which LTP might occur in learning brains, and, at the very least, can help to investigate synaptic plasticity under more realistic conditions by ruling out experimental conditions that cannot be considered physiologic.

Pike and coauthors state that LTP is an attractive model for processes that underlie learning and memory, yet unfortunately the wide range of results from studies that investigated the relation of LTP to memory have produced a rather confusing mess of contradictions and inconsistencies. One reason for this might be that artificially induced LTP is too removed from natural processes that occur during learning. The firing patterns of neurons in the hippocampus are different from HFS patterns. Clearly, it is better to record actual neuronal activity during learning to find out what changes actually occur in the brain, and what firing patterns are actually observed. Complex spike activity is observed in active brains, along with field oscillations such as theta rhythm. Also, place cell activity is also seen in the hippocampus.

Postsynaptic bursts comparable to complex spike firing can facilitate the induction of synaptic plasticity *in vitro* and perhaps play an important role in learning. Action potentials can back-propagate to dendrites and therefore prime postsynaptic sites for synaptic potentiation. The model proposed by Pike et al. is that during bursting in the hippocampus, information is acquired ("read-in") and during simple spike activity the information is recalled ("read-out").

Maroun and coauthors suggest that LTP in the amygdala and the hippocampus is still a valid model for learning, but LTP alone is not sufficient. It is important to keep the overall properties of neuronal circuits in the processing of information in mind. GABA interneurons greatly modulate network activity and therefore play an important role in the induction of synaptic plasticity.

Frequency-dependent inhibition (FDI) in the dentate is a good example of modulation of local inhibition and of local circuit plasticity. There also is an important age-related factor that changes FDI properties. Old rats display FDI that is not affected by tetanic stimulation, whereas in younger rats stimulation reduces FDI. Theta-burst stimulation (TBS) is another example for such dynamic network processes of modulation of neuronal transmission.

In contrast to the hippocampus, it was possible to show that field EPSPs in the amygdala were increased after learning. This suggests that LTP might be a mechanism for memory formation in the amygdala. Here, paired-pulse depression can be reduced in the basal amygdaloid nucleus after TBS. LTP of field EPSPs can also be readily induced by TBS. This type of LTP is as likely the result of the reduction of local inhibition as it is of the upregulation of excitatory synaptic transmission. Hence, it is important to keep the circuit properties in mind when analyzing changes that might occur after learning and that might encode information. Changes at individual synapses might not reflect the full extent of system plasticity.

In agreement with other authors in this book, Hölscher states that long trains of HFS do not resemble neuronal firing patterns seen in living brains. Using a more physiologic protocol of bursts of few stimuli in the presence of theta activity can facilitate the induction of LTP if the right time window for stimulation is chosen. Theta rhythm is produced by several generators, including local negative feedback circuits between inhibitory interneurons and excitatory pyramidal neurons. The oscillations increase and reduce inhibition of pyramidal neurons. This naturally occurring process focuses neuronal firing within a small time window of lowest inhibition and bundles firing of neurons into bursts. Such focusing of neuronal activity in time secures the arrival of input onto other neurons within a relatively short time of each other, which increases the chance of inducing synaptic plastic processes (compared with input that is distributed over time). Additionally, these bursts arrive at a time of lowest inhibition of target neurons, when postsynaptic polarization is already reduced. This mechanism would make the induction of a "natural" type of LTP feasible. However, it is important to realize that the actual stimulation intensity employed is very low and localized, very different from HFS stimulation. LTP that might be induced during learning could have completely different properties than LTP induced by comparatively powerful stimulation such as HFS. Additionally, there are intrinsic dynamic regulatory mechanisms at work in the nervous system that greatly change the system parameters of the neuronal networks. These network properties greatly affect information processing, memory formation, and memory retrieval, and add important qualities to network activity that go beyond the basic mechanism of alteration of synaptic transmission. These mechanisms should be taken into account or ideally, utilized in experiments, rather than ignored.

Munk also emphasizes the importance of network properties in his chapter. When analyzing how the central nervous system processes information, it has not been appreciated how such networks could cooperate in information processing, and how the separately encoded properties of objects are brought together in a holistic picture. Neuronal network theories suggest that large populations of neurons process information in a parallel rather than linear process. In order to synchronize the neurons that cooperate in processing the same piece of information (and to distinguish them from other neurons that do not cooperate with them), gamma oscillations and theta oscillations could be used to functionally bind such networks together.

There is ample empirical evidence that support this assumption; for example, oscillations that are produced in the retina and can be measured in the lateral geniculate body and also in the primary visual cortex. In addition, neuronal areas that collaborate in processing information are synchronous in the gamma-frequency band, but are not synchronous if they do not collaborate in analyzing the

same object. Gamma oscillation also facilitates the induction of neuronal plasticity: Stimulation of the mesencephalic reticular formation (MRF) facilitated onset
of gamma oscillation in the cortex after the presentation of a visual stimulus. After
conditioning the system, the visual stimulus alone induced the onset of gamma
oscillations. This suggests that there is some mechanism of neuronal plasticity
involved, which could be LTP of synaptic transmission, but does not have to be.
Oscillations disinhibit neurons and facilitate firing of neurons within defined time
windows and neurons tend to receive their excitatory input within a small time
window during which they are already disinhibited. This would favor the induction of synaptic plasticity according to Hebb, and the induction of LTP-like
processes (e.g., via the activation of NMDA receptors). However, other mechanisms appear to play a role. For example, the temporal profile of pyramidal neuronal activity in the neocortex has been observed to change the depolarization
properties of post- and presynaptic sites without affecting the gain of synaptic
transmission. Detailed investigations showed that at least three parameters other
than synaptic strength determine the transmission capacity of frequency-dependent synapses (alteration of firing probability, change of firing patterns to burst
mode rather than single spikes, or change of recovery time). Could there be more?

The data clearly show that neuronal networks in living animals follow highly
complex and dynamic rules. HFS-induced LTP as studied in an *in vitro* preparation cannot do this justice and, therefore, results obtained with this technique are
prone to producing artifacts. Clearly, the recording of neuronal activity in living
brains will tell us more about the parameters that govern information processing
in the brain.

Lisman and coauthors postulate that the hippocampus can be seen to play the
role of a short-term memory buffer. Mossy-fiber synapses undergo nonassociative
LTP and could therefore potentially store nonassociative memory. The hippocampus is perhaps not required for long-term memory but for short-term memory
(STM) storage, as the data from patients with hippocampal damage suggest. Lists
kept in STM appear to be in some sort of buffer memory, and adding to a list of
items to be learned increases retrieval times in a linear fashion. Adding an item to a
list of numbers to be kept increases retrieval time by approximately 40 msec. This
time is roughly equivalent to one cycle of gamma oscillation. Five to seven gamma
cycles could fit into one theta cycle. If STM is limited by theta activity, five to seven
items would be a "natural" limit to the STM buffer system in humans. Theta activity was measured in the temporal lobe in a task- and load-dependent manner. This
correlation suggests that theta is directly involved in STM development.

In their model of hippocampal functions, contextual input arrives at CA3 via
the entorhinal cortex (EC), and the dentate and area CA3 consist of recurrent neuronal networks. Theta-gamma oscillations could serve as a buffer to keep information in memory for longer time. Intention or motivation could facilitate
memory formation by activating cholinergic projections from basal brain nuclei
and thereby facilitating LTP.

Cain discusses the experimental evidence for LTP as a memory mechanism.
He points out that the hippocampal slice technique has limitations in answering

the questions related to LTP and learning mechanisms. He sums up recent studies that show that understanding the exact relations between LTP and learning or memory is not a simple and straightforward undertaking. Many investigations of the correlation between LTP and learning use the water maze task. However, as he discusses in detail, water maze tasks are not a purely spatial task, and drugs or other manipulations have been shown to interfere with the animals' abilities to learn the task that are not related to spatial learning. Some drugs such as NMDA antagonists can induce ataxia and impair the animals' performance. Detailed analysis of behavior in the water maze has indicated a need to distinguish among different components of this seemingly simple task. Nonspatial pretraining allows for the separation of behavioral strategy learning and learning the spatial location of the hidden platform. Nonspatially pretrained rats can learn the location of a hidden platform as quickly as controls despite being treated with any of a variety of pharmacologic agents. Therefore, when a water maze task of average difficulty is used, nonspatially pretrained rats given an NMDA receptor antagonist to block hippocampal LTP can learn the location of the hidden platform as quickly as controls.

Such results should caution us about taking water maze tasks as clear evidence for spatial impairments. The correlation between LTP and learning can be tenuous, and further research is required to investigate what animals actually learn in such spatial tasks, and how LTP might play a role in memory formation.

Jeffery discusses the phenomenon of place cells in the rat hippocampus. She finds that the theory that LTP is the basis for memory has been the subject of much debate, and the amount of contradictory results in the literature makes it virtually impossible to make a decision one way or the other.

In the hippocampus, pyramidal neurons were found to fire predominantly when the animal is in a particular location (place cells). Clearly, the occurrence of such specialized place cell firing patterns requires some form of plasticity to emerge. The technical limitation is that we cannot measure synaptic strength in single cell recordings. However, it is possible to change the sensory input (visual input, head direction sensory input, etc.) used by place cells to develop their place field firing patterns. Changing external cues changes (most) place fields, a form of learning that has to be based on some form of neuronal plasticity. Because place fields change quickly when the animal is brought into a new environment and might change back to the original place fields when brought back to the original surroundings, there is a very dynamic process at work that does not resemble artificially induced LTP in a slice, but more a reversible dynamic learning type of plasticity that reverses plastic changes (an "anti-Hebb" process, e.g., LTD) while still retaining previous traces.

Jeffery concludes that LTP as induced artificially *in vitro* or *in vivo* might still be a valuable technique for studying mechanisms of synaptic plasticity if one keeps its clear limitations in mind. It is, however, preferable to study the activity of neurons in living, behaving animals, and models of how the brain actually lays down memory traces can only come from recording experiments of neuronal assemblies in the living and exploring brain.

Diamond and coauthors agree with McNaughton and question that the role of the hippocampus is primarily that of storing memory. They postulate that the role of the hippocampus is to regulate stress and stress responses. This is demonstrated by the observation that manipulation of the hippocampus modulates glucocorticoid release and effects of stress. Also, stress blocks the induction of LTP in the hippocampus and the formation of memory. However, stress can also increase the formation of memory in some cases. To resolve this confusion we have to look to other brain areas. The amygdala plays a crucial role in learning of emotional learning and its association with environmental stimuli. Stimulating the amygdala enhances emotional memory formation, and also increases LTP in the hippocampus. The amygdala and the hippocampus therefore could work together to form and retrieve memory. In conditions of high stress the amygdala could store information, at least temporarily, that is then transferred and interpreted by the hippocampus. From the hippocampus it then will be transferred to other long-term memory systems. The cellular mechanism for memory formation could be an LTP-like process, but LTP could be more directly involved in modulation of stress responses, affecting memory formation in a more indirect way.

Rose and Diamond are of the opinion that although learning impairments often go hand in hand with reduced LTP inducibility, one cannot infer from this that LTP is memory. We do not know enough about learning or LTP to make specific statements.

LTP induction is usually accomplished by using long trains of 100 to 400 Hz, which cannot be considered physiologic. Imitating more natural firing patterns is a better way, and LTP can be induced using such patterns. Theta rhythm is an important factor in learning, and using theta-type stimulation protocols induces LTP. Also, making use of the local network disinhibition induced by theta rhythm helps to induce LTP. One should keep in mind that LTP is not a single process; there are many types and stages (e.g., a late-stage LTP has been described that is dependent on PKA activation). This makes a simple correlation between the inducibility of LTP and memory formation more complex. When analyzing the correlation between LTP and learning in aged rats one is faced with more contradictory results. Some researchers did not find an effect of aging on the inducibility of LTP. Others described deficits of LTP in the dentate gyrus in aged animals. Other studies showed deficits in LTP induction in aged animals when using theta-patterned stimulation patterns. NMDA-dependent LTP appears to decline, while voltage-dependent calcium channel–dependent LTP is facilitated. Late-stage LTP appears to be affected also. When comparing young with aged rats in studies that correlated LTP and learning, LTP decayed earlier in aged rats and forgetting was quicker. Several studies appeared to show a correlation between learning, LTP, and aging, although the correlation coefficients are not high.

Improving age-related decay of LTP and learning was shown in some studies. However, there are many pitfalls and there are many types of LTP that might play different roles. The authors conclude that more research is required, and until then LTP and learning studies can be a helpful tool for designing pharmaceutical tools to ameliorate aging processes.

Where Do We Go from Here?

We can draw several conclusions from this presentation of observations, concepts, and predictions.

■ **What Type of LTP?** A number of misunderstandings are based on the fact that researchers discuss the concept of LTP on different levels. LTP as a concept is the idea that neuronal communication can change after learning and this concept is an idea (like the idea of a perfect circle that does not exist in reality) that includes a number of different physiologic processes via which neuronal communication (synaptic or not) can be altered. Few people will have a problem with the idea of LTP as such, and it is pratically impossible to prove or disprove the idea as such. When researchers reject the idea that LTP is a method for storing information within a neuronal network they almost certainly refer to experimental results, to a physically existing form of LTP. It is possible to prove or disprove that a certain type of LTP does or does not play a role in learning. As has been described in various chapters it is possible to show that some types of LTP do not correlate with learning abilities of animals. Such results, of course, strongly reduce the interest of some researchers in the idea of LTP. However, there are potentially limitless types of LTP.

■ **LTP: A Learning Mechanism for Some Areas Only?** It is of interest to note that researchers who work in the area of fear conditioning and the role of the amygdala do not have a problem with LTP as a model for memory mechanisms. Here, all predictions about what should be observed if LTP was a model for learning have come true. Crucial anatomic projections in the limbic system and the amygdala (and the afferences) are capable of expressing (HFS-induced) LTP. Blocking LTP in the amygdala did show learning impairments in fear conditioning tasks, and most important, field EPSPs in one pathway of the circuit involved showed a naturally induced LTP after fear conditioning. Here, LTP is a powerful and convincing model for memory storage. If research had started in this area in 1973 maybe no problems and doubts would ever have arisen.

There are still a number of crucial questions to be answered in this field: Is there naturally occurring LTD? Is there a ceiling effect of natural LTP after several fear conditioning tasks? How long does this type of LTP last? Is modulation of synaptic efficacy the only mechanism for memory formation? Are intraamygdala projections upregulated also? However, it is safe to conclude at the moment that LTP is a strong candidate for the memory mechanism that is responsible for retention of fear conditioning experiences.

■ **What Does the Hippocampus Really Do?** Scientists who work in the hippocampus are more mixed in their opinions. Here, the basic predictions about what one would see if LTP was the model for memory formations have not come through in a convincing manner. In particular, there never has been shown an upregulation of field EPSPs *in vivo* after spatial learning tasks. Many authors noted that there is much evidence to show that the hippocampus seems to be involved in the acquisition, but not storage, of memory. Perhaps the hippocampus is the wrong area to look for long-term changes of neuronal activity. The hippocampus had been chosen as a main area for memory research purely for historical reasons, since the temporal lobe was the first area that appeared to be linked to severe deficits in memory consolidation.

Furthermore, several authors noted that even if LTP is a mechanism that is used in the hippocampus, perhaps the architecture is such that we cannot see synaptic changes in field EPSPs. If there is a sparse coding network in the hippocampus we would have problems identifying the synapses that change in a spatial task. Single cell recordings of space cells show that there are processes of neuronal plasticity in the hippocampus. Changes occur quickly and can be altered just as quickly. How could we find out if LTP is the process that makes these changes possible?

Ideally one would record from single synapses in the living brain. This is technically challenging, but it is possible to record from single cells. With the use of advanced software it can be determined, for example, which neurons in the dentate drive neurons in area CA3. The more neurons recorded from the higher the chance to record from neuronal pairs that change their responses after learning. If one also records local field potentials in area CA3 it might be possible to estimate the contribution of afferent neurons to the size of the field potential, and therefore the synaptic efficacy. As mentioned earlier, in additional to modulation of synaptic efficacy, other mechanisms could be responsible for neuronal plastic changes. If neurons changed their firing probability or firing rates (e.g., changing after excitatory input from single firing mode to burst firing mode), it could account for changes observed in place cell recordings. These parameters could be measured in single cell recording setups. If synaptic efficacy is not changed, perhaps firing rates are.

Because we know that LTP might play different roles in different areas, it would be of importance to conduct such experiments in as many areas as possible. A negative result in area CA3 would not rule out the possibility of a positive result in a different area.

A number of authors noted that the hippocampus is not involved only in the processing of spatial information and in the acquisition of episodic memories. Because the hippocampus is part of the limbic system it is suggested that emotional aspects do play a role in hippocampal activity. The emotional state of the animal is crucial for memory formation. The acquisition of declarative memory could go hand in hand with the modulation of emotional states. Munk showed that stimulation of the MRF facilitates onset of gamma oscillations, suggesting that these oscillations are intrinsically linked to attention, perhaps motivation, and not just to information processing. The onset of theta activity is correlated with novelty, importance, or complexity of tasks. Perhaps motivation and attention affects neuronal activity and memory formation directly by activating local oscillations that improve information processing and set the stage for neuronal plasticity. If this is the case the fact that stress can block learning and that motivation can improve learning is not surprising.

■ **Neuronal Circuit Activity: More Than the Sum of Its Parts?** Several authors showed that looking at changes of individual synapses alone will not give us the complete answer to how the brain processes and stores information. Neuronal circuits are more than just the sum of their neurons, and the system properties are crucial in understanding how the brain works. Taking together the contributions of the various authors one could tentatively sketch a model of how the hippocampus could process information.

The chapters by Munk, Hölscher, Lisman et al., and Rose et al. describe how the anatomic architecture of the cortex and of the hippocampus favor the establishment of oscillations, especially via disinhibition feedback loops with local interneurons. Oscillations disinhibit neurons and facilitate firing of neurons within defined time windows. This means that neurons tend to receive their excitatory input within a small time window during which they are already disinhibited. This could functionally "bind" neuronal groups together and would favor the induction of synaptic plasticity according to Hebb and the induction of LTP-like processes (e.g., via the activation of NMDA receptors).

The chapters by Maroun et al. and Hölscher show that bursts are more efficient in inducing synaptic changes. Rolls describes that from a theoretical viewpoint, postsynaptic bursts of depolarization are potentially more efficient in encoding information in a neuronal network. Pike et al. show that postsynaptic depolarization in bursts actually induces LTP easier. In natural settings, action potentials can back-propagate to dendrites and therefore prime postsynaptic sites for synaptic potentiation by synchronous presynaptic activity.

Munk describes in detail how synchronized responses cause improved transmission of a signal. The precision of synchronized firing could determine the speed of neuronal signal transmission and the strength of synaptic efficacy changes. Hölscher also describes similar processes and mentions the mechanism of paired pulse facilitation that would improve signal transmission compared with single pulses. As suggested by Pike et al., read-out of the information would be via single spikes that would enable the previously active network to be reactivated but would not induce synaptic plasticity.

If one takes these observations together one can come up with a model in which afferent input is delivered to the hippocampus and cause hippocampal neurons to respond in bursts, partly due to the architecture of the nervous system, and partly due to firing properties of individual neurons. If theta rhythm is simultaneously activated in the hippocampus (e.g., via novelty-dependent activation of basal nuclei) and gamma oscillation (vial local network oscillations), the firing of hippocampal neurons would be bursts that are focused in time windows of low inhibition, and thereby increase the probability of the induction of synaptic plasticity. This process would be enforced even further by paired pulse facilitation, and if action potentials of neurons that have been successfully activated can travel back antidromically to their dendrites. This should greatly enhance the probability of synaptic plasticity after a couple of initial spikes that prime and synchronize the system. The LTP induced in this manner would be localized (sparse coding) and potentially small, not reaching saturation values. If the exact conditions are not met (e.g., no theta activity, asynchronous input, or no antidromic postsynaptic depotentiation because pyramidal neurons had not been activated), no network plasticity would be induced.

If this model is correct, LTP could be induced with very little effort, and HFS requires such powerful stimulation to induce LTP because it overrides the system's safety mechanisms.

In conclusio

LTP research has come a long way since 1973. We now know much more about how the brain operates in learning conditions and that the original concept of LTP as a memory mechanism as expressed in a slice preparation after HFS is a far too simplistic and mechanistic concept. Not surprisingly, neuronal systems operate according to multilevel and highly complex rules and use a number of network principles and mechanisms to process information that have to be taken into account. On the other hand, there has been evidence for synaptic plastic processes in some areas of the living brains, and LTP (of synaptic efficacy or of different parameters) is a likely candidate for mechanisms through which the neuronal system alters communication. It is possible that LTP is only one of many memory mechanisms used by the brain, and that it is not used by all areas.

Modern techniques have been developed that nobody would have dreamt of 25 years ago, and these enable us to analyze in finer detail how neuronal systems work. Inducible transgenic constructs that can be limited in their expression to defined brain areas will tell us more about the role of individual molecules and brain areas in learning, and multiarray single cell recording in learning animals will inform us about how the neuronal networks actually work in learning situations. Whether or not LTP will one day be shown to be the memory mechanism used by the brain, the theory will have been an important catalyst in making researchers ask the tough and detailed questions and develop new techniques that enable us to find out in further detail how the brain actually works. The journey continues.

Index